MW00377419

Requisites in
DERMATOLOGY
General Dermatology

For Elsevier

Commissioning Editor: Thu Nguyen
Development Editor: Claire Bonnett
Project Manager: Jess Thompson and Krishnan Balakrishnan
Designer: Stewart Larking
Illustration Manager: Kirsteen Wright
Illustrator: Richard Prime

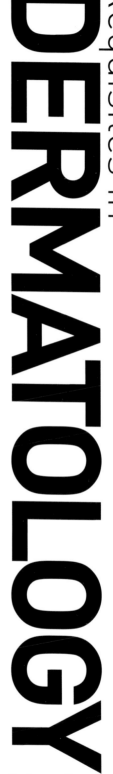

Requisites in **DERMATOLOGY**

General Dermatology

Edited by

Kathryn Schwarzenberger, MD
Associate Professor of Medicine
Director, Dermatology Residency Program
University of Vermont College of Medicine
Division of Dermatology
Burlington, VT, USA

Andrew E Werchniak, MD
Associate Physician,
Brigham & Women's Hospital
Instructor in Dermatology,
Harvard Medical School,
Boston, MA, USA

Christine J Ko, MD
Assistant Professor of Dermatology
and Pathology Yale University
School of Medicine
New Haven, CT, USA

Series editor
DIRK M ELSTON

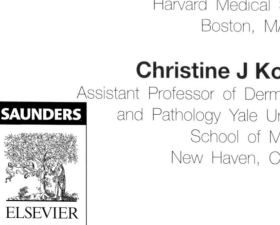

SAUNDERS

ELSEVIER

Edinburgh London New York Oxford Philadelphia St Louis Sydney Toronto 2008

SAUNDERS

ELSEVIER

An imprint of Elsevier Limited

First published 2009

ISBN: 978-0-7020-3093-2

British Library Cataloguing in Publication Data
A catalogue record for this book is available from the British Library

Library of Congress Cataloging in Publication Data
A catalog record for this book is available from the Library of Congress

Notice

Medical knowledge is constantly changing. Standard safety precautions must be followed, but as new research and clinical experience broaden our knowledge, changes in treatment and drug therapy may become necessary or appropriate. Readers are advised to check the most current product information provided by the manufacturer of each drug to be administered to verify the recommended dose, the method and duration of administration, and contraindications. It is the responsibility of the practitioner, relying on experience and knowledge of the patient, to determine dosages and the best treatment for each individual patient. Neither the Publisher nor the author assume any liability for any injury and/or damage to persons or property arising from this publication.

The Publisher

Printed in China

Contents

Contributors

David R Adams, MD, PharmD
Associate Professor of Dermatology
Penn State Hershey Medical Center
Hershey, PA, USA

April W Armstrong, MD
Assistant Professor of Dermatology
Department of Dermatology
University of California Davis Health Systems
Davis, CA, USA

Kimberly Bohjanen, MD
Clinical Associate Professor
Department of Dermatology, University of
Minnesota Medical School,
Minneapolis, MN, USA

Katy Burris, MD
Department of Dermatology, State University
New York Health Science Center at Brooklyn
Brooklyn, NY, USA

David F Butler, MD
Chair, Department of Dermatology
Scott and White Clinic
Texas A&M University College of Medicine
Temple, TX, USA

Melvin W Chiu, MD
Assistant Clinical Professor
Division of Dermatology, Department of
Medicine
David Geffen School of Medicine at UCLA
Los Angeles, CA, USA

Steven Chow, MD, MS
Department of Dermatology,
University of Minnesota Medical School,
Minneapolis, MN, USA

Jonathan Cotliar, MD
Assistant Clinical Professor
Associate Residency Program Director
Director of Inpatient Dermatology Services
Division of Dermatology, Department of
Medicine
David Geffen School of Medicine at UCLA
Los Angeles, CA, USA

Richard Devillez, MD
Staff Dermatologist
Wilford Hall Medical Center
Lackland, TX, USA

David Doyle, Jr., MD
Assistant Chief of Dermatology
Dwight D. Eisenhower Army Medical Center
Fort Gordon, GA, USA

Lisa C Edsall, MD, PhD
Clinical Instructor
Department of Dermatology
Virginia Commonwealth University
Dermatology Associates of Virginia, P.C
Richmond, VA, USA

Dirk M Elston, MD
Director, Department of Dermatology
Geisinger Medical Center Laboratory Medicine
Danville, PA, USA

Laura Korb Ferris, MD, PhD
Assistant Professor of Dermatology
Department of Dermatology
University of Pittsburgh School of Medicine
Pittsburgh, PA, USA

Robin P Gehris, MD
Chief, Pediatric Dermatologic Surgery
Children's Hospital of Pittsburgh
Clinical Assistant Professor of Dermatology
and Pediatrics
University of Pittsburgh School of Medicine
Pittsburgh, PA, USA

Robert T Gilson, MD
Program Director of Dermatology
Wilford Hall Medical Center
Lackland, TX, USA

Whitney A High, MD
Assistant Professor
Dermatology and Dermatopathology
University of Colorado School of Medicine
Denver, CO, USA

Jenny C Hu, MD, MPH
Division of Dermatology, Department of
Medicine
David Geffen School of Medicine at UCLA
Los Angeles, CA, USA

Maria Yadira Hurley, MD
Assistant Professor of Dermatology and
Pathology
Director of Dermatopathology, Department
of Dermatology
Saint Louis University School of Medicine
Saint Louis, MO, USA

Sharon E Jacob, MD
Assistant Professor of Medicine and
Pediatrics (Dermatology),
University of California,
San Diego; Voluntary Clinical
Associate Professor of Dermatology and
Dermatologic Surgery,
University of Miami, FL, USA

Juan P Jaimes, MD, MS
Department of Dermatology
University of Minnesota
Minneapolis, MN, USA

Jonette E Keri, MD, PhD
Assistant Professor
Chief, Dermatology Services at Miami VA
Hospital
Miami Veterans Affairs Medical Center
University of Miami/Jackson Memorial
Medical Center
Miami, FL, USA

Christine J Ko, MD
Assistant Professor of Dermatology and
Pathology
Yale University School of Medicine
New Haven, CT, USA

Eve J Lowenstein, MD, PhD
Associate Professor and Director of Clinical
Research,
Department of Dermatology
SUNY Health Science Center at Brooklyn
Brooklyn, NY, USA

Jared Lund, MD
Marshfield Clinic
Marshfield, WI, USA

Donald Miech, MD
Clinical Professor of Medicine, Dermatology,
University of Wisconsin Madison
Assistant Clinical Professor, Dermatology,
University of Minnesota-Minneapolis
Marshfield Clinic
Marshfield, WI, USA

Linda S Nield, MD
Associate Professor
West Virginia University
School of Medicine
Morgantown, WV, USA

Julia R Nunley, MD
Professor, Department of Dermatology
Virginia Commonwealth University
Richmond, VA, USA

Geeta K Patel, DO
Intern
New York College of Osteopathic Medicine
New York, NY, USA

Arturo P Saavedra, MD, PhD
Instructor in Dermatology, Harvard Medical
School
Instructor in Medicine, Brigham and Women's
Hospital,
Boston, MA, USA

Papri Sarkar, MD
Associate Physician
Brigham & Women's Hospital
Instructor in Dermatology,
Harvard Medical School,
Boston, MA, USA

Elizabeth Satter, MD, MPH
Staff Dermatologist and Head of
Dermatopathology for Residency Program
Department of Dermatology, Naval Medical
Center
San Diego, CA, USA

Brooke N Shadel, MD, PhD
Department of Dermatology, School of
Medicine
Secondary Professor, School of Public Health
Saint Louis University
Saint Louis, MO, USA

Christopher B Skvarka, MD
Department of Dermatology
Drexel University College of Medicine,
Philadelphia, PA, USA

James E Sligh, MD, PhD
Dermatology Section Chief
University of Arizona
Tucson, AZ, USA

Stefani Takahashi, MD
Assistant Clinical Professor, Division of
Dermatology, Department of medicine
David Geffen School of Medicine at UCLA
Los Angeles, CA, USA

Donna Marie Vleugels, MD
Department of Dermatology
Washington University
Saint Louis, MO, USA

Oliver J Wisco, DO
Staff Dermatologist
Wilford Hall Medical Center
Lackland, TX, USA

Clarissa Yang, MD
Associate Physician,
Brigham & Women's Hospital
Instructor in Dermatology,
Harvard Medical School
Boston, MA, USA

Also in the series

Requisites in
DERMATOLOGY

Series Editor: **Dirk M Elston, MD**

Dermatopathology
Dirk M Elston and Tammie Ferringer

Cosmetic Dermatology
Murad Alam, Hayes B Gladstone,
and Rebecca C Tung

Pediatric Dermatology
Howard B Pride, Albert C Yan,
and Andrea L Zaenglein

Dermatologic Surgery
Allison T Vidimos, Christie T Ammirati,
and Christine Poblete-Lopez

General Dermatology
Kathryn Schwarzenberger, Andrew E Werchniak,
and Christine J Ko

Series foreword

The ***Requisites in Dermatology*** series of textbooks is designed around the principle that learning and retention are best accomplished when the forest is clearly delineated from the trees. Topics are presented with an emphasis on the key points essential for residents and practicing clinicians. Each text is designed to stand alone as a reference or to be used as part of an integrated teaching curriculum. Many gifted physicians have contributed their time and energy to create the sort of texts we wish we had had during our own training and each of the texts in the series is accompanied by an innovative online module. Each online module is designed to complement the text, providing lecture material not possible in print format, including video and lectures with voice-over. These books have been a labor of love for all involved. We hope you enjoy them.

Series dedication

This series of textbooks is dedicated to my wife Kathy and my children, Carly and Nate. Thank you for your love, support, and inspiration. It is also dedicated to the residents and fellows it has been my privilege to teach and to the patients who have taught me so much.

Dirk M Elston

Preface

When Dirk Elston first approached me about editing a new general dermatology textbook, my first response was to wonder if we really needed another book. Certainly, there are several outstanding dermatology textbooks on my bookshelf, and it was hard to imaging improving on them. In talking with Dirk, however, it became clear that the Requisites series was intended to help identify essential knowledge and present it in an easily readable format. We asked our authors to be generous in their use of tables, charts, and algorithms, and some of them responded in a very creative way. Because of this, you may note that some of the chapters "read" a bit differently than others. We chose to leave the chapters in the format conceived by the authors, and we hope you like the outcome as much as we do. Enjoy the book. We hope that it makes your learning, whether you are a beginning student or a more "seasoned" practitioner of dermatology, a bit easier.

Kathy Schwarzenberger, MD

Acknowledgments

The editors and authors would like to thank the editorial and publication team at Elsevier without whom these texts would not have been possible; Jess Thompson, Krishnan Balakrishnan, Claire Bonnett, Thu Nguyen and not forgetting Joanne Husovski, Karen Bowler and Sue Hodgson who were invaluable in the planning stages of the Series. Dr. Elston provided many of the clinical and histologic images. Those produced while he was a full time federal employee are in the public domain.

Dedication

With love and gratitude to my husband Roger and son Jackson, for their never-ending support and for accepting without complaint the time spent away from them working on this and other projects; for my Dad, with sincere thanks for his unwavering encouragement, and in loving memory of my Mom, who always believed me to be better than I ever could hope to be.

Kathryn Schwarzenberger

To my wife Jeanine and my children for their love, support, and encouragement.

Andrew E Werchniak

To my family.

Christine J Ko

Urticaria and other reactive erythemas

1

Elizabeth Satter

Urticartia

Clinical presentation

Key Points

- Characterized by wheal and flare reaction
- Acute urticaria
  - Individual lesions last < 24 hours
  - One-time event or intermittent episodes lasting <6-weeks
  - Identifiable triggers include infections, insect stings, medications, or foods
- Chronic urticaria
  - Individual lesions last < 24 hours
  - Urticarial episodes extend beyond 6 weeks
  - More frequently occurs in middle-aged women

Ten to 30% of the general population have urticaria at some point in their lifetime. They are characterized by transient cutaneous edema (wheals) accompanied by surrounding blanchable erythema (flares). The lesions are polymorphous and often form irregular, intensely pruritic plaques (Figure 1-1).

Urticaria have been classically subclassified into two categories based on the duration of the episodes. They are considered acute when a patient experiences hives either as a one-time event or has intermittent episodes that self-resolve within 6-weeks. Chronic urticaria, in contrast, are defined as urticarial episodes that persist beyond 6-weeks. Other variants include persistent "neutrophilic" urticaria which consist of refractory urticarial lesions that persist beyond 24 hours; papular urticaria associated with insect bites; urticaria due to hormonal changes (autoimmune progesterone dermatitis); or urticaria that occur in association with syndromes such as Muckle–Wells syndrome (urticaria, amyloidosis, deafness).

Diagnosis

Key Points

- Urticarial lesions are pruritic, evanescent and migratory
- They may be circinate, papular, annular, or polycyclic
- Urticarial lesions often have dusty centers which can be misinterpreted as erythema multiforme.
- Lesions that last longer than 24-hours, burn or resolve with purpura require a biopsy.

Urticaria are a reaction pattern that may occur in response to an ingested or inhaled allergen or direct mast cell degranulator. Common triggers include opiates, polymyxin B, radiocontrast dye, aspirin, other nonsteroidal anti-inflammatory drugs (NSAIDs), tartrazine, tubocurarine, and sodium benzoate. Aspirin exacerbates chronic urticaria in about 30% of patients. Individuals with aspirin sensitivity often have cross-sensitivity to tartrazine, natural salicylates, and benzoic acid derivatives, which are common food additives and preservatives. Monosodium glutamate (MSG) commonly produces flushing, but rarely causes urticaria. Although urticaria may occur in response to infection, connective tissue diseases, or an inherited syndrome, more than 50% of chronic urticaria are idiopathic. Infectious causes include hepatitis, upper respiratory infections, dental abscesses, sinusitis, vaginitis, and parasitic infestations. Physical urticarias account for about 10% of cases of chronic urticaria.

The first step in the evaluation of urticaria is to determine the type and duration of individual lesions (Figure 1-2). Lesions that last longer than 24 hours require a biopsy to rule out urticarial vasculitis, an urticarial allergic eruption (dermal hypersensitivity response), or the urticarial stage of an immunobullous disorder. Those that burn or heal with purpura also suggest urticarial vasculitis and require a biopsy (Figure 1-3).

The second step in evaluation is to determine the frequency of occurrences, as the pattern of recurrence correlates with different causes of urticaria (Figure 1-4). Physical urticarias are a distinct subset of urticaria triggered by physical stimuli, including scratching, pressure, vibration, cold, galvanic current, or solar radiation. Most physical urticarias can be recognized by the temporal association with the trigger, duration, and location of lesions (Table 1-1).

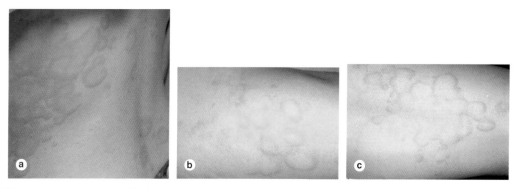

Figure 1-1 a–c Appearance of urticaria

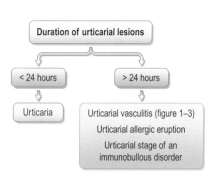

Figure 1-2 Algorithm to determine the type and duration of individual lesions

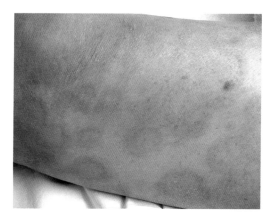

Figure 1-3 Urticarial vasculitis

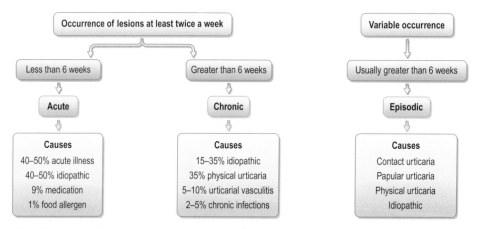

Figure 1-4 Algorithm to determine frequency of occurrence of urticaria

Differential diagnosis

> ### Key Points
>
> * Urticarial lesions that last longer than 24 hours should be biopsied
> * Urticarial lesions of autoinflammatory syndromes may burn or resemble cellulitis

Several dermatological conditions can mimic urticaria, including bullous pemphigoid, dermatitis herpetiformis, erythema multiforme, urticaria pigmentosa, pruritic urticarial papules and plaques of pregnancy, dermatomyositis, eosinophilic cellulitis (Well's syndrome), polymorphous light eruption, acute contact dermatitis, granuloma annulare, necrobiosis lipoidica (Figure 1-5), tinea (Figure 1-6), systemic lupus erythematosus, annular lesions of neonatal lupus erythematosus (Figure 1-7), and morbilliform drug eruptions (Box 1-1).

Urticaria may be a component of several syndromes (Table 1-2). Urticarial vasculitis must be differentiated from urticaria and serum sickness.

Table 1-1 Types of physical urticarias

Type of urticaria by frequency of occurrence	Stimulus	Location	Onset	Duration	Associated angioedema	Special findings
Dermatographism	Stroking skin	Trunk and extremities	5–10 minutes	15–20 minutes	No	Seen in 2–5% of healthy people
Cholinergic (Figure 1-8)	Rise in core temperature: exercise, stress, fever, shower	Upper trunk and arms	2–5 minutes	Up to 1 hour	Rare, but a subset of cases may present with exercise-induced anaphylaxis	2–3 mm uniform wheals with prominent flare
Acquired cold urticaria (Figure 1-9)	Rewarming after cold exposure	Any area of contact	2–5 minutes	1–2 hours	30–50% of patients	Associated underlying disease, most commonly infection
Familial cold urticaria	Generalized cooling	Any area of contact	2–18 hours	Up to 48 hours		Autoinflammatory syndrome, AD mutation in a pyrin-like protein on 1q44; associated systemic symptoms
Delayed-pressure urticaria	Deep prolonged pressure	Any area of contact	4–6 hours	Up to 48 hours	Rare	Associated systemic symptoms
Solar urticaria	Exposure to wavelengths between 290 and 800 nm, often with a defined action spectrum	Less involvement of the face and hands	Less than 30 minutes	Minutes to hours	Rare	Pruritus and stinging common
Aquagenic urticaria	Exposure to water	Areas of contact	Variable	Variable	Rare	Non temperature dependent, resembles cholinergic urticaria but with fewer lesions.
Vibratory urticaria	Provoked by vibration	Areas subject to vibration	Variable	Variable	Rare	Localized edema and erythema, can be familial
Galvanic urticaria	Reported after iontophoresis	Areas exposed to current	Variable	Variable	Not reported	

Laboratory testing

Key Points

- Testing is directed by signs and symptoms
- Acute urticaria
  - History is more likely than lab testing to reveal cause
- Chronic urticaria
  - 33–50% of cases of chronic urticaria occur as a result of circulating autoimmune antibodies; 27% of these patients have been shown to have other associated autoimmune diseases (Figure 1-10)
- Radioallergosorbent tests (RAST) may be of value when history suggests food or latex allergy
- There is a risk of anaphylaxis with prick or scratch testing, especially in patients with a suspected latex allergy

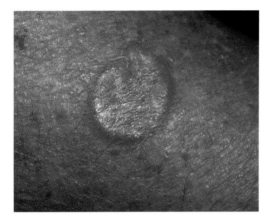

Figure 1-5 Annular necrobiosis lipoidica

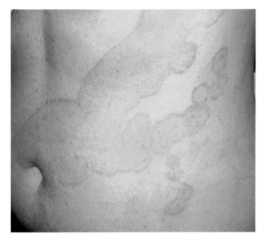

Figure 1-6 Tinea corporis

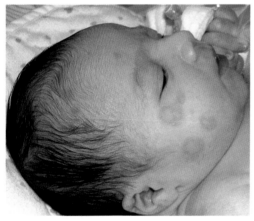

Figure 1-7 Neonatal lupus erythematosus

Acute urticaria typically occur in younger patients and triggers such as infections, insect stings, medications, or foods can often be identified. Since most cases of acute urticaria are self-limited, diagnosis is usually based on history and clinical evaluation alone, without the need for further testing.

> ### BOX 1-1
>
> **Differential diagnosis: mimickers of urticaria**
>
> Urticarial stage of various immunobullous disorders
>
> Erythema multiforme
>
> Urticaria pigmentosa
>
> Pruritic urticarial papules and plaques of pregnancy
>
> Systemic lupus erythematosus
>
> Dermatomyositis
>
> Eosinophilic cellulitis (Well's syndrome)
>
> Polymorphous light eruption
>
> Acute contact dermatitis
>
> Morbilliform drug eruptions

Table 1-2 Syndromes associated with chronic urticaria and/or angioedema

Syndrome	Symptoms
Muckle–Wells syndrome	Episodic attacks of urticaria, malaise, fever, leukocytosis, deafness, and amyloidosis
Chronic infantile neurological, cutaneous, and articular or CINCA syndrome	Urticarial skin eruption, fever, chronic meningitis, uveitis, sensorineural hearing loss, and a characteristic deforming arthropathy
Schnitzler's syndrome	Chronic urticaria and/or angioedema, intermittent fever, arthralgia or bone pain, elevated erythrocyte sedimentation rate and monoclonal IgM gammopathy
Episodic angioedema with eosinophilia	Episodic fever, weight gain, myalgia, peripheral blood eosinophilia, and elevated major basic protein
Serum sickness	Urticaria, facial edema, vasculitis, fever, lymphadenopathy, arthralgias, gastrointestinal manifestations, glomerulonephritis, and peripheral neuropathy

Chronic urticaria, on the other hand, are more complicated. Some cases are associated with chronic infections, including dental, sinus, and parasitic infections. Recent studies have shown that 33–50% of cases of chronic urticaria occur as a result of circulating autoimmune antibodies, and such patients may develop hives in response to injection of their own serum. Dermatographism can produce a hive with any injected liquid, so such testing should be interpreted cautiously. To test for autoantibodies to FcεRIa, intradermal

Figure 1-8 Cholinergic urticaria

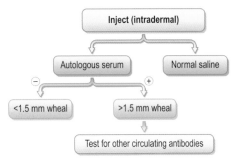

Figure 1-10 Testing for FcεRIa autoantibodies

extensive testing is low in the absence of specific signs and symptoms.

Provocative tests can be performed to diagnose some physical urticarias. RAST testing may be helpful in the evaluation of allergic causes of urticaria.

Pathogenesis

Key Points

- The mast cell is the primary effector cell in urticaria
- Mast cell degranulation has both immunologic and nonimmunologic triggers
- Acute urticaria are the result of a type I immunoglobulin E-mediated hypersensitivity reaction and are triggered by various stimuli or direct mast cell degranulation
- Chronic urticaria can be caused by infection or ingestants, but also have a strong association with the major histocompatibility complex alleles, human leukocyte antigen (HLA)-DR4 and HLA-DQ8 and the formation of autoimmune antibodies

Acute urticaria result from a type I hypersensitivity reaction triggered by various stimuli. They typically occur in younger patients and affect 10–30% of the general population at some point in their lifetime. Chronic urticaria, on the other hand, affect 0.1% of population and most frequently occur in middle-aged women. They are strongly associated with the major histocompatibility complex alleles, HLA-DR4 and HLA-DQ8, and the formation of autoimmune antibodies.

Regardless of whether urticaria are acute or chronic or are associated with angioedema, (Table 1-3) the mast cell is the primary effector cell. The mast cell contains numerous preformed vasoactive mediators and, upon stimulation, synthesizes others, resulting in local vasodilatation and tissue edema (Table 1-4).

The pathogenesis of urticarial vasculitis differs from that of urticaria in that it is due to a type III hypersensitivity reaction (Table 1-3). It results from deposition of immune complexes in the cutaneous vasculature, which leads to complement activation and neutrophil chemotaxis.

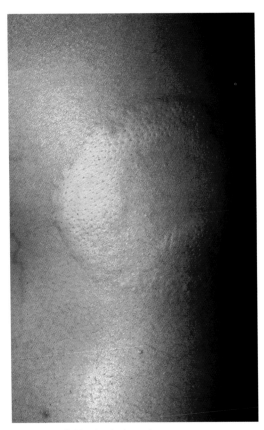

Figure 1-9 Cold urticaria, ice cube test

injection of autologous serum is compared to normal saline; a test is positive when a 1.5 mm or greater wheal is produced (Figure 1-10). Since 27% of these patients have been shown to have other associated autoimmune diseases, serum testing for other circulating antibodies should be performed in this subgroup of patients. Rarely, chronic urticaria may result from a subclinical infection, and a complete blood count, thyroid testing, and sinus and dental X-rays are advocated by some. However, in general the yield of

Table 1-3 Mechanisms of mast cell degranulation in urticaria and angioedema

Mechanisms	Causes
Type I Immediate hypersensitivity reaction, IgE mediated	Foods, drugs (antibiotics, especially penicillin and cephalosporins) latex, viral illnesses, insect stings or bites
Type II Autoimmune hypersensitivity reaction, IgG mediated	Anti-FcεRI antibodies, anti-IgE antibodies
Type III Immune complex or complement-related hypersensitivity reaction	Blood products. Low complement levels associated with hereditary angioedema and urticarial vasculitis
Nonimmunologic: mast cell degranulation	Radiocontrast dyes, curare, opiates, alcohol, neurohormones (neurotensin, substance P, adenosine triphosphate)
Nonimmunologic: other	Aspirin, nonsteroidal anti-inflammatories, angiotensin-converting enzyme inhibitors and physical stimuli, nettle stings
Idiopathic	

Ig, immunoglobulin.

Table 1-4 Mast cell-derived mediators

Preformed mediators	Newly synthesized from arachidonate acid metabolism
Histamine	Cyclooxygenase: prostaglandin D_2 (PGD_2), PGE_2, PGF_2, PGI_2
Heparin	Thromboxane A and B
Eosinophilic chemotactic factor of anaphylaxis (ECF-A)	Lipooxygenase: hydroxyeicosatetraenoic acids (HETEs) or hydroperoxyeicosatetraenoic acids (HPETEs)
Neutrophilic chemotactic factor	Slow-reacting substances of anaphylaxis (SRS-A): leukotriene C, D, and E
Proteases	Platelet-activating factor (PAF)
Cytokines	

Treatment

Key Points

- Eliminate any identifiable triggering factors and substances known to cause mast cell degranulation
- 40–50% of patients will flare when given aspirin and NSAIDS; therefore should be avoided
- Antihistamines are the mainstay of treatment
- Labeled doses of antihistamines may be inadequate and higher doses are frequently needed
- Doxepin can be effective in treatment of refractory chronic urticaria, including cold urticaria
- Autoimmune urticaria commonly require immunosuppressive therapy

Treatment of urticaria includes elimination of any identifiable triggering factors and substances known to cause mast cell degranulation. In addition, since 40–50% of patients will experience a flare when given aspirin and NSAIDS, patients should be advised to avoid all medications that contain these products. The initial pharmacologic treatment should consist of continuous, suppressive doses of an antihistamine. The best antihistamine for a given patient should maximize response, while minimizing side-effects. The mainstay of therapy for most patients is a long-acting, nonsedating antihistamine. The more sedating antihistamines should be reserved for patients refractory to second-generation antihistamines and/or for nighttime use in patients who do not need to drive or operate machinery. As an alternative to sedating antihistamines, refractory patients may benefit from the addition of H_2 antagonists or the use of doxepin, a tricyclic antidepressant with potent H_1 antihistamine properties. Although acute urticaria can be suppressed with a 3–5-week course of prednisone when needed, the long-term toxicity of prednisone precludes its use in chronic urticaria. Patients who have autoimmune chronic urticaria commonly require methotrexate or cyclosporine (Figure 1-11; Table 1-5). Plasmapheresis, calcium channel blockers, and intravenous immune globulin have occasionally been used.

Controversies

Key Points

- Urticarial allergic eruption
  - Lesions often persist beyond 24 hours
  - Causes include medications, arthropod bites and stings, autoimmune progesterone dermatitis, various syndromes
- It has become common practice to increase the daily dose of the second-generation antihistamines beyond that recommended by the package insert
- Data are mixed as to whether use of H_2 antihistamines provides any additional benefit beyond that of H_1 antihistamines

It has become common practice to increase the daily dose of the second-generation antihistamines beyond that recommended by the package insert. Some produce clinically significant sedation at higher doses and patients must be cautioned about this.

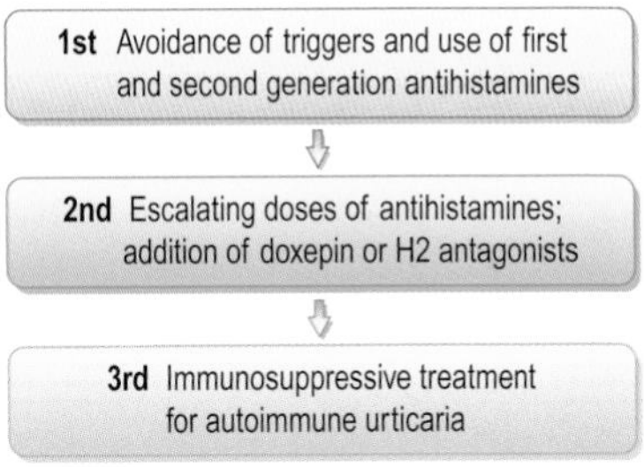

1st Avoidance of triggers and use of first and second generation antihistamines

⇩

2nd Escalating doses of antihistamines; addition of doxepin or H2 antagonists

⇩

3rd Immunosuppressive treatment for autoimmune urticaria

Figure 1-11 Treatment of urticaria

Angioedema

Clinical presentation

Key Points

- Nonpitting, nonpruritic, deep subcutaneous and submucosal edema
- Preferentially affects cutaneous areas with loose connective tissue, such as the face, eyelids, lips, tongue, and genital region
- Occurs in association with urticaria in 40% of cases
- HAE occurs *without* urticaria
- Associated with systemic findings including edema of the gastrointestinal mucosa and upper respiratory tract, resulting in abdominal pain, dysphagia, hoarseness, or shortness of breath

Angioedema that occurs without associated urticaria suggests the possibility of hereditary angioedema (HAE), whereas co-occurrence of urticaria virtually excludes this diagnosis. There are five major types of angioedema. Angioedema associated with allergic reactions is the most common and occurs in approximately 40% of patients with urticaria. Angioedema that occurs secondary to medications, such as angiotensin-converting enzyme (ACE) inhibitors is rare with an incidence of 1–2 cases per 1000 persons. Hereditary angioedema (HAE) is another rare form of angioedema with a reported incidence of 1 per 150, 000 persons. It is divided into three subtypes. The most common type, referred to as type I HAE, occurs in patients with insufficient levels of C1-esterase inhibitor (C1-INH). In type II HAE, the amount of C1-INH is normal but the enzyme is dysfunctional. In type III HAE, both the levels and function of C1-INH are normal. Patients in the latter category have normal levels and functioning of C1-INH. The rarest form of angioedema is acquired angioedema (AAE), which is separated into two categories. Type I AAE is caused by excess activation of complement resulting in consumption of C1-INH, whereas type II AAE is caused by autoantibodies directed against C1-INH. When none of the above etiologies can be attributed to the cause of angioedema it is referred to as idiopathic angioedema.

Differential diagnosis

Key Points

- Submucosal edema in angioedema can clinically mimic an asthmatic attack, acute chest or acute abdominal pain, and must be differentiated from those conditions

Laboratory testing

Key Points

- HAE is an autosomal-dominant condition that is not associated with urticaria
- In HAE C1-INH can be low or absent or dysfunctional and C4 is depressed both during and between attacks, but C1q is usually normal. (Figure 1-12 and Table 1-6).
- In acquired angioedema there is excessive consumption of C1 esterase inhibitor, with reduction of C1q, C2, and C4 during the attack (Table 1-6)
- In rare situations, patients with AAE have autoimmune antibodies directed against C1 esterase inhibitor and an immunoblot assay can be performed to look for a 95-kDa cleavage product
- For cases of acquired angioedema, it is important to determine if the patient has used an ACE inhibitor.
- Patients with lymphoproliferative disorders can develop anti-idiotype antibodies leading to consumption of C1-INH and angioedema

The screening test of choice for types I and II HAE is a C4 level. C4 will usually be less than 40% of normal, even between attacks as a result of continuous activation and consumption. Patients with types I and II angioedema may also have low C1, C1q, and C2 levels. C1 esterase inhibitor is a labile protein, and sample decay is common. A low C1 esterase inhibitor in the presence of normal C4 levels suggests sample decay, rather than true HAE.

In rare situations, patients may have autoimmune antibodies directed against C1 esterase inhibitor. In these cases, an immunoblot assay can be performed to look for a 95-kDa cleavage product. It is important to perform all the above tests on fresh serum that is less than 4 hours old for the most accurate results.

Pathogenesis

Key Points

- Histamine plays no pathogenic role in angioedema not associated with urticaria, but rather it occurs as a result of insufficient, or a dysfunctional C1 esterase inhibitor, which is central to the regulation of the complement, coagulation, and contact (kinin-forming) system proteases
- ACE inhibitors can cause angioedema

Table 1-5 Summary of common treatments of urticaria and angioedema

Drug category	Generic name	Brand name	Adult dosage	Pediatric dosage	Pregnancy category	Special indications
First-generation H₁-antihistamine	Diphenhydramine	Benadryl	25–50 mg q6–8 hours	2–5 years: 6.25 mg po q4 hours (max. = 25 mg/day) 6–12 years: 12.5 mg po q4 hours (max. = 50 mg/day) Chewable tabs Liquid	B	
	Cyproheptadine	Periactin	4–8 mg q8–12 hours	2–6 years: start: 2 mg bid–tid (max. = 12 mg/day) Syrup	B	Cold urticaria
	Hydroxyzine	Atarax	12.5–50 mg tid–qid	<6 years: 50 mg/day divided qid >6 years: 50–100 mg/day divided qid Syrup	Unrated	
	Chlorpheniramine	Chlor-Trimeton	4–8 mg tid	6–11 years: 2 mg po q4–6 hours (max 12 mg/day) 2–5 years: 1 mg q4–6 hours (max. 6 mg/day) Syrup	B	
Second-generation H₁-antihistamine	Desloratadine	Clarinex	5 mg daily	6–11 months:1 mg qd 1–5 years:1.25 mg qd 6–11 years: 2.5 mg qd Fast-dissolve reditabs Syrup	C	
	Cetirizine	Zyrtec	10–20 mg qd	6–23 months: 2.5 mg qd 2–5 years: 2.5 mg qd-bid Chewable tabs Syrup	B	
	Loratadine	Claritin	10 mg qd	2–5 years: 5 mg qd Fast-dissolve tabs Syrup	B	
	Fexofenadine	Allegra	Labeled dose 180 mg qd, but tolerated over a broad range of doses	6–12 years: 30 mg bid (tabs, caps)	C	

Class	Generic	Brand	Dose	Pediatric dose	Category	Indication
Tricyclic	Doxepin	Sinequan	10–100 mg HS	Not approved in children under 12 years	B	Chronic urticaria / Cold urticaria
H_2-receptor antagonist	Cimetidine	Tagamet	300 mg qid	20–40 mg/kg per day	B	Used in conjunction with an H_1 antagonist
	Famotidine	Pepcid	20 mg bid	0.5 mg/kg qd	B	
	Nizatidine	Axid	150 mg bid		B	
	Ranitidine	Zantac	150 mg bid	1–4 mg/kg qd	B	
Leukotriene receptor antagonist	Monteleukast sodium	Singulair	10 mg qd	5 mg qd	B	Aspirin sensitivity-associated urticaria
	Zafirlukast	Accolate	20 mg bid	10 mg bid	B	Aspirin sensitivity-associated urticaria
Other	Prednisone	Deltasone	1 mg/kg per day with a reduction by half in dose each week		C	Refractory cases of acute urticaria
	Methylprednisolone	Medrol			C	Refractory cases of acute urticaria
	Colchicine		0.6 mg bid		D	Refractory neutrophilic urticaria
	Dapsone		50–100 mg qd		C	Refractory neutrophilic urticaria
	Danazol	Danocrine	2 mg PO tid. Maintenance dose of 2 mg/day PO or 2 mg PO qod after 1–3 months	<6 years: 1 mg/day PO; 6–12 years: 2 mg/day PO; >12 years: Administer as in adults	X	Hereditary angioedema

Continued

Table 1-5 Summary of common treatments of urticaria and angioedema—cont'd

Drug category	Generic name	Brand name	Adult dosage	Pediatric dosage	Pregnancy category	Special indications
	Aminocaproic acid	Amicar	8 g q4 hours IV, then 16 g/day in acute attacks	8–10 g/day PO	C	Hereditary
			6–10 g/day PO maintenance	Syrup		Angioedema
	Cromolyn sodium	Gastrochrome	200 mg q 6 hours	2–12 years:100 mg qid	B	Mastocytosis
	Epinephrine 1:1000	EpiPen	0.3 mg/dose SQ		C	Anaphylaxis, angioedema allergic angioedema (HAE and AAE will not respond to epinephrine)
	Epinephrine 1:2000	EpiPen Jr		0.15 mg/dose SQ	C	Anaphylaxis, angioedema allergic angioedema (HAE and AAE will not respond to epinephrine)
	Cyclosporine	Neoral	2–5 mg/kg per day for 4–8 weeks		C	Chronic autoimmune urticaria
	Methotrexate	Rheumatrex	15 mg/week			Chronic autoimmune urticaria
	Intravenous immunoglobulin	Gammagard	2 g/kg total over 5 days		C	Chronic autoimmune urticaria

Dosing: qd, once a day; bid, twice a day; every 12 hours; tid, three times a day; every 8 hours; qid, four times a day; every 6 hours; IV, intravenously; PO, orally; SQ, subcutaneous injection; qod, every other day.

Pregnancy drug risk categories: X, contraindicated during pregnancy; D, positive evidence that risk can occur to a fetus; C, human studies lacking, animal studies may or may not show risk; B, no risk to humans, despite possible animal risk, or no risk to animals but no human studies done; A, controlled human studies show no fetal risk; Unrated, no pregnancy category has been assigned.

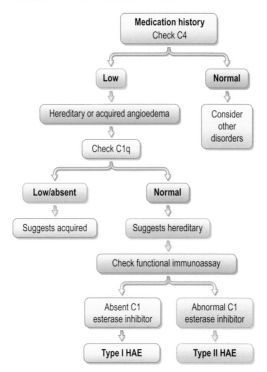

* Perform all the above tests on fresh serum less than four hours old for the most accurate results

Figure 1-12 Angioedema without urticaria*. HAE, hereditary angioedema

* The uncontrolled activation of the complement system eventuates in the excess production bradykinin which in turn results in vasodilation and edema of subcutaneous or submucosal tissues
* Although the exact mediator for angioedema is unknown, bradykinin appears to play an essential role
* Type III HAE differs from Type I and II HAE in that it is an estrogen-dependent HAE that occurs exclusively in women that have normal functional and quantitative levels of C1-INH. Currently the pathogenesis is unknown

Treatment

Key Points

* Patients with C1 esterase inhibitor deficiency should receive C1 esterase inhibitor concentrate or fresh frozen plasma in emergency situations and anabolic steroids such as danazol for maintenance
* In children who do not suffer from frequent or severe attacks of angioedema, no maintenance therapy is usually indicated; for children who are symptomatic, the literature suggests that antifibrinolytics (such as aminocaproic acid (Amicar)) should be the first drug of choice, since anabolic steroids are associated with numerous side-effects

The treatment of choice for acute HAE types I and II is replacement therapy, with either concentrates or fresh frozen plasma. Estrogens may precipitate attacks and should be avoided. The antifibrinolytic tranexamic acid, a drug related to epsilon-aminocaproic acid, has also been studied. Type III does not respond to C1 inhibitor replacement, but may respond to danazol.

Urticarial vasculitis

Clinical presentation

Key Points

* Erythematous plaques that may reveal nonblanching purpura with diascopy
* Lesions last longer than 24 hours and are more painful than itchy
* Lesions resolve with postinflammatory pigmentation
* Typically located on the lower extremities or at pressure points
* May present as an acute single event, or become chronic representing 5–10% of cases of chronic "urticaria"
* Can be associated with autoimmune diseases and/or hypocomplementemia or cryoglobulinemia

Urticarial vasculitis is associated with systemic findings such as transient and migratory arthralgia (49%), angioedema (42%), obstructive lung disease (21%), abdominal pain (17%), fever (10%), Raynaud's phenomenon (6%), and uveitis (4%). Some patients eventually meet criteria for systemic lupus erythematosus.

Differential diagnosis

Key Point

* Urticarial vasculitis must be differentiated from other vasculitides and serum sickness

Laboratory testing

Key Points

* Urticarial plaques lasting greater than 24 hours, or those that burn and/or resolve with purpura necessitate a biopsy.

If urticarial vasculitis is suspected, a punch biopsy should be performed to confirm the presence of leukocytoclastic vasculitis (endothelial cell swelling, neutrophilic infiltrate with some nuclear dust, extravasated erythrocytes, and fibrinoid deposits around the affected vessels). If the biopsy confirms the diagnosis, a complete blood count, erythrocyte sedimentation rate, complement levels (C1q, C3, C4, CH50), urinalysis and antinuclear antibody

Table 1-6 Angioedema: laboratory testing

	C1-INH	C1q	C2	C4
Hereditary angioedema type I	Low	Normal	Low	Low*
Hereditary angioedema type II	Normal	Normal	Low	Low*
Acquired angioedema type I	Low	Low	Low	Low
Acquired angioedema type II	Low	Low	Low	Low

*C4 levels are low both during and between attacks.

test should be performed as initial screening tests. Further testing is based on these results.

Pathogenesis

Key Points

- Secondary to a type III hypersensitivity reaction (Table 1-3)
- Immune complexes are deposited in the cutaneous vasculature, leading to complement activation and neutrophil chemotaxis
- May be secondary to connective tissue diseases, viral disorders, neoplasms, medications

Treatment

Key Points

- Use of NSAIDs and/or corticosteroids leads to improvement in 50% of patients
- In cases refractory to the above treatment or requiring chronic therapy, colchicine, dapsone, or an antimalarial may be beneficial

Gyrate or annular erythemas

Clinical presentation

Key Points

- Heterogeneous group of conditions
- Erythematous annular and polycyclic lesions that expand centrifugally with central clearing

Gyrate or figurate erythema refers to a heterogeneous group of recurrent annular lesions that most frequently arise on the trunk and extremities. These lesions begin as erythematous macules that expand centrifugally with central clearing. The lesion can show epidermal alterations such as a fine trailing border of scale or may simply have an indurated border. The superficial form, erythema annular centrifugum (Figure 1-13), demonstrates a trailing scale. Deeper forms lack scale. Other forms of gyrate erythemas include erythema gyratum repens (which presents with a wood-grain pattern and is strongly associated with rheumatic fever), erythema marginatum (an evanescent eruption associated with rheumatic fever), and erythema chronicum migrans (a manifestation of Lyme disease).

Diagnosis

Key Points

- Erythema annulare centrifugum (EAC) has a trailing scale
- Deep gyrate erythema has an indurated border without scale
- The two have similar associations, although EAC may be more likely to be associated with dermatophyte infections

The gyrate erythemas have been divided into two general groups. EAC, or superficial gyrate erythema, is characterized by a tight perivascular lymphohistiocytic infiltrate with a "coat sleeve" appearance that involves the superficial to mid dermal vascular plexus. There is epidermal spongiosis and parakeratosis, which clinically correspond to the trailing scale. The perivascular infiltrate in superficial gyrate erythemas may vary slightly in its intensity and type of inflammatory cells present, depending upon the antigenic stimulus, the patient's immunological response, and/or the timing of the biopsy. The second type of gyrate erythema, deep gyrate erythema, consists of a more dense perivascular lymphohistiocytic

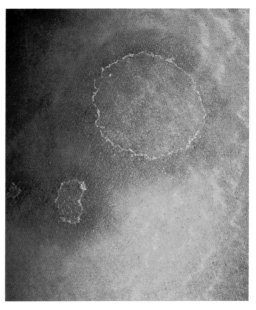

Figure 1-13 Erythema annulare centrificum

Table 1-7 Gyrate erythemas

Name	Clinical findings	Symptoms	Antigenic stimulus	Histological findings
Erythema annulare centrifugum (EAC) (superficial variant of gyrate erythema) (Figure 1-7)	A gradually expanding erythematous plaque with a trailing border of scale. Lesions are often recurrent and appear on the trunk and proximal extremities of a middle aged person	± Pruritus	The exact etiology is unknown, but it is hypothesized to represent a hypersensitivity reaction to a variety of antigens tinea, ingestion of blue cheese, tomatoes, and medications as possible triggers.	Superficial and mid dermal tight (coat-sleeve) perivascular lymphohistiocytic infiltrate associated with focal epidermal spongiosis and parakeratosis
Annular erythemas of infancy (Figure 1-8)	Resembles EAC, but occurs at a much younger age typically from infancy until adolescence	± Pruritus	The etiology is unknown although some cases may be familial	Superficial and deep dermal perivascular lymphohistiocytic infiltrate. The epidermis can be spongiotic with parakeratosis, and eosinophils may be present in the infiltrate
Deep gyrate erythema (Figure 1-9)	Erythematous plaque with an indurated border, but no epidermal alteration		Although the etiology remains enigmatic some cases may be related to autoimmune diseases	Superficial and deep tight lymphohistiocytic perivascular infiltrate with no epidermal alteration
Erythema gyratum repens (EGR)	Multiple expanding erythematous plaques with a peripheral rim of scale that forms a wood-grain pattern. The plaque enlarges at a rate of 1 cm/day. 85–90% have an underlying malignancy		Epidermal antibodies are hypothesized to cross-react with tumor antigens	Superficial perivascular lymphohistiocytic infiltrate with focal epidermal spongiosis and associated parakeratosis
Erythema marginatum rheumatica (EMR)	Peripherally expanding evanescent plaques that lack scale and enlarge by 0.2–1.2 cm/day	Fever, carditis, migratory polyarthralgia, Syndenham's chorea, and subcutaneous nodules	Serum antibodies to *Streptococcus*	Scant superficial perivascular infiltrate consisting primarily of neutrophils with a few lymphocytes and eosinophils
Erythema chronicum migrans (ECM)	In 50–75% of patients with Lyme disease, an expanding annular erythema develops at site of tick bite reaching up to 6 cm in diameter	Fatigue, headache, arthralgia, myalgia, and fever	Serum antibodies to *Borrelia*. Warthin–Starry stains spirochetes in the upper papillary dermis in 50% of cases	Superficial and deep perivascular and interstitial infiltrate of lymphocytes, with scattered plasma cells and eosinophils

infiltrate that involves the superficial and deep dermal vascular plexus without epidermal alteration. The other gyrate erythemas have similar histologic findings varying slightly by the degree of inflammatory infiltrate, the type of inflammatory and the location of the inflammation (Table 1-7).

Differential diagnosis

Key Points

- A multitude of conditions can assume an annular appearance

- Many of these conditions remain relatively fixed, and as a whole, can be differentiated from gyrate erythemas by characteristic histological findings (Table 1-8)

Laboratory testing

Key Points

- Gyrate erythema is a diagnosis of exclusion, since no specific diagnostic test exists
- EGR, EMR and ECM can be differentiated by clinical symptoms and serologic tests

Table 1-8 Differential diagnosis of annular eruptions differentiated based upon histopathological patterns

Histological pattern	Circinate or annular eruptions
Vasculopathic	Erythema elevatum diutinum Purpura annulare telangiectoides Acute hemorrhagic edema of infancy Sweet's syndrome Urticarial vasculitis
Granulomatous	Granuloma annulare Palisading neutrophilic and granulomatous dermatitis Sarcoidosis Necrobiosis lipoidica diabeticorum Leprosy
Vesiculobullous	Eosinophilic folliculitis (Ofugi's disease) Chronic bullous disease of childhood or linear IgA bullous dermatoses Sneddon–Wilkinson disease IgA pemphigus
Interface	Erythema multiforme Fixed drug Connective tissue diseases*
Lymphomatous/ pseudolymphomatous	Mycosis fungoides Palpable arciform migratory erythema Jessner's lymphocytic infiltrate Hodgkin's disease
Other	Elastosis perforans serpiginosa Porokeratosis Lichen planus Nummular eczema Psoriasis Dermatophytosis Secondary syphilis Lyme disease

Ig, immunoglobulin.
*Especially connective tissue diseases associated with antibodies to anti-Ro and anti-La such as neonatal lupus, subacute cutaneous lupus, Rowell's syndrome, and annular erythema of Sjögren's syndrome.

Table 1-9 Reactive erythemas and annular eruptions differentiated by the four hypersensitivity reactions as originally described by Gell and Coombs

Type of reaction	Serology	Histology-perivascular accumulation	Example
Type I: IgE-dependent immediate hypersensitivity	Elevated IgE and eosinophils	Early few PMNs, then lymphocytes + scattered eosinophils.	Urticaria
Type II: Cytotoxic-cytolytic antibody	± Lymphopenia	Lymphocytes, PMNs and NK cells, leukocytoclasis	Neonatal lupus
Type III: Arthus reaction, circulating immune complex	± Consumption of complement	Early PMNs, then replaced by lymphocytes	Urticarial vasculitis, Rowell's syndrome, possibly erythema marginatum rheumatica
Type IV: Delayed hypersensitivity	Activated T cells and macrophages	Lymphocytes and histiocytes	GA, leprosy, sarcoidosis, possibly gyrate erythemas

Ig, immunoglobulin; PMNs, polymorphonuclear leukocytes; NK, natural killer; GA, granuloma annulare.

Pathogenesis

Key Points

* Hypersensitivity reaction to a variety of antigens

All types of gyrate erythemas are hypothesized to represent a hypersensitivity reaction to a particular antigen; that antigen, however, is often unknown (Table 1-9). The annular configuration seen clinically is hypothesized to occur due to localized interactions between various cytokines and adhesion molecules with neighboring blood vessels, inflammatory cells, and the epidermis.

Treatment

Key Points

* Treatment is directed toward symptomatic relief
* Most lesions are asymptomatic and spontaneously regress within a few weeks
* Look for triggers in patients with recurrent lesions

Treatment is directed toward symptomatic relief. Fortunately, most lesions are asymptomatic and spontaneously regress within a few weeks; therefore, treatment is not necessary for many patients. For those with pruritus, corticosteroids and antihistamines may be of some benefit. Topical steroids may reduce the erythema and decrease the superficial inflammation, but the limited benefits must be weighed against the potential side-effects. A trigger can be identified and eliminated in some patients.

Further reading

Ackerman AB. Histologic Diagnosis of Inflammatory Skin Diseases. Philadelphia: Lea and Febiger, 1978: 169–175, 180, 231–233, 284.

Bressler GS, Jones RE, Jr. Erythema annulare centrifugum. J Am Acad Dermatol 1981;4: 597–602.

Burgdorf WHC. Erythema annulare centrifugum and other figurate erythemas. In: Fitzpatrick TB, Eisen AZ, Wolff K, et al., eds. Dermatology in General Medicine, 4th edn. vols I–II. New York: McGraw-Hill, 1993: 1183–1186, 2411–2413, 193–194.

Cox NH, McQueen A, Evans TJ, et al. An annular erythema of infancy. Arch Dermatol 1987;123:510–513.

Espana A. Erythemas. In: Bolognia JL, Jorrizzo JL, Rapini RP, eds. Dermatology. Edinburgh: Mosby, 2003:303–311.

Grattan CE, Black AK. Urticaria and angioedema. In: Bolognia JL, Jorrizzo JL, Rapini RP, eds. Dermatology. Edinburgh: Mosby, 2003:287–302.

Greaves MW. Antihistamines. In: Wolverton SE, ed. Comprehensive Dermatologic Drug Therapy. Philadelphia: WB Saunders, 2001:360–372.

Haas N, Hermes B, Henz BM. Adhesion molecules and cellular infiltrate: histology of urticaria. J Invest Dermatol Symp Proc 2001;6:137–138.

Hebert AA, Esterly NB. Annular erythema of infancy. J Am Acad Dermatol 1986;14:339–343.

Jorizzo JL. Dermatologic Clinics: Urticaria and the Reactive Inflammatory Vascular Dermatoses. Philadelphia: WB Saunders, 1985.

Jung MA. The clinical and histopathologic spectrum of "dermal hypersensitivity reactions," a nonspecific histologic diagnosis that is not very useful in clinical practice, and the concept of a "dermal hypersensitivity reaction pattern." J Am Acad Dermatol 2002;47:898–907.

Kaplan AP. Chronic urticaria: Pathogenesis and treatment. J Allergy Clin Immunol 2004;114: 465–474.

Kim KJ, Chang SE, Choi JH, et al. Clinicopathologic analysis of 66 cases of erythema annulare centrifugum. J Dermatol 2002;29:61–67.

Kossard S, Hamann I, Wilkinsion B. Defining urticarial dermatitis: a subset of dermal hypersensitivity reaction pattern. Arch Dermatol 2006;142:29–34.

Krishnaswamy G, Youngberg G. Acute and chronic urticaria: challenges and considerations for primary care physicians. Postgrad Med 2001;109:107–123.

Peterson AO, Jarratt M. Annular erythema of infancy. Arch Dermatol 1981;117:145–148.

Toonstra J, de Wit FE. 'Persistent' annular erythema of infancy. Arch Dermatol 1984;120:1069–1072.

Weedon D. Skin Pathology, 2nd edn. London: Churchill Livingstone, 2002:227–230, 242–246.

Weyers W, Diaz-Cascajo C, Weyers I. Erythema annulare centrifugum: results of a clinicopathologic study of 73 patients. Am J Dermatopathol 2003;25:451–462.

Pruritus 2

David F. Butler

Pruritus may be defined as the uneasy sensation that provokes the desire to scratch. Patients who present with diffuse pruritus in the absence of a primary skin disorder should be evaluated for the possibility of an internal disorder.

Key Points

- When presented with an itchy patient, it is essential to determine if the itch is the result of a primary skin condition, or if the itching (and resultant scratching) is the cause of the skin lesions
- Consider systemic causes for itching in the absence of primary skin disorder
- Underlying causes can include renal insufficiency, cholestasis, endocrine and hematologic disorders, human immunodeficiency virus (HIV), and internal malignancy
- Diagnosis requires thorough history, physical exam, and laboratory evaluation (Table 2-1)
- Endogenous opioids play an important role in pathophysiology
- Treatment may require topical, oral, or ultraviolet light therapies (Table 2-2)

Clinical presentation

The key to diagnosing pruritus caused by an underlying systemic disease is first to recognize the absence of a "primary" skin lesion. Primary skin lesions are those characteristic of the skin disease itself, and may consist of papules, nodules, vesicles, bullae, pustules, and/or wheals. The skin lesions themselves are itchy, and unaffected skin may or may not itch. Pruritic systemic disorders, on the other hand, make the skin itself itch, and the resultant scratching produces the "secondary" skin lesions, which may include excoriations, lichenification, prurigo nodules, and hypo/hyperpigmentation. Skin that has not been scratched should appear normal.

Primary skin disorders with itching as prominent clinical feature

- Atopic dermatitis
- Bullous disorders: pemphigoid, dermatitis herpetiformis, linear immunoglobulin (Ig) A dermatosis
- Connective tissue diseases (dermatomyositis)
- Dermatoses of pregnancy
- Dermatographism
- Infections: dermatophytosis, folliculitis, varicella, parasites
- Infestations: scabies, lice
- Insect bites: mosquitos, fleas, bedbugs
- Lichen planus
- Mastocytosis
- Mycosis fungoides
- Photodermatitis
- Psoriasis
- Sarcoidosis
- Urticaria
- Xerosis

One of the most common causes of itchy skin, especially in older persons, is xerosis (dry skin). Xerosis normally resolves with adequate hydration of the skin, avoidance of harsh soaps, and use of emollients. Primary skin disorders associated with HIV, such as seborrheic dermatitis, eosinophilic folliculitis, and skin infections, may also itch, and both HIV infection as well as acquired immunodeficiency syndrome (AIDS) can be associated with generalized pruritus.

Secondary changes caused by scratching

- Excoriations (Figure 2-1)
- Lichenification: lichen simplex chronicus (Figure 2-2)
- Prurigo nodularis (Figure 2-3)
- Secondary bacterial infection
- "Butterfly sign": skin spared on mid back (Figure 2-4)
- Hypopigmentation
- Hyperpigmentation

Diagnosis

See Table 2-1. Evaluation may include history and physical exam to exclude primary skin disease, review of systems regarding internal disorders, laboratory studies, skin biopsy for histology ± immunofluorescence.

Table 2-1 Evaluation and treatment algorithm for diffuse pruritus

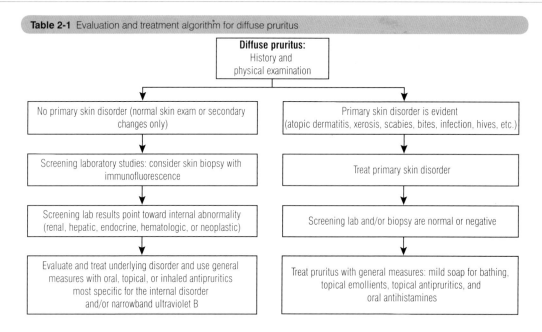

History

History should include onset, duration, severity, location, provoking factors (including pressure, water, heat), and relationship to activities such as bathing, as well as personal and family history of skin disease.

Carry out a review of systems, particularly pertaining to renal, hepatic, endocrine, and hematologic disorders and the potential for internal malignancy. Take a medication history, including illicit drug use and history of alcohol intake.

- Renal pruritus: symptoms may range from paroxysmal discomfort to continuous itching. 46% of patients with renal pruritus claim to have daily episodes of itching. Pruritus may be localized to the back, abdomen, head, or shunt arm. The vertex of the scalp is often affected
- Cholestatic pruritus: symptoms are intermittent and mild, initially with insidious onset and most often become generalized. Pruritus is typically worse on the hands and feet and under tight-fitting clothing. Primary biliary cirrhosis often presents with pruritus and fatigue
- Endocrine pruritus is most often generalized and may be associated with other symptoms of endocrine disease, such as tachycardia and weight loss due to hyperthyroidism, depression and constipation due to hypothyroidism and scalp itching due to the peripheral neuropathy of diabetes
- Hematologic pruritus: iron-deficiency pruritus is most often generalized but occasionally localized to perianal or genital area;

polycythemia vera may demonstrate pruritus after a hot bath or shower
- Malignancy-associated pruritus: often generalized or located on extensor surfaces with lymphoreticular malignancies; nasal pruritus has been associated with brain tumors. Pruritus may precede the development of lymphoma by 5 years

Physical exam: skin signs associated with the underlying systemic disease

- Renal insufficiency
  - Xerosis
  - Half and half (Lindsey) nails (Figure 2-5)
  - Scalp excoriations
- Cholestasis (Figure 2-6)
  - Jaundice
  - Spider angiomas
  - Dupuytren contractures
  - Gynecomastia
  - Xanthelasma
  - Terry's nails
  - Hepatosplenomegaly
  - Ascites
- Endocrine disorders
  - Hypothyroidism
  Brittle hair and nails
  Xerosis
  - Hyperthyroidism
  Warm, smooth skin
  Exophthalmos (Figure 2-7)
  Tachycardia
  Urticaria

Table 2-2 Medications used in the treatment of pruritus

Drug	Adult dosage	Uses	Comments/side-effects
Activated charcoal	6 g/day in divided doses	Hepatic and renal pruritus	May decrease effectiveness of co-administered medications; diarrhea and black stools
Cholestyramine	4–16 g/day in divided doses	Hepatic pruritus	Inhibits absorption of other drugs, constipation
Doxepin	10–25 mg every 8 hours	Histamine-related, renal and endocrine pruritus	Potent antihistamine, blocks both H1 and H2 receptors, some drug interactions may exacerbate cardiac and central nervous system disorders and urinary retention. Also available as a topical cream (Zonalon)
Ursodeoxycholic acid	10–16 mg/kg per day	Intrahepatic cholestasis of pregnancy	GI distress, diarrhea, constipation
Rifampin	150 mg PO qd. Increase to 300–600 mg/day	Hepatic pruritus	Inhibits reuptake of hepatic bile acids and induces hepatic enzymes that detoxify bile acids
Ondansetron	8 mg PO qd or bid	Hepatic pruritus	Hydroxytryptamine-3 antagonist
Mirtazapine	15–30 mg PO qd	Hepatic, renal, lymphoma	Alpha-2 adrenergic antagonist, antidepressant
Paroxetine	10–20 mg PO qd	Malignancy	Potent selective inhibitor of neuronal serotonin reuptake
Naltrexone	Initial 12.5 mg PO qd, maintenance 25–100 mg PO qd	Hepatic, renal, and hematologic pruritus	Opioid antagonist may induce opioid withdrawal; monitor liver function
Butorphanol	Initial 1 mg (1 spray) intranasal at bedtime, may increase to 2 mg at bedtime	Hepatic, renal, and hematologic pruritus	Mu opioid antagonist; kappa agonist; potential somnolence, nausea, and vomiting. Risk of dependence

qd, once a day; bid: twice a day, every 12 hours; PO, orally.

- Hematologic disorders
  - Anemia
    Skin pallor
    Angular cheilitis
    Glossitis
  - Polycythemia
    Ruddy complexion
    Hypertension
    Splenomegaly
- Lymphoreticular malignancy (especially Hodgkin's disease)
  - Lymphadenopathy
  - Hepatosplenomegaly
  - Herpes zoster
  - Ichthyosis (Figure 2-8)
  - Hyperpigmentation

Laboratory testing

- Complete blood count with differential
- Serum iron, ferritin, and total iron-binding capacity
- Serum creatinine and blood urea nitrogen
- Liver transaminases (aspartate aminotransferase/alanine aminotransferase), alkaline phosphatase, bilirubin (direct and indirect), antimitochondrial antibodies (if primary biliary cirrhosis is suspected), hepatitis B and C serologies
- Serum tryptase
- Thyroid-stimulating hormone and thyroxine
- Fasting glucose
- Stool for occult blood, ova, and parasites
- HIV antibodies (if risk factors are present)
- Serum protein electrophoresis
- 24-hour urine for hydroxyindoleacetic acid if clinically indicated
- Skin biopsy for routine histology and immunofluorescence (if indicated)

Other studies

- Chest radiography and computed tomography scan should be considered to evaluate the possibility of mediastinal lymphadenopathy

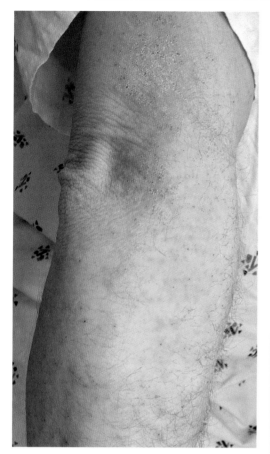

Figure 2-1 Excoriated, eczematous patch on the arm

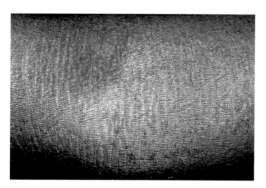

Figure 2-2 Lichenified skin

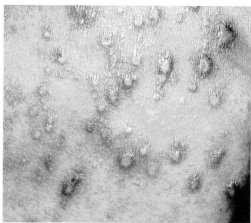

Figure 2-3 Prurigo nodules

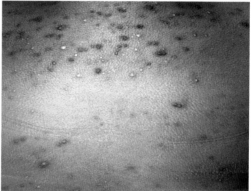

Figure 2-4 Butterfly sign: relative sparing of center of back

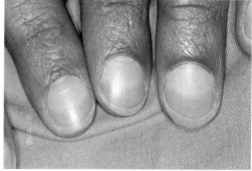

Figure 2-5 Half and half nails of renal insufficiency

- Ultrasound of the liver could be considered to evaluate the biliary system

Pathogenesis

General

Within the skin, nerve impulses of pruritus are transmitted through slow-conducting C polymodal and possibly type A delta nocioceptive neurons. These nerves have free nerve endings at the dermal–epidermal junction or within the epidermis. Histamine, substance P, serotonin, bradykinin, proteases such as tryptase, and endothelin may activate these nerve endings. Systemic disorder may cause "central" pruritus through a variety of mediators not directly involving the skin.

Renal pruritus occurs in the setting of chronic renal insufficiency. It typically does not occur in

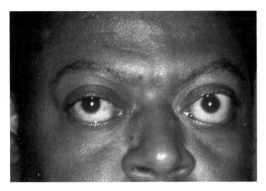

Figure 2-6 Exophthalmos due to Graves disease (hyperthyroidism)

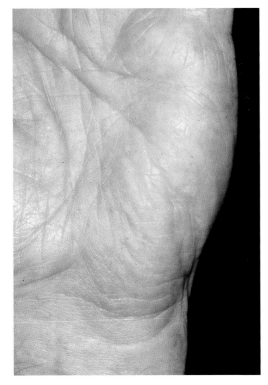

Figure 2-7 Palmar erythema of liver disease

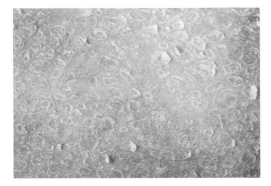

Figure 2-8 Acquired ichthyosis as a sign of lymphoreticular malignancy

acute renal insufficiency and therefore is not directly related to elevated serum urea or creatinine. Elevated levels of several mediators or other factors have been proposed:

- Histamine (responds only marginally to antihistamines)
- Parathyroid hormone (may respond to parathyroidectomy if elevated)
- Divalent ions: calcium, magnesium phosphate
- Serotonin
- Serum bile acids
- Peripheral neuropathy
- Endogenous opioids (stimulation of mu receptors)
- Interleukin-2 (overexpression of activated TH1 helper T cells)
- Ferritin
- Xerosis

Cholestatic pruritus results from obstruction of the biliary tract and retention of bile salts and acids. Indirect (unconjugated) hyperbilirubinemia does not cause itching. Several mediators of pruritus have been proposed:

- Bile salts
- Histamine
- Pruritogenic substance from damaged hepatocytes
- Endogenous opioids
- Combination of the above

Hematologic pruritus may be related to iron deficiency even in the absence of anemia. Polycythemia is associated with a basophilia and increased tissue mast cells which may liberate histamine and prostaglandin metabolites, resulting in platelet release of serotonin. Products of eosinophils such as major basic protein, cationic protein, peroxidase, and neurotoxin are known to cause itching. The mediators of pruritus occurring in leukemia and myelodysplasia remain unknown.

Endocrine pruritus may be seen in hyperthyroidism, hypothyroidism, hyperparathyroidism, and diabetes. Excess thyroid hormone may activate kinins from accelerated tissue metabolism or reduce itch threshold due to skin warmth and vasodilatation. Hypothyroidism may result in severe xerosis. Calcium seems to mediate the pruritus of hyperparathyroidism. Autonomic dysfunction, anhydrosis, and neuropathy may cause itching in diabetes.

Malignancy-associated pruritus currently has no known mediators, although several theories have been suggested. These theories center on the immune response to the tumor or a release of a chemical mediator by the tumor. In Hodgkin's disease, leukopeptidase and bradykinin are released in an immune response to malignant lymphoid cells. Serotonin is associated with pruritus found in carcinoid syndrome. Inter-leukin-2 may play a role in the pruritus of T-cell lymphomas.

Treatment

General measures

- Avoidance of skin irritants (e.g., wool clothing, hot showers/baths)
- Use of oilated soap such as Dove or Cetaphil for bathing
- Emollients applied immediately after bath to reduce xerosis
- Lotion with 0.25% camphor and menthol, pramoxime, or both
- Oral antihistamines such as hydroxyzine or diphenhydramine 10–25 mg every 6–8 hours for histamine-mediated itch and for sedation at bedtime
- Opiate antagonists
- Gabapentin for localized neuropathic itch

Physical modalities

Narrowband ultraviolet B (NBUVB) phototherapy delivers a more specific wavelength of light (311–313 nm) which results in greater efficacy and fewer adverse effects than broadband ultra-violet B light (290–320 nm). UVB therapy has proven to be particularly effective in the treatment of renal, hepatic, hematologic, and HIV-associated pruritus.

Psoralen plus ultraviolet light A (PUVA) is effective in the treatment of pruritus related to polycythemia and myelofibrosis.

Medications

Table 2-2 demonstrates a variety of medications available for the treatment of pruritus. Some are relatively specific for a particular type of pruritus. Please refer to the package insert for detailed pre-scribing information.

Further reading

Adams SJ. Iron deficiency and other hematological causes of generalized pruritus. In: Bernhard JD, ed. Itch: Mechanisms and Management of Pruritus. New York: McGraw Hill, 1994;243–250.

Bergasa NV. Pruritus in chronic liver disease: mechanisms and treatment. Curr Gastroenterol Rep 2004;6:10–16.

Bernhard JD. General principles, overview, and miscellaneous treatments of itching. In: Bernhard JD, ed. Itch: Mechanisms and Management of Pruritus. New York: McGraw Hill, 1994:367–381.

Blachley JD, Blankenship DM, Menter A, et al. Uremic pruritus: skin divalent ion content and response to ultraviolet phototherapy. Am J Kidney Dis 1985;5:237–241.

Cho YL, Liu HN, Huang TP, et al. Uremic pruritus: roles of parathyroid hormone and substance P. J Am Acad Dermatol 1997;36:538–543.

Dawn AG, Yosipovitch G. Butorphanol for treatment of intractable pruritus. J Am Acad Dermatol 2006;54:527–531.

Ghent CN. Cholestatic pruritus. In: Bernhard JD, ed. Itch: Mechanisms and Management of Pruritus. New York: McGraw Hill, 1994:229–242.

Greaves MW. Itch in systemic disease: therapeutic options. Dermatol Ther 2005;18:323–327.

Hampers CL, Katz AI, Wilson RE, et al. Disappearance of "uremic" itching after subtotal parathyroidectomy. N Engl J Med 1968;279: 695–697.

Hundley JL, Yosipovitch G. Mirtazapine for reducing nocturnal itch in patients with chronic pruritus: a pilot study. J Am Acad Dermatol 2004;50:889–891.

Kantor GR. Diagnostic evaluation of the patient with generalized pruritus. In: Bernhard JD, ed. Itch: Mechanisms and Management of Pruritus. New York: McGraw Hill, 1994:337–346.

Lebwohl M. Phototherapy of pruritus. In: Bernhard JD, ed. Itch: Mechanisms and Management of Pruritus. New York: McGraw Hill, 1994;399–411.

Lidstone V, Thorns A. Pruritus in cancer patients. Cancer Treat Rev 2001;27:305–312.

Manenti L, Vaglio A, Costantino E. Gabapentin in the treatment of uremic itch: an index case and a pilot evaluation. J Nephrol 2005;18:86–91.

Palma J, Reyes H, Ribalta J, et al. Ursodeoxycholic acid in the treatment of cholestasis of pregnancy: a randomized, double-blind study controlled with placebo. J Hepatol 1997;27:1022–1028.

Pederson JA, Matter BJ, Czerwinski AW, et al. Relief of idiopathic generalized pruritus in dialysis patients treated with activated oral charcoal. Ann Intern Med 1980;93:446–448.

Schwartz IF, Iaina A. Management of uremic pruri-tus. Semin Dial 2000;13:177–180.

Ständer S, Steinhoff M, Schmelz M, et al. Neuro-physiology of pruritus: cutaneous elicitation of itch. Arch Dermatol 2003;139:1463–1470.

Terg R, Coronel E, Sorda J, et al. Efficacy and safety of oral naltrexone treatment for pruritus of cholestasis, a crossover, double blind, placebo-controlled study. J Hepatol 2002;37:717–722.

Yosipovitch G, Fleischer A. Itch associated with skin disease: advances in pathophysiology and emerging therapies. Am J Clin Dermatol 2003;4:617–622.

Erythema multiforme, Stevens–Johnson syndrome, and toxic epidermal necrolysis

April W. Armstrong

Although some scholars regard erythema multiforme (EM) (Figure 3-1), Stevens–Johnson syndrome (SJS) (Figure 3-2), and toxic epidermal necrolysis (TEN) (Figure 3-3) as entities of the same disease spectrum, it is important to appreciate the differences in etiology, clinical presentation, and prognosis among these three diseases. EM is a distinct clinical entity often associated with infectious agents. In contrast, SJS and TEN have considerable overlap in histology and clinical presentation, and are associated with *Mycoplasma* and medications.

Erythema multiforme

Key Points

- Most commonly associated with herpes simplex virus (HSV) infection
- Typical clinical presentation includes "target" lesions
- Oral mucosa, dorsal hands, or palms frequently involved
- Episodes are recurrent and self-limited

EM, an acute and self-limited cutaneous eruption, is most commonly associated with HSV infection. The distinctive clinical morphology of EM is that of target skin lesions with a dusky or bullous center. Lesions run a benign, self-limited course and resolve without long-term sequelae. Most cases of EM do not require specific treatment; however, long-term, suppressive, antiviral therapy reduces the recurrence rate of HSV-associated EM.

Pathogenesis

HSV infection, specifically HSV-1, is the most frequent precipitating factor in EM. Over 50% of cases of EM are associated with preceding orolabial HSV infection. EM can occur before, during, or after the clinical appearance of herpetic lesions.

However, in most cases, EM lesions follow the outbreak of herpes by 3–14 days, with an average onset of 10 days after lesions appear. EM caused by HSV is commonly limited to the oral mucosa or the hands and feet.

Other inciting factors associated with EM include infection by other organisms, radiation, contact dermatitis (poison ivy), and, rarely, medications. Orf, *Histoplasma capsulatum*, and Epstein–Barr virus have been implicated in the development of EM. Infection by *Mycoplasma pneumoniae* appears to be associated more commonly with SJS than with EM. Radiation is an infrequent but recognized cause of EM, especially in neurosurgical patients receiving prophylactic phenytoin and systemic corticosteroids for whole-brain radiation. As steroids are tapered in these patients, EM lesions first appear at radiation ports, progress to involve the rest of the body, and potentially evolve into SJS. In the rare cases of drug-induced EM, the cutaneous eruption tends to be more extensive than that induced by infectious agents, and the eruption has the potential to evolve into TEN. Drugs that are implicated in EM are the same agents associated with SJS and TEN (see below). The majority of idiopathic EM cases, in which no clear precipitating factors can be identified, are now thought to be associated with recurrent HSV infection.

Clinical presentation

Key Points

- Most common in young adults
- Target lesions are classic
- Lips may be involved
- Self-limited, usually resolving over 2 weeks

HSV-associated EM affects young adults during spring and fall. It undergoes a self-limited – albeit

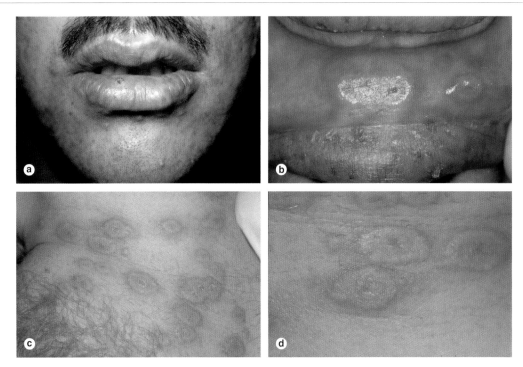

Figure 3-1 **a** Erythema multiforme. **b** Oral erythema multiforme. **c, d** Target lesions of erythema multiforme

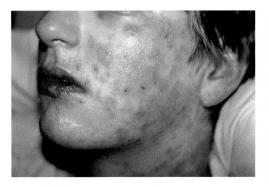

Figure 3-2 Stevens–Johnson syndrome

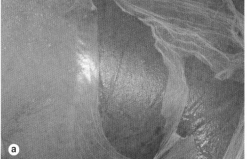

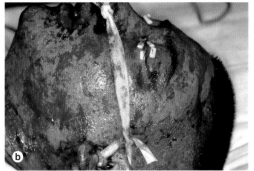

Figure 3-3 **a** Toxic epidermal necrolysis.
b Anticonvulsant-induced toxic epidermal necrolysis

recurrent – course that lasts 1–4 weeks. Almost all cutaneous lesions appear during the first 24–48 hours and cause a mildly pruritic or burning sensation. The hallmark of EM is the target or "iris" lesion. A target lesion is strictly defined as a lesion with three concentric zones of color: a center of dusky purpura, encircled by a pale, edematous ring, surrounded by an outer zone of macular erythema. The center of a target lesion typically demonstrates evidence of epidermal damage; the dusky purpura of the center seen at early stages can evolve into a bulla or crust during later stages. Koebner phenomenon can occur with EM lesions. EM lesions tend to favor extensor limbs, elbows, knees, palms, soles, and dorsal feet, with limited involvement of the trunk.

Mucosal involvement occurs in up to 25% of cases, and is typically mild and limited to the mouth. Few oral erosions may be present on the lips, buccal mucosa, or the tongue, and rarely, crusted erosions on the lips may resemble those of SJS. However, involvement of multiple mucosal surfaces, such as the conjunctiva, genitourinary epithelium, respiratory tract, or the gastrointestinal tract, is not seen. Additionally, constitutional signs and symptoms of fever, hepatosplenomegaly, and lymphadenopathy are also absent in EM.

The target lesions are usually fixed for 7 days, and an episode of EM typically lasts 2 weeks. Recurrences are common, averaging approximately 2–3 episodes per year. Long-term antiviral therapy has been shown to reduce the number of recurrences in HSV-associated EM, whereas corticosteroids may increase the frequency of recurrences.

Pathology

Key Points

- Individual necrotic keratinocytes (satellite necrosis) under a basket-weave stratum corneum
- Interface change

Skin biopsy helps distinguish EM from other diseases that share similar clinical features. Characteristic biopsy findings of an EM lesion include scattered, necrotic keratinocytes and hydropic degeneration of the epidermal basal layer, with occasional subepidermal blister formation. The papillary dermis is often edematous, and there are perivascular or interface lymphocytes.

Differential diagnosis

The differential diagnosis of EM includes other diseases with annular, circinate or "target-like" lesions. These conditions include multifocal fixed drug eruptions, erythema annulare centrifugum, urticarial vasculitis, subacute lupus erythematosus, bullous arthropod reactions, autoimmune and paraneoplastic bullous diseases, and granuloma annulare. Urticaria often develops dusky centers and is often confused with EM. Histology and response to antihistamines will distinguish the two.

Treatment

Most cases of EM are self-limited and do not require specific treatment. Mixtures of kaolin, viscous lidocaine, and diphenhydramine elixir may provide symptomatic relief of oral lesions.

In HSV-associated EM, prevention of herpes outbreaks may reduce the incidence of EM. Lip balms containing broad-spectrum sunscreen help prevent ultraviolet B-induced outbreaks of orolabial HSV. Chronic suppressive antiviral therapy is effective in reducing recurrences in 90% of HSV-associated EM. Intermittent antiviral therapy is usually ineffective, as is the initiation of antiviral therapy after the appearance of herpetic or EM lesions. The use of oral corticosteroids is controversial, as they may increase the frequency as well as the duration of subsequent attacks.

Stevens–Johnson syndrome and toxic epidermal necrolysis

SJS and TEN overlap in clinical presentation, histology, and treatment. They are frequently considered entities in the same disease spectrum. SJS is associated with *Mycoplasma* and sulfa whereas TEN is frequently associated with anticonvulsants and nonsteroidal anti-inflammatory drugs (NSAIDs). Both are increased in severity when there is concomitant human immunodeficiency virus (HIV) infection. All patients with SJS have involvement of two or more mucosal surfaces and a variable degree of cutaneous involvement, but mucosal involvement is also common in TEN. SJS is sometimes defined as having less than 10% of total body surface area (TBSA) with epidermal detachment; SJS–TEN overlap is then defined as having 10–30% of TBSA with epidermal detachment, and TEN is defined as having greater than 30% of TBSA with epidermal detachment. These divisions are somewhat arbitrary. Treatment of SJS and TEN involves prompt discontinuation of the offending drug and attentive supportive care to prevent both short-term and long-term sequelae.

Pathogenesis

Key Points

- Most commonly secondary to medications
- Also associated with *Mycoplasma* infection

In addition to medications, SJS has been associated with certain infections (Table 3-1), most notably *Mycoplasma pneumoniae*. *M. pneumoniae* infection is a common cause of SJS in children, leading to characteristic oral and conjunctival erosions. Drugs commonly associated with SJS and TEN include NSAIDs, sulfonamides, anticonvulsants, penicillins, and tetracyclines (Table 3-2). Currently, no laboratory test is available for rapid and accurate identification of inciting drugs.

Genetic differences in detoxification of reactive, intermediate drug metabolites may play a role in the development of SJS and TEN. Patients with human leukocyte antigen (HLA)-B12 genotype are more susceptible to SJS and TEN than the general population. Molecular levels of epoxide hydrolases, enzymes responsible for converting epoxides to *trans*-dihydrodiols, appear to be deficient in individuals susceptible to SJS and TEN. Fas-Fas ligand (FasL) interactions have been implicated in the pathogenesis of SJS/TEN. Lesional skin of patients with SJS and TEN has an increased expression of Fas ligand. Binding of FasL to Fas initiates cytolytic activities that result

Table 3-1 Associated factors in Stevens–Johnson syndrome

Drugs	See Table 3-2
Bacterial infections	*Mycoplasma pneumoniae*
	Chlamydia
	Mycobacterium tuberculosis
	Treponema pallidum
	Yersinia
	Less commonly, *Streptococcus, Pneumococcus, Salmonella typhi,* Enterobacteria
	Others
Viral infections	Adenoviruses
	Enteroviruses
	Influenza
	Measles
	Mumps
	Others
Fungal infections	Histoplasmosis
	Coccidioidomycosis
	Others
Vaccines	Bacille Calmette-Guérin (BCG)
Inflammatory bowel disease	
Radiation therapy	

Table 3-2 Drugs commonly associated with Stevens–Johnson syndrome and toxic epidermal necrolysis

Nonsteroidal anti-inflammatory drugs	Ibuprofen, naproxen, piroxicam, phenylbutazone
Sulfonamides	Trimethoprim-sulfamethoxazole, sulfadoxine-pyrimethamine, sulfadiazine, sulfasalazine
Anticonvulsants	Carbamazepine, phenytoin, phenobarbital, lamotrigine, valproic acid
Penicillins	Penicillin, aminopenicillins, cephalosporins
Tetracyclines	Doxycycline, tetracycline
Others	Allopurinol, barbiturates, chlormezanone, nevirapine

in apoptosis of keratinocytes. Blockade of the FasL and Fas interaction serves as a molecular rationale for the use of intravenous immunoglobluin (IVIg) in SJS and TEN patients.

Clinical presentation

Key Points

- Diagnosis of SJS requires involvement of two or more mucosal surfaces, with < 10% body surface area involved
- Diagnosis of TEN requires > 30% body surface area involvement
- Ocular involvement can result in significant morbidity

SJS occurs at approximately 1.2–6 events per million person-years, whereas TEN occurs at 0.4–1.2 events per million person-years. SJS affects children predominantly, and SJS is far more common than EM in childhood. The majority of patients with TEN are adults, and the incidence increases with age. There is a 1.5:1 female predominance for the development of TEN. Patients susceptible

to developing SJS and TEN include those with concomitant HIV infection, slow acetylator genotype, and those with brain tumors undergoing radiotherapy and receiving antiepileptic agents. Average mortality with SJS is 5% and 30–35% with TEN.

SJS is frequently preceded by an upper respiratory illness, characterized by a prodrome of fever, chills, cough, rhinitis, and sore throat. This prodrome is followed 1–14 days later by the development of mucosal erosions and a rash. Two or more mucosal surfaces must be involved to classify the eruption as SJS, and oral mucosa and conjunctiva are the most frequent sites of involvement. Extensive erosion and crusting commonly develop on the lips and oral mucosa. Conjunctiva are inflamed with an exudative discharge. The rash on the torso and extremities begin as erythematous, round macules and patches that have an atypical, targetoid morphology. The centers of these lesions are often dusky and purpuric, and they can evolve into coalescing bullae with extensive epidermal necrosis. When the bullae are sheared, the underlying dermis becomes clinically visible as areas of epidermal detachment (see Figure 3-1). The skin is tender to touch. SJS is commonly accompanied by fever, lymphadenopathy, arthralgia or arthritis, and hepatitis. Laboratory abnormalities may include elevated erythrocyte sedimentation rate, leukocytosis, eosinophilia, and elevated transaminases. The development of urinary pain, vaginal pain, difficulty swallowing, gastrointestinal bleeding, and/or shortness of breath may indicate progression of the disease to involve genitourinary, alimentary, and respiratory tracts.

The condition is termed TEN when the epidermal detachment involves more than 30% of the TBSA. TEN typically occurs 7–21 days after the initiation of the causative drug, and it runs an unpredictable course with high mortality. Affected skin is extremely tender. The cutaneous eruption progresses from the trunk to the neck, face, mucosal surfaces, and extremities. Involved skin is erythematous with dusky gray macules arising in areas of epidermal necrosis. As the eruption progresses, extensive bullae may develop, and full-thickness denudation of the skin occurs, often in areas of friction. A positive Nikolsky sign is elicited when lateral, mechanical, shearing pressure on erythematous skin splits the skin at the dermal–epidermal junction. Patients with TEN commonly have high fevers as well as difficulty eating or drinking. TEN involves the respiratory epithelium in 25% of cases, and these patients often require mechanical ventilation.

Mortality from TEN is often due to infection, acute respiratory distress syndrome, and massive fluid loss. Staphyloccoccal and pseudomonal skin infections leading to bacteremia and sepsis are among the common causes of death. The management of bacteremia can be especially challenging when antibiotics are suspected as the causative agent for TEN. Re-epithelialization of the epidermis begins within days and can be complete by 3 weeks. Long-term potential sequelae of SJS and TEN include scarring of the involved skin, contracture of joints underlying the scarred skin, and potential permanent loss of nails. A number of important ocular complications can result from SJS and TEN. Corneal scarring can lead to blindness; pseudomembrane formation can lead to symblepharon, entropion, and immobility of the eyelids; scarring of the lacrimal ducts results in severe xerophthalmia due to a lack of tear production. Vaginal involvement in women can result in synechiae formation with scarring.

Pathology

The histopathology of SJS and TEN is essentially the same. In early TEN, numerous necrotic keratinocytes are seen along the basal and suprabasalar layers of the epidermis. A sparse perivascular lymphocytic infiltrate is usually present in the dermis. In a fully developed lesion, there is full-thickness epidermal necrosis, often with a subepidermal blister. This is the histopathological hallmark of SJS and TEN.

Differential diagnosis

The main differential diagnoses for SJS and TEN include staphylococcal scalded-skin syndrome (SSSS), acute generalized exanthematous pustulosis (AGEP), and severe graft-versus-host disease. In SSSS, staphylococci secrete epidermolysin, which targets desmoglein-1 and causes a subcorneal split in the skin. The plane of split in SSSS is much more superficial than SJS and TEN, and the exfoliation typically reveals an intact epidermis below. Mucosal surfaces, palms, and soles are usually spared in SSSS. AGEP, a skin condition commonly caused by medications, presents as large, confluent areas of blanching erythema with numerous 1–3-mm white to yellow pustules. Clinical identification of these pustules, in combination with histological finding of subcorneal and intraepidermal neutrophilic infiltrates, aids in establishing the diagnosis of AGEP. Some cases of acute, severe graft-versus-host disease can be clinically and histologically indistinguishable from TEN; however, the clinical context is helpful in establishing the correct diagnosis.

Treatment

Key Points

- Discontinue any potential medication causes
- Supportive care
- Some studies support the use of IVIg, although data are mixed
- Ophthalmologic consultation should be sought in patients with ocular involvement

Because of the significant morbidity and mortality of SJS and TEN, patients should be cared for in an acute care setting by medical staff familiar with these diseases. Factors that have been shown to reduce mortality in patients with TEN include admission to a burn unit or intensive care unit, prompt discontinuation of the causative drug, and short half-life of the causative drug. Rapid diagnosis, prompt discontinuation of the causative drug, and meticulous supportive care are critical. The medication list for the patient should be minimized to avoid complicating the clinical presentation, and drugs with a shorter half-life are preferred.

Supportive care should be directed at correcting fluid and electrolyte imbalances, meticulous skin care to prevent bacteremia, pulmonary care, ophthalmologic care, nutritional support, and physical therapy. Denuded areas can be covered with petrolatum-impregnated gauze or silver dressings. Ophthalmologic and/or gynecologic consultation should be obtained for patients with conjunctival and/or vaginal involvement.

The use of immunosuppressive agents in SJS and TEN is an area of active investigation, and their risks and benefits are actively debated. IVIg, purported to act by blocking the interaction between Fas and FasL, has been used to manage severe cases of SJS and TEN. If used, IVIg should be initiated early in the course of the disease. Recommended dosing of IVIg includes either 1 g/kg per day for 3 days, or 0.75 g/kg per day for 4 days, to yield a total of at least 3 g/kg. Thromboembolic phenomena are a recognized complication of therapy. Cyclosporine, tumor necrosis factor (TNF) antagonists, and N-acetylcysteine have been anecdotally successful in some cases of TEN, but data are mixed. Thalidomide, which has anti-TNF effects, worsens the course of the disease. The use of systemic corticosteroids is highly controversial, and, like the use of other immuno-suppressive agents, requires further study. If used, they should be used at high dose, early in the course of the disease, and for less than 48 hours.

For survivors of SJS and TEN, the average time for epidermal healing is 3 weeks. Physical therapy is helpful to prevent contractures that could develop as a result of scarring over joints.

Further reading

Brice SL, Huff JC, Weston WL. Erythema multiforme. Curr Probl Dermatol 1990;II:3–26.

Brice SL, Stockert SS, Bunker JD, et al. The herpes-specific immune response of individuals with herpes-associated erythema multiforme compared with that of individuals with recurrent herpes labialis. Arch Dermatol Res 1993;285:193–196.

Halebian PH, Corder VJ, Madden MR, et al. Improved burn center survival of patients with toxic epidermal necrolysis managed without corticosteroids. Ann Surg 1986;204:503–512.

Kim PS, Goldfarb IW, Gaisford JC, et al. Stevens–Johnson syndrome and toxic epidermal necrolysis: a pathophysiologic review with recommendations for a treatment protocol. J Burn Care Rehabil 1983;4:91–100.

Paul C, Wolkenstein P, Adle H, et al. Apoptosis as a mechanism of keratinocyte death in toxic epidermal necrolysis. Br J Dermatol 1996;134:710–714.

Prins C, Kerdel FA, Padilla RS, et al. Treatment of toxic epidermal necrolysis with high-dose intravenous immunoglobulin: multicentric retrospective analysis of 48 consecutive cases. Arch Dermatol 2003;139:26–32.

Roujeau JC, Huynh TN, Bracq C, et al. Genetic susceptibility to toxic epidermal necrolysis. Arch Dermatol 1987;123:1171–1173.

Rzany B, Correia O, Kelly JP, et al. Risk of Stevens–Johnson syndrome and toxic epidermal necrolysis during the first weeks of antiepileptic therapy: a case control study. Lancet 1999;353:2190–2194.

Stevens AM, Johnson FC. A new eruptive fever associated with stomatitis and ophthalmia. Am J Dis Child 1922;24:526–533.

Sullivan JR, Shear NH. The drug hypersensitivity syndrome. What is the pathogenesis? Arch Dermatol 2001;137:357–364.

Tan AW, Thong BY, Yip LW, et al. High-dose intravenous immunoglobulins in the treatment of toxic epidermal necrolysis: an Asian series. J Dermatol 2005;32:1–6.

Tatnall FM, Schofield JK, Leigh IM. A double-blind, placebo-controlled trial of continuous acyclovir therapy in recurrent erythema multiforme. Br J Dermatol 1995;132:267–270.

Viard I, Wehrli P, Bullani R, et al. Inhibition of toxic epidermal necrolysis by blockade of CD95 with human intravenous immunoglobulin. Science 1998;282:490–493.

Weston WL. What is erythema multiforme? Pediatr Ann 1996;25:106–109.

Wolkenstein P, Carriere V, Charue D, et al. A slow acetylator genotype is a risk factor for sulphonamide-induced toxic epidermal necrolysis and Stevens–Johnson syndrome. Pharmacogenetics 1995;5:255–258.

Wolkenstein P, Charue D, Laurent P, et al. Metabolic predisposition to cutaneous adverse drug reactions. Role in toxic epidermal necrolysis caused by sulfonamides and anticonvulsants. Arch Dermatol 1995;131:544–551.

Panniculitis and lipodystrophies **4**

Papri Sarkar

Panniculitides

Clinical presentation

Key Points

- Panniculitis is inflammation of the subcutaneous fat
- Due to the deep location of the lesions in the skin, different forms of panniculitis share similar clinical features
- In general, lesions are tender, erythematous, subcutaneous nodules on the lower extremities
- Lesions are most often bilateral and symmetric
- The physical location of lesions may help generate a preliminary differential diagnosis for this condition (Table 4-1). For example, erythema nodosum usually presents on the distal extensor lower extremities, whereas lupus panniculitis is more common on the trunk, shoulders, and face
- Etiology of lesions may be differentiated by histology and systemic symptoms (Box 4-1)

Clinical presentation of selected panniculitides

See Table 4-1.

Diagnosis

Key Points

- Histology is the gold standard for diagnosis of all panniculitides
- Ideally, a deep wedge or excisional biopsy extended into affected fat should be obtained for optimal histological diagnosis
- For the discussion in this chapter, the types of panniculitis are classified into four main histological patterns. These categories include: (1) septal panniculitis without vasculitis; (2) septal panniculitis with vasculitis; (3) lobular panniculitis without vasculitis; and (4) lobular panniculitis with vasculitis. While inflammation spills over into the lobule in septal panniculitis, the lobule is not necrotic. In contrast, fat necrosis is seen in lobular panniculitis
- A useful tip is always to polarize the histology slide to check for refractile foreign material, which may be present in factitial or foreign-body panniculitis

- Given the similar clinical presentation of many of the panniculitides, diagnosis must be made by corroborating the clinical picture with the histology. Some diagnostic hints are listed in Table 4-2. This table should be used in conjunction with Table 4-1, which lists typical distribution and systemic signs associated with various disorders

Discussion of major panniculitides

Septal panniculitis with vasculitis

Cutaneous polyarteritis nodosa

- **Clinical**: bilateral tender, erythematous nodules, livedo reticularis, ulceration of the lower limbs
- Mild constitutional symptoms often present but usually no systemic involvement (in contrast to systemic polyarteritis nodosa)
- **Histology**: early neutrophilic infiltrate which progresses to include lymphocytes and histiocytes
- Vasculitis of the medium-sized arteries and arterioles of the septa over time may cause a target-like appearance of the vessel
- **Treatment** options may include nonsteroidal anti-inflammatory drugs (NSAIDS) or low-dose prednisone

Superficial migratory thrombophlebitis

- **Clinical**: erythematous, tender subcutaneous cord-like nodules along veins of the lower extremity, which migrates from location to location
- Classically associated with an underlying hypercoagulable state, but may simply be due to venous insufficiency
- Trosseau's sign: hypercoagulable state secondary to underlying malignancy
- Malignancies most commonly associated with this disorder include pancreas, stomach, lung, prostate, colon, ovary, and bladder

Table 4-1 Clinical presentation of selected panniculitides

Panniculitis	Location	Associated findings
Erythema nodosum (EN) (Figure 4-1)	Bilateral pretibial areas	Fever, arthralgia, malaise
Subacute nodular migratory panniculitis (EN migrans)	Nodules on legs, often unilateral	Streptococcal or thyroid disease
Erythema induratum/nodular vasculitis	Posterior lower legs	Ulceration and drainage
Alpha-1 antitrypsin deficiency	Lower trunk and proximal extremities	Ulceration and drainage
Pancreatic panniculitis	Legs, abdomen, chest, arms, scalp	Fever, arthritis, abdominal pain
Lupus panniculitis	Face, proximal extremities, trunk	Lupus (especially discoid lupus erythematosus)
Cytophagic histiocytic panniculitis	Extremities and trunk	Fever, hepatosplenomegaly, pancytopenia, liver failure, hemorrhage
Lipodermatosclerosis (stasis panniculitis) (Figure 4-2)	Legs, champagne-bottle deformity	Accompanying changes of stasis dermatitis clinically or histologically

- Behçet's disease may also be associated with this phenomenon
- **Histology** shows a mild septal panniculitis with thrombophlebitis of the large veins of the upper subcutis
- Diagnostic work-up should include search for malignancy
- **Treatments** include exercise for prophylaxis, dressings, and referral to vascular surgery if significant venous insufficiency is found. If a malignancy is found, anticoagulation may be considered.

Septal panniculitis without vasculitis

Erythema nodosum

- Erythema nodosum is the most common type of panniculitis (Box 4-2)
- **Clinical**: tends to occur in second to fourth decade of life, predominantly in women
- Sudden onset of symmetric, tender, erythematous nodules on the lower extremities, usually overlying the shins
- May be associated with fever, fatigue, cough, headache, abdominal pain, vomiting

- Multiple etiologies (see mnemonic in Box 4-1), the most common of which is streptococcal infection in children and drugs, sarcoidosis, or inflammatory bowel disease in adults
- **Pathophysiology**: believed to be a hypersensitivity response to various sources
- Lofgren's syndrome: fever, arthritis, hilar adenopathy, and erythema nodosum. Form of acute sarcoidosis that generally has a short-lived course and is associated with a good prognosis
- **Histology**: Meischer's radial granulomas: histiocytes surrounding septal cleft-like spaces may be present on histology
- **Treatment** options include bedrest, NSAIDS, potassium iodide, and systemic corticosteroids

Necrobiosis lipoidica (diabeticorum)

- **Clinical**: well-defined yellow-brown indurated plaques with an erythematous perimeter and an atrophic center with telangiectasias
- Most commonly on the anterior lower legs
- May be associated with long-standing diabetes
- **Histology**: palisading granulomas consisting of histiocytes and giant cells surrounding degenerated collagen of the dermis that may extend into the subcutaneous fat
- Histology may resemble "layers of a cake" with alternating bands of inflammatory cells and fibrosis
- **Treatments** include intralesional steroids, aspirin, dipyridamole, pentoxyfylline and antitumor necrosis factor agents.

Lobular panniculitis with vasculitis

Erythema induratum of Bazin/nodular vasculitis

- **Clinical**: typically affects middle-aged women, more common in obese persons
- Tender, erythematous to violaceous subcutaneous nodules and plaques on the posterior calves. These may ulcerate. May also arise in other fatty areas such as thighs, buttocks, arms
- Heal with scarring and may recur in crops
- Similar to erythema nodosum, this is thought to be a reactive process to an underlying factor. Initially was associated with *Mycobacterium tuberculosis* infection, but has also been shown to be a reaction to other infectious agents, drugs, etc.
- **Histology** shows mixed inflammatory lobular infiltrate with neutrophils, lymphocytes, histiocytes, giant cells and vasculitis of small to medium-sized vessels
- **Treatment**: supportive therapy includes bedrest, compresssion bandages, and treatment of underlying venous insufficiency

BOX 4-1

Primary panniculitis and entities with secondary involvement of the fat

Septal panniculitis with vasculitis

- Cutaneous polyarteritis nodosa
- Polyarteritis nodosa
- Superficial migratory thrombophlebitis
- Leukocytoclastic vasculitis

Mnemonic: septal panniculitis with vasculitis: "CUPS"

CUtaneous polyarteritis nodosa

Polyarteritis nodosa

Superficial migratory thrombophlebitis

Septal panniculitis without vasculitis

- Scleroderma
- Erythema nodosum
- Eosinophilic fasciitis (although inflammation must involve the fascia, as well)
- Necrobiosis lipoidica
- Rheumatoid nodule
- Subcutaneous granuloma annulare
- Necrobiotic xanthogranuloma
- Morphea profunda

Mnemonic: septal panniculitis without vasculitis: "SEEN"

Scleroderma

Erythema nodosum

Eosinophilic fasciitis

Necrobiosis lipoidica (diabeticorum)

Lobular panniculitis with vasculitis

- Nodular vasculitis/erythema induratum
- Erythema nodosum leprosum

- Neutrophilic lobular panniculitis associated with rheumatoid arthritis
- Crohn's disease

Mnemonic "ENN"

Erythema nodosum leprosum

Nodular vasculitis

Neutrophilic lobular panniculitis associated with rheumatoid arthritis

Lobular panniculitis without vasculitis

- Sclerema neonatorum
- Subcutaneous fat necrosis of the newborn
- Cold panniculitis
- Paraffinoma
- Pancreatic panniculitis
- Alpha-1 antitrypsin deficiency
- Cytophagic histiocytic panniculitis
- Poststeroid panniculitis
- Lupus panniculitis
- Panniculitis in dermatomyositis
- Calciphylaxis
- Oxalosis
- Lipodermatosclerosis
- Infectious panniculitis
- Sarcoidosis
- Factitial panniculitis
- Lipoatrophy
- Gout panniculitis
- Crystal-storing histiocytosis
- Postirradiation pseudosclerodermatous panniculitis

- If secondary to an underlying disorder, the etiologic factor should be treated. Otherwise, treatment options include potassium iodide, tetracycline, gold, NSAIDS, and corticosteroids.

Erythema nodosum leprosum

- **Clinical**: affects patients with borderline or lepromatous leprosy
- Painful erythematous to violaceous nodules on extremities, accompanied by constitutional symptoms including fever, arthralgia, neuritis, and leukocytosis
- **Pathophysiology:** immune complex-mediated vasculitis of dermis and fat
- **Histology**: inflammation in dermis and subcutaneous fat composed of lepra cells,

abundant neutrophils, and adjacent vasculitis. Lepra cells are histiocytes that have engulfed the acid-fast bacilli

- **Treatment** of choice is thalidomide. If unable to use thalidomide, may consider clofazimine

Lobular panniculitis without vasculitis
(Tables 4-3–4-5)

Lipodermatosclerosis (aka stasis panniculitis, sclerosing panniculitis, hypodermitis sclerodermiformis)

- **Clinical**: woody, indurated plaques with erythema, edema, telangiectasia, and hyperpigmentation on the distal lower extremities. Chronic venous stasis dermatitis changes

Table 4-2 Diagnostic clues and buzzwords

Diagnosis	Histology or important association/clinical finding	Buzzword
Cutaneous polyarteritis nodosa	Septal panniculitis with vasculitis of medium-sized arteries	
Superficial migratory thrombophlebitis	May be associated with underlying malignancy, especially pancreatic	
Erythema nodosum	May be associated with Lofgren's syndrome	Meischer's radial granulomas
Necrobiosis lipoidica diabeticorum	Palisaded granulomas	Histology resembles "layers of a cake"
Scleroderma	Diffuse sclerosis of collagen and loss of periadnexal fat; may lead to obliteration of adnexal structures	
Subcutaneous granuloma annulare	Necrobiosis and mucin surrounded by palisading granulomas in septa	
Rheumatoid nodule	Large areas of necrobiosis and fibrin surrounded by palisading granulomas of the dermis and fat	
Necrobiotic xanthogranuloma	Necrobiosis alternating with granulomas, Touton giant cells, cholesterol crystals at center of degenerated collagen	
Sclerema neonatorum	Very mild inflammation	Radially arranged needle-shaped clefts in adipocytes
Subcutaneous fat necrosis of the newborn	Patchy fat necrosis surrounded by moderate granulomatous infiltrate	Giant cells and adipocytes with radially arranged needle-shaped clefts
Oxalosis	Yellow-brown radially oriented needle or rectangular crystals	
Lupus panniculitis	Lesions are proximally distributed	May see lymphoid follicles on histology
Pancreatic panniculitis	Oily brown discharge from very tender subcutaneous plaques	Elevated lipase, amylase, or trypsin
Alpha-1 antitrypsin-deficiency panniculitis	Neutrophilic panniculitis with splaying of neutrophils between collagen bundles. Severe fat necrosis with skip areas of normal histology	
Infective panniculitis	Bacterial or fungal (multiple organisms; see Table 4-4)	Direct inoculation or hematogenous spread. Most commonly due to hematogenous spread from respiratory tract
Paraffinoma or sclerosing lipogranuloma	May be associated with hepatosplenomegaly and pulmonary fibrosis. 66% develop autoimmune findings	"Swiss-cheese"-like histology (empty spaces of various sizes due to removal of fat during processing)
Silicone granuloma	Foamy histiocytes and multinucleated giant cells surrounding polygonal translucent angulated foreign bodies	
Artecoll granuloma	Uniform, round vacuoles enclosing translucent, nonbirefringent foreign bodies with perimeter of sclerotic stroma.	
Vitamin K granulomas	Sclerosis of collagen, lymphocytic and plasma cell infiltrate	Resembles subcutaneous morphea histologically
Cytophagic histiocytic panniculitis	Often associated with T-cell lymphoma	Beanbag cells: enlarged macrophages containing red blood cells, lymphocytes, and nuclear debris

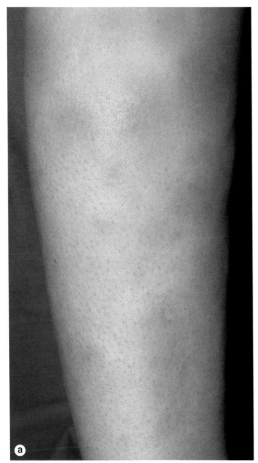
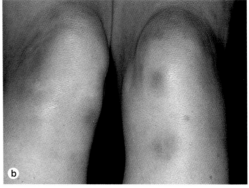

Figure 4-1 a, b Erythema nodosum

- Classically said to resemble an "inverted wine bottle"
- Closely associated with chronic venous insufficiency. Patient may also have history of arterial ischemia or thrombophlebitis
- **Histology** varies according to age of lesion. Early in course, a lymphocytic infiltrate and lobular necrosis are seen. As the condition becomes chronic, the septa thicken and become fibrotic with resultant fat atrophy. Eventually the classic but nonspecific finding of lipomembranous change is seen. This refers to eosinophilic material within areas of fat necrosis that have an undulating border or "corrugated" appearance
- **Treatment** for this condition is challenging and often unrewarding. Venous insufficiency should be treated, in the absence of significant arterial disease, with compression stockings. In addition, stanazolol, oxandrolone, pentoxyfylline, ultrasound, and phlebectomy have been tried, with some beneficial results

Calciphylaxis

- **Clinical**: associated with chronic renal failure, obesity, and poor nutrition

- Painful violaceous, retiform (net-like) plaques and nodules with ischemic necrosis, which often ulcerate and may blister. Common locations include the distal extremities, buttocks, or thighs
- **Pathophysiology**: thought to be secondary to abnormal calcium and phosphorus metabolism. Hypothesized to be related to the secondary hyperparathyroidism seen in many chronic renal failure patients
- **Histology** shows characteristic calcium deposits in small to medium vessels of the deep dermis and fat. Neutrophils, lymphocytes, and histiocytes are also present
- **Treatment**: prognosis is extremely poor and treatment is mainly supportive. Wound care, electrolyte management, and surgical debridement are standards of care. In addition, parathyroidectomy, binding agents, and low-calcium hemodialysis have been shown to be of benefit in some. Anecdotal reports cite hyperbaric oxygen and prednisone followed by cimetidine, as well as use of sodium thiosulfate, as being beneficial

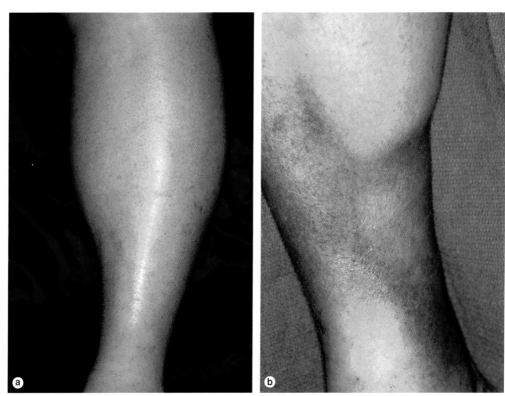

Figure 4-2 a, b Lipodermatosclerosis, "champagne-bottle" deformity

---

Lupus panniculitis (lupus erythematosus profundus)

- **Clinical**: occurs in fewer than 5% of patients with lupus erythematosus. Affects mostly females and adults
- Tender, erythematous nodules and plaques on the face, lateral upper arms, shoulders, trunk, and hips. More proximal distribution than other panniculitides. Overlying skin may resemble discoid lesions. Heals with atrophy and scarring
- Often precipitated by trauma
- **Histology** may show characteristic changes of discoid lupus in the epidermis/dermis, including epidermal atrophy, vacuolar change at the dermoepidermal junction, thickened basement membrane, interstitial mucin, and follicular plugging. Deeper sections will show lobular panniculitis with a predominantly lymphocytic inflammatory infiltrate. Characteristic, but nonspecific, lymphoid follicles with peripheral plasma cells may be appreciated. Fibrin is prominent
- **Treatment** options include topical or systemic corticosteroids, hydroxychloroquine, dapsone, cyclophosphamide, or thalidomide
- Subcutaneous lymphoma may mimic lupus panniculitis or may evolve in the setting of lupus panniculitis

Pancreatic panniculitis

- **Clinical**: occurs in 2–3% of patients with pancreatic disorders, including pancreatitis, pancreatic carcinoma (especially acinar type), pancreatic divisum or pseudocysts, vasculopancreatic fistulas
- Exquisitely tender erythematous brown subcutaneous nodules that ulcerate and drain an oily, brown material. Usually present on distal lower extremities. May also be found on the thighs, buttocks, calves, arms, and abdominal skin

Table 4-3 Other important lobular panniculitides without vasculitis

Diagnosis	Epidemiology/ etiology	Clinical	Associations	Treatment
Primary oxalosis	Hereditary (autosomal-recessive enzyme defect)	Livedo reticularis and acral gangrene	Renal failure	In vitro fertilization, alkalinization
Secondary oxalosis	Excessive oxalate or glycolic acid ingestion, ethylene glycol poisoning, intravenous glycerol or xylitol infusion, etc.	Firm papules and nodules on palmar fingers	Renal failure	Renal transplant
Sclerema neonatorum	Severely ill premature neonate	Yellow-white woody induration of buttocks and thighs; visceral fat may be involved	Severe underlying disease (sepsis, pneumonia, congenital heart defect, etc.)	Treatment of underlying disease, exchange transfusions, very poor prognosis
Subcutaneous fat necrosis of the newborn	Healthy infants, usually in first 4 weeks of life	Smooth, localized subcutaneous plaques on cheeks, shoulders, buttocks	Hypercalcemia or thrombocytopenia	Self-limited, must be vigilant for high calcium and treat if present
Cold panniculitis	Infants, children after cold exposure	Subcutaneous plaques in areas of cold exposure (cheeks, etc.)	Icecubes, popsicles, etc.	Rewarming, heals without scarring
Equestrian panniculitis	Women equestrians who ride in cold	Subcutaneous plaques of the upper outer thighs		Loose clothing, rewarming, avoid cold
Pancreatic panniculitis	Patients with pancreatitis, pancreatic carcinoma, pseudocysts, etc.	Erythematous subcutaneous nodules on distal lower extremity which ulcerate and drain oily brown substance	Joint pain, pleural effusion, ascites, pericardial effusion, elevated lipase, amylase, trypsin	Treat underlying etiologic pancreatic disorder
Alpha-1 antitrypsin deficiency panniculitis	Homozygous alpha-1 antitrypsin-deficient patients only	May initially look like cellulitis with oily discharge → subcutaneous nodules LE, arms, trunk, face. Heals with atrophic scarring	Emphysema, hepatitis, cirrhosis, vasculitis, angioedema	Dapsone, alpha-1 protease inhibitor concentrate, liver transplant. Avoid debridement
Factitial panniculitis	Self-inflicted, usually from injection into subcutaneous fat	Tender or nontender subcutaneous nodules; may be localized anywhere	Psychiatric disturbance	Cease injections
Cytophagic histiocytic panniculitis	Young and middle-aged adults	Erythematous ± tender subcutaneous nodules or diffuse ill-defined hemorrhagic plaques on trunk or extremities. May get ulceration or persistent drainage posttrauma	Many with T-cell lymphoma	Prednisone, cyclosporine, dapsone. Chemo if associated with lymphoma

- May be accompanied by acute arthritis, secondary to necrosis of periarticular fat tissue. Rarely associated with necrosis of abdominal fat, bone marrow fat, pleural effusions, mesenteric thrombosis, and leukemoid reaction and eosinophilia

- **Pathophysiology:** hypothesized that pancreatic enzymes from the inflamed pancreas spread hematogenously to cause subcutaneous fat necrosis. However, pancreatic panniculitis is extremely rare and has occurred in patients with normal pancreatic enzyme levels

Table 4-4 Causes of infective panniculitis

Bacteria	Mycobacteria	Fungi
Streptococcus pyogenes	Atypical mycobacteria	Cryptococcus neoformans
Staphylococcus aureus	Mycobacterium tuberculosis	Sporothrix schenckii
Pseudomonas species		Fusarium species
Klebsiella species		Aspergillus fumigatus
Nocardia species		Chromomycosis species
Actinomyces israelii		Histoplasma capsulatum
		Candida species

Table 4-5 Syndromes associated with panniculitis

Lofgren's syndrome	Erythema nodosum, fever, arthritis, hilar adenopathy. Form of sarcoidosis	Associated with good prognosis
Marshall's syndrome	Alpha-1 antitrypsin deficiency panniculitis and Sweet's syndrome	Leads to acquired cutis laxa

- **Histology**: characteristic coagulative necrosis of adipocytes leading to loss of adipocyte nuclei. Because of the loss of nuclei, they are called "ghost cells." Calcium deposition or saponification can result from dystrophic calcification in ghost cells from hydrolytic action of pancreatic enzymes on fat followed by calcium deposition
- **Treatment** requires treatment of the underlying pancreatic disorder and, in appropriate clinical contexts, may include octreotide, pancreatic stents, or surgery

Laboratory testing

Key Points

- The most important diagnostic test for panniculitis is an adequate tissue biopsy. A generous excisional sample, extending deep into the fat, is ideal. This should be analyzed by hematoxylin and eosin and, in the appropriate clinical context, microbial stains and tissue culture
- Many of the panniculitides are due to an underlying disorder. In these cases, lab testing is directed by the etiology of the condition

Lipodystrophies

Clinical presentation

Key Points

- Lipodystrophies are characterized by localized or generalized alteration of subcutaneous body fat (Tables 4-6 and 4-7). Although many are associated with loss of body fat, hypertrophy of body fat is also seen
- Lipodystrophies may be congenital or acquired (Tables 4-8 and 4-9)
- Many syndromic forms of lipodystrophy are associated with metabolic or systemic abnormalities that significantly affect patient morbidity
- In general, there is a direct correlation between the amount of subcutaneous tissue lost and the severity of the metabolic changes

Pathogenesis

Key Points

- Normal adipocytes function as endocrine organs and secrete the hormone leptin
- Leptin is derived from the Greek word "leptos," meaning thin. Leptin has been shown to have important functions in regulating body weight, metabolism, and reproductive function
- Patients with inherited and acquired lipodystrophy syndromes have been shown to have decreased leptin levels. It is hypothesized that decreased levels of this important hormone lead to the metabolic derangements found in these patients. However, the exact pathogenesis of most lipodystrophies is unclear
- Human immunodeficiency virus (HIV)-related lipodystrophy is most commonly seen in patients who have been on antiretroviral therapy, specifically protease inhibitors and nucleoside analogue inhibitors of viral reverse transcriptase. It is thought that these two categories of drugs, especially in combination, alter the transcription, secretion, and mitochondrial function of adipocytes.

Laboratory testing

Key Point

- If there is any concern for a syndromic form of lipodystrophy, a metabolic work-up should be pursued. Parameters to be considered include complete blood count, full chemistry panel, including liver transaminases, fasting lipid profile, glucose tolerance testing, a lupus panel, thyroid-stimulating hormone, C3, C3 nephritic factor, and HIV status.

Treatment

Key Points

- In general, treatment options for lipodystrophy are few and disappointing

Table 4-6 Classification of lipodystrophy syndromes

Age of onset/distribution	Generalized	Partial	Localized
Congenital	Berardinelli–Seip syndrome	Koebberling–Dunnigan syndrome	
Acquired	Lawrence syndrome	Barraquer–Simons syndrome Protease inhibitor-associated	Trauma, pressure, injections, connective tissue disease, idiopathic, postpanniculitides

Table 4-7 Familial lipodystrophy syndromes

Familial lipodystrophy syndromes	Epidemiology	Inheritance	Gene	Clinical	Laboratory	Systemic
Congenital generalized lipoatrophy (Berardinelli–Seip syndrome)	Birth	Autosomal-recessive	Type I: AGPAT2 gene Type II: seipin gene (more severe phenotype)	Loss of fat of face, body, limbs, viscera	Diabetes mellitus, high triglycerides and metabolic rate	Hypertrophic cardiomyopathy, liver and renal failure, organomegaly, Type II associated with mental retardation
Familial partial lipodystrophy (Koebberling–Dunnigan syndrome)	Puberty, >females	Autosomal-dominant	LMNA gene	Dunnigan: loss of fat from limbs only. ± excess fat of face and neck. Koebberling: face spared	Diabetes mellitus, high triglycerides and insulin resistance. Low high-density lipoproteins	Pancreatitis, diabetes mellitus and cardiovascular complications
Mandibuloacral dysplasia: type I		Autosomal-recessive	LMNA	Mandibular and clavicular hypoplasia, acro-osteolysis, joint contractions, mottled pigmentation. Loss of fat trunk and limbs	Diabetes mellitus, high triglycerides, insulin resistance in some	
Mandibuloacral dysplasia: type II		Autosomal-recessive	ZMPSTE24 gene (more severe)	Same as above plus generalized lipoatrophy and progeroid features	Diabetes mellitus, high triglycerides, insulin resistance in some	Renal failure

- Fat transfer surgery or soft-tissue augmentation may address aesthetic concerns
- Metabolic derangements may be treated with hypoglycemic or lipid-lowering medications. In addition, when insulin resistance is identified, insulin sensitizers such as thiazolidinediones or metformin may be helpful. Patients should be counseled regarding proper nutrition and exercise
- Close follow-up with specialty services such as endocrinology, cardiology, gastroenterology, and nephrology is recommended for patients at risk for insulin resistance, premature cardiovascular disease, cardiomyopathy, liver or renal failure
- Genetic counseling should be offered for patients with inherited lipodystrophy syndromes
- Patients with HIV-associated lipodystrophy may require a change in their HIV medication regimen. Metabolic abnormalities should be closely monitored and treated. Metformin has been specifically shown to help decrease insulin resistance in these patients.

Table 4-8 Acquired lipodystrophy syndromes

Acquired lipodystrophy syndromes	Onset	Clinical	Laboratory	Associated data
Acquired generalized lipoatrophy (Lawrence syndrome)	Childhood-puberty, >females	Face, body, extremities	Diabetes mellitus, high triglycerides, insulin resistance	Varices and liver failure, one-third with preceding autoimmune disease or infection
Acquired partial lipodystrophy (Barraquer–Simons syndrome)	Childhood-puberty, >females	Wasting of face, trunk, extremities. Hypertrophy of LE	Low C3, high C3 nephritic factor, +antinuclear antibodies	Prodromal fever, associated with autoimmune disease, glomerulonephritis
Human immunodeficiency virus (HIV)-related lipodystrophy	Variable	Wasting of face and limbs, excess fat of neck/upper back, abdomen and breasts	Insulin resistance, high triglycerides, glucose, and cholesterol	HIV. ± Protease inhibitors or nucleoside reverse transcriptase inhibitors

Table 4-9 Localized lipodystrophies

Localized lipodystrophy	Onset	Clinical	Associations
Lipoatrophia semicircularis	20–30-year-old females	Semicircular band-like atrophy of lower extremities	Posttraumatic
Insulin-related lipodystrophy	Variable	Lipohypertrophy	Insulin therapy (especially nonpurified)
Involutional lipoatrophy	Women	Tender lipoatrophy of extremities, buttocks, scalp	Intramuscular or intra-articular injections
Atrophic connective tissue disease	Variable	Limbs	Autoimmune disease
Annular lipoatrophy	Variable	Tender band-like atrophy of arm or ankle	Arthritis ± associated with autoimmune disease
Lipodystrophia centrifugalis abdominalis infantalis	Asians, childhood	May start with erythema + scale, centrifugal enlargement of lesion on groin, axilla, abdomen, chest	Lymphadenopathy
Progressive hemifacial atrophy (Parry–Romberg syndrome)	Childhood to young adult	Progressive unilateral facial atrophy of skin, subcutaneous, muscles, bones	Epilepsy, trigeminal neuralgia, headache, ± central nervous system lesions, thought to be form of scleroderma

Further reading

Brodell RT, Mehrabi D. Underlying causes of erythema nodosum. Postgrad Med 2000;108:147–149.

Camilleri MJ, Su WPD. Panniculitis. In: Freedberg IM, Eisen AZ, Wolff K, et al., eds. Fitzpatrick's Dermatology in General Medicine, 6th edn. Philadelphia: McGraw-Hill, 2003:1047–1061.

Capeau J, Magre J, Lascols O, et al. Diseases of adipose tissue: genetic and acquired lipodystrophies. Biochem Soc Trans 2005;33:1073–1077.

Eberhard BA, Ilowite NT. Panniculitis and lipodystrophy. Curr Opin Rheumatol 2002;14:566–570.

Epstein EH, Lipodystrophy. In: Freedberg IM, Eisen AZ, Wolff K, et al., eds. Fitzpatrick's Dermatology in General Medicine, 6th edn, Philadelphia: McGraw-Hill, 2003:1063–1066.

Junkins-Hopkins JM, Avram AS. Lipodystrophies. In: Bolognia JL, Jorrizo JL, Rapini RP, eds: Dermatology, Philadelphia: Elsevier Mosby, 2003:1575–1585.

McKee PH, Calonje E, Granter SR. Pathology of the Skin with Clinical Correlation, 3rd edn. Philadelphia: Elsevier Mosby, 2005:341–384 .

Patterson JW. Panniculitis. In: Bolognia JL, Jorrizo JL, Rapini RP, eds. Dermatology. Philadelphia: Elsevier Mosby, 2003:1551–1573.

Raquena L, Sanchez Yus ES. Panniculitis. Part II. Mostly lobular panniculitis. J Am Acad Dermatol 2001; 45:325–361.

Raquena L, Yus ES. Panniculitis. Part I. Mostly septal panniculitis. J Am Acad Dermatol 2001;45: 163–183.

Blistering dermatoses

Brooke N. Shadel and Maria Yadira Hurley

Vesiculobullous lesions result from a defect in cohesion between keratinocytes or between the epidermis and the underlying basement membrane zone. In this chapter, the blistering dermatoses will be categorized primarily by the anatomic level of split and secondarily by the mechanism responsible for the split, specifically whether it is acquired or congenital.

When a blistering disorder is suspected, an early, intact lesion with adjacent skin should be biopsied to ensure that an accurate histopathological diagnosis is made (Table 5-1). If autoimmune blistering dermatoses are being considered (Table 5-2), an additional biopsy for direct immunofluorescence (DIF) should be performed. For immunobullous disease, the ideal specimen for DIF is taken from normal-appearing, perilesional skin. Other special studies such as salt-split skin immunofluorescence, indirect immunofluorescence, and electron microscopy may be useful adjuncts.

It should be noted that the recommended use of medications in the treatment of the majority of the blistering dermatoses is off-label. These drugs are not approved by the Food and Drug Administration for the treatment of blistering disorders, and evidence-based practice guidelines are generally lacking. Treatment is based upon published evidence, expert opinion, and consensus.

INTRACORNEAL AND SUBCORNEAL BLISTERS

Pemphigus foliaceus (Box 5-1)

Clinical presentation

- Recurrent crops of vesicles or pustules that easily rupture, leaving crusted erosions
- Patients may rarely be erythrodermic
- Usually found on the head, neck, and upper trunk, but may be widespread
- Mucous membranes are rarely involved
- Adults are most commonly affected, usually during midlife
- Associations: other autoimmune diseases and thymoma
- Rare clinical presentations: pemphigus herpetiformis (herpetiform pemphigus)

Pemphigus foliaceus (Figure 5-1) represents 10–20% of all pemphigus cases and is a less severe form of the disease than is pemphigus vulgaris. Patients present with very superficial blisters that easily rupture, leaving erosions, especially on the upper body. Rarely, the entire body is involved. The Nikolsky sign is positive. Light rubbing of unaffected skin adjacent to a blister or erosion will cause separation of the skin. Drug-induced pemphigus often has this pattern.

Pemphigus herpetiformis is a rare presentation in which patients have generalized lesions that clinically resemble dermatitis herpetiformis. Patients have widespread pruritic vesicles that are often clustered. Although histologic findings can vary, the diagnosis is confirmed by DIF showing intercellular deposits of immunoglobulin.

Diagnosis

- Lesional biopsy for histopathology (Figure 5-2): superficial blister with split in the granular layer or directly beneath the stratum corneum
- Perilesional biopsy for DIF (Figure 5-3): intercellular staining for immunoglobulin (Ig) G and C3, rarely IgA

Differential diagnosis

See Box 5-2.

Laboratory testing

- Indirect immunofluorescence on guinea pig lip or esophagus (weaker reaction or absent on monkey esophagus)

Pathogenesis

- Autoantibodies IgG_4 subclass to desmoglein-1 (160 kDa), which is a transmembrane glycoprotein present in desmosomes

Table 5-1 Blistering diseases – target antigens

Disease	Major target antigen (molecular weight)	Site of antigen	Autoimmune (A) or genetic (G)
Pemphigus foliaceus	Desmoglein 1 (160 kDa)	Desmosomes of upper epidermis	A
Pemphigus erythematosus	Unknown		
Immunoglobulin A pemphigus	Subcorneal pustular dermatosis type – desmocollin 1	Desmosome	A
	Intraepidermal neutrophilic type – desmoglein 1 (160 kDa) or desmoglein 3 (130 kDa)		
Pemphigus vulgaris (vegetans)	Desmoglein 3 (130 kDa)	Desmosomes of lower epidermis	A
	Also desmoglein 1 and desmocollins		
Paraneoplastic pemphigus	Desmoglein 1 (160 kDa)	Cytoplasmic dense plaques	A
	Desmoglein 3 (130 kDa)		
	HD1/plectin (>500 kDa)		
	Desmoplakin I (250 kDa)		
	BP230		
	Desmoplakin II (210 kDa)		
	Envoplakin (210 kDa)		
	Periplakin (190 kDa)		
	170 kDa unknown antigen		
Epidermolysis bullosa acquisita	Collagen VII (290 kDa)	Anchoring fibrils	A
Epidermolysis bullosa simplex	K5, K14	Keratin intermediate filaments of lower epidermis	G
Epidermolysis bullosa with muscular dystrophy	Plectin	Hemidesmosomal dense plaque	G
Epidermolysis bullosa with pyloric atresia	Alpha6-beta4-integrin	Hemidesmosomal dense plaque	G
Junctional epidermolysis bullosa	Laminin 5	Lamina lucida	G
Dystrophic epidermolysis bullosa	Collagen VII (290 kDa)	Anchoring fibrils	G
Lichen planus pemphigoides	BP230	Hemidesmosome	A
	BP180	Hemidesmosomal transmembrane protein	
Bullous pemphigoid	BP230 (BPAg1)	Hemidesmosome	A
	BP180 (Ag2)	Hemidesmosomal transmembrane protein	
Pemphigoid (herpes) gestationis	BP230	Hemidesmosome	A
	BP180	Hemidesmosomal transmembrane protein	
Dermatitis herpetiformis	Maybe tissue transglutaminase (tG3)	Gut and maybe skin	A
Linear immunoglobulin A bullous dermatosis (chronic bullous disease of childhood)	BP180	Hemidesmosomal transmembrane protein	A
	LAD-1 (120 kDa) and LABD (97 kDa): degradation products of BP180		
	Collagen VII (290)	Anchoring fibrils	
Ocular cicatricial pemphigoid	Beta4-integrin	Conjunctiva	A

Table 5-1 Blistering diseases – target antigens—cont'd

Disease	Major target antigen (molecular weight)	Site of antigen	Autoimmune (A) or genetic (G)
Mucous membrane (cicatricial) pemphigoid	BP230	Hemidesmosome	A
	BP180	Hemidesmosomal transmembrane protein	
	Laminin 5 (Epiligrin)	Lamina lucida	
	Laminin 6	Lamina lucida	
	Collagen VII (290 kDa)	Anchoring fibrils	
Bullous lupus erythematosus	Collagen VII (290 kDa)	Anchoring fibrils	A

- Drug-induced form is most commonly caused by penicillamine and captopril (thiol-containing drugs) (Box 5-3)
- Other implicated drugs include penicillins, cephalosporins, enalapril, rifampin, and interferon

Adult mucosal surfaces contain enough desmoglein-3 to compensate for disruption of desmoglein-1 attachments, and the mucosa are not involved in the blistering process. A similar compensation is believed to protect the growing fetus from maternal autoantibodies against desmoglein-1.

Treatment

- Medication options are similar to those used for pemphigus vulgaris (see below) but there is some role for dapsone alone (100 mg daily) or the addition of hydroxychloroquine (200 mg daily)

Fogo selvagem

Clinical presentation

- Flaccid blisters, crusted erosions, occasional erythroderma
- "Burned" appearance of the skin ("fogo selvagem" means "wildfire" in Portuguese)
- May have associated fever, malaise, and arthralgias
- Initially involves head and neck before spreading to rest of body
- Children, young adults

Fogo selvagem is the endemic form of pemphigus foliaceus that is mainly found in rural areas of Brazil, Colombia, El Salvador, Paraguay, and Peru. A hallmark of the disease is a sensation of burning of the skin. Erosions have a corresponding burned look. Patients are usually children or young adults. Like pemphigus foliaceus, erythroderma is possible.

Diagnosis

See pemphigus foliaceus section, above.

Pathogenesis

- The epidemiology of endemic pemphigus foliaceus strongly suggests an environmental factor
- As in pemphigus foliaceus, antibodies are directed against desmoglein-1

Urbanization eradicates endemic foci, and the blackfly (Simuliidae) has been implicated as the vector in rural areas.

Treatment

- Oral corticosteroids
- Hydroxychloroquine

Pemphigus erythematosus

Clinical presentation

- Erythematous, scaly plaques
- Butterfly distribution over the nose and malar areas of the face, as well as other seborrheic areas
- Adults; rare in children
- Associated with other autoimmune diseases, including thymoma, myasthenia gravis and, rarely, systemic lupus erythematous

Pemphigus erythematosus is also known as Senear–Usher syndrome. It represents about 10% of all cases of pemphigus and is considered a variant of pemphigus foliaceus with features of lupus erythematosus. Sunlight may worsen the disease. The course is generally chronic.

Diagnosis

- Lesional biopsy for histopathology: subcorneal blister containing rare acantholytic cells, as in pemphigus foliaceus, and a lichenoid tissue reaction
- Perilesional biopsy for DIF: IgG and/or C3 intercellular and linear granular IgM and/or IgG and C3 along the dermoepidermal junction

Table 5-2 Autoimmune blistering diseases

Disease	Direct immuno-fluorescence (DIF)	Indirect immunofluorescence	Collagen IV by immunohistochemistry	Salt split skin at lamina lucida
Pemphigus foliaceus	IC IgG and C3	IC IgG Substrate: guinea-pig lip		
Pemphigus erythematosus	IC IgG and C3 BMZ: linear/granular IgM ± IgG and C3	IC IgG ANA		
IgA pemphigus	IC IgA	IC IgA (in 50%)		
Pemphigus vulgaris (vegetans)	IC IgG and C3	IC IgG Substrate: monkey esophagus		
Paraneoplastic pemphigus	IC IgG and C3 BMZ: linear/granular IgG and C3 May have cytoid bodies with IgM	IC IgG BMZ: linear/granular IgG Substrate: rat bladder epithelium		
Epidermolysis bullosa acquisita	BMZ: linear IgG and C3 (occasional IgA or IgM)	BMZ: linear IgG (in 50%)	Epidermal/roof of blister	Dermal pattern
Porphyria cutanea tarda (not a true autoimmune disorder; however, has DIF findings)	Vessels: IgM and C3 BMZ: weak, thick linear BMZ			
Lichen planus pemphigoides	BMZ: linear IgG and C3 plus cytoid bodies with IgM Shaggy BMZ with fibrinogen	BMZ: linear IgG (in 50%)	Dermal pattern/floor of blister	Epidermal pattern
Bullous pemphigoid	BMZ: linear IgG and C3	BMZ: linear IgG (in 75%)	Dermal pattern/floor of blister	Epidermal pattern
Pemphigoid (herpes) gestationis	BMZ: linear C3 and IgG (uncommon)	BMZ: uncommon IgG	Dermal pattern/floor of blister	Epidermal pattern
Linear IgA bullous dermatosis/chronic bullous disease of childhood	BMZ: linear IgA, may have IgG, IgM, and C3	BMZ: linear IgA more common in chronic bullous disease of childhood		Epidermal, dermal or combined
Dermatitis herpetiformis	BMZ: granular IgA with deposition of dermal papillae	IgA antiendomysial antibodies (normal diet)		
Mucous membrane (cicatricial) pemphigoid	BMZ: linear IgG, IgA, or C3	BMZ: linear IgG (in 20–30%)		Epidermal, dermal (antiepiligrin), or combined
Bullous lupus erythematosus	BMZ: linear IgG, IgA and/or IgM, and C3	ANA	Epidermal pattern/roof of blister	Dermal pattern

IC, intercellular (intraepidermal cell surface); Ig, immunoglobulin; BMZ, basement membrane zone; ANA, antinuclear antibodies.

BOX 5-1

Diseases with an intracorneal/subcorneal split

Pemphigus foliaceus
  Fógo selvagem
Pemphigus erythematosus
Subcorneal pustular dermatosis
Immunoglobulin A pemphigus
Acute generalized exanthematous pustulosis
Impetigo
Staphylococcal/streptococcal scalded-skin syndrome
Dermatophytosis
Infantile acropustulosis
Erythema toxicum neonatorum
Transient neonatal pustular melanosis
Miliaria crystallina

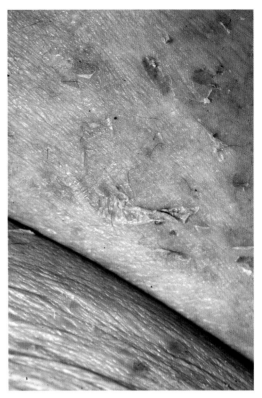

Figure 5-1 Pemphigus foliaceus

Differential diagnosis

The differential diagnosis includes pemphigus foliaceus, seborrheic dermatitis, and lupus erythematosus.

Laboratory testing

- Indirect immunofluorescence: intercellular IgG
- Antinuclear antibodies present in 30%, but antibodies to DNA usually absent
- Enzyme-linked immunosorbent assay (ELISA): detection of antidesmoglein-1 antibodies

Pathogenesis

- Drug-induced form is most commonly caused by penicillamine
- A few case reports associated with antihypertensive medications

Treatment

- Oral prednisone (lower dose than that needed for pemphigus foliaceus)
- Case reports of successful treatment with systemic corticosteroids with or without immunosuppressants or dapsone
- Avoid sunlight, as it may adversely affect course

Subcorneal pustular dermatosis

Clinical presentation

- Flaccid, sterile pustules
- Predilection for the trunk, especially axillae, groin, neck and flexor surfaces

- Spares face and mucous membranes
- Most common in women in their fourth to fifth decades
- Acute episodes do not have associated fever
- Benign, chronic, relapsing course
- Associations: IgA monoclonal gammopathy associated with some cases, lymphoproliferative disorders, or pyoderma gangrenosum

Subcorneal pustular dermatosis is also known as Sneddon-Wilkinson disease. Patients present with flaccid, sterile pustules, sometimes in an annular arrangement, primarily on the trunk and flexural surfaces. The face and mucous membranes are never involved. The pustules characteristically have yellowish fluid in the dependent half with clearer fluid in the top half of the lesion. Women are most commonly affected. IgA pemphigus may have a similar appearance.

Diagnosis

- Lesional biopsy for histopathology: subcorneal pustule filled with neutrophils and occasional eosinophils
- Perilesional biopsy for DIF: usually negative

Differential diagnosis

See Box 5-4.

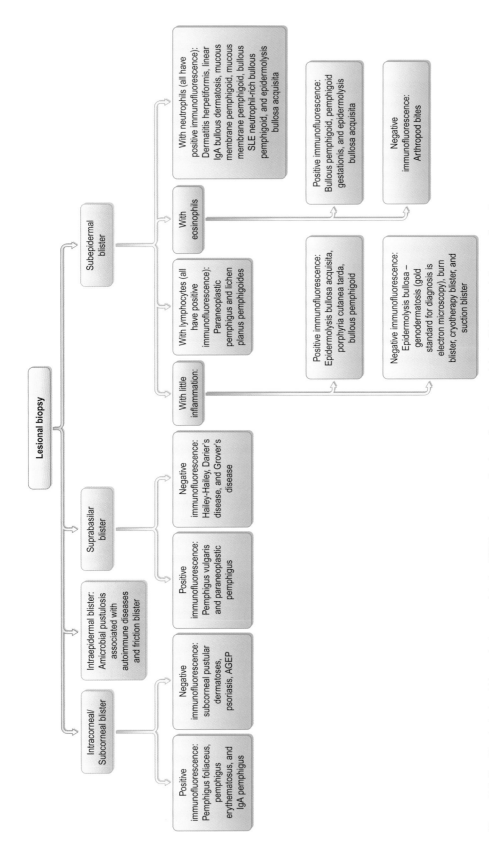

Figure 5-2 Algorithm for lesional biopsy. Ig, immunoglobulin; AGEP, acute generalized exanthematous pustulosis; SLE, systemic lupus erythematosus

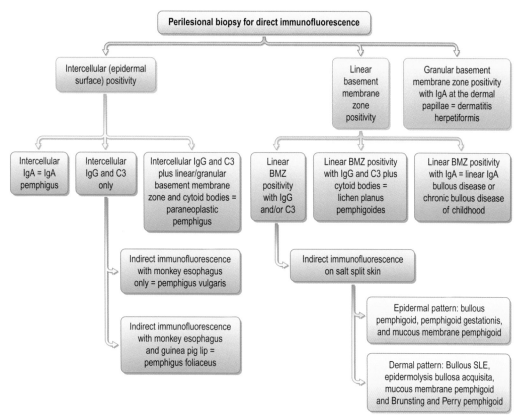

Figure 5-3 Algorithm for perilesional biopsy for direct immunofluorescence. Ig, immunoglobulin; BMZ, basement membrane zone; SLE, systemic lupus erythematosus

Laboratory testing

- Indirect immunofluorescence: usually negative
- Serum protein electrophoresis and DIF may be repeated every few years

Pathogenesis

- Unknown

Treatment

- Dapsone 50–150 mg daily (adult dose)
- If dapsone-intolerant, can use sulfapyridine 500 mg bid and increase slowly
- Acitretin for those intolerant of both dapsone and sulfapyridine
- Colchicine 1.5 mg daily and other immuno-suppressants have been anecdotally successful for treatment of recalcitrant disease

Controversies

This disease is viewed by some authorities as a variant of pustular psoriasis. Some cases previously diagnosed as subcorneal pustular dermatosis had demonstrable intercellular IgA and have been re-classified as IgA pemphigus.

IgA pemphigus

Clinical presentation

- Flaccid vesicles on erythematous or normal skin
- Annular or circinate pattern with central crusting
- Lesions observed on axilla and groin > trunk, extremities, abdomen
- Average age of onset 45 years, reported cases in children and elderly
- Associations: IgA antibodies present in approximately 50% cases; 20% have an IgA monoclonal gammopathy
- Two distinct groups:
  - IgA confined to upper epidermis (subcorneal pustular dermatosis, SPD type)
  - IgA throughout the epidermis (intraepidermal pustules, IEN type)

IgA pemphigus (Figure 5-4) may have some clinical overlap with subcorneal pustular dermatosis. Subcorneal pustular dermatosis and the SPD type of IgA pemphigus present with similar

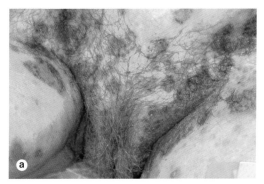

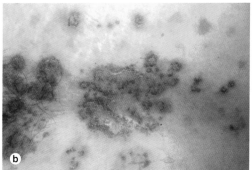

Figure 5-4 a, b Immunoglobulin A pemphigus

annular, crusted vesicles and pustules in the axilla and groin. The IEN type of IgA pemphigus may preferentially involve the trunk, rather than the intertriginous areas. IgA pemphigus has a slightly increased frequency of an associated IgA monoclonal gammopathy than does subcorneal pustular dermatosis.

Diagnosis

- Lesional biopsy for histopathology: subcorneal or intraepidermal split with neutrophils underlying the split; early lesions show neutrophil exocytosis and neutrophils at the dermoepidermal junction
- Perilesional biopsy for DIF:
  - SPD type: intercellular IgA deposition in the upper epidermis
  - IEN type: intercellular IgA in the lower epidermis or throughout

Differential diagnosis

See Box 5-4.

Laboratory testing

- Indirect immunofluorescence is unreliable; only 50% have detectable circulating IgA

Pathogenesis

- Antibodies to desmocollin 1 (SPD type) and desmoglein-1 or 3 (IEN type)

Treatment

- Dapsone 25–100 mg daily
- Alternatively, if dapsone-intolerant: start sulfapyridine 500 mg bid and increase slowly

Controversies

Some cases were previously diagnosed as subcorneal pustular dermatosis with IgA deposition. There are cases with overlap features of the SPD type and IEN type, suggesting variable disease expression.

Acute generalized exanthematous pustulosis (See also Chapter 23)

Clinical presentation

- Pin-sized, nonfollicular pustules
- Most patients have a fever and a history of a recently added medication

Acute generalized exanthematous pustulosis (AGEP) is a pustular eruption also known as toxic pustuloderma and pustular drug rash. The eruption begins as acute, erythematous edema on the face or intertriginous areas and is quickly followed by numerous pin-sized nonfollicular pustules with an intertriginous accentuation. Mucous membranes may be involved in about 20% of cases. Most patients have a fever above 38°C. The eruption usually resolves in a few days, although rarely patients may have a more prolonged course with systemic involvement. AGEP is uncommon in children.

Diagnosis

- Lesional biopsy for histopathology: spongiform subcorneal/intraepidermal pustule, papillary dermal edema, may have exocytosis of eosinophils, single dyskeratotic keratinocytes, and occasionally vasculitis
- Perilesional biopsy for DIF: negative

Differential diagnosis

See Table 5-3.

Laboratory testing

- Leukocytosis mostly due to high neutrophils counts
- Eosinophilia in one-third of patients

Pathogenesis

- 90% are drug-induced with an onset of hours (antibiotics) to 3 weeks (other drugs)
- Drugs associated with AGEP:
  - Antibiotics: aminopenicillins, macrolides, cephalosporins
  - Antimycotics: terbinafine
  - Other: calcium channel blockers, carbamazepine
- Minority of cases linked to viral infections

Treatment

- Remove offending drug
- Antipyretics as needed
- Supportive care

INTRAEPIDERMAL BLISTERS

See Box 5-5.

Table 5-3 Differential diagnosis of acute generalized exanthematous pustulosis

Disease	Differentiating points
Acute generalized exanthematous pustulosis	Flexural, compatible drug history, short duration
Pustular psoriasis	Diffuse; history of psoriasis
Subcorneal pustular dermatosis	Larger, circinate pustules; nonacute
Pustular vasculitis	Biopsy
Drug hypersensitivity syndrome	Eosinophilia, organ involvement (liver, kidney)
Toxic epidermal necrolysis	More than one mucous membrane involved, severely ill patients

---

BOX 5-5

Disease with an intraepidermal split

Amicrobial pustulosis associated with autoimmune diseases

Friction blister

Spongiotic diseases

Palmoplantar pustulosis

Viral blistering

Amicrobial pustulosis associated with autoimmune diseases

Clinical presentation

- Acute and recurring pustules
- Predilections for scalp and flexures
- Mostly young to middle-aged females
- Associations: autoimmune diseases

This entity is also known as pustular dermatosis, follicular impetigo, and pyodermatitis vegetans. This is a rare disorder in which there is acute onset and a recurring course of pustules involving the scalp, external auditory canal, and flexures. Follicular and nonfollicular pustules coalesce into erosive areas. It is associated with autoimmune diseases, mainly lupus erythematosus, but also celiac disease, myasthenia gravis, and idiopathic thrombocytopenia purpura.

Diagnosis

- Lesional biopsy for histopathology: intraepidermal spongiform pustule with a neutrophilic infiltrate in the dermis

- Perilesional biopsy for DIF: negative
- Bacterial culture is negative

Differential diagnosis

See Box 5-5.

Laboratory testing

- Culture of pustules is negative for bacterial organisms, unless secondarily infected
- Check zinc levels

Pathogenesis

- Unknown relationship to autoimmune diseases
- Possible relationship to zinc deficiency

Treatment

- Prednisone (1 mg/kg) and/or zinc supplementation

Friction blister

Clinical presentation

- Noninflamed blister
- More likely to occur in skin that has a thick horny layer held tightly to underlying dermis (e.g., palms or soles)
- The most commonly affected sites include the tips of the toes, the balls of the feet, and the posterior heel
- Occurs in vigorously active populations

Diagnosis

- History and location
- Lesional biopsy for histopathology: necrosis just below the stratum granulosum in the upper stratum spinosum

Differential diagnosis

The differential diagnosis is epidermolysis bullosa simplex.

Pathogenesis

- Development is linked to magnitude of frictional force and number of cycles across the skin

Treatment

- Maintain blister roof intact to speed healing time; larger lesions may need to be drained
- Prevention – avoid friction through use of acrylic socks, closed-cell neoprene insoles, thin polyester sock combined with thick wool or propylene sock

SUPRABASILAR BLISTERS

See Box 5-6.

BOX 5-6

Diseases with a suprabasilar split

Pemphigus vulgaris

Pemphigus vegetans

Paraneoplastic pemphigus

Grover's disease

Hailey–Hailey disease

Darier's disease

Pemphigus vulgaris

Clinical presentation

- Flaccid bullae break to form painful erosions
- Oral involvement occurs first in 60% of cases, followed by the skin
- Other mucosal surfaces may be involved
- Commonly involves trunk, groin, axillae, pressure points, scalp and face
- Average age at presentation fifth or sixth decade
- More common in Jewish/Mediterranean populations
- Associations: other autoimmune disorders (myasthenia gravis and thymoma)

Pemphigus vulgaris (Figure 5-5) is the most common form of pemphigus, representing 70% or more of all subtypes. It is more common in older adults and Ashkenazi Jews. It is the most common type of pemphigus in children. In contrast to bullous pemphigoid, pemphigus vulgaris often involves mucosal surfaces and creates flaccid bullae on the skin that quickly erode. Bullae may arise on nonerythematous skin. Pemphigus vulgaris is the classic disease associated with the Nikolsky sign, in which light friction on perilesional skin induces a blister. The Asboe–Hansen sign, in which pressure on the surface of a bulla causes the blister to spread laterally, is also positive. Lesions usually heal with hyperpigmentation, but without scarring. Prior to the widespread use of systemic corticosteroids, mortality was very high.

Diagnosis

- Lesional biopsy for histopathology: suprabasal bullae with acantholysis, tombstone appearance of basal cells
- Perilesional biopsy for DIF: intercellular staining between keratinocytes for IgG and C3; upper layers may be spared

Although the classic biopsy findings are suprabasilar acantholysis with a "tombstone" intact basal layer, early lesions may show eosinophilic or neutrophilic spongiosis. In contrast to Hailey–Hailey

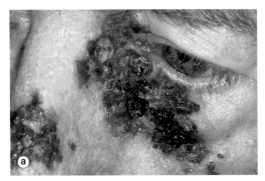

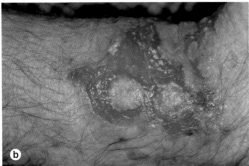

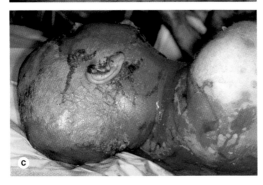

Figure 5-5 **a** Crusted lesions of pemphigus. **b** Pemphigus vulgaris erosions. **c** Pemphigus vulgaris

Table 5-4 Treatment of pemphigus vulgaris

Medication	Suggested dosage
Prednisone	1 mg/kg per day for 6–10 weeks, then taper by 10 mg to 20 mg every 2–4 weeks until 40 mg daily, then 40 mg every other day, alternating with 35 mg and decreasing the second day's dose by 5 mg every 2–4 weeks to a dose of 5 mg; followed by a similar taper for the first day's dose. If no recurrence, then maintenance regimen of 5 mg daily for up to several years
Azathioprine	2.5 mg/kg per day if thiopurine methyltransferase is high (majority of population)
Mycophenolate mofetil	35–45 mg/kg per day
Cyclophosphamide	1–3 mg/kg per day or monthly intravenous pulse
Cyclosporine	5 mg/kg per day

Laboratory testing

- Indirect immunofluorescence: intercellular IgG
- Antibody titer to desmoglein-3 parallels disease activity

Pathogenesis

- Both humoral and cell-mediated mechanisms contribute
- Autoantibodies of the predominantly IgG_4 subclass target desmoglein-3 early and later cross-react with desmoglein-1
- Many different drugs have precipitated this disease, especially those with thiol groups, although pemphigus foliaceus is more commonly induced

The autoantibodies against desmoglein-3 are pathogenic. Mouse studies have shown that injection of antibodies against desmoglein-3 induces blister formation. Although IgG_4 autoantibodies are the most common, IgA and IgE classes have also been detected.

In the adult, desmoglein-3 is concentrated in the basal and suprabasal layers of the epidermis and in mucosal surfaces. Patients with pemphigus vulgaris may also have antibodies to desmoglein-1 and/or desmocollins.

Treatment (Table 5-4)

- Goal is to decrease or eliminate circulating antidesmoglein antibodies and then the bound antibodies in the skin
- Treatments include prednisone, with transition to steroid-sparing immunosuppressive agents such as azathioprine or mycophenolate mofetil

---

BOX 5-7

Differential diagnosis of oral erosions

Pemphigus vulgaris

Acute herpetic stomatitis

Erythema multiforme

Aphthous ulcers

Erosive lichen planus

Cicatricial pemphigoid

---

disease, acantholysis in pemphigus vulgaris involves hair follicles.

Differential diagnosis

See Box 5-7.

Controversies

Plasmapheresis may increase the response to cyclophosphamide. Extracorporeal photopheresis is being evaluated.

Pemphigus vegetans

Clinical presentation

- Vesicles or pustules that become vegetating plaques
- Axillae/groin (flexural), oral mucosa
- Mean age at onset: fifth decade

Pemphigus vegetans is a variant of pemphigus vulgaris. Since erosions in flexural areas in pemphigus vulgaris tend to form vegetating plaques, some patients with pemphigus vulgaris seem to manifest both diseases. Pemphigus vegetans has traditionally been classified into Neumann and Hallopeau types. In the Neumann type, lesions typically begin as typical flaccid blisters of pemphigus vulgaris, become eroded, and form vegetating plaques. Plaques are often studded with pustules. In the Hallopeau type, pustular lesions evolve into vegetating plaques. The Hallopeau type may be more benign and remit spontaneously; whereas the Neumann type tends to have a chronic course.

Diagnosis

- Biopsy shows epidermal hyperplasia and intraepidermal eosinophilic abscesses with sometimes minimal acantholysis
- The differential diagnosis includes Hailey–Hailey disease and infections
- DIF is identical to pemphigus vulgaris
- Differential diagnosis (Box 5-8)

Paraneoplastic pemphigus

Clinical presentation

- Polymorphic skin lesions with features of both erythema multiforme and pemphigus vulgaris
- Cutaneous lesions are necrotic, erosive, and progressive
- Mucosal, trunk/extremities, palmoplantar involvement is characteristic
- Mean age at onset: fifth decade
- Associations: internal neoplasms, especially non-Hodgkin's lymphoma

Paraneoplastic pemphigus (Figure 5-6) has some overlap features with erythema multiforme and lichen planus pemphigoides. Patients have intractable oral stomatitis with polymorphous skin lesions that include tense blisters, targetoid and lichenoid lesions, and erosions. Some cases have been

---

BOX 5-8

Differential diagnosis of pemphigus vegetans

Hailey–Hailey disease

Iododerma/bromoderma

Syphilitic condyloma

Granuloma inguinale

Leishmaniasis

Condyloma acuminata

Deep fungal infection

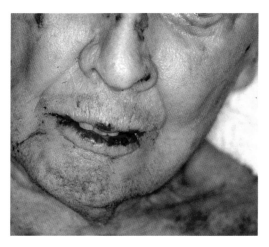

Figure 5-6 Paraneoplastic pemphigus

described following treatment with interferon or radiation. Morbidity and mortality are high, and 30–40% develop pulmonary injury. A variety of internal malignancies are associated with paraneoplastic pemphigus, with non-Hodgkin's lymphoma being the most common. Other associations include chronic lymphocytic leukemia, Castleman's disease, thymoma, poorly differentiated sarcoma, Waldenström's macroglobulinemia, inflammatory fibrosarcoma, bronchogenic squamous cell carcinoma, round cell liposarcoma, Hodgkin's disease, T-cell lymphoma, and treatment with fludarabine. In some cases, resection of the underlying malignancy results in disease remission.

Diagnosis

- Lesional biopsy for histopathology: suprabasilar acantholysis, exocytosis of lymphocytes, dyskeratotic and necrotic keratinocytes, basal cell vacuolization
- Perilesional biopsy for DIF: intercellular and basement membrane staining with C3 and/or IgG similar to pemphigus erythematosus
- Differential diagnosis: erythema multiforme, bullous pemphigoid, pemphigus vulgaris

Laboratory testing

- Evaluate for an occult neoplasm
- Indirect immunofluorescence: intercellular staining; for best screening results use rat bladder epithelium

Pathogenesis

- Autoantibodies to envoplakin and periplakin, desmoplakin-1 and 2, desmoglein-1 and 3, bullous pemphigoid antigen-1 (BPAg1), and plectin
- Epitope spreading may be responsible for the diverse clinicopathologic findings and large number of antibodies

Treatment

- Includes treatment of underlying neoplasm and immunosuppression
- Complete resolution is rare
- Glucocorticoids 1–2 mg/kg per day
- Adjunctive immunosuppressive drugs as needed (cyclophosphamide, azathioprine, mycophenolate, rituximab)
- Plasmapheresis may be initiated

Grover's disease

Clinical presentation

- Excoriated papules and papulovesicles
- Trunk
- Middle-aged to older adults

Grover's disease, also know as transient acantholytic dermatosis, is a relatively common disorder that presents with excoriated papules and papulovesicles on the trunk. There are three variants: transient eruptive, persistent pruritic, and chronic asymptomatic. There is often coexistence with other dermatoses, including asteatotic eczema and psoriasis.

Diagnosis

- Confirmed with a biopsy for histology
- DIF is negative

Four histologic patterns can be seen – Darier-like, Hailey–Hailey-like, pemphigus vulgaris-like, and spongiotic.

Pathogenesis

- Unknown, but linked to heat and sweating

Treatment

- Potent topical steroids
- Isotretinoin 0.5 mg/kg for 2–6 months in refractory cases
- Some reports of success with psoralen with ultraviolet A (PUVA) and dapsone

SUBEPIDERMAL BLISTERS

See Box 5-9.

Bullous lymphedema

Clinical presentation

- Tense bullae on edematous skin (Figure 5-7)

Treatment

- Compression and diuretics

Bullous pemphigoid

Clinical presentation

- Tense bullae on normal or erythematous skin, urticarial/eczematous lesions
- Lower abdomen, shins
- Mucosal involvement in up to 20%
- Onset usually in adults older than 65, but young adult and pediatric cases occur

Bullous pemphigoid (Figure 5-8) is the most common subepidermal bullous disease. There is often a prodrome that lasts weeks to months, in which

---

BOX 5-9

Diseases with a subepidermal split

Bullous pemphigoid

Cicatricial pemphigoid

Lichen planus pemphigoides

Pemphigoid gestationis

Epidermolysis bullosa acquisita

Dermatitis herpetiformis

Linear immunoglobulin A bullous dermatosis

Bullous systemic lupus erythematosus

Arthropod bite

Cryotherapy blister

Burn blister

Suction blister

Drug overdose bullae

Bullous lesions in diabetes mellitus

Epidermolysis bullosa

Porphyria cutanea tarda

Toxic epidermal necrolysis

Bullous drug reactions

Erythema multiforme

Bullous fixed drug

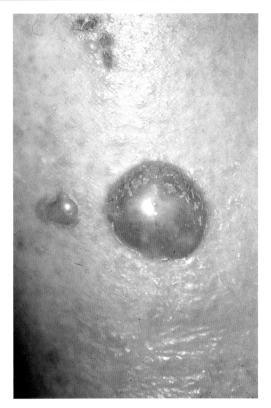

Figure 5-7 Bullous lymphedema

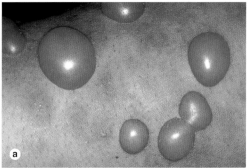

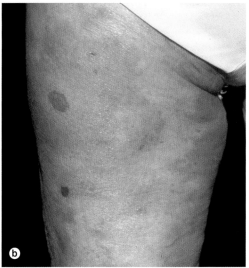

Figure 5-8 a Bullous pemphigoid. **b** Urticarial lesions of bullous pemphigoid

patients present with urticarial or eczematous lesions. Blisters are tense and heal without scarring. Milia are sometimes present. Patients tend to have a chronic course with remission after about 6 years. The childhood form often remits after 1 year. Morbidity and mortality are low with treatment. Several clinical variants have been described (Table 5-5).

Diagnosis

- Lesional biopsy for histopathology: subepidermal blister with a predominance of eosinophils; early lesions may show only eosinophilic spongiosis
- Perilesional biopsy for DIF: linear C3 (in close to 100%) and/or IgG (in ~80%) at basement membrane zone; sometimes IgA and IgM
- Differential diagnosis: other blistering disorders

Laboratory tests

- Indirect immunofluorescence: IgG_4 antibasement membrane zone antibodies positive in 75% of cases (n-serrated pattern)
- Salt-split skin: positive epidermal pattern in 70–80% of cases; type IV collagen will map to the roof
- Peripheral eosinophilia common

Pathogenesis

- Autoantibodies to BPAg1 and BPAg2
- Etiology of the development of autoantibodies is not entirely known; however, some cases suggest drugs, trauma, or burns

Autoantibodies of the IgG, IgE, and IgA subclasses bind to both a polypeptide in the basal cell hemidesmosome (BPAg1) and a transmembrane glycoprotein (BPAg2) that interacts with the anchoring filaments. BPAg2 is also known as type XVII collagen. Only IgG_1 can fix complement, and it is believed that IgG_1 that is bound at the basement membrane activates complement, leading to chemotaxis of neutrophils and eosinophils which release proteolytic enzymes responsible for the blister formation. Medications implicated in the cause of bullous pemphigoid include furosemide, sulfasalazine, penicillins, penicillamine, and captopril Box 5-10. Many of these medications contain thiol groups. Bullous pemphigoid has also been described after treatment with ultraviolet light, PUVA, and radiation.

Table 5-5 Variants of bullous pemphigoid

Variant	Presentation
Pemphigoid nodularis	Simulates prurigo nodularis; generalized or localized to shins; blisters rare
Localized	On extremities. Sometimes progresses to rest of body
Localized vulvar	Young girls with nonscarring blistering of vulva
Localized oral	Isolated desquamative gingivitis, no skin lesions
Pemphigoid vegetans	Intertriginous hypertrophic plaques with peripheral pustules and blisters
Lichen planus emphigoides	Blisters in a patient with lichen planus arising on skin that is not involved with lichen planus
Vesicular pemphigoid	Tense, small blisters; sometimes grouped
Dyshidrosiform pemphigoid	Localized vesicles on soles
Anti-p105 pemphigoid	Variant of pemphigoid with autoantibodies directed against p105
Anti-p200 pemphigoid	Variant of pemphigoid with autoantibodies directed against p200

Treatment

- Steroids and immunosuppressants
- Tetracycline and nicotinamide

Many patients can be successfully managed with topical use of class I steroids such as clobetasol; this often provides relief with a lower risk of side-effects than do systemic immunosuppressants. Patients requiring systemic treatment are usually started on prednisone 0.5–1 mg/kg daily. After cessation of new lesions and healing of old lesions, the dose can be slowly tapered to an every-other-day regimen to minimize steroid side-effects. Immunosuppressants/immunomodulatory drugs may be used in patients who do not tolerate corticosteroids or as an adjunct for severe disease; these include methotrexate, cyclosporine, mycophenolate mofetil, azathioprine, leflunomide, rarely cyclophosphamide or chlorambucil. Some patients can be adequately controlled on tetracycline and nicotinamide, which are thought to work through their anti-inflammatory effects. Localized lesions may be treated with intralesional steroids such as triamcinolone suspension 10 mg/mL monthly or class I topical steroids twice daily.

Controversies

- Bullous pemphigoid is associated with an increased rate of internal malignancy (up to 5–6%) in Japan and China
- Although azathioprine was commonly used as a treatment in the past, recent reports document potential increased mortality with this treatment. It may simply be that all systemic treatments have greater toxicity than topical treatments

Cicatricial or mucous membrane pemphigoid

Clinical presentation

- Rare, tense bullae; crusted erosions
- Lesions tend to recur in the same area
- Scarring may result in adhesions and strictures
- Predilection for oral (85% of cases) and ocular mucous membranes that scar
- Other mucous membranes may be affected as well
- Skin lesions (25% of cases), with scalp, head, neck, upper trunk most common
- Predominance in older adult females
- Chronic and progressive course
- Associations: autoimmune disorders

Oral lesions are the most common manifestation of this condition. Patients present with desquamative gingivitis, erythema, ulcers, and vesicles. The gingival and buccal mucosa, tongue, palate, and tonsillar pillars may be involved. Ocular involvement begins with bilateral erythema and vesicles that eventuate in xerosis, fibrosis, and scarring. Ankyloblepharon, symblepharon, and blindness are end-stage sequelae.

Skin lesions are seen in about 25% of patients. Blisters resemble those of bullous pemphigoid and may be on the head, neck, or extremities. Patients sometimes have generalized bullae. A localized variant of cicatricial pemphigoid, referred to as Brunsting–Perry disease, consists of recurrent blisters on the head and neck that heal with scarring. These patients generally have no mucosal involvement.

Diagnosis

- Lesional biopsy for histopathology:
  - Mucosal: subepidermal bullae with mixed infiltrate
  - Skin: subepidermal bullae with mostly neutrophils and eosinophils; dermal scarring
- Perilesional biopsy for DIF: linear IgG and C3 linear at basement membrane zone; presence of IgA may help differentiate from bullous pemphigoid

Laboratory testing

- Indirect immunofluorescence: linear basement membrane zone with IgG and IgA in 20%
- Salt-split skin: epidermal, dermal, or combined
- Antiepiligrin cicatricial pemphigoid has an increased risk for solid cancers; therefore, screening is indicated

Pathogenesis

- Suspected that molecular mimicry results in development of autoantibodies that target different autoantigens (BPAg1 and 2, laminin 5 and 6, integrin subunit beta 4; antigens of 120 kDa, 160 kDa, 45 kDa)

Because of the many different target antigens found in cicatricial pemphigoid patients, it may be that this disorder represents a disease phenotype rather than a single entity.

Treatment

- Mild disease limited to mouth may respond to topical glucocorticosteroid applied with dental appliances overnight or elixir for swish and spit of dexamethasone
- Treatment of chronic lesions may include intralesional triamcinolone acetonide (10 mg/mL, 0.25–0.5 mL/site)
- Topical tetracycline or cyclosporine are alternative treatments
- Severe disease: if ocular, laryngeal, or urogenital epithelia are scarred: aggressive treatment with glucocorticoids 1 mg/kg per day along

with other immunosuppressants, such as cyclophosphamide. Alternatives include intravenous immunoglobulin with or without plasmapheresis
- Refer to ophthalmologist for even mild conjunctival disease
- Minimize loss of gingival tissue and teeth through good oral hygiene
- Irrigation of sinuses twice daily followed by nasal lubricant if nasal involvement

Ocular cicatricial pemphigoid

Clinical presentation

- Rare blisters, erosions, ulcers with subsequent conjunctival and corneal scarring
- Scarring is predominant with fornix obliteration and symblepharon formation that leads to ankyloblepharon

Ocular cicatricial pemphigoid (Figure 5-9) is also known as ocular mucous membrane pemphigoid. It is a subcategory of mucous membrane pemphigoid. Squamous metaplasia with keratinization of the ocular surface epithelium results in blindness.

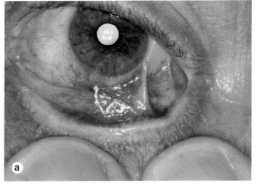

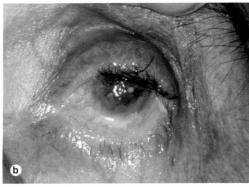

Figure 5-9 a Cicatricial pemphigoid. **b** Advanced cicatricial pemphigoid

Diagnosis

- Perilesional biopsy for DIF from conjunctiva: linear basement membrane zone IgG and/or IgA in conjunctival biopsies
- Differential diagnosis: paraneoplastic pemphigus, mucous membrane pemphigoid

Pathogenesis

- IgA antibodies against the intraepidermal portion of the beta-4 subunit of alpha6-beta4 integrin

Treatment

- Oral low-dose weekly methotrexate is a useful first-line treatment for mild-to-moderate ocular cicatricial pemphigoid
- Systemic cyclophosphamide with short-term adjunctive high-dose prednisolone is the preferred treatment for severe and/or rapidly progressing ocular cicatricial pemphigoid

Localized cicatricial pemphigoid

Clinical presentation

- Also known as Brunsting–Perry-type cicatricial pemphigoid
- Predominance in older adult males
- Rare disease with one or more scarring lesions on the head or neck without mucous membrane involvement
- Flaccid blisters with adjacent erythema

Diagnosis

- Lesional biopsy for histopathology: subepidermal bullae with mostly neutrophils, lymphocytes, and eosinophils; microabscesses develop in less than 2 days
- Perilesional biopsy for DIF: IgG and C3 linear at basement membrane zone
- Indirect immunofluorescence: negative
- Differential diagnosis: bullous pemphigoid that heals without scarring, mucous membrane pemphigoid that has mucosal involvement, and epidermolysis bullosa acquisita

Pathogenesis

- Unknown

Treatment

- Treatment of chronic lesions may include intralesional triamcinolone acetonide every 2–4 weeks (10 mg/mL, 0.25–0.5 mL/site)
- Topical tetracycline or cyclosporine are alternative treatments
- For recalcitrant or more aggressive disease: follow treatment algorithm for epidermolysis bullosa acquisita (see below)

Controversies

Some authorities consider this to be a localized form of epidermolysis bullosa acquisita

Lichen planus pemphigoides

Clinical presentation

- Rare disorder characterized by bullae on skin uninvolved by lesions of lichen planus
- Usually less severe than bullous pemphigoid; may have recurrent lesions of lichen planus only

Diagnosis

- Lesional biopsy for histopathology: subepidermal blister with rare eosinophils and neutrophils
- Perilesional biopsy for DIF: linear basement membrane zone positivity with IgG and C3 and cytoid bodies
- Differential diagnosis: bullous pemphigoid, bullous lichen planus, epidermolysis bullosa acquisita

Pathogenesis

- Antigens with molecular weight of 230 kDa and 180 kDa, which are consistent with bullous pemphigoid antigens, have been identified

It has been proposed that damage to the basal cells in lichen planus unmasks or creates neoantigens, leading to antibody formation and induction of bullous pemphigoid. Drug-induced cases have been associated with cinnarizine, captopril, ramipril, and PUVA therapy.

Treatment

- Same as bullous pemphigoid

Controversies

- Question if lichen planus pemphigoides represents coexistence of lichen planus and bullous pemphigoid or is a distinct entity

Epidermolysis bullosa acquisita

Clinical presentation

- Four clinical presentations:
  - Noninflammatory (65%): mechanobullous, acral distribution with scarring and milia formation, scarring alopecia, loss of nails, esophageal stenosis
  - Inflammatory (25%): inflammatory bullous eruption involving trunk, skin folds, and extremities; lacking skin fragility, scarring, and milia (may resemble pemphigoid)

- Mucous membrane involvement predominant (10%): erosions and scars on mucosal surfaces including buccal, conjunctival, gingival, nasopharyngeal, esophageal, rectal, and genital
- Head and neck involvement predominant (rare): bullous eruption localized to head and neck with scarring, minimal mucosal involvement
- Onset usually in adulthood, but can occur at any age, including childhood
- Associations: inflammatory bowel disease, systemic lupus erythematosus, rheumatoid arthritis, amyloidosis

Epidermolysis bullosa acquisita may have a diverse clinical presentation. Classic cases present with noninflammatory bullae. Trauma contributes to blister formation, especially on the extensor surfaces of elbows, knees, ankles, and buttocks. Periods of remission and exacerbation are common. Other presentations overlap with bullous pemphigoid and cicatricial pemphigoid. African Americans residing in southeastern United States may be at increased risk for this disorder.

Diagnosis

- Lesional biopsy for histopathology: subepidermal bullae with eosinophils and neutrophils or cell poor
- Perilesional biopsy for DIF: linear IgG deposits in basement membrane zone (u-serrated pattern), sublamina densa and can observe deposits of IgA, IgM, and C3
- Immunoelectron microscopy: gold standard; split sublamina densa and decreased anchoring fibrils
- Differential diagnosis: bullous pemphigoid, cicatricial pemphigoid, linear IgA dermatosis, porphyria cutanea tarda, bullous systemic lupus erythematosus (usually on sun-exposed skin in a patient with a history of lupus, good response to dapsone, DIF may show a more granular than linear pattern)

Laboratory testing

- Indirect immunofluorescence: linear basement membrane IgG in 50% of cases
- Salt-split skin: dermal pattern linear IgG
- ELISA: autoantibody against NC1 domain of type VII collagen

Pathogenesis

- Autoantibody to type VII collagen in sublamina densa, the major component of anchoring fibrils that connect the basement membrane to dermal structures
- These antibodies activate complement

Treatment

- Generally resistant to therapy
- Minimize trauma to skin and, if mucous membranes are involved, avoid hard brittle foods or those with high acid content
- Dapsone started at 50 mg daily and increased by 50 mg weekly until remission occurs, usually at a dose less than 250 mg/day. Maintain at remission dose for several months, then decrease slowly until the drug can be discontinued
- Variable response to colchicine and glucocorticoids if unresponsive to dapsone
- If no response to glucocorticoids, consider cyclosporine at 4 mg/kg per day divided into two doses, which usually produces a rapid response
- Noninflammatory variant is more resistant to treatment and may require intravenous immunoglobulin, plasmapheresis, or extracorporeal photochemotherapy

Dermatitis herpetiformis

Clinical presentation

- Chronic, pruritic small papules and vesicles, often with excoriations
- Predilection for extensor surfaces; symmetrical distribution, especially on elbows, knees, buttocks
- Mucous membrane are rarely involved
- Onset age 20–40 most common, but may occur at any age, including childhood
- Associations: 95% of cases have gluten-sensitive enteropathy; thyroid disease, small-bowel lymphoma, non-Hodgkin's lymphoma also associated

Dermatitis herpetiformis (Figure 5-10) is an extremely pruritic disorder that presents with clustered vesicles that are quickly excoriated. Vesicles arise in crops and are distributed symmetrically on the scalp, sacrum, and extensor extremities. Some patients, especially children, may have palmar involvement. The disease course is usually lifelong; spontaneous remissions occur in up to 10% of patients. Patients with dermatitis herpetiformis commonly have gluten-sensitive enteropathy or "celiac sprue."

Diagnosis

- Three criteria for diagnosis:
  - Pruritic, papulovesicular eruption of extensor surfaces
  - Vesicle formation at the dermoepidermal junction and infiltration of dermal papillary tips with neutrophils
  - Granular IgA at the dermoepidermal junction

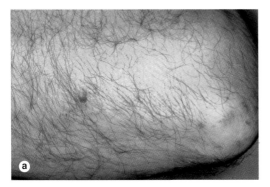

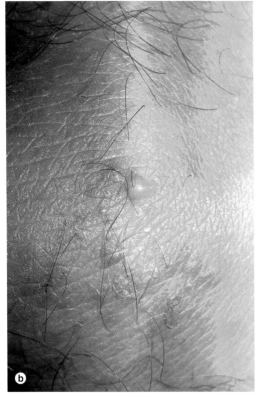

Figure 5-10 a Dermatitis herpetiformis. **b** Intact vesicles are rare in dermatitis herpetiformis

- Lesional biopsy for histopathology: subepidermal blister, microabscesses in dermal papillae with collection of neutrophils and rare eosinophils
- Perilesional biopsy for DIF: granular IgA deposits in papillary dermal tips, sometimes C3
- Differential diagnosis: linear IgA bullous dermatosis, atopic dermatitis, bullous pemphigoid, scabies, contact dermatitis, bites

Laboratory testing

- Serum antibodies: antiendomysial IgA, antireticulin, thyroid microsomal, antinuclear, tissue transglutaminase
- Human leukocyte antigen (HLA)-B8 in 80%

Pathogenesis

- Uncertain pathogenesis, but may be due to tissue transglutaminase
- Granular deposition of IgA in the dermal papillae, activation of complement system, chemotaxis of neutrophils followed by release of enzymes that alter or destroy laminin and type IV collagen contributing to the formation of blisters
- Iodine and nonsteroidal anti-inflammatory drugs may exacerbate disease in susceptible patients

Treatment

- Gluten-free diet is the preferred treatment for both the skin and gastrointestinal disease. Long-term adherence decreases risk of lymphoma
- Skin often responds rapidly to dapsone: adult initial dose 25–50 mg daily or children 0.5 mg/kg, average adult maintenance dose 100 mg daily. Lesions return abruptly upon discontinuation. Gastrointestinal disease is not adequately controlled with dapsone
- Alternative if dapsone-unresponsive or allergic: sulfapyridine 500 mg three times daily up to 2 g three times daily
- Occasional application of topical steroids to control lesions
- Lifelong treatment is needed

Linear IgA bullous dermatosis

Clinical presentation

- Discrete bullae that often occur in clusters: "cluster of jewels" or "string of pearls"
- Lesions in adults are predominantly on the trunk and limbs
- Facial and perineal lesions more common in the childhood form
- Mucosal involvement common
- Bimodal age distribution with two forms of the disease
  - Linear IgA bullous dermatosis occurs in older adults
  - Chronic bullous disease of childhood occurs in children
- Circulating IgA antibodies in only 20% of adult cases
- Associations: ulcerative colitis, lymphoma

Linear IgA bullous disease (Figure 5-11) includes both adult and childhood forms. The disease in children begins around age 2–3 and usually remits by puberty. Facial/perineal lesions are common, with blisters often sausage-shaped and arranged in flower-like arrangements. In adults, mucosal involvement is more common, and blisters more often develop on the trunk and limbs. The disease

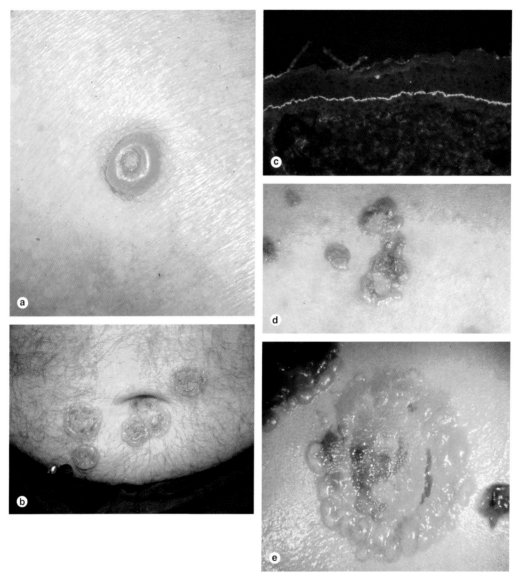

Figure 5-11 **a** Vancomycin-induced linear immunoglobulin (Ig) A. **b** Linear IgA disease (courtesy of Julie Hodge MD).
c Linear IgA direct immunofluorescence. **d** Linear IgA disease. **e** Chronic bullous disease of childhood

may resemble bullous pemphigoid or dermatitis herpetiformis. Adults generally have a chronic course, but the disease can go into remission after many years.

Diagnosis

- Lesional biopsy for histopathology: subepidermal blister with neutrophils, often indistinguishable from dermatitis herpetiformis; sometimes the blister is cell-poor or with numerous eosinophils
- Perilesional biopsy for DIF: linear-pattern IgA basement membrane zone, in 20% of cases IgG or IgM
- Differential diagnosis: bullous pemphigoid, cicatricial pemphigoid, herpes simplex and zoster, dermatitis herpetiformis, pemphigus vulgaris

Laboratory testing

- Indirect immunofluorescence: linear IgA antibodies in 33–50% (70% in chronic bullous disease of childhood)

Pathogenesis

- Linear IgA bullous dermatosis-1 (LAD-1:120kDa) antigen and linear IgA bullous dermatosis (LABD: 97kDa) antigen which are breakdown products of the transmembrane protein collagen XVII/BPAg2 (180 kDa)
- Rare cases in which the antigen is collagen VII of the anchoring fibril

- Chemotaxis of neutrophils and eosinophils, along with release of enzymes, results in tissue lesions
- Drug-induced form is most commonly due to vancomycin (remits several weeks after cessation of the drug) and diclofenac

Other implicated medications include lithium, amiodarone, captopril, penicillins, PUVA, furosemide, oxaprozin, interleukin-2, interferon-alpha, and phenytoin.

Treatment

- Response usually seen in 48–72 hours with dapsone or sulfonamides
- Dapsone 100 mg (0.5–1.4 mg/kg in children) daily usually controls eruption, but higher doses or the addition of prednisone up to 40 mg daily may be needed
- Resistant cases may need immunosuppression with agents described in bullous pemphigoid section
- Cyclophosphamide recommended to prevent scarring if there is ocular involvement

Controversies

The rare cases with antibodies against collagen VII may best be classified as epidermolysis bullosa acquisita.

Bullous systemic lupus erythematosus (BSLE)

Clinical presentation

- Herpetiform vesicles or, more often, large, tense fluid-filled to hemorrhagic bullae
- Usually on sun-exposed skin
- Bullous lupus erythematosus (Figure 5-12) is a rare presentation of systemic lupus erythematosus. Patients generally meet criteria for systemic lupus erythematosus. Bullae arise on sun-exposed skin on a noninflammatory or inflammatory base. Lesions resemble dermatitis herpetiformis histologically

Diagnosis

- Histopathology: subepidermal blister with neutrophils without interface changes
- DIF: linear basement membrane zone staining with IgG, IgA and/or IgM, and C3
- Differential diagnosis: rule out an associated primary blistering disorder or blistering that results from severe vacuolization at the basement membrane zone in lupus erythematosus

Laboratory testing

- Indirect immunofluorescence: negative
- Salt-split skin:

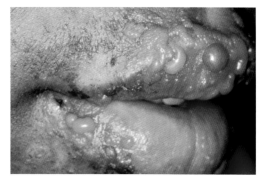

Figure 5-12 Bullous lupus erythematosus

- Antibodies to type VII collagen classically stain the dermal side (BSLE type 1)
- Patients fulfilling the criteria for BSLE without circulating antibodies to type VII collagen are classified as having BSLE type 2
- Patients with epidermal binding should not be excluded from a diagnosis of BSLE; a recent classification revision includes type 3, which includes patients with classical, clinical and histological features whose sera binds to an epidermal epitope

Pathogenesis

- Autoantibodies to type VII collagen (290 kDa protein) in the anchoring fibrils
- Autoantibodies are identical to those of epidermolysis bullosa acquisita

Treatment

- Dapsone (100 mg/day in an adult)
- Combination of dapsone with prednisone is the treatment of choice for severe or recalcitrant disease

Arthropod bite

Arthropod bites can cause subepidermal blisters. Clinically, the typical presentation is urticarial papules or blisters, sometimes in groups (e.g., the "breakfast, lunch, and dinner" lesions seen with bed bugs). The lesional biopsy for histopathology shows, in addition to the subepidermal blister, some spongiosis and a superficial and deep perivascular infiltrate with numerous eosinophils. Treatment with class I topical steroids is usually sufficient and prevention is encouraged.

Bullous lymphedema

- Tense blisters
- Pitting edema
- Subepidermal blister

Cryotherapy blister

Clinical presentation

- Tense blister at site of prior cryotherapy

Cryotherapy is a very common, effective, and rapid destructive treatment for benign and malignant skin diseases. The usual coolant is liquid nitrogen at a temperature of −196°C. This is applied via cotton applicators or using a hand-held spray gun.

Diagnosis

- Clinical history is key
- May consider lesional biopsy for histopathology: subepidermal blister with little to no inflammation

Differential diagnosis

- Could consider other blistering disorder; however, clinical history is usually sufficient to rule these out
- Contact dermatitis if allergen or irritant was applied to area after cryotherapy

Pathogenesis

Therapeutic doses of liquid nitrogen produce moderate to severe inflammation of the skin with a subsequent subepidermal blister. The mechanism is complex and not well understood, but edema appears shortly after treatment. The blister occurs in the lamina lucida.

Treatment

- No treatment is usually required
- Topical steroids (clobetasol propionate)
- Oral and topical nonsteroidal anti-inflammatory drugs

Burn blisters

Clinical presentation

Blistering can develop in second-degree thermal burns and following electrodesiccation therapy. Blisters may develop months after the initial burn.

Diagnosis

- Clinical history is key
- May consider lesional biopsy for histopathology: subepidermal blister with an overlying necrotic epidermis, vertical elongation of keratinocytes, and fusion of collagen bundles are distinctive features
- Differential diagnosis: could consider other blistering disorder; however, clinical history is usually sufficient to rule these out

Pathogenesis

- Unclear, but disturbance of the basement membrane zone may be a contributing factor. Epidermal necrosis is present

Treatment

- Cool the burn
- May drain blister, but keep roof intact to help prevent infection
- Nonsteroidal inflammatory agents

Cantharidin blisters

- From blister beetles or medical cantharidin
- Suprabasilar acantholysis

Suction blisters

Clinical presentation

Blisters may be iatrogenically induced for grafting, especially for the treatment of stable vitiligo, or can arise by accidental or factitial trauma, particularly in children.

Diagnosis

- Lesional biopsy for histopathology: cell-poor subepidermal blister with preservation of the dermal papillae
- Split occurs in lamina lucida
- Differential diagnosis: epidermolysis bullosa simplex

Pathogenesis

- A pressure of 300–500 mmHg is needed to cause the blister

Treatment

- Treatment algorithm: may drain blister, but keep roof intact to help prevent infection

"Coma bullae"

Clinical presentation

- Bullae, erosions, and dusky erythematous plaques
- Lesions arise in sites of pressure in patients who have been in a deep coma

The coma may be drug-induced or secondary to carbon monoxide poisoning and rarely as a consequence of other neurologic disorders. Patients may also develop neuropathy as a sequela.

Diagnosis

- Clinical history of coma
- Lesional biopsy for histopathology: subepidermal blister or intraepidermal spongiotic

vesicle with focal necrosis of keratinocytes adjacent to acrosyringium; sweat gland necrosis beneath bullae is key to diagnosis
- Differential diagnosis: could consider other blistering disorder; however, clinical history is usually sufficient to rule these out

Pathogenesis

- Result of tissue ischemia secondary to local pressure necrosis and systemic hypoxia

Treatment

- Supportive and pressure relief.

Bullous lesions in diabetes mellitus

Clinical presentation

- Noninflammatory bullae that are tense and vary in diameter from small to very large

Bullous lesions in diabetes mellitus are a rare complication of long-standing diabetes mellitus. These lesions are also known as diabetic bullae or bullosis diabeticorum. Lesions heal within several weeks without scarring and may become dark as they dry up.

Diagnosis

- Clinical history of diabetes mellitus
- Lesional biopsy for histopathology: subepidermal blister with a sparse perivascular infiltrate in early lesions. Later lesions show intraepidermal blisters with surrounding spongiosis, which likely represents healing. There may be associated diabetic microangiopathy
- Perilesional biopsy for DIF: negative
- Differential diagnosis: bullous pemphigoid, which is more common in patients with diabetes mellitus

Pathogenesis

- Association with diabetic nephropathy and/or peripheral vascular disease

Treatment

- Supportive

Controversies

This disorder may not be a uniform entity. There may be some overlap with bullous pemphigoid, as these patients have an increased frequency of diabetes mellitus.

Further reading

Dart J. Cicatricial pemphigoid and dry eye. Semin Ophthalmol 2005;20:95–100.

Mutasim DF, Bilic M, Hawayek LH, et al. Immunobullous diseases. J Am Acad Dermatol 2005;52:1029–1043.

Sitaru C, Dahnrich C, Probst C, et al. Enzyme-linked immunosorbent assay using multimers of the 16th non-collagenous domain of the BP180 antigen for sensitive and specific detection of pemphigoid autoantibodies. Exp Dermatol 2007;16:770–777.

Solomon LW, Helm TN, Stevens C, et al. Clinical and immunopathologic findings in oral lichen planus pemphigoides. Oral Surg Oral Med Oral Pathol Oral Radiol Endod 2007;103:808–813.

Vassileva S. Bullous systemic lupus erythematosus. Clin Dermatol 2004;22:129–138.

Yancey KB. The pathophysiology of autoimmune blistering diseases. J Clin Invest 2005;115: 825–828.

Zhu X, Zhang B. Paraneoplastic pemphigus. J Dermatol 2007;34:503–511.

Cutaneous histiocytoses

Arturo P. Saavedra

The term "histiocytosis" applies to disorders in which specific kinds of cells infiltrate the skin and other organs. As more is learned about these disorders, classification has become more elaborate. It is now accepted that "histiocytes," which are derived from a similar progenitor (CD34+ cells), may differentiate into different cell types including dendritic cells, interstitial dendrocytes and monocyte/macrophages. Despite new data, all of these cells still continue to be grouped under the general term "histiocyte."

Traditionally, these disorders have been separated into two broad categories: Langerhans cell histiocytosis (LCH) and non-Langerhans cell histiocytosis (non-LCH). Langerhans cells are antigen-presenting cells that migrate to lymph nodes but do not recirculate back to the skin. They stain for a specific immunohistochemical marker (CD1a) and contain ultrastructural components resembling tennis rackets called Birbeck granules. On the other hand, non-Langerhans histiocytes do not stain for CD1a and lack Birbeck granules. Though they can also present antigens, they are mostly phagocytic in nature. A third category, indeterminate cell histiocytosis, is applied to those disorders in which histiocytes stain for CD1a but do not exhibit Birbeck granules on electron microscopy (Table 6.1).

Non-Langerhans cell histiocytosis

Clinical presentation

Key Points

Juvenile xanthogranuloma (JXG)

- JXG (Figure 6-1) is the most common form of non-LCH
- One-half to two-thirds of patients present before 6 months of age, but disease has also been reported in adults (adult xanthogranuloma)
- Male predominance has been suggested
- Over 90% of cases present as a single, yellow to orange or tan dome-shaped papule measuring up to 1 cm

- The disease is most common on the face or upper torso
- Spontaneous regression is the rule for cutaneous lesions, but disseminated cutaneous disease, as well as systemic involvement in the upper airways, eyes, and visceral tissue has been reported
- Erdheim–Chester disease is the association of multiple xanthogranulomas and sclerotic bony lesions
- Multiple xanthogranulomas have also been associated with neurofibromatosis and juvenile myelomonocytic leukemia

Necrobiotic xanthogranuloma (NXG)

- NXG is a rare disease
- It affects a wide range of ages (17–85 years) and has no gender predilection
- Red-orange papules and nodules coalesce into plaques that show central atrophy and telangiectasia
- NXG favors the face and trunk. In 50% of cases, periocular manifestations are observed
- It is associated with immunoglobulin (Ig) G paraproteinemias, myeloma, cryoglobulinemia, arthritis, biliary cirrhosis, and thyroid disease
- Clinical course is usually progressive, despite available treatment with steroids or chemotherapy for disease related to neoplasia

Reticulohistiocytoma and multicentric reticulohistiocytosis

- Solitary reticulohistiocytic granulomas (reticulohistiocytomas) are not rare, but multicentric reticulohistiocytosis is a rare disease
- No clear gender predilection
- Reticulohistiocytoma is a solitary lesion and presents as a nontender, brown to yellow nodule, particularly on the face and hands
- The disease remits after several years (mean duration of 8 years)
- When disease presents with multisystem involvement, termed multicentric reticulohistiocytosis, about 25% of cases are associated with malignancy
- Patients are older (average 43 years), usually female and Caucasian, and a larger number of lesions are noted
- These lesions, which exhibit the same morphology as a single reticulohistiocytoma, tend to cluster around the nailbed ("coral bead sign") and prognosis may depend on associated comorbidities

Table 6-1 Classification of the histiocytoses

Disease	CD1a	S100	Birbeck granules	"Histiocyte" infiltrating the skin
Langerhans cell histiocytosis	+	+	+	Dendritic cell
Indeterminate cell histiocytosis	+	+	–	Unclear, but likely dermal dendrocytes
Non-Langerhans cell histiocytosis (except Rosai–Dorfman disease and multicentric reticulohistiocytosis)	–	–	–	Dermal/interstitial dendrocyte (interstitial dendritic cells)
Rosai–Dorfman, multicentric reticulohistiocytosis	–	+	–/+	Likely macrophage

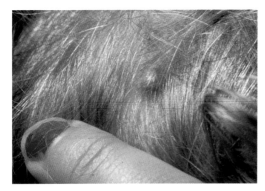

Figure 6-1 Juvenile xanthogranuloma

- About half of patients present with mucous membrane involvement and possibly visceral involvement
- This disease is associated with arthritis that is destructive (arthritis mutilans) and usually irreversible ("opera-glass hand")
- Vasculitis may be seen

Sinus histiocytosis with massive lymphadenopathy (Rosai–Dorfman syndrome)

- Rosai–Dorfman syndrome (Figure 6-2) is an extremely rare disease.
- Most patients are under 20 years of age
- There is predilection in blacks and slight sexual predilection for males
- Disease limited to the skin is more common in Caucasians and Asians
- Patients present with fever, night sweats, painless lymphadenopathy, flu-like symptoms and rarely (< 10%) with cutaneous disease in the form of polymorphic, red to brown macules, papules, plaques, and tumors that may ulcerate
- The face (eyelids and malar region) is commonly affected and there is predilection for cervical lymphadenopathy
- There may be systemic involvement of viscera, joints, immunologic and nervous systems
- The clinical course is benign with spontaneous resolution most of the time

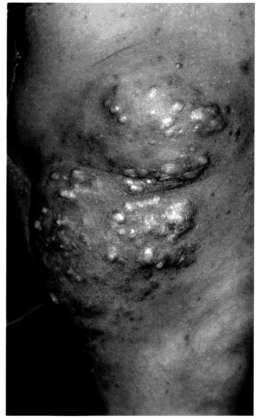

Figure 6-2 Rosai–Dorfman disease

Other rare forms of non-Langerhans cell histiocytosis (fewer than 150 cases reported for each) (Table 6.2)

These disorders are normolipemic and information regarding their clinical presentation and clinical course exists mostly as case reports. They include:
- Xanthoma disseminatum
- Generalized eruptive histiocytoma
- Benign cephalic histiocytosis

Table 6-2 Uncommon subtypes of non-Langerhans cell histiocytosis

Subtype	Frequency	Sex and age predilection	Clinical presentation	Body site predilection	Clinical course	Other
Xanthoma disseminatum (Montgomery's syndrome)	Fewer than 150 cases reported	Males > females; most cases under 25 years of age	Generalized and eruptive; hundreds of yellow-brown papules, nodules, and plaques	Flexural areas, but can also generalize and become confluent; mucosa, upper airways, and viscera can be affected	May remit, persist (most common), or progress	Diabetes insipidus is associated in 40% of cases, as well as myeloma; central nervous system symptoms may occur; normal lipids are the rule
Generalized eruptive histiocytoma	Fewer than 50 cases described	Unclear sex predilection; 3–60 years (mostly adults)	Symmetric, firm, yellow to red to brown and blue papules	Trunk and proximal extremities; mucous disease is rare; no visceral disease	Spontaneous resolution after several years but disease may be recurrent	Normal health; considered an early form of xanthoma disseminatum
Benign cephalic histiocytosis	Fewer than 50 cases reported	Males > females, mean age is 13.5 months; onset is during the first 3 years of life	Round to oval, yellow-brown macules and papules; early lesions may show erythema	Upper face; always spares mucous membrane and viscera; may involve trunk and buttocks rarely	Spontaneous resolution without scarring in 2–8 years	Normal health; some believe this is an early version of juvenile xanthogranuloma
Progressive nodular histiocytosis	Extremely rare	Males = females; 40–60 years of age	Hundreds of diffuse papules and nodules, 0.2–5 cm	Generalized, no clustering around flexures	Can be deforming without resolution; resistant to therapy	Normal health; rarely chronic myeloid leukemia; growth failure
Papular xanthoma	Fewer than 30 cases reported	Females > males; under 1 year of age (males are affected most commonly when single lesions are noted)	Yellow to brown papules and nodules that do not coalesce into plaques	Generalized; mucous involvement but spares flexures; no visceral involvement	In children, regression within 5 years; may persist in adults	Diabetes insipidus is not reported
Hereditary progressive mucinous histiocytosis	Fewer than 20 cases reported	Females only	Skin-colored or red nodules that do not ulcerate	Spares the mucosa and the viscera	Progressive and resistant to therapy	Normal health; familial inheritance reported

- Progressive nodular histiocytosis
- Papular xanthoma
- Hereditary progressive mucinous histiocytosis.

The term "non-Langerhans cell histiocytosis" incorporates a group of disorders in which "histiocytes" predominantly infiltrate the dermis. These histiocytes fail to fulfill the criteria for Langerhans cells based on their differentiation into dermal dendrocytes or macrophages, their lack of staining for markers such as CD1a, S100, and Langerin, and the lack of Birbeck granules on electron microscopy. This group contains several disorders, some of which are very rare and are listed in Table 6-2. The more prevalent disorders of this category are discussed below.

The non-LCHs have been subclassified into several disorders, though some authors suggest that they are all part of the same disease spectrum. Some proponents separate these disorders into those of dermal/interstitial dendrocytes (the JXG family) and those derived from monocytes/macrophages. With the current advances in molecular and immunological techniques, our understanding of clinical pathogenesis and response to therapy will undoubtedly improve. In the meantime, careful study of morphology, clinical course, and histopathology has led to the description of discrete disorders.

The most common type of non-LCH is JXG. This disease is most common in children but can also be seen in adults (and termed adult xanthogranuloma). JXG usually presents as an asymptomatic yellow to red solitary lesion that varies from 0.5 to 2 cm in diameter over 80–90% of the time. It is important to note that exceptions (giant variants > 2 cm, ulcerated forms, and clustered lesions) have been documented. In these cases, biopsy for histopathologic examination is suggested. Disseminated cutaneous disease and systemic involvement of nearly every organ have been reported. The disease may present in the subcutis and in the soft tissues, primarily in children. Particularly in patients with multiple lesions, it is important to rule out eye involvement, most commonly of the iris. However, an extensive evaluation beyond a thorough history and physical examination is not suggested for every patient who presents with cutaneous disease.

JXG usually appears abruptly and lesions can continue to appear. They often resolve spontaneously. Association with hyperlipidemia or diabetes has not been established. Therefore, treatment is usually supportive unless organ compromise is noted from either compression or tissue infiltration. If treatment is needed, surgical approaches are preferable for cutaneous disease, but recurrences have been reported. Systemic disease usually requires radiotherapy or chemotherapy, particularly for unresectable lesions.

NXG, though less common than JXG, is associated with potentially lethal disease and is therefore important to recognize. Lesions tend to favor the face, particularly the periorbital region, and present as yellow or red-orange papules that may coalesce into plaques. This is a disorder of dermal infiltration that may cause dermal atrophy and result in visible telangiectasias. Occasionally lesions may become ulcerated. Unlike JXG, adults are most frequently affected, with an equal incidence in males and females. Over 90% of cases are associated with paraproteinemias/monoclonal gammopathies and therefore appropriate laboratory testing, including electrolytes, complete blood count, liver function tests and serologies, thyroid panel, erythrocyte sedimentation rate, serum and urine electrophoresis and occasionally bone marrow biopsy are recommended. These tests are required in order to rule out multiple myeloma, Waldenström's hypergammaglobulinemia, as well as other associated disorders that include cryoglobulinemia, arthropathies, Graves disease, and biliary cirrhosis. Clinical course is usually progressive and prognosis is related to the associated disorder uncovered during work-up.

Finally, reticulohistiocytomas may be encountered in clinical practice. These lesions may be single or multiple, and present as asymptomatic, dome-shaped papulonodules, distributed mostly on the face and hands. Occasionally, pruritus may be noted. Periungal disease, often resembling "coral beads," is noted in cases where multiple lesions exist. Isolated or multiple reticulohistiocytomas occur most commonly in adult men. Multicentric reticulohistiocytosis, however, is a disease of older women, often associated with mutilating arthritis. About 50% of patients also have mucosal disease and systemic disease has been reported involving visceral, neural, and skeletal tissues. Importantly, multicentric reticulohistiocytosis may be associated with hyperlipidemia, thyroid disease, and collagen vascular diseases. Paraneoplastic disease associated with colon and breast cancer is most commonly reported, but melanoma, lymphoma, and sarcoma can also occur. It is important to follow patients closely, as most cancers occur during or after the development of skin disease.

Diagnosis/histopathology

Key Points

Juvenile xanthogranuloma

- There is a dermal infiltrate of foamy histiocytes with Langhans (wreath) and Touton (lipidized wreath) giant cells (Figure 6-3). Spindle cells may also be seen
- Extension into reticular dermis or subcutaneous tissue has been noted
- The early stage is composed of uniform nonlipidized histiocytes
- Neutrophils, lymphocytes, and eosinophils are variably present

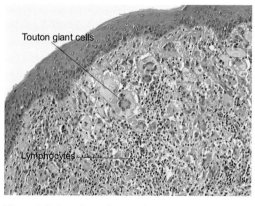

Figure 6-3 Juvenile xanthogranuloma

- In advanced cases, the epidermis may be involved and can ulcerate
- Like in other non-LCH, CD1a and S100 stains are negative, but factor XIIIa and CD68 are positive
- Cellular atypia is absent and mitoses are rarely observed

Necrobiotic xanthogranuloma

- A granulomatous dermal and subcutaneous infiltrate is noted
- Langhans and foreign-body giant cells, and Touton giant cells surround a central devitalized (necrobiotic) area with nuclear debris and cholesterol clefts (Figure 6-4)
- The epidermis is usually not involved unless the lesion is progressive and ulcerative

Reticulohistiocytoma and multicentric reticulohistiocytosis

- There is a dermal and subcutaneous infiltrate of mononuclear histiocytes with two-tone (dark and pale) eosinophilic cytoplasm that mimics "ground glass" and stains positive for periodic acid–Schiff (Figure 6-5)
- Cells may appear large and atypical
- Vacuolated spindle cells and lipid-laden mononuclear cells are often seen

Unlike other non-LCH groups, cells are factor XIII-negative in multicentric reticulohistiocytosis. It has been suggested that the pathology of isolated reticulohistiocytoma is different in that cells are much larger and do stain for factor XIIIa and HHF35, in comparison to those of multicentric reticulohistiocytosis, which do not stain for these markers.

Sinus histiocytosis with massive lymphadenopathy (Rosai–Dorfman syndrome)

- The epidermis is usually unaffected
- Within the dermis or subcutaneous tissue, there are sheets of histiocytes with nodular mononuclear cell aggregates visible at low power

- Histiocytes often fill lymphatics in skin and sinusoids in lymph nodes
- Rosai–Dorfman cells are described as having a pale, "water-clear" cytoplasm
- Unlike in other non-LCH, cells in Rosai–Dorfman are S100-positive and occasionally CD68-positive. Rare reports showing CD1a-positive staining are available
- No nuclear atypia is seen and there is no evidence for clonal disease
- Neutrophils, eosinophils, plasma cells, and lymphocytes may be seen
- Lymph node pathology is similar, but also includes dilation of sinuses, occasional mitotic figures, and Reed–Sternberg-like cells
- Lymphophagocytosis (degenerating lymphocytes and plasma cells present within phagolysosomes in the cytoplasm of histiocytes) and emperipolesis (intact mononuclear cells, simply "passing through" the cytoplasm of histiocytes) may be seen, particularly in skin (Figure 6-6)
- Search for infectious organisms such as Epstein–Barr virus, human herpesvirus (HHV)-6 and -8 has revealed inconsistent findings

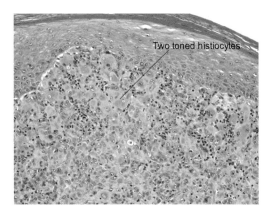

Figure 6-5 Reticulohistiocytosis

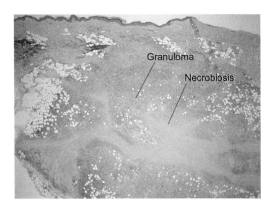

Figure 6-4 Necrobiotic xanthogranuloma

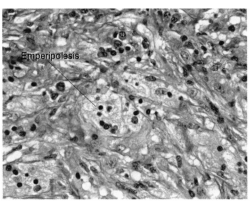

Figure 6-6 Rosai–Dorfman disease

Other rare forms of non-Langerhans cell histiocytosis

- *Xanthoma disseminatum*: foamy cells have angulated borders with round vesicular nuclei that predominate over Touton giant cell. Histiocytes contain microvilli under electron microscopy
- *Generalized eruptive histiocytosis*: histiocytes are arranged around vessels; worm-like bodies may be seen under electron microscopy
- *Benign cephalic histiocytosis*: "comma-shaped" bodies have been described under electron microscopy in the cytoplasm of histiocytes in up to 30% of cases, but are not pathognomonic

Clinical differential diagnosis

Juvenile xanthogranuloma

- Benign cephalic histiocytosis
- Nodular LCH
- Xanthomas
- Spitz nevi
- Dermal nevi
- Dermatofibroma
- Solitary mastocytosis
- Cysts

Necrobiotic xanthogranuloma

- Necrobiosis lipoidica diabeticorum
- Granuloma annulare
- Xanthoma
- Reticulohistiocytoma
- Non-LCH
- Sarcoidosis

Reticulohistiocytoma and multicentric reticulohistiocytosis

- Dermatofibroma
- Other non-LCH, including Rosai–Dorfman disease
- Xanthoma
- Xanthogranuloma
- Rheumatoid nodules, rheumatoid arthritis
- Sarcoidosis
- Spitz nevi
- Lymphoma
- Adnexal tumors
- Histiocytic sarcoma

Sinus histiocytosis with massive lymphadenopathy (Rosai–Dorfman syndrome)

- Extensive differential
- Eruptive xanthoma
- LCH
- Human immunodeficiency virus infection
- Localized infection by many organisms such as *Streptococcus*, *Staphylococcus*, *Bartonella*, tularemia, *Klebsiella*, *Toxoplasma*, and others

- Large number of "inflammatory" conditions, including sarcoid, granuloma annulare, xanthogranuloma and reticulohistiocytoma, and Kikuchi's disease
- Malignancy, including lymphoma, parasagittal meningioma, metastatic adenocarcinoma of unknown primary, and hematophagocytic syndromes

Laboratory testing

Juvenile xanthogranuloma

Extensive laboratory evaluation after a complete history and physical exam is not required unless review of systems suggests extracutaneous involvement. If so, imaging and blood work are indicated, depending on the tissue affected. Though data are only suggestive but not confirmatory, for children with neurofibromatosis-1 who are also noted to have JXG, complete work-up to rule out juvenile myelogenous leukemia is important to consider. This will require complete blood counts and referral to oncology for potential bone marrow evaluation. Referral to ophthalmology may also be considered in children with several lesions or those under the age of 2 years, as cases have rarely led to blindness from glaucoma or hyphema.

Necrobiotic xanthogranuloma

Complete physical examination is essential. Given its association with paraproteinemia, work-up should include electrolytes, including calcium, erythrocyte sedimentation rate, liver function tests, serum and urine electrophoresis, and potential bone marrow biopsy. Rare associations with cryoglobulinemia have been reported and complement levels may be decreased. If a monoclonal gammopathy is uncovered, oncologic referral is beneficial. There has been a suggestion in the literature that patients with NXG may have a higher risk of developing atherosclerosis. Patients should be referred for cardiovascular evaluation if other risk factors for heart disease are present or if review of systems suggests that such investigations are warranted. On autopsy, cardiac NXG has been documented.

Reticulohistiocytoma and multicentric reticulohistiocytosis

Solitary lesions do not require any additional evaluation. The association of multicentric lesions with arthritis is important to remember, particularly as it is erosive and usually irreversible if untreated. Physical examination should focus on evaluation of joints, with attention to the hands. Rheumatoid factor is negative. Complete blood count with differential, erythrocyte sedimentation rate, and cryoglobulins should be considered. Lipids may be elevated and a large number of patients may have a positive tuberculin test. The risk of malignancy is also important to remember, but like arthritis, malignancy can present before, during, or after the diagnosis of reticulohistiocytosis. Therefore, patient follow-up is as important as the initial visit. Additionally, age-appropriate screening for malignancy appears to be the best approach at this time, but associations include carcinoma of the breast, cervix, lung, and colon as well as melanoma and leukemia. Autoimmune disorders, including Sjögren's syndrome, have been occasionally linked to multicentric reticulohistiocytosis.

Sinus histiocytosis with massive lymphadenopathy (Rosai–Dorfman syndrome)

Complete blood count, erythrocyte sedimentation rate, and serum/urine electrophoresis are suggested given associations with gammopathies (though they are usually polyclonal). Lymphoma has rarely been reported as well. Titers for infectious organisms are not usually helpful and are not recommended.

Other rare forms of non-Langerhans cell histiocytosis

Lipid studies may be helpful when ruling out xanthomatous disorders with hyperlipidemic syndromes. Benign cephalic histiocytosis, generalized eruptive histiocytosis, papular xanthoma, and xanthoma disseminatum are normolipemic states. Particularly in xanthoma disseminatum, work-up for associated diabetes insipidus and paraproteinemia is indicated.

Pathogenesis

Juvenile xanthogranuloma

JXG is considered to be a reactive granulomatous process stimulated by either infectious or physical agents. Though these etiologies remain unproven, proliferation of interstitial dendrocytes or plasmacytoid monocytes is the currently accepted model. Recently, expression of MS-1, a protein specific for sinusoidal endothelial cells, has been noted in JXG and other non-LCH disorders, but not in LCH. Many authors believe that non-LCH disorders represent clinical spectra of one pathological entity.

Necrobiotic xanthogranuloma

Pathogenesis remains unclear, but a role for deposition of immunoglobulins in giant cells has been suggested. These immunoglobulins may activate monocytes, which leads to intracellular accumulation of lipoprotein-derived lipids. In one case, the activation of monocytes led to hypocholesterolemia. A role for complement reactions and increased levels of monocyte colony-stimulating factor has been postulated.

Reticulohistiocytoma and multicentric reticulohistiocytosis

Pathogenesis is poorly understood but a role for mycobacteria, immune or neoplastic mechanisms has been suggested, without confirmatory results.

Sinus histiocytosis with massive lymphadenopathy (Rosai–Dorfman syndrome)

Infectious agents, including HHV-6, -8, Epstein–Barr virus, and *Klebsiella* among others, have been suggested as potential etiological agents. However, polymerase chain reaction analysis and culture have yielded inconsistent results. Immunologic mechanisms are also postulated, involving the cell-mediated arm of the immune response. The disease is polyclonal.

Other rare forms of non-Langerhans cell histiocytosis

Benign cephalic histiocytosis, generalized eruptive histiocytosis, xanthoma disseminatum, and progressive nodular histiocytosis have been considered part of the same disease spectrum as JXG but with variable cellular morphologic differentiation (from xanthomatous to spindled). It has been noted that hereditary progressive mucinous histiocytosis may be an inherited form of a poorly characterized storage/deposition disease.

Treatment

Juvenile xanthogranuloma

Lesions may resolve spontaneously and therapy beyond shave biopsy is not required unless tissue is compromised either by extrinsic compression or by parenchymal obliteration. In such cases, surgical approaches have been most successful, though recurrences after complete excision have been reported. Topical, intralesional, and systemic steroids have been used for ocular lesions. Radiotherapy, chemotherapy, and cyclosporine are alternatives for surgery, but can also be used when surgical approaches are not possible (central nervous system involvement, for instance). Of note, although JXG is less common in adults, when it occurs, the course may be persistent and more difficult to treat. Otherwise, prognosis in children is favorable and most are in general good health.

Necrobiotic xanthogranuloma

Topical and intralesional steroids have been used for localized disease, but systemic involvement or potential risk to any organ (e.g., eye), may require systemic corticosteroids. Hydroxychloroquine has also been used. Though melphalan, chlorambucil, and plasma exchange have successfully treated NXG, they do not prevent progression to multiple myeloma. Radiotherapy has also been employed. Surgical approaches are not generally successful and should be avoided.

Reticulohistiocytoma and multicentric reticulohistiocytosis

For solitary lesions, no treatment beyond shave biopsy is required. For multiple lesions, if any signs of malignancy are documented, referral to oncology is paramount. Arthritis can be managed in conjunction with rheumatologists, and the use of alendronate and etanercept has been reported. Systemic disease or destructive cutaneous disease can be treated with corticosteroids and antimalarials, but escalation to cytotoxic medication and immunosuppressives or surgical approaches may be required in recalcitrant cases. Of note, some authors believe that treatment is not helpful.

Sinus histiocytosis with massive lymphadenopathy (Rosai–Dorfman syndrome)

Lesions tend to regress spontaneously so treatment is not usually indicated. In a recent literature review, about half of patients did not require any treatment. Localized disease may be treated with surgical excision. The use of antibiotics or antituberculous medication is not fruitful. If disease becomes progressive or infiltrative, successful treatment with systemic glucocorticoids, cyclophosphamide, and immunosuppressive agents has been reported. Recalcitrant cases have been treated with chemotherapy (vinca alkaloids, anthracyclines, alkylating agents), radiotherapy, surgery, or a combination of the above.

Other rare forms of non-Langerhans cell histiocytosis

Few case reports appear in the literature, but as many of these disorders may be self-limited, conservative management is recommended. Localized disease may be treated with surgical excision. However, it is unclear if these disorders respond to medical therapy, and in the case of progressive nodular histiocytosis, disease is typically recalcitrant to all forms of treatment. In xanthoma disseminatum, vasopressin may be needed if diabetes insipidus is diagnosed. Referral to oncology for evaluation and management of paraproteinemias is helpful.

Controversies

A link between neurofibromatosis and JXG with the development of juvenile myelomonocytic leukemia has been reported in children, but remains poorly understood. Males appear to be overrepresented in this group of patients.

Langerhans cell histiocytosis and indeterminate cell histiocytosis

Clinical presentation

Key Points

Indeterminate cell histiocytosis

- This is a rare disease with fewer than 100 reported cases
- Adults (most common) and children are affected, with male preponderance
- Lesions may be symmetrical, yellow to brown firm papules and may progress to form nodules and plaques
- Rarely, visceral involvement has been reported

Langerhans cell histiocytosis

- LCH may present in an adult, child (most common), or congenitally
- Most congenital cases have varicelliform, papulovesicular morphology (Figure 6-7)
- Erosions and ulcers may occur which become superinfected and painful
- Seborrheic-like widespread dermatitis with surrounding petechiae can be seen in the scalp, particularly in children (Figure 6-8). In severe cases, alopecia may be seen
- Flexures may also be involved, including the groin, the perianal region (Figure 6-9), and inframammary folds
- Disease may occur near genitalia, more commonly in women. Involvement of the genitalia in men is rare
- Nail involvement is considered a poor prognostic sign
- Disease is comprised of several clinical presentations, now thought to be part of one disease spectrum (Table 6-3)

LCH describes a proliferation of epidermal Langerhans cells into the dermis and other organs. Though cutaneous disease is most often diagnosed by dermatologists, significant visceral involvement has been noted in virtually every organ. The disease can manifest in children and adults, and a congenital variant is also recognized. Disease can present as papules, nodules, plaques, and ulcers, usually with yellow to orange discoloration. The congenital form has been described as varicelliform given its resemblance to chickenpox, which is an important entity to consider in the differential diagnosis. Rarely, the disease has been reported in twins, as well as in different members of the same family, suggesting a potential genetic or heritable subset of cases. Bone and lung involvement are most common when the disease has systemic effects. The skull and the proximal femur are the most commonly affected bones.

Several variants have been described in the literature, depending on the extent of involvement and the age of the patient (see Table 6-3). LCH can erupt as one isolated lesion, multiple lesions, or as disseminated, systemic disease. Usually the extremes of age and those with extensive or disseminated involvement tend to have the worse

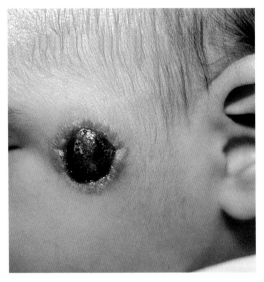

Figure 6-7 Congenital self-healing Langerhans cell histiocytosis

prognosis. However, it is now believed that these variants represent different stages of the same disease, and less importance is placed on the variant. In fact, limited cutaneous disease can go on to become disseminated, and disseminated cutaneous disease may progress to involve the viscera. Progression of disease is very difficult to predict, and careful and frequent patient follow-up is required. For historical reasons, variants are described in Table 6-3, though currently the main classification groups patients into three sets: localized, disseminated, and systemic disease with organ dysfunction.

Pathologic evaluation is essential in establishing the diagnosis. Diseases such as chickenpox, non-LCH, lymphomas, severe drug eruptions, mastocytosis, and disseminated infection are important to consider. Langerhans cells contain a reniform nucleus with sparse chromatin that appears to fold on to itself. There is ample eosinophilic cytoplasm and cells are large. In ulcerative variants, these cells may be found in the ulcer bed. Immunohistochemistry is invaluable in establishing that these are S100+ and CD1a+, which readily distinguishes this group of disorders from the rest. Ultrastructurally, Birbeck granules are observed; these have been described to resemble tennis rackets. It is important to note, however, that only "the handle" of the racket may be observed as a pentalaminar dense structure under electron microscopy. Though still controversial,

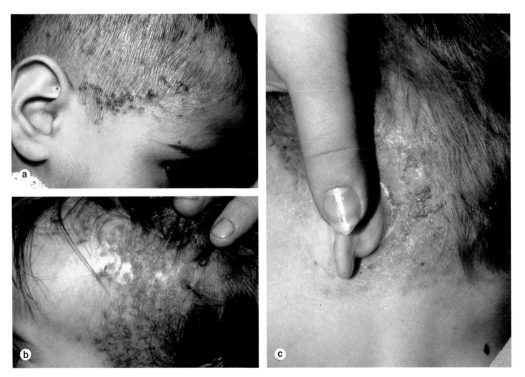

Figure 6-8 a-c Langerhans cell histiocytosis. (courtesy of Geisinger Medical Center Teaching file)

these structures are thought to represent fragments of endocytosed cytosolic membrane.

A rare and unusual form of LCH has been reported. Fewer than 100 cases are found in the literature. Though lesions stain for S100 and CD1a, albeit less strongly than other LCH, histiocytes do not contain Birbeck granules. This disorder has been termed "intermediate cell histiocytosis."

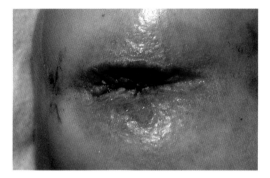

Figure 6-9 Langerhans cell histiocytosis (courtesy of Geisinger Medical Center Teaching file)

Therapy of LCH depends on patient characteristics, the extent of involvement, and the location of lesions. Disease limited to the cutaneous surface portends a better prognosis. Cutaneous disease has been treated with both topical and systemic steroids, methotrexate, psoralen with ultraviolet A (PUVA), and topical mustard. Isolated bone lesions respond to radiotherapy and local excision. Once disease disseminates or compromises visceral function, systemic agents like methotrexate and chemotherapeutic agents, including etoposide and vinblastine, are commonly used in conjunction with an oncologist.

Diagnosis/histopathology

Key Points

Indeterminate cell histiocytosis

Histiocytes infiltrate the dermis and stain for S100 and variably for CD1a. Birbeck granules are not noted on electron microscopy. Otherwise, histopathology resembles that of LCH.

Table 6-3 Langerhans cell histiocytosis and clinical variants

Variant	Patient characteristics	Morphology	Associated symptoms	Prognosis
Eosinophilic granuloma (unifocal disease)	Usually between 5 and 30 years of age, with male predominance	Swelling and tenderness over bony lesion; rarely a nodule or ulcer above bone involvement is noted; may also occur in lung and lymph nodes	Pruritus; uncommon systemic symptoms but localizes to bone causing pain and fractures	Benign, can heal spontaneously
Hand–Schüller–Christian disease	Usually under the age of 30, but disease also reported in those over 60	Papulosquamous over seborrheic distribution; purpuric and necrotic lesions; mucosa may be involved with nodules and ulcers	Skull lesions, proptosis, and diabetes insipidus form classic triad, but uncommon to find all in the same patient (< 10%); may involve lung and cause pneumothorax; also involves teeth and ear	Lung involvement is poor prognostic sign; can be fatal in up to 50% of cases; otherwise may be chronic and progressive
Letterer–Siwe disease	Usually under the age of 2 but congenital cases and adult cases are reported	Disseminated red, discrete papules and pustules with coalescence in intertriginous zones; crusting and ulceration are common; translucent papules can be initial lesion but macules that ulcerate are also common	Ill-appearing child, disseminated cutaneous eruption, multisystem disease with fever, weight loss, hepatosplenomegaly, lymphadenopathy, and malabsorption; disease is acute and fulminant	Most aggressive with fulminant course
Hashimoto–Pritzker syndrome (congenital self-healing reticulohistiocytosis)	Presents at birth or develops in the first weeks of life	Like Letterer–Siwe, but nodules may be the predominant morphology; mucous membranes are not involved	Children are usually in normal health; no visceral involvement	Benign, can heal spontaneously

Langerhans cell histiocytosis

Findings may reveal epidermal hyperkeratosis, parakeratosis and crusting. There is a dermal proliferation of Langerhans cells that show round, pale and granular eosinophilic cytoplasm and kidney-shaped nucleus (Figure 6-10). Cells have dispersed chromatin and lack prominent dendritic extensions. Cells may infiltrate the epidermis and form abscesses. They stain for S100, CD1a, CD207 (Langerin), adenosine triphosphatase (ATPase), peanut agglutinin, placental alkaline phosphatase, and interferon-γ receptor. A variable number of admixed eosinophils, basophils, mast cells, and neutrophils is often present. In late lesions, macrophages may replace Langerhans cells and the disease may be confused with a granulomatous process. Marked edema, red cell extravasation, and infiltration around vessels of the lower dermis may be noted. Granulomatous and xanthomatous variants are reported. Electron microscopy reveals cytoplasmic Birbeck granules.

Differential diagnosis

- Extensive differential diagnosis
- Non-LCH, including sinus histiocytosis with massive lymphadenopathy
- Eczema and atopic dermatitis
- Scabies
- Varicella
- Seborrheic dermatitis
- Intertrigo
- Miliaria
- Lichen niditus
- Guttate psoriasis
- Pytiriasis rosea
- Gingivitis, periodontitis
- Grovers' disease, Hailey–Hailey, and Darier's disease
- Mastocytosis and urticaria pigmentosa
- Leukemia, lymphoma (including mycosis fungoides), and multiple myeloma

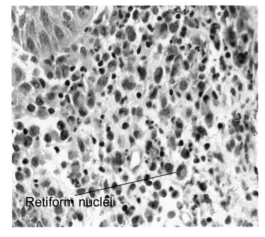

Retiform nuclei

Figure 6-10 Langerhans cell histiocytosis

Laboratory testing

- Complete blood count with differential, coagulation studies, electrolytes, liver function tests, and erythrocyte sedimentation rate are commonly obtained
- A complete history, physical exam, and review of systems are required in order to tailor further radiologic testing
- Because the lung is most commonly involved, particularly in smokers, baseline chest radiography is helpful. X-ray findings have been described as "honeycombing." Depending on the level of disease, further pulmonary work-up may be necessary, including but not limited to chest computed tomography scan, pulmonary function tests with spirometry, and biopsy
- For those with pituitary gland involvement, brain magnetic resonance imaging, urinary electrolytes, and plasma/urine osmolarity are important to consider. Endocrine consultation and hormonal profiles may be necessary
- Finally, given the risk of bone marrow involvement, oncologic consultation for potential bone marrow biopsy is helpful in those with disseminated and/or congenital disease. There is an association with leukemia, particularly in children. Data in adults is sparse

Pathogenesis

- There is an unknown stimulus for clonal Langerhans cell proliferation, but cytokines are released which are responsible for most tissue damage
- Langerhans cells are arrested at an earlier stage and interact aberrantly with T lymphocytes, creating inappropriate and high concentrations of cytokines
- Particularly, granulocyte–macrophage colony-stimulating factor and tumor necrosis factor-α have been shown to induce differentiation of Langerhans cells from CD34+ progenitors
- Eosinophils, lymphocytes, and macrophages also appear to be dysregulated
- No evidence exists to suggest a viral etiology for this disease
- In adults, the disease is still considered an "orphan" disease

Treatment

- Topical nitrogen mustard, PUVA, and thalidomide have been used for localized cutaneous disease. Oral isotretinoin, carbon dioxide laser, curettage, and systemic steroids may also be options
- Evidence exists for the use of trimethoprim-sulfamethoxazole for 1–3 months in children in the setting of cutaneous disease

- Methotrexate, vinblastine, and etoposide are used for systemic involvement, if corticosteroids do not work. Particularly in children, combination therapy with prednisolone and vinblastine is the treatment of choice. On the other hand, adults may respond to etoposide more favorably. Busulphan and cyclophosphamide have also been used
- Data suggest that maintenance with azathioprine for a year after "remission" prevents morbidity from disseminated disease
- Excision and radiotherapy have been used for isolated lesions, particularly in eosinophilic granuloma of bone. Intralesional steroids have been used in children to avoid surgical defects and risk for development of secondary malignancy
- For those with diabetes insipidus, vasopressin is the treatment of choice
- Dental care for those with "floating teeth" may be beneficial
- Finally, severe and recalcitrant disease has been treated with bone marrow or lung transplantation

Controversies

- Whether LCH is a clonal or reactive process is still the subject of debate. Viral and bacterial etiologies have not been proven. In the lung, however, relationship to smoking suggests a reactive process. Recent clustering in families, DNA aneuploidy, and cell cycle disruption argue for a neoplastic etiology

Further reading

Arico M. Langerhans cell histiocytosis in adults: more questions than answers? Eur J Cancer 2004;40:1467–1473.

Caputo R. Cutaneous nonhistiocytosis X. In: Goldsmith LA, Katz SI, Gilchrest BA, et al., eds. Dermatology in Internal Medicine, 6th edn. New York: McGraw-Hill, 2003:1590–1598.

Caputo R. Langerhans cell histiocytosis. In: Goldsmith LA, Katz SI, Gilchrest BA, et al., eds. Dermatology in Internal Medicine, 6th edn. New York: McGraw-Hill, 2003:1581–1589.

Chang MW. Update on juvenile xanthogranuloma: unusual cutaneous and systemic variants. Semin Cutan Med Surg 1999;18:195–205.

Chu A. Langerhans cell histiocytosis. In: Lebwohl MG, Heymann WR, Berth-Jones J, et al., eds. Treatment of Skin Disease: Comprehensive Therapeutic Strategies, 2nd edn. London: Elsevier Mosby, 2006:3324–3327.

Gianotti F, Caputo R, Ermacora E, et al. Benign cephalic histiocytosis. Arch Dermatol 1986;122:1038–1043.

Goodman WT, Barrett TL. Histiocytoses. In: Bolognia JL, Jorizzo JL, Rapini RP, eds. Dermatology. London: Mosby, 2003:1429–1445.

Hernandez-Martin A, Baselga E, Drolet BA, et al. Juvenile xanthogranuloma. J Am Acad Dermatol 1997;26:355–367.

Holubar K. Multicentric reticulohistiocytosis. In: Goldsmith LA, Katz SI, Gilchrest BA, et al., eds. Dermatology in Internal Medicine, 6th edn. New York: McGraw-Hill, 2003:1599–1602.

Jaffe R. The histiocytoses. Clin Lab Med 1999;19:135–155.

James WD, Berger TG, Elston DM. The histiocytoses. In: James WD, Berger TG, Elston DM, eds. Clinical Dermatology, 10th edn. Philadelphia: WB Saunders, 2006:714–724.

Laman JD, Leenen PJM, Annels N, et al. Langerhans-cell histiocytosis 'insight into DC biology.' TRENDS Immunol 2003;24:190–196.

McKee PH, Calonje E, Granter SR. Cutaneous lymphoproliferative diseases and related disorders. In: McKee PH, Calonje E, Granter SR, eds. Pathology of the Skin with Clinical Correlations 3rd edn. London: Elsevier Mosby, 2005: 1457–1484.

Moschella SL. An update of the benign proliferative monocyte–macrophage and dendritic cell disorders. J Dermatol 1996;23:805–815.

Munn S, Chu AC. Langerhans cell histiocytosis of the skin. Hematol Oncol Clin North Am 1998;12:269–286.

Pulsoni A, Anghel G, Falcucci P, et al. Treatment of sinus histiocytosis with massive lymphadenopathy (Rosai–Dorfman disease): Report of a case with literature review. Am J Hematol 2002;69:67–71.

Valderrama E, Kahn LB, Festa R, et al. Benign isolated histiocytosis mimicking chicken pox in a neonate: report of two cases with ultrastructural study. Pediatr Pathol 1985;3:103–113.

Weitsman S, Jaffe R. Uncommon histiocytic disorders: the non-Langerhans cell histiocytosis. Pediatr Blood Cancer 2005;45:256–264.

Wood GS, Chung-Hong H, Beckstead JH, et al. The indeterminate cell proliferative disorder: report of a case manifesting as an unusual cutaneous histiocytosis. J Dermatol Surg Oncol 1985;11:1111–1119.

Woolf K, Johnson RA, Suurmond D. Langerhans cell histiocytosis. In: Woolf K, Johnson RA, Suurmond D, eds. Color Atlas and Synopsis of Clinical Dermatology. 5th edn. New York: McGraw-Hill, 2005: 515–518.

Mastocytosis

Jenny C. Hu and Stefani Takahashi

Clinical presentation

Mastocytosis consists of a heterogeneous group of diseases characterized by an accumulation of mast cells in various organs, including the heart, lung, gastrointestinal tract, liver, spleen, bone marrow, lymph nodes, and skin. Mastocytosis most often presents as cutaneous disease, which can be accompanied by systemic involvement. However, it can also present as a systemic disease without cutaneous involvement. A consensus classification by Valent et al. proposes the following categories for mastocytosis: cutaneous mastocytosis, indolent systemic mastocytosis, systemic mastocytosis with associated clonal hematological nonmast cell lineage disease, mast cell leukemia, and mast cell sarcoma (Box 7-1). Cutaneous mastocytosis consists of four clinical types: UP (Figure 7-1), mastocytoma, diffuse cutaneous mastocytosis, and TMEP (Figure 7-2). More recently, Hartmann and Henz proposed a revised classification of cutaneous mastocytosis

with the following clinical types: maculopapular mastocytosis (to replace UP), plaque-type mastocytosis, nodular mastocytosis/mastocytoma, diffuse mastocytosis, and telangiectatic mastocytosis (to replace TMEP).

Cutaneous mastocytosis can develop during either childhood or adulthood (Table 7-1). Childhood-onset cutaneous mastocytosis is the more common presentation and often manifests as mastocytoma or UP, whereas adult-onset cutaneous mastocytosis usually presents as UP or TMEP. From several series of pediatric patients, the prevalence of cutaneous mastocytosis ranges from 1:500 to 1:800 for first-time pediatric visits or from 1:200 to 1:8000 for dermatology visits. Familial occurrence of the disease is rare, but has been reported.

Urticaria pigmentosa

UP, also known as maculopapular mastocytosis, is the most common form of cutaneous mastocytosis and is seen in both children and adults. It accounts for approximately 65–90% of cutaneous mastocytosis cases observed in children and usually develops within the first 2 years of life, although there is a clear peak of incidence in the first year of life. In adults, UP can develop at any age; the median age in one study was approximately 30 years of age. UP does not typically have systemic involvement. UP usually presents as multiple reddish-brown macules, papules, or plaques symmetrically distributed on the trunk and often spares the scalp, face, palms, and soles. Mucous membranes may also be involved. Lesions of UP vary in size from several millimeters to several centimeters in diameter, although lesions in children tend to be larger and more widespread compared to adults. The lesions can number from tens to hundreds and sometimes reach confluence when numerous. They usually arise over a period of 1–2 months, but can

BOX 7-1

Classification of mastocytosis

Cutaneous mastocytosis

    Urticaria pigmentosa (UP)

    Mastocytoma

    Diffuse cutaneous mastocytosis

    Telangiectasia macularis eruptiva perstans (TMEP)

Indolent systemic mastocytosis (ISM)

    Bone marrow mastocytosis (BMM)

    Smoldering systemic mastocytosis (SSM)

Systemic mastocytosis with associated clonal hematological nonmast cell lineage disease (SM-AHNMD)

    Systemic mastocytosis with myelodysplastic syndrome (SM-MDS)

    Systemic mastocytosis with myeloproliferative syndrome (SM-MPS)

    Systemic mastocytosis with acute myeloid leukemia (SM-AML)

    Systemic mastocytosis with non-Hodgkin's lymphoma (SM-NHL)

Aggressive systemic mastocytosis (ASM)

    Lymphadenopathic mastocytosis with eosinophilia

Mast cell leukemia (MCL)

    Classical MCL

    Aleukemic variant of MCL

Mast cell sarcoma (MCS)

Extracutaneous mastocytoma

Modified from Valent P, Horny HP, Escribano L, et al. Diagnostic criteria and classification of mastocytosis: a consensus proposal. Leuk Res 2001;25: 603–625.

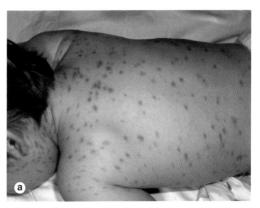

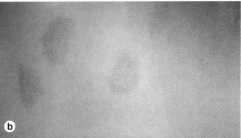

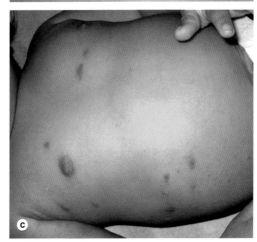

Figure 7-1 a–c Urticaria pigmentosa (courtesy of the Victor Newcomer MD collection at UCLA and Logical Images Inc)

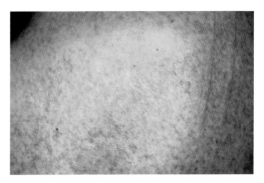

Figure 7-2 Telangiectasia macularis eruptiva perstans

continue to erupt over years. Bullous lesions occasionally form, particularly in children younger than 2 years of age. The clinically diagnostic Darier's sign (Figure 7-3), in which stroking or rubbing a cutaneous lesion causes urtication with erythema, edema, and pruritus, can be elicited in the majority of cases. In combination with clinical findings, Darier's sign may be more accurate for diagnosing mastocytosis than biopsy. However, a negative Darier's sign does not rule out mastocytosis. (Darier's sign is highly specific, but not completely sensitive.) Patients often experience concomitant pruritus and sometimes flushing due to the release of mast cell mediators, particularly histamine. Patients with UP do not seem to have higher incidences of atopy compared to a healthy population.

The prognosis of UP is associated with the age of onset. UP that develops before 10 years of age resolves either partially or completely by adolescence in 55–90% of patients. UP that develops after the age of 10 continues into

Table 7-1 Clinical presentation of cutaneous mastocytosis

Cutaneous mastocytosis	Age predominance	Clinical features
Urticaria pigmentosa (UP)	0–2 years old	Multiple reddish-brown macules, papules, or plaques symmetrically distributed on the trunk and often sparing the scalp, face, palms, and soles
Mastocytoma	0–1 years old	Single or several erythematous and yellow or brown macules, nodules, or plaques, which sometimes have a leathery or peau d'orange texture
Diffuse cutaneous mastocytosis	Birth or early infancy	Generalized edema and thickening of the skin, giving the skin a leathery or doughy appearance and accentuating the skin folds; often with spontaneous blistering
Telangiectasia macularis eruptiva perstans	Adulthood	Generalized red to brown poorly demarcated macules with visible telangiectasias
Associated systemic involvement	–	Bone marrow disorders, skeletal abnormalities, hematological disorders, gastrointestinal involvement, hepatosplenomegaly, and central nervous system involvement

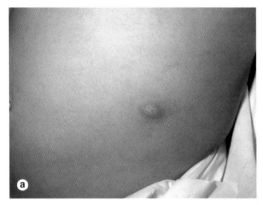

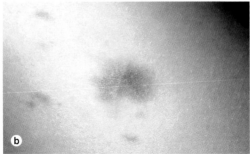

Figure 7-3 a, b Mastocytoma with Darier's sign (courtesy of Nancy Esterly MD collection and Logical Images Inc)

adulthood in 90% of patients. Of these, 15–30% will develop systemic involvement. In adult-onset UP, the lesions usually persist throughout life and may even progressively worsen. A poorer prognosis is associated with extensive cutaneous involvement, bullous lesions, and systemic involvement.

Mastocytoma

Mastocytomas are the second most common form of childhood-onset mastocytosis, accounting for approximately 10–51% of cases

developing in children. They often develop within the first year of life and are rarely found in adults. They typically present as a single or several erythematous and yellow or brown macules, nodules, or plaques, which sometimes have a leathery or peau d'orange texture. Macular lesions may have a bruise-like appearance, which can be mistaken for child abuse. Mastocytomas range in size from 0.5 to 3 cm and most often involve the extremities, but may also occur on the scalp, face, neck, and trunk. Rarely, the lesions occur on the palms and soles. They have also been reported to occur on the vulva and at vaccination sites. Blisters can develop spontaneously in areas that experience pressure, such as beneath edges of clothing, or following stroking of the lesion. The formation of blisters, in conjunction with tenderness, can also occur following abrupt temperature changes. Flushing may also be an associated clinical feature. Darier's sign is also often present in patients with mastocytoma. Mastocytomas are benign and generally involute spontaneously either completely or partially by adolescence, although they have been reported to persist into adulthood. Although uncommon, mastocytomas may be associated with asthma or extracutaneous symptoms, including pruritus, flushing, headaches, and gastrointestinal complaints. The range of these symptoms typically depends on the extent of the mast cell disease and the organs involved.

Diffuse cutaneous mastocytosis

Diffuse cutaneous mastocytosis is rare and becomes apparent either at birth or during early infancy. It typically presents as generalized edema and thickening of the skin, giving the skin a leathery or doughy appearance and with accentuation of the skin folds. The palms and soles may also be involved. Spontaneous widespread blistering often develops and may be the initial presentation of the disease. Blisters may show hemorrhage, erosion, and/or crusting. The sometimes extensive blistering presentation of diffuse cutaneous mastocytosis may be mistaken for staphylococcal scalded-skin syndrome. Varying degrees of erythroderma may also be present, ranging from a red to reddish-yellow appearance. Marked dermographism is often present and Darier's sign is usually prominent and frequently associated with blister formation. Diffuse cutaneous mastocytosis is known to resolve spontaneously during childhood, although dermographism and diffuse hyperpigmentation may persist into adulthood.

Diffuse cutaneous mastocytosis may be associated with more severe systemic complications, including flushing, hypotension, syncope, shock, diarrhea, and gastrointestinal bleeding, as a result of the widespread mast cell infiltration in the skin. Elevated plasma histamine levels are frequently demonstrated in children with diffuse cutaneous mastocytosis and can be useful for identifying those who are at risk for gastrointestinal bleeding. Fatalities have been reported in this type of cutaneous mastocytosis.

Telangiectasia macularis eruptiva perstans

TMEP, also known as telangiectatic mastocytosis, is the rarest form of cutaneous mastocytosis. Although it typically occurs in adults, especially in women, TMEP has recently been reported in children. The clinical features of TMEP somewhat overlap with those of UP. TMEP usually presents as generalized red to brown poorly demarcated macules with visible telangiectasias. The lesions range in size from 2 to 10 mm and are not frequently accompanied by Darier's sign or blisters. Although uncommon, TMEP has been reported to occur in a unilateral distribution. It may also be associated with pruritus, dermographism, flushing, and occasional generalized redness following stressful situations. Very few patients with TMEP have concomitant systemic disease involving the bone marrow, spleen, and gastrointestinal tract.

Systemic involvement

Patients with cutaneous mastocytosis can present with symptoms of systemic involvement, but may not necessarily meet criteria for the diagnosis of systemic mastocytosis. Systemic mastocytosis can be classified as indolent systemic mastocytosis, systemic mastocytosis with associated clonal hematological nonmast cell lineage disease (SM-AHNMD), and aggressive systemic mastocytosis.

Indolent systemic mastocytosis typically presents with UP-like lesions and bone marrow involvement, without hematologic abnormalities or progressive organ destruction. This type of systemic mastocytosis is usually low- to intermediate-grade and is associated with a good prognosis. In SM-AHNMD, myeloid and rarely lymphoid neoplasms can develop. In aggressive systemic mastocytosis, cutaneous lesions are infrequently present. Patients exhibit progressive organ dysfunction, usually possess hematologic abnormalities, and have a poor prognosis.

Cutaneous mastocytosis can be associated with systemic involvement, including bone marrow disorders, skeletal abnormalities, hematological disorders, gastrointestinal involvement, hepatosplenomegaly, and central nervous system involvement. Recurrent syncope and anaphylaxis have also been reported. In children with cutaneous mastocytosis, systemic involvement is rare, is typically benign, and usually resolves spontaneously. Systemic involvement in adults with cutaneous mastocytosis, however, usually follows a chronic and progressive course associated with increased morbidity and mortality. In addition, there is a well-established association between UP and systemic involvement, with approximately 56–100% of patients with systemic mastocytosis exhibiting UP lesions. Furthermore, adults with a high density of cutaneous lesions and longer durations of UP are more likely to have severe bone marrow abnormalities, lymphadenopathy, hepatomegaly, and splenomegaly, as well as experience constitutional symptoms such as fatigue and musculoskeletal pain.

The bone marrow of patients with cutaneous mastocytosis often shows increased mast cell infiltrates, even in the absence of any systemic symptoms. In a series of 13 adult patients with cutaneous mastocytosis (most of whom were diagnosed with UP) with no symptoms of systemic involvement, an increased number of mast cells in the bone marrow was detected in all but one patient. This finding was consistent, although at a higher incidence, with previous studies reporting bone marrow involvement in approximately 46–60% of adult patients with cutaneous mastocytosis. Children with cutaneous mastocytosis have lower incidences of bone marrow involvement, and there is little evidence that results of bone marrow biopsy alter management in the absence of signs or symptoms. The bone marrow of affected patients often shows nodular, granuloma-like, or diffuse mast cell accumulation. In addition, increases in bone marrow angiogenesis and vascular endothelial growth factor expression have been found in patients with systemic mastocytosis. The accumulation of mast cells within the bone marrow can occasionally lead to complications, including bone pain, osteoporosis, early skeletal decalcification, spontaneous fractures, and hematological disorders that may be premalignant or malignant in nature. Osteoporosis is thought to be caused by mast cell mediators, particularly histamine, that increase bone turnover. Hematological abnormalities, due to extensive fibrosis within the bone marrow, include anemia, thrombocytopenia, leukocytosis, leukopenia, and eosinophilia. Children rarely exhibit lymphoproliferative or myeloproliferative disorders associated with systemic mastocytosis.

Gastrointestinal involvement occurs in 16–80% of adults and up to 40% of children with mastocytosis. Symptoms include nausea, vomiting, abdominal pain, diarrhea, malabsorption, peptic ulcers, and gastrointestinal bleeding. Children with mastocytosis rarely develop peptic ulcer disease or gastrointestinal bleeding. These gastrointestinal symptoms are due to the release of mast cell mediators in patients with mastocytosis. In addition, hepatomegaly is observed in 12–84% of adults and splenomegaly is observed in 11–86% of adults with cutaneous mastocytosis. In contrast, only approximately 17% of affected children have hepatomegaly and 7% have splenomegaly.

Diagnosis

Key Points

- Histopathological sections show mast cell infiltrates, which are better visualized with Wright–Giemsa, toluidine blue, chloroacetate esterase, and aminocaproate esterase; immunohistochemical stains include tryptase and CD117 (c-kit)
- Serum total tryptase levels is an important marker for systemic mastocytosis
- A complete blood cell count with differential and peripheral smear should be performed to rule out associated hematological disorders
- Urinary N-methylhistamine > 300 µmol/mol creatinine should be an indicator for obtaining a bone marrow biopsy in patients with mastocytosis suspected of having bone marrow involvement
- Hepatomegaly and splenomegaly should be sought during the physical examination and liver transaminases should be checked in adults and symptomatic children

The differential diagnosis for UP includes urticaria. For mastocytoma, the differential includes juvenile xanthogranuloma, Spitz nevus, pseudolymphomas, and arthropod bites. The differential diagnoses for diffuse cutaneous mastocytosis include urticaria, histiocytosis X, nonhistiocytosis X of childhood, secondary syphilis, generalized eruptive histiocytoma, and papular sarcoidosis. When bullae are present in diffuse cutaneous mastocytosis, the differential also includes herpes simplex, bullous impetigo, bullous pemphigoid, bullous linear immunoglobulin A disease, dermatitis herpetiformis, staphylococcal scalded-skin syndrome, and toxic epidermal necrolysis.

Although cutaneous mastocytosis may be diagnosed on clinical presentation, skin biopsy will aid in the definitive diagnosis. Histopathological findings include a mast cell infiltrate that is better visualized with basic cytochemical stains, including Wright–Giemsa, toluidine blue, chloroacetate esterase, and aminocaproate esterase. The Wright–Giemsa stain helps to identify the basophilic granules of mast cells and accompanying eosinophilic reactions, whereas the toluidine blue stain confirms the metachromatic granules of mast cells. Chloroacetate esterase is abundant in mast cells; thus, this stain helps to identify mast cells. However, this enzyme is also present in neutrophilic myelocytes. Staining for aminocaproate esterase is more specific for mast cells, but requires special tissue preparations. Immunohistochemical stains, including tryptase and CD117 (c-kit), further aid in identifying mast cells on paraffin sections. The immunohistochemical stain for tryptase is a sensitive and specific marker for mast cells in paraffin sections. It has also been found to be of greater diagnostic value in diagnosing aggressive systemic mastocytosis than the conventional Wright–Giemsa and chloroacetate esterase stains in systemically affected tissue. The CD117 stain has been useful in diagnosing mastocytosis, since mutations in the proto-oncogene c-kit are believed to be involved in the pathogenesis of mast cell disorders. However, it may be more useful in detecting patients with systemic mastocytosis, in which CD117 positivity has been demonstrated in both normal and abnormal mast cells of bone marrow biopsy sections.

The distribution of the mast cell infiltrate on histological sections partially correlates with the clinical appearance of cutaneous mastocytosis. In UP, a perivascular and interstitial infiltrate of mast cells is often seen, particularly involving the papillary and middle dermis. In patients with lesions that are more nodular or confluent, as in some cases of UP and in mastocytoma, the mast cell infiltrate may appear nodular or involve the entire dermis and occasionally the subcutis. In addition, mastocytomas have shown tumor-like aggregations of mast cells throughout the dermis. In patients with diffuse cutaneous mastocytosis and in some with UP, a diffuse or sheet-like pattern of mast cell infiltrate within the papillary and upper reticular dermis may be found. Histopathological findings of patients with TMEP show a perivascular pattern of mast cells accompanied by vascular dilatation, though the increase in mast cell number may be subtle. Although an increased number of mast cells is usually found in only lesional skin, patients with UP have been reported to demonstrate increased mast cell numbers in nonlesional skin biopsies as well. Eosinophils are found in lesions that have degranulated in response to trauma. Sometimes, more than one biopsy may be needed to confirm the diagnosis. Furthermore, in some cases of TMEP, the number of mast cells may fall within the normal range and relative increases in mast cells may be best appreciated when compared to nonlesional skin. The presence of large hyperchromatic spindled mast cells is typical for TMEP.

The diagnosis of cutaneous mastocytosis relies mainly on clinical findings and histopathological evidence of increased numbers of mast cells. However, a diagnostic workup should also be performed if systemic involvement may be suspected (Figure 7-4). Serum total tryptase levels are important markers for systemic mastocytosis and reflect the total burden of mast cells in the body. Normal patients have total tryptase levels of approximately 5 ng/mL, whereas patients with systemic mastocytosis typically have total tryptase levels exceeding 20 ng/mL. Patients with cutaneous mastocytosis or limited systemic mastocytosis usually have total tryptase levels < 20 ng/mL. Although serum total tryptase levels are usually normal or only slightly elevated in patients with cutaneous mastocytosis, they have been shown to correlate with the number of mast cells in the skin, as well as with the severity of cutaneous disease. In adults with cutaneous mastocytosis, the density of cutaneous lesions, rather than the extent of skin lesions appears to be a better reflection of serum total tryptase levels. Adult patients with skin involvement of greater than 50% body surface area and a maximum density of skin lesions exceeding 10% may require a more thorough evaluation, including screening for organomegaly and a bone marrow biopsy. In addition, increased levels of serum interleukin-6 have been demonstrated in patients with systemic mastocytosis and are associated with more severe mastocytosis with organomegaly and osteoporosis. Interleukin-6 is a multifunctional cytokine that is involved in the regulation of hematopoiesis, immune response, and inflammation. It has been found to correlate with serum total tryptase levels and, therefore, may serve as an additional surrogate marker of systemic mastocytosis.

In addition to serum total tryptase levels, a complete blood cell count with differential and peripheral smear should be performed to rule out possible associated hematological disorders, including anemia, eosinophilia, leukopenia, leukocytosis, or thrombocytopenia. Urinary N-methylhistamine, particularly levels > 300 μmol/mol creatinine, have been demonstrated to be an indicator of bone marrow involvement in adult mastocytosis. Abnormal findings in either the complete blood cell count or urinary N-methyl-

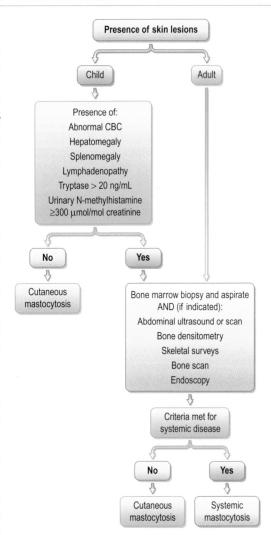

Figure 7-4 Diagnostic algorithm for cutaneous versus systemic mastocytosis. CBC, complete blood count (modified from Akin C, Metcalfe DD. Systemic mastocytosis. Annu Rev Med 2004;55:419–432; and Hartmann K, Henz BM. Mastocytosis: recent advances in defining the disease. Br J Dermatol 2001;144:682–695).

histamine levels should be followed with a bone marrow biopsy. Patients with abnormal bone marrow findings and with progressive disease should be followed regularly. It is important to note that bone abnormalities found in children with cutaneous mastocytosis are usually transient and asymptomatic.

Patients should be examined for hepatomegaly and splenomegaly during the physical examination and liver transaminases should be checked. Most authors recommend that invasive diagnostic procedures should only be performed in patients with hematologic abnormalities, persistent and localized bone pain, persistent severe gastrointestinal symptoms, or biochemical evidence of hepatic insufficiency.

Criteria to diagnose systemic mastocytosis

Diagnosis of systemic mastocytosis requires major criteria + one minor criteria *or* three minor criteria

Major criteria

Multifocal dense infiltrates of mast cells, with the mast cell number exceeding 15 in each infiltrate, in sections of bone marrow or other extracutaneous organs

Minor criteria

1. Presence of >25% abnormal spindle-shaped mast cells in sections of the bone marrow or other extracutaneous organs or >25% atypical mast cells in bone marrow smears
2. Presence of a *c-kit* point mutation at codon 816 in the bone marrow, blood, or other extracutaneous organs
3. Presence of Kit+ mast cells coexpressing CD2 and/or CD25 in the bone marrow, blood, or other extracutaneous organs
4. Persistently elevated serum total tryptase concentration >20 ng/mL

Modified from Valent P, Horny HP, Escribano L, et al. Diagnostic criteria and classification of mastocytosis: a consensus proposal. Leuk Res 2001;25:603–625.

The diagnosis of systemic mastocytosis is based on the fulfillment of one major and minor criteria or three minor criteria from the recent consensus proposal of Valent et al. (Box 7-2). The major criterion for systemic mastocytosis is the finding of multifocal dense infiltrates of mast cells, with the mast cell number exceeding 15 in each infiltrate, in sections of bone marrow or other extracutaneous organs. The minor criteria include the following: (1) presence of >25% abnormal spindle-shaped mast cells in sections of the bone marrow or other extracutaneous organs or >25% atypical mast cells in bone marrow smears; (2) presence of a c-kit point mutation at codon 816 in the bone marrow, blood, or other extracutaneous organs; (3) presence of Kit+ mast cells coexpressing CD2 and/or CD25 in the bone marrow, blood, or other extracutaneous organs; and (4) a persistently elevated serum total tryptase concentration >20 ng/mL.

Pathogenesis

Key Points

- Activating c-kit mutations have been found to be associated with mastocytosis, including the more recognized Asp816Val mutation (in codon 816) detected in the majority of adult-onset mastocytosis
- The antiapoptotic bcl-2 and bcl-xL proteins have been implicated in dysregulating apoptosis in mast cells

Table 7-2 Pathogenesis of mastocytosis

	Type of mastocytosis
***c-kit* mutations**	
Asp816Val	Majority of adult-onset systemic mastocytosis (regardless of type or prognosis)
	Childhood-onset cutaneous mastocytosis
Asp816Phe	Childhood-onset cutaneous mastocytosis
Val560Gly	Adult-onset mastocytosis
	Aggressive mastocytosis
Asp820Gly	Aggressive mastocytosis
Gly839Lys	Childhood-onset mastocytosis
Ala533Asp	Familial diffuse cutaneous mastocytosis
Overexpression of antiapoptotic proteins	
Bcl-2	Cutaneous mastocytosis (found in mast cells of cutaneous lesions)
	Mast cell leukemia (found in mast cells of bone marrow)
Bcl-xL	Systemic mastocytosis (found in mast cells of bone marrow)

Although the cause of increased mast cell numbers in mastocytosis is still unknown, recent findings have offered several hypotheses regarding the pathogenesis of mastocytosis. These hypotheses include activating c-kit mutations and dysregulation in mast cell apoptosis (Table 7-2).

C-KIT mutations

Mutations in the proto-oncogene c-kit have been detected in adult-onset and rarely in childhood-onset cutaneous mastocytosis. The c-kit proto-oncogene codes for KIT, which is a transmembrane tyrosine kinase expressed by several cell types, including mast cells and melanocytes. KIT is activated by binding of the mast cell growth factor known as stem cell factor. This ligand-binding leads to a sequence of events that may affect cell proliferation and differentiation. The activation of KIT has been shown to stimulate proliferation and inhibit apoptosis of mast cells in vitro and in vivo. Although most known c-kit mutations cause loss of KIT function, such as in piebaldism, the c-kit mutations found associated with mastocytosis result in ligand-independent constitutive phosphorylation and subsequent activation of the KIT receptor.

Thus far, several activating c-kit mutations have been identified in patients with mastocytosis, including the more recognized mutation in codon 816. The Asp816Val mutation, which substitutes aspartate for valine in codon 816, has been detected in the majority of adult-onset systemic mastocytosis, regardless of the classification or prognosis of their disease. It has also been shown to cause disease similar to mastocytosis in vivo, providing a causal link between the Asp816Val mutation and mast cell neoplasia. This mutation, however, has not been found in familial mastocytosis and has only rarely been detected in children with extensive or progressive disease. However, a recent report by Zhao et al. (2007) demonstrated codon 816 mutations, either Asp816Val or Asp816Phe, in 83% of a series of 12 children with cutaneous mastocytosis (9 with UP, 2 with solitary mastocytoma, and 1 with diffuse cutaneous mastocytosis). In addition, the Asp816Val mutation, as opposed to the Asp816Phe mutation, was detected in 70% of children with codon 816 mutations. Furthermore, children with Asp816Phe mutation developed cutaneous mastocytosis at an earlier age compared to children with the Asp816Val mutation. Although previous findings regarding the Asp816Val mutation suggest that childhood-onset mastocytosis is a different disease entity from persisting and adult-onset mastocytosis, the more recent findings of the codon 816 mutations in childhood-onset mastocytosis may suggest that the codon 816 mutation may be responsible for earlier-onset mastocytosis and an indication of an indolent and transient clinical course.

Other c-kit mutations detected in patients with mastocytosis include Val560Gly, which has been found in several adult patients and in a patient with aggressive mastocytosis and Asp820Gly, also found in aggressive mastocytosis. In addition to the c-kit mutation in codon 816, a Gly839Lys mutation was detected in a pediatric patient, though the incidence of this mutation is unknown. Furthermore, although a codon 816 c-kit mutation has not been identified in patients with familial mastocytosis, the germline mutation Ala533Asp has been detected in all affected members of three generations with familial diffuse cutaneous mastocytosis.

Dysregulation of mast cell apoptosis

The increased number of mast cells in mastocytosis may also be due to inhibition apoptosis. Mast cells in cutaneous mastocytosis lesions have been shown to exhibit decreased apoptosis compared to healthy skin. In addition, bcl-2 and bcl-xL are proteins that inhibit apoptosis by blocking cytochrome C. A recent study by Hartmann et al. (2003) found that bcl-2 is overexpressed in mast cells of cutaneous mastocytosis lesions, although the related bcl-xL protein was comparable to healthy controls. However, in the same patients with cutaneous lesions who had systemic mastocytosis, the mast cells of bone marrow lesions showed overexpression of bcl-xL but not bcl-2. A previous study also showed similar results with regard to normal expression of bcl-2 in the bone marrow of systemic mastocytosis, but demonstrated an overexpression of bcl-2 in bone marrow mast cells of a patient with mast cell leukemia. Moreover, activation of c-kit led to an upregulation of bcl-2, but not bcl-xL, in human mast cell cultures.

These findings suggest that the dysregulation of apoptosis in mast cells contributes to the development of mastocytosis, in both cutaneous and bone marrow lesions, although through different antiapoptotic proteins. Also, these results may help explain the pathogenesis of mastocytosis in patients with and without c-kit mutations.

Treatment

Key Points

- Patients should be counseled on avoiding mast cell mediator-releasing triggers
- General symptomatic treatment in patients with cutaneous mastocytosis includes antihistamines for pruritus, flushing, wheal formation, and gastrointestinal symptoms as well as disodium cromoglicate for diarrhea and abdominal cramping
- Treatments for UP include diluted topical corticosteroids under wet wraps, oral psoralen plus ultraviolet A (PUVA) therapy, and UVA1 therapy
- Treatments for mastocytoma include potent topical corticosteroids either with or without occlusive dressings, intralesional corticosteroids, and surgical excision as a last resort
- Treatments for diffuse cutaneous mastocytosis include bath and oral PUVA, topical corticosteroids, and oral corticosteroids
- Treatments for TMEP include oral PUVA therapy and the 585-nm flashlamp-pumped dye laser

Treatment for patients with cutaneous mastocytosis consists mainly of avoidance of mediator-releasing triggers and symptomatic treatment (Table 7-3).

Avoidance of mediator-releasing triggers

Patients should be counseled on avoiding triggers known to cause release of mast cell mediators, including friction, physical exertion, sudden cold temperature, heat, emotional stress, alcohol, mechanical irritation (such as vigorous toweling),

Table 7-3 Treatment of cutaneous mastocytosis

	Recommendation/treatment
Mediator-releasing triggers	Avoid friction, physical exertion, sudden cold temperature, heat, emotional stress, alcohol, mechanical irritation, particular drugs (nonsteroidal anti-inflammatory medications, codeine, narcotic analgesics, morphine, dextran, sympathomimetics, muscle relaxants, polymyxin B, radiological contrast media), and animal venoms
	Anaphylaxis may occur with bacterial toxins, infections, and certain foods such as fish, lobster, and crabs
General symptoms	
Pruritus, flushing, wheal formation	H_1-antihistamines:
	Cetirizine 5–10 mg PO qd
	Loratadine 10 mg PO qd
	Hydroxyzine 25 mg PO q6–24 hours prn
	Add H_2-antihistamines as needed:
	Cimetidine 400 mg PO qhs
	Ranitidine 150 mg PO bid
Abdominal pain, gastrointestinal symptoms	H_2-antihistamines:
	Cimetidine 400 mg PO qhs
	Ranitidine 150 mg PO bid
Diarrhea, abdominal cramps	Cromolyn sodium 200 mg PO qid
Headache, musculoskeletal pain, central nervous system complaints	Cromolyn sodium 200 mg PO qid
Urticaria pigmentosa	Diluted topical corticosteroids under wet wraps (not recommended for children in puberty)
	Oral psoralen plus ultraviolet A (PUVA) therapy
	Medium-dose or high-dose ultraviolet A1 (UVA1) therapy
Mastocytoma	Potent topical corticosteroids, with or without occlusive dressings
	Intralesional corticosteroid
	Surgical excision (last resort)
Diffuse cutaneous mastocytosis	Oral PUVA
	Bath PUVA (for infants)
	Topical corticosteroids (for bullae)
	Oral corticosteroids (for more severe bullae)
Telangiectasia macularis eruptiva perstans	Oral PUVA
	585-nm flashlamp pumped dye laser

particular drugs (nonsteroidal anti-inflammatory medications, codeine, narcotic analgesics, morphine, dextran, sympathomimetics, muscle relaxants, polymyxin B, radiological contrast media), and animal venoms. Anaphylaxis may occur with bacterial toxins, infections, and certain foods such as fish, lobster, and crabs. Severe anaphylactic reactions, including near-fatal reactions, have also been reported in patients with cutaneous mastocytosis and indolent systemic mastocytosis following insect stings, particularly *Hymenoptera* stings. Therefore, patients with mastocytosis should also be counseled on the signs and symptoms of anaphylaxis. Furthermore, patients with mastocytosis and a known history of anaphylaxis may benefit from carrying antihistamines, corticosteroids, and injectable epinephrine with them regularly. Of note, elevated serum baseline levels of mast cell tryptase (> 13.5 μg/L) and mastocytosis appear to increase a patient's risk for severe allergic reactions to stings.

General symptomatic treatment

Antihistamines are useful for the symptomatic treatment of mastocytosis. H_1-antihistamines (such as hydroxyzine or the less sedating cetirizine and loratadine) help relieve pruritus, flushing, and wheal formation. In general, the nonsedating antihistamines may be tried first. H_2-antihistamines, including cimetidine and ranitidine, may be added if H_1-antihistamines are insufficient or if there is concomitant abdominal pain or gastrointestinal symptoms, particularly those of gastritis and peptic ulcer disease. Disodium cromoglicate has also been shown to help alleviate diarrhea and abdominal cramping as well as headache, musculoskeletal pain, and central nervous system complaints.

Urticaria pigmentosa

Diluted topical corticosteroids under wet wraps have been shown to be helpful in children with UP, although strict checks of weight, growth, and cortisol levels are indicated. This treatment should not be used in children undergoing puberty, since there is an increased risk of developing striae. Undiluted topical corticosteroids, whether or not used under occlusion, are also not recommended due to the resultant local atrophy, potential systemic effects, and frequent increase in mast cell numbers following steroid treatment.

Oral PUVA therapy has been shown to be effective in controlling pruritus and cutaneous wheals, although it should be used with caution in children. It is also effective in reducing numbers of mast cells and histamine and leukotriene levels in the skin. However, UP symptoms and lesions frequently recur within several weeks or months of cessation of therapy. Bath PUVA appears to be ineffective. Also, both medium-dose and high-dose ultraviolet A1 (UVA1) therapy appear to be equally helpful in alleviating pruritus, as well as reducing the number of mast cells in adult patients with UP. Although UVA1 therapy does not reduce the number of cutaneous lesions, patients receiving UVA1 therapy may show continued improvement for at least 6 months following cessation of the treatment. While some authors found oral PUVA to be superior to UVA1 therapy, others have found the two treatments to be similarly effective.

Mastocytoma

Potent topical corticosteroids, either with or without occlusive dressings, can be effective in treating solitary mastocytomas, particularly if the lesion is persistent or causes severe symptoms. Prolonged application of the topical corticosteroids may cause atrophy and possibly adrenal suppression. In addition, intralesional corticosteroid has been shown to be helpful in reducing the lesion and associated symptoms. Surgical excision should be reserved as a last resort, since most mastocytomas involute spontaneously.

Diffuse cutaneous mastocytosis

Both bath and oral PUVA have been shown to be helpful in the treatment of cutaneous lesions and associated pruritus and flushing in patients with diffuse cutaneous mastocytosis. However, it appears that oral PUVA may be more effective. Bath PUVA may be more practical in infants who are too young to be able to take the necessary protective measures before and after UVA exposure. Patients presenting with bullae may benefit from topical corticosteroids. In more severe bullous disease, oral corticosteroids can be used until most lesions subside, at which time topical corticosteroids can be used to control occasional new lesions.

Telangiectasia macularis eruptive perstans

The management of patients with TMEP consists mainly of symptomatic treatment. Oral PUVA therapy has been shown to be beneficial with respect to the reducing cutaneous lesions and pruritus. Temporary treatment has also been reported with the 585-nm flashlamp-pumped dye laser.

Further reading

Akin C, Metcalfe DD. Systemic mastocytosis. Annu Rev Med 2004;55:419–432.

Almahroos M, Kurban AK. Management of mastocytosis. Clin Dermatol 2003;21:274–277.

Azana JM, Torrelo A, Mediero IG, et al. Urticaria pigmentosa: a review of 67 pediatric cases. Pediatr Dermatol 1994;11:102–106.

Brockow K, Metcalfe DD. Mastocytosis. Curr Opin Allergy Clin Immunol 2001;1:449–454.

Brockow K, Akin C, Huber M, et al. Assessment of the extent of cutaneous involvement in children and adults with mastocytosis: relationship to symptomatology, tryptase levels, and bone marrow pathology. J Am Acad Dermatol 2003;48:508–516.

Brockow K, Akin C, Huber M, et al. IL-6 levels predict disease variant and extent of organ involvement in patients with mastocytosis. Clin Immunol 2005;115:216–223.

Fearfield LA, Francis N, Henry K, et al. Bone marrow involvement in cutaneous mastocytosis. Br J Dermatol 2001;144:561–566.

Hannaford R, Rogers M. Presentation of cutaneous mastocytosis in 173 children. Australas J Dermatol 2001;42:15–21.

Hartmann K, Henz BM. Mastocytosis: recent advances in defining the disease. Br J Dermatol 2001;144:682–695.

Hartmann K, Artuc M, Baldus SE, et al. Expression of Bcl-2 and Bcl-xL in cutaneous and bone marrow lesions of mastocytosis. Am J Pathol 2003;163:819–826.

Horny HP, Sillaber C, Menke D, et al. Diagnostic value of immunostaining for tryptase in patients with mastocytosis. Am J Surg Pathol 1998;22:1132–1140.

Li CY. Diagnosis of mastocytosis: value of cytochemistry and immunohistochemistry. Leuk Res 2001;25:537–541.

Longley BJ Jr, Metcalfe DD, Tharp M, et al. Activating and dominant inactivating c-KIT catalytic domain mutations in distinct clinical forms of human mastocytosis. Proc Natl Acad Sci USA 1999;96:1609–1614.

Marone G, Spadaro G, Granata F, et al. Treatment of mastocytosis: pharmacologic basis and current concepts. Leuk Res 2001;25:583–594.

Schwartz LB. Clinical utility of tryptase levels in systemic mastocytosis and associated hematologic disorders. Leuk Res 2001;25:553–562.

Topar G, Staudacher C, Geisen F, et al. Urticaria pigmentosa: a clinical, hematopathologic, and serologic study of 30 adults. Am J Clin Pathol 1998;109:279–285.

Valent P, Horny HP, Escribano L, et al. Diagnostic criteria and classification of mastocytosis: a consensus proposal. Leuk Res 2001;25:603–625.

Viscasillas XB, Puigdemont GS, Salvador CA. A slowly enlarging, unilateral, erythematous macular lesion. Arch Dermatol 2006;142:641–646.

Wolff K, Komar M, Petzelbauer P. Clinical and histopathological aspects of cutaneous mastocytosis. Leuk Res 2001;25:519–528.

Yanagihori H, Oyama N, Nakamura K, et al. *c-kit* Mutations in patients with childhood-onset mastocytosis and genotype–phenotype correlation. J Mol Diagn 2005;7:252–257.

Zhao W, Bueso-Ramos CE, Verstovsek S, et al. Quantitative profiling of codon 816 KIT mutations can aid in the classification of systemic mast cell disease. Leukemia 2007;21:1574–1576.

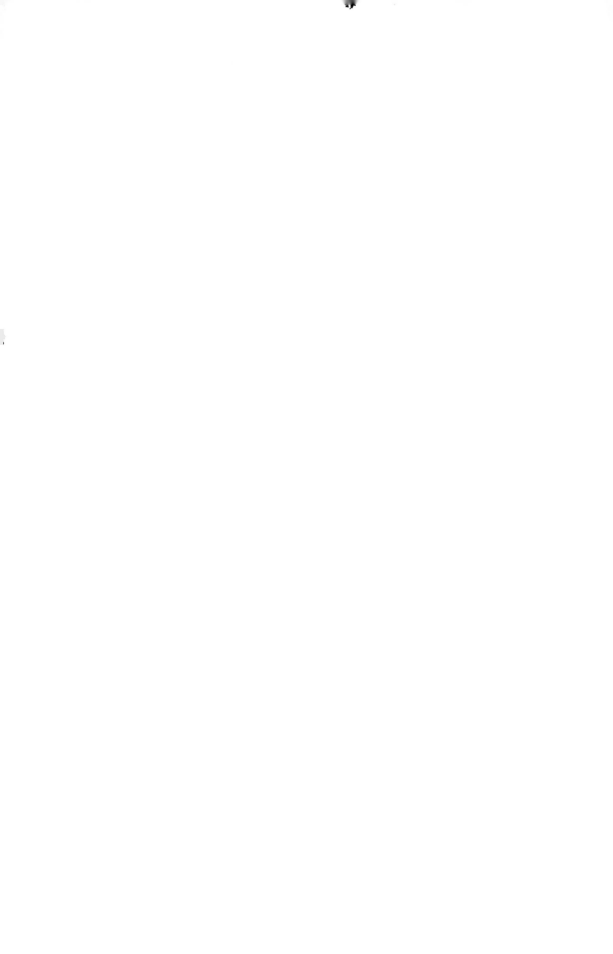

Cutaneous infections

8

Whitney A. High

VIRAL INFECTIONS

Molluscum contagiosum

Clinical presentation

Key Points

- Molluscum contagiosum is caused by a DNA poxvirus of the *Molluscipox* genus
- In healthy patients, molluscum is mainly a disease of children
- Molluscum infection produces smooth, dome-shaped, umbilicated papules
- Papules may grow in a linear configuration following autoinoculation
- The host immune response may cause surrounding eczematous dermatitis
- Immunocompromised patients may have larger lesions or a recalcitrant course

Four viral subtypes of molluscum virus are recognized: MCV1, MCV2, MCV3, and MCV4. MCV1 causes 75–90% of lesions in healthy persons. Children are affected more frequently than adults. When molluscum does infect adults, it may be a sexually transmitted disease or it may occur in association with human immunodeficiency virus (HIV)/acquired immunodeficiency syndrome (AIDS). The prevalence of molluscum contagiosum in HIV patients may be as high as 5–18%, and it is associated with declining CD4 counts. Molluscum is more prevalent in communities with overcrowding, poor hygiene, and poverty, but any child may be infected. Direct contact or shared fomites often spread the disease among siblings or within social groups.

Molluscum has an incubation period of 2–7 weeks. Typical lesions appear as small, dome-shaped, umbilicated papules (Figure 8-1). Favored sites include the axillae, antecubital and popliteal fossae; or in the case of sexual transmission, the genitals.

Up to 10% of patients develop a surrounding dermatitis ("molluscum eczema"). Immunocompromised patients, particularly those with HIV and diminished CD4 counts, may manifest larger lesions ("giant molluscum"), often on the face.

Diagnosis/differential diagnosis

Key Points

- The diagnosis of molluscum is usually based on the clinical appearance and historical information
- Histologic examination reveals intracytoplasmic inclusions within keratinocytes (Henderson–Paterson bodies; Figure 8-2)

In children, molluscum may be confused with verruca, benign nevi, Spitz nevi, or even juvenile xanthogranuloma. Molluscum on the genitals may be misdiagnosed as condyloma. In immunocompromised patients (HIV/AIDS), molluscum may be confused with cryptococcosis, histoplasmosis, and penicilliosis; in this situation, a biopsy may be indicated. Histologic examination of molluscum reveals characteristic intracytoplamic inclusions within keratinocytes that are eosinophilic in the lower layers of the epidermis, but become basophilic as they migrate upward.

Treatment

Key Points

- Molluscum contagiosum is a self-limited disease in healthy patients
- Destructive or medical therapies may hasten resolution (Table 8-1).

Molluscum may be protracted in those with atopic dermatitis or in immunocompromised individuals. Picking and scratching should be discouraged, as this may lead to autoinoculation and scarring. The decision to treat depends upon the patient's needs, the extent of disease, and the likelihood of sequelae, such as scarring or dyspigmentation.

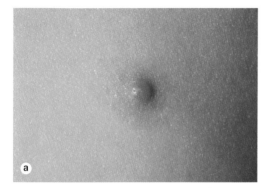

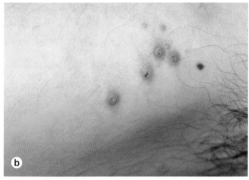

Figure 8-1 a, b Molluscum contagiosum

Table 8-1 Methods of treatment for molluscum contagiosum

Destructive modalities	Medical modalities
Liquid nitrogen/cryosurgery	Topical imiquimod (often requires occlusion on thick skin)
Sharp curettage	
Tricarboxylic acid	Topical tretinoin
Cantharidin	Oral cimetidine (limited evidence of antiviral properties)
Podophyllin	
	Topical or intralesional cidofovir (high cost limits use)

Table 8-2 Human papillomavirus (HPV) subtypes and associated clinical lesions

HPV subtype	Associated clinical lesion
1	Plantar warts (verruca plantaris, verruca palmaris)
2, 4	Common warts (verruca vulgaris)
3, 10	Flat warts (verruca planae)
5, 8, 20	Epidermodysplasia verruciformis
6, 11	Low-risk genital warts (condyloma)
7	Butcher's warts
16, 18, 31, 33, 51	High-risk genital warts (including cervical neoplasia)
16	Digital squamous cell carcinoma
13,32	Heck's disease

* Over 100 HPV subtypes have been characterized
* Different viral subtypes tend to produce different clinical lesions (Table 8-2).
* Immunocompromised patients may have larger or more recalcitrant warts
* Up to 80% of women are infected with sexually transmitted strains of HPV, although most cases are subclinical and are never detected

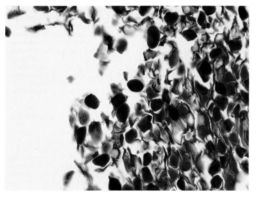

Figure 8-2 Molluscum bodies

Destructive modalities are performed in the office and may be repeated until a satisfactory response is achieved. Medical options include topical medications, oral medications, and intralesional cidofovir. The high cost of cidofovir limits use of this modality to only the most recalcitrant cases.

Verruca and condyloma (Warts)

Clinical presentation

Key Points

* Warts are caused by human papillomavirus (HPV), a ubiquitous DNA virus

Warts affect 7–12% of the population, but among school-aged children, the prevalence may exceed 10–20%. A common wart (verruca vulgaris) presents as a scaling, often filiform or digitate papule. Flat warts (verruca plana) are flat-topped, flesh-colored papules that often grow in linear configurations following autoinoculation. Occasionally, women who shave their legs with a contaminated razor may develop hundreds of lesions. Plantar or palmar warts (verruca plantaris/palmaris) are end-ophytic and may be distinguished from clavi by their interruption of skin lines and thrombosed capillaries in the center of warts (Figure 8-3).

Genital warts (condylomata acuminata) are the most common venereal disease. They have a

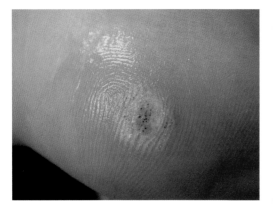

Figure 8-3 Punctate clotted vessels in plantar wart

variable appearance, ranging from scaly and papular to smooth and flesh-colored. Perhaps it is the location on the penis, vulva, or perianal area that is most distinguishing (Figure 8-4). HPV-6 and 11 cause 90% of genital warts, whereas uncommon variants like HPV-16, 18, 31, and 33 are associated with an increased risk of cervical cancer. Condylomata may grow rapidly during pregnancy. Genital warts in neonates and infants can be acquired from the mother, therefore, child abuse should not necessarily be immediately suspected in children under the age of 2 who have perianal warts.

Diagnosis/differential diagnosis

Key Points

* Warts are usually diagnosed by their clinical appearance and history
* Histologic examination of warts may reveal koilocytes within the epidermis
* The differential diagnosis for extremely large warts includes verrucous carcinoma, an unusual form of squamous cell carcinoma

Most warts are easily diagnosed by their clinical appearance and historical information. Larger lesions may be concerning for a malignant process and, in this situation, a biopsy is indicated. Condyloma may be confused with molluscum, although umbilication and surrounding dermatitis distinguishes the latter. Histologic examination of warts reveals characteristic features, including acanthosis, hypergranulosis, or koilocyte formation, the latter being indicative of HPV-infected keratinocytes.

Treatment

Key Points

* Most warts are self-limited in healthy patients
* Destructive or medical modalities may hasten resolution

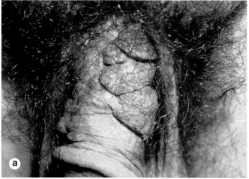

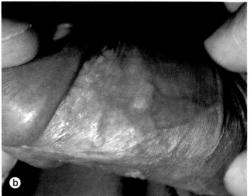

Figure 8-4 a, b Condylomata acuminata

* Treatment must always be tailored to the site involved
* *Some* condylomata are associated with an increased risk of cervical cancer

Most verrucas in healthy persons resolve spontaneously, but treatment may hasten the process (Table 8-3). Destructive modalities for common warts include cryosurgery, focal tricarboxylic acid, cantharidin, laser destruction, or surgical removal. Medical treatment options include topical salicylic acid, oral cimetidine, imiquimod, or intralesional *Candida* antigen. Injection of intralesional *Candida* antigen stimulates a local, delayed-type immune response, which is thought to trigger serendipitously an immune response to the nearby wart. Even simple duct tape occlusion has been reported to be effective, probably due to skin maceration that leads to clearance of virally infected keratinocytes.

The location of the wart should be considered when choosing the best therapeutic approach. For example, periungual verruca overlying the nail matrix should not be treated aggressively with liquid nitrogen, as damage to the matrix may cause permanent nail dystrophy. Intralesional *Candida* in digits should also be avoided, as edema from a particularly aggressive immune

Table 8-3 Methods of treatment for verruca and condyloma

Destructive modalities	Medical modalities
Duct tape occlusion	Topical imiquimod (often requires occlusion on thick skin)
Salicylic acid plaster/liquid	
Liquid nitrogen/cryosurgery	Oral cimetidine (limited evidence of antiviral properties)
Tricarboxylic acid	
Cantharidin	
Podophyllin	Intralesional *Candida* antigen (limited evidence of efficacy)
	Intralesional bleomycin or 5-fluorouracil (rarely used)

Table 8-4 Information on Gardasil

Indication	Prevention or infection with human papillomavirus (HPV) 6, 11, 16, 18
	(HPV 16 and 18 are implicated in 70% of cervical cancer)
Patient population	Girls and women 9–26 years old*
Administration	Intramuscular injection to upper arm or upper thigh (3 doses)
Dosing schedule	Dose 1 – elected date
	Dose 2 – 2 months after initial dose
	Dose 3 – 6 months after initial dose
Adverse reactions (decreasing frequency)	Pain
	Swelling
	Erythema
	Fever
	Pruritus
Contraindications	Hypersensitivity to any of the ingredients
	Aluminum is the added adjuvant
	Patients with hypersensitivity should not receive further doses

*Approved for ages 11–26 years old, but may be administered to 9–10-year-olds at discretion of physician.

response can cause compartment syndrome. The endophytic nature of plantar warts makes them very recalcitrant to treatment. As a general rule, plantar warts are not surgically removed because of a high risk of recurrence along the incision. Plantar warts are often treated with repeated and prolonged application of salicylic acid followed by manual paring. Cryotherapy may also be used.

Condylomata may respond to destruction with liquid nitrogen or podophyllin. Topical application of imiquimod may also be effective. Imiquimod increases local production of interferon, a natural inhibitor of viral growth and replication. It is effectively absorbed on the thin skin of the genitalia, but may be less well absorbed on thicker skin, limiting the effectiveness of its use for other types of warts. Patients with condylomata should be counseled regarding other sexually transmitted diseases.

In June 2006, the Food and Drug Administration (FDA) approved a quadrivalent vaccine (Gardasil) for the prevention of infection with HPV-6, 11, 16, and 18 (Table 8-4). In trials, this vaccine, comprising a capsid protein and adjuvant, decreased the incidence of infection with these types of HPV by 90% over a 3-year span. While the administration of the vaccine does not require prior HPV testing or a Papanicolaou (Pap) smear, the vaccine has been approved for prevention only and the effect of the vaccine on women with concurrent HPV infection is unclear. A history of an abnormal Pap smear is not a contraindication.

Herpesvirus infections

Clinical presentation

Key Points

- Cutaneous herpes infection is caused by a DNA virus
- Cutaneous herpes simplex infections have two common forms:
  - Herpes labialis – "cold sores" or "fever blisters" around the mouth (Figure 8-5)
  - Herpes genitalis – sexually transmitted lesions of the genital region
- Herpes usually presents as small, fluid-filled vesicles on an erythematous base
- Following primary herpes infection, the virus lies dormant in nervous tissue, but may recur at the original site of infection
- Chronic ulcerative herpes infection occurs in patients with immunosuppression (Figure 8-6)

Two subtypes of herpes simplex virus are recognized: HSV1 and HSV2. HSV1 causes > 80% of perioral lesions, whereas HSV2 causes > 80% of genital lesions; however, significant overlap may occur. All age groups may develop herpes labialis. Any slight diminution in immunity, such as a low-grade fever from a coincidental infection, may cause quiescent herpes labialis to relapse; this led to the term "fever blisters." Sexually active persons may acquire herpes genitalis.

During primary infection, herpes simplex virus has an incubation period of 2–7 days. Regardless of location, lesions of herpes initially appear as small, fluid-filled vesicles on an erythematous base. Lesions more than several days old may

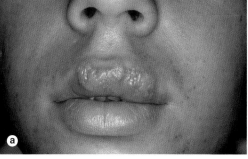
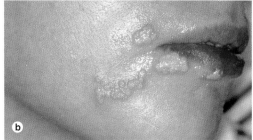
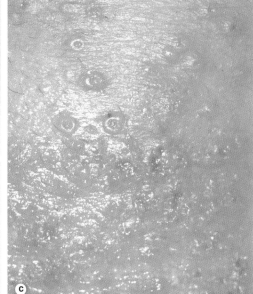

Figure 8-5 a Herpes labialis. **b, c** Herpes simplex

evolve into crusted papules or small, punched-out ulcers. Initial HSV infections may have multiple, widespread lesions, whereas recurrences are characteristically a single cluster of vesicles in the distribution of the infected sensory nerve. HSV-2 tends to be more virulent, and primary infections caused by this subtype are more likely to cause severe pain or even systemic symptoms, such as fever and lymphadenopathy.

After the primary infection clears, the virus lies dormant in the dorsal root ganglia of the central nervous system. Secondary eruptions occur with varying frequency, depending upon the individual and viral subtype, with HSV-2 infections tending to recur more frequently than HSV-1. A prodrome of pain or burning often precedes the eruption. Secondary eruptions are generally more limited in severity and duration than are primary infections.

Diagnosis/differential diagnosis

Key Points

- HSV is usually diagnosed on the basis of clinical appearance and historical information
- Supportive diagnostic modalities include:
  - Tzanck preparation from an intact vesicle
  - Direct fluorescent antibody (DFA) examination from an intact vesicle
  - Viral culture
  - Histologic analysis of a skin biopsy

A Tzanck preparation obtained from a freshly un-roofed vesicle may show diagnostic features of infection with HSV or varicella-zoster virus (VZV),

including multinucleated keratinocytes and cytopathic effect (Figure 8-7). The Tzanck does not distinguish between herpes simplex and herpes zoster infection. In experienced hands, a Tzanck preparation has a sensitivity of around 80%, but the technique is not useful for crusted lesions. DFA testing, viral culture, Polymerase chain reaction (PCR) testing, and even a biopsy represent additional diagnostic modalities that may be used to make a diagnosis. Serum antibodies to HSV are not useful in the clinical setting.

Treatment

Key Points

- Oral antiviral agents (Table 8-5) are used to treat primary and secondary herpes genitalis and often moderate-to-severe herpes labialis
- Patients with frequent recurrences (≥ 6/year) may benefit from continuous suppressive therapy
- Patients without active lesions can asymptomatically shed virus and are capable of infecting others

There is no cure for herpes and all infected patients have the potential for recurrent disease. Primary outbreaks are treated with oral acyclovir or related derivatives, such as valacyclovir or famcilovir. These latter medications have a greater bioavailability that allows for less frequent dosing. Topical acyclovir offers little benefit. Topical long-chain alcohols, such as n-docasonol, modestly shorten the course of disease and are available over the counter. Recurrent HSV may be treated

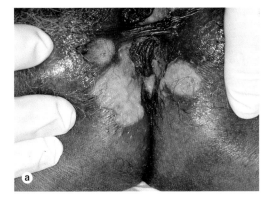

Table 8-5 Treatment for genital herpes simplex virus (HSV) infection*

Primary HSV	Secondary HSV (episodic treatment)	Prophylaxis
Acyclovir	**Acyclovir**	**Acyclovir**
400 mg tid × 7–10 days	400 mg tid × 5 days	400 mg bid
200 mg 5× /day × 7–10 days	200 mg 5× /day × 5 days	**Valacyclovir**
Valacyclovir	800 mg bid × 5 days	500 mg qd
1 g bid × 7–10 days	**Valacyclovir**	1.0 g qd
Famciclovir	500 mg bid × 3–5 days	**Famciclovir**
250 mg tid × 7–10 days	1.0 g qd × 5 days	250 mg bid
	Famciclovir	
	125 mg bid × 5 days	

*Minor cases of herpes may not require treatment. Severe herpes of any kind occurring in an immunocompromised patient may require intravenous medication.

bid, twice a day, every 12 hours; tid, three times a day, every 8 hours; qd, once a day.

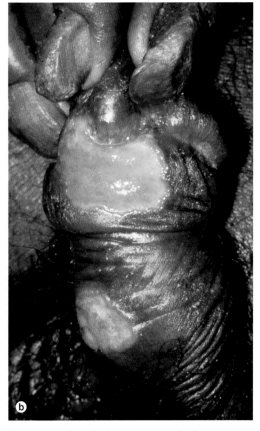

Figure 8-6 a Chronic ulcerative herpes simplex in a patient with ovarian carcinoma. **b** Chronic ulcerative herpes simplex in patient with lymphoma

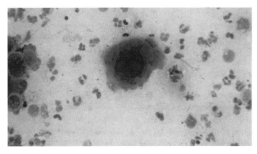

Figure 8-7 Tzanck preparation

with the same medications, although the duration of treatment is shorter. Acyclovir is well tolerated unless the patient has severe renal insufficiency. In this situation the drug may crystallize within renal tubules and reduced doses are indicated.

Patients with frequent recurrences of herpes genitalis or severe herpes labialis (typically ≥ 6 episodes/year) may benefit from continuous suppressive oral therapy. Suppressive therapy reduces the frequency of genital herpes recurrences by 70–80%, and many patients report no symptomatic outbreaks. Asymptomatic viral shedding may lead to infection in sexual partners, and for this reason, the economic and societal benefit of suppressive therapy which reduces, but does not completely eliminate shedding, is debated. Pregnant women with a history of genital herpes are often placed on suppressive treatment from 36 weeks' gestation until delivery. The presence of active lesions or a prodrome at the time of delivery is an indication for cesarean section.

Varicella-Zoster

Clinical presentation

Key Points

- VZV is a DNA virus from the Herpesviridae family that causes two forms of cutaneous disease:
  - Primary infection – "chickenpox"
  - Recrudescence – "shingles" or "zoster"

- Chickenpox usually presents in children as a diffuse eruption of pruritic papulovesicles with a truncal predominance
- Zoster most frequently presents as a painful, vesicular eruption confined to a single dermatome in an elderly or immunocompromised patient

Primary infection with VZV, which is transmitted in areorespiratory droplets, causes chickenpox, a common disease in children. Over 90% of chickenpox occurs before the age of 10 years. After a 2-week incubation period, chickenpox erupts in "crops" (groups of lesions in different phases of evolution) of pruritic papules and/or vesicles primarily on the trunk. Each lesion is a distinct umbilicated vesicle (Figure 8-8) or crust.

Once an effective immune response has been mounted, the exanthem clears and the disease becomes latent within dorsal root ganglia. With advancing age, intercurrent infection, or immunosuppression, cell-mediated immunity to VZV may weaken, allowing the latent virus to reactivate. The proliferating virus travels down axons to the skin, yielding the characteristic painful, dermatomal eruption of zoster (Figure 8-9). The cumulative lifetime risk of zoster in the entire population is about 10–20%. Recrudescence serves as a "booster" to the immune system and most patients will have only a single episode of zoster in a lifetime. Some patients, particularly older patients and those who experience significant pain with the eruption, may develop postherpetic neuralgia that persists, by definition, more than 30 days after resolution of the skin lesions. The incidence of postherpetic neuralgia in patients with zoster who are > 60 years old is about 40%, whereas the incidence in those less < 60 years old is about 10%.

A vaccine for primary VZV infection was approved for use in the United States in 1995. Prior to this, nearly all children were infected with chickenpox, leaving them vulnerable to the development of zoster later in life. The duration of immunity provided by the vaccination is not known with certainty, and concern has been raised that immunized persons may be susceptible to the development of primary varicella later in life. Some experts have hypothesized that exogenous exposure to VZV will serve as a booster and these vaccinated patients may never have zoster. Even with vaccination, "breakthrough" cases of chickenpox may occur in otherwise healthy patients, although such disease is typically milder and more limited than that in nonimmunized persons. More recently, a secondary vaccine for the prevention of zoster in older adults has become available (see below).

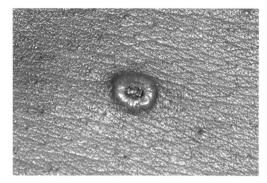

Figure 8-8 Varicella (chickenpox)

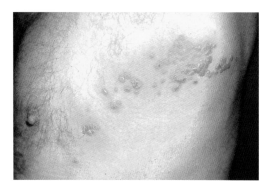

Figure 8-9 Zoster (shingles)

Diagnosis/differential diagnosis

Key Points

- The diagnosis of chickenpox or zoster is usually based on clinical appearance and historical information
- Diagnostic modalities for zoster include:
  - Tzanck preparation from an intact vesicle
  - DFA examination from a intact vesicle
  - Skin biopsy for histologic evaluation
  - Viral culture

A Tzanck preparation performed on cells scraped from the base of a freshly unroofed blister may reveal diagnostic epidermal changes, including multinucleated keratinocytes and cytopathic effect. These are common to both HSV and VZV infections. Clinical information and/or viral DFA or PCR testing may then be used to discriminate between the two conditions. Viral culture may also be performed, but it is advisable to inform the lab of the clinical suspicion; VZV culture is technically demanding and has a relatively low sensitivity. For this reason, VZV DFA or PCR analysis are the preferred tests and should be obtained whenever possible if diagnostic confirmation is needed.

The recent threat of bioterrorism has renewed the importance of being able to distinguish chickenpox from smallpox (Table 8-6).

Table 8-6 Distinguishing chickenpox from smallpox

Category	Chickenpox	Smallpox
Prodrome	Moderate – occurs commensurate with rash	Severe – prodrome present 2–3 days before onset of rash
Appearance of lesions	"Crops" of lesions in different phases of development	Monomorphic lesions all essentially in the same phase of development
Stability of lesions	Lesions easily collapse with rupture	Lesions are resistant to rupture and do not easily collapse
Distribution of lesions	Centripetal – truncal predominance	Centrifugal – predominate on extremities, often with palmoplantar involvement

Treatment

Key Points

- Chickenpox occurring in young children is self-limited and requires no treatment, but symptomatic care may be provided to reduce associated pruritus
- Chickenpox in patients > 12 years of age is of greater concern and oral antiviral agents are advised if they are started in the first 24 hours
- Zoster may be treated with oral antiviral agents, started ideally within 72 hours of the onset of symptoms
- Prednisone may help decrease the incidence of postherpetic neuralgia
- Postherpetic neuralgia may be treated with tricyclic antidepressants, gabapentin, or pregabalin

Treatment for varicella depends on the disease form and the age of the patient (Table 8-7). Chickenpox in an otherwise healthy child is self-limited and requires no treatment. Patients older than 12 have a greater risk of developing complications of VZV, including pneumonitis and/or hepatitis, and should be treated with acyclovir or related compounds within the first 24 hours of symptoms. The other related antiviral compounds appear to be equally efficacious, but only acyclovir is FDA-approved for the treatment of chickenpox.

Treatment of zoster is more controversial, but acyclovir or other antiviral medications are often employed. For the best response to treatment, therapy should be started within the first 72 hours of the onset of symptoms. Elderly patients and those with severe pain at the outset are more likely to develop persistent postherpetic neuralgia following clearance of the skin lesions. For this reason, many patients with zoster are concomitantly treated with prednisone (40–60 mg/day) followed by a rapid taper over 2–3 weeks. Postherpetic neuralgia may be treated with tricyclic antidepressants, gabapentin, or a related compound, pregabalin. Topical capsaicin may have modest benefit in treating postherpetic neuralgia.

In May 2006, the FDA approved a new live attenuated varicella vaccine (Zostavax) that is 14-fold more potent than that of the varicella vaccine used in children (Table 8-8). In nearly 40 000 patients ≥ 60 years of age enrolled in the vaccine trial, the burden of zoster dropped 61% in the comparison to the control group, and the incidence of postherpetic neuralgia dropped 67%. According to data available to date, the vaccine offers protection for at least 4 years, but it is not yet known whether it will completely prevent zoster or possibly just delay its onset. Nevertheless, this vaccine is an available option for elderly adults who wish to reduce their risk of developing zoster later in life.

Variola (Smallpox)

Clinical presentation

Key Points

- Smallpox was eradicated as a human disease as of December 1979
  - Two international laboratories maintain small quantities of frozen smallpox virus for research purposes
- Smallpox classically begins with severe systemic symptoms that precede the rash by 2–3 days
- The rash of smallpox consists of monomorphic papulopustules and is accentuated upon the extremities

Smallpox (variola), once a major cause of human mortality, has decimated entire cultures throughout history. Development of an effective vaccine has led to its presumed eradication; the last naturally occurring case was reported in Somalia in 1977. Small quantities of this DNA virus have been retained at two research institutions; the Centers for Disease Control and Prevention (CDC) in Atlanta, Georgia, and the Institute of Virus Preparations in Siberia, Russia. There is a concern that unknown quantities of the virus may be possessed or stolen and could potentially be used as a weapon of bioterrorism.

Smallpox is highly contagious and has an incubation period of 7–17 days. Constitutional symptoms, such as malaise, fever, rigors, vomiting, headache, and backache, precede development of the rash by 2–3 days. The cutaneous eruption consists of papulovesicles, which are predominantly

Table 8-7 Treatment of varicella-zoster infections

| | Chickenpox (primary disease) | | Zoster (recrudescence) |
	Young children (<12 years)	Older children and adults	
Antiviral medication	None	**Acyclovir**	**Acyclovir**
		800 mg 5×/day × 7 days	800 mg 5×/day × 7–10 days
			Valacyclovir
			1 g tid × 7 days
			Famciclovir
			500 mg tid × 7-10 days
			Foscarnet*
			40mg/kg IV q8 hours × 14–21 days
Symptomatic or adjunctive care	Calamine lotion	Calamine lotion	**Prednisone†**
	Pramoxine gel	Pramoxine gel	40–60 mg qd with 3-week taper
	Colloidal oatmeal baths	Colloidal oatmeal baths	
	Oral antihistamines	Oral antihistamines	

*For use in acyclovir-resistant varicella-zoster virus (rare).

†For prevention of postherpetic neuralgia in those > 60 years of age, or those with severe pain at the outset of disease.

tid, three times a day; IV, intravenously; qd, once a day.

Table 8-8 Information on Zostavax

Indication	Prevention of zoster (*not* to be used for treatment)
Patient population	Men and women >60 years old
Administration	Subcutaneous injection
Dosing schedule	One-time dose
Adverse reactions (decreasing frequency)	Erythema
	Pain
	Swelling
	Hematoma
	Pruritus
	Warmth
Contraindications	History of hypersensitivity or anaphylaxis to gelatin, neomycin, or any other component of the vaccine
	Current immunosuppressive medication(s)
	History of an immunodeficient state (live vaccine)
	Active untreated tuberculosis (live vaccine)
	Pregnancy (live vaccine)

located on the extremities. These monomorphic lesions are all in the same stage of development. Typical smallpox occurring in individuals without immunity is associated with a mortality rate of around 30%; with particularly virulent forms, mortality may approach 100%.

Diagnosis/differential diagnosis

Key Points

- Any suspected case of smallpox should be immediately reported to local, state, and national health officials
- Vaccinated and specially trained personnel should obtain samples from the oropharynx or open skin lesions to confirm or refute the diagnosis
- Smallpox may be differentiated from chickenpox based on the clinical appearance and historical information

Any suspected case of smallpox should be immediately reported to local and state health officials and to the CDC (24-hour Rash Hotline: (770) 488-7100). An interactive algorithm to assess the risk of smallpox in a patient, as well as additional information regarding smallpox, is available on the CDC website (http://www.bt.cdc.gov/agent/smallpox/diagnosis).

State or local health departments should alert local vaccinated and specially trained personnel to obtain samples that will be examined using electron microscopy, PCR analysis immunohistochemical analysis, or viral culture. Serologic testing may be performed to detect neutralizing antibodies, but the results cannot differentiate smallpox infection from infection with other orthopoxvirus species, such as monkeypox.

Treatment

Key Points

- Initial treatment of smallpox involves strict respiratory and contact isolation
- Vaccination during the early incubation period may attenuate or prevent disease in persons known to be exposed
- Supportive care includes adequate hydration and nutrition, eye care, and prevention of secondary infection within skin lesions
- Laboratory evidence indicates that cidofovir may be beneficial if provided early in the course of disease, but this has not been proven in humans

The most important initial management strategy is strict respiratory and contact isolation. The patient should be placed in a negative-pressure room to minimize the possibility of aerorespiratory dispersion. Supportive measures include adequate nutrition and hydration, eye care, and prevention of secondary infection. Vaccinia immune globulin does not offer a survival benefit when given to patients during the incubation period or in active disease.

Vaccination with a related attenuated virus, vaccinia, was once standard practice in the United States. Discontinuation of this practice in 1971 has left up to 50% of the current population without immunity to variola. Persons vaccinated 30 or more years ago may retain partial immunity. Current bioterrorism response plans include vaccination of first-responders, and in times of an emergency, mass vaccination of the population using serial dilutions from current vaccinia stock. Contraindications to vaccination with vaccinia include immunosuppression, pregnancy, or a history of eczema, atopic dermatitis, or another acute, chronic, or exfoliative skin condition.

Erythema infectiosum

Clinical presentation

Key Points

- Erythema infectiousm is a DNA virus infection with different presentations in children or adults:
  - Children – erythema of the cheeks ("slapped-cheek syndrome")
  - Adults – variable skin eruption with symmetric polyarthropathy
  - Unusual forms – pruritic papular and petechial glove–stocking syndrome
- Immunocompromised patients, pregnant women, or patients with chronic anemia may suffer significant morbidity

Erythema infectiosum (fifth disease) is caused by human parvovirus B19. This common infection usually occurs in late winter or early spring, with cyclical peaks every 4–7 years. Sixty percent of adults demonstrate antibodies to parvovirus B19 by 20 years of age. Manifestations of infection depend in large part upon the age and health of the individual.

Healthy children infected with parvovirus B19 develop brightly erythematous cheeks following a subtle viral prodrome. This common form of parvovirus infection is often referred to as "slapped-cheek syndrome." A characteristic reticulated erythema is noted on the trunk (Figure 8-10) and proximal extremities. Cutaneous manifestations in adults are more varied, but a symmetric polyarthropathy of the hands, wrists, knees, and ankles is common. Unusual presentations of parvovirus infection include sharply demarcated papules, petechiae, and pruritus or pain localized to a glove–stocking distribution of the distal upper and lower extremities (Figure 8-11).

Complications with parvovirus B19 infection are rare, but potentially severe. Pregnant women infected during the first trimester have up to a 30% incidence of hydrops fetalis. The virus itself tends to infect erythroid cells, yielding a reticulocytopenia for 7–10 days. In patients with decreased red blood cell survival, such as a hemolytic anemia, sickle-cell anemia, thalassemia, or glucose-6-phosphate dehydrogenase deficiency, an aplastic crisis may ensue.

Diagnosis/differential diagnosis

Key Points

- In children, erythema infectiosum is inconsequential and is usually diagnosed on clinical grounds alone
- Adult cases or unusual presentations of parvovirus infection may be confirmed with serological testing that identifies immunoglobulin (Ig) M antibodies

Treatment

Key Points

- Erythema infectiosum in healthy patients is self-limited and requires no treatment
- Analgesics or anti-inflammatory agents are useful for those with arthralgias
- Pruritus may respond to oral antihistamines
- Pregnant women should be referred to an obstetrician for fetal monitoring
- Pregnant teachers may consider leaving the classroom during an outbreak
- Children with the rash are no longer contagious

The vast majority of cases of erythema infectiosum require no specific treatment. Adult patients with arthralgias may be treated with analgesics.

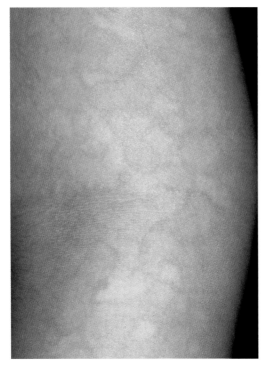

Figure 8-10 Erythema infectiosum.

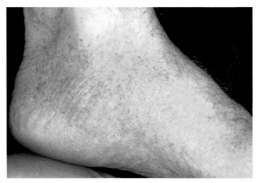

Figure 8-11 Purpuric gloves and socks syndrome (parvovirus B19)

Oral antihistamines may be useful in those with pruritus. A pregnant woman with IgM antibodies to parvovirus B19 should be monitored by her obstetrician for complications using maternal alpha-fetoprotein levels and serial ultrasound. Patients with potential for an aplastic crisis should be closely followed and may require blood transfusions or other supportive care.

Roseola infantum (Exanthem subitum)

Clinical presentation

> **Key Points**
>
> * Roseola infantum is a viral illness likely caused by infection with human herpesvirus type 6 or type 7
> * Roseola infantum initially presents as a mild upper respiratory infection with a high fever that lasts about 3 days
> * Rapid defervescence on the third day is followed by development of a subtle morbilliform exanthem

The classic patient with roseola infantum is a 9–12-month-old infant with abrupt onset of a high fever (> 40°C) and minor upper respiratory symptoms. Febrile seizures may occur in up to 15% of patients. Rapid defervescence occurs on the third day and a subtle pink, morbilliform exanthem follows. In about two-thirds of patients, characteristic erythematous papules on the oral mucosa may present on the fourth day.

Diagnosis/differential diagnosis

> **Key Points**
>
> * Roseola infantum is usually diagnosed based on clinical and historical information alone
> * No widely accepted or available diagnostic test exists

Treatment

> **Key Points**
>
> * Treatment for roseola infantum is supportive
> * Antiepileptic medications are generally not needed in patients who have a related febrile seizure

Orf and milker's nodules

Clinical presentation

> **Key Points**
>
> * Orf and milker's nodules are animal-borne infections caused by parapoxviruses
> * They usually occur in patients exposed to livestock
> * Lesions of orf and milker's nodules most often occur on the hands

Orf and milker's nodules are related conditions. These parapoxviruses are endemic to sheep and cows, respectively. The virus is transmitted to humans by direct inoculation or from fomites. After an incubation period of 5–7 days, erythematous, slightly tender papules develop at sites of infection. The papules enlarge over time, resolving within 3–6 weeks. Orf and milker's nodules are well recognized by farm workers and many cases are never brought to medical attention.

Diagnosis/differential diagnosis

Key Points

- The diagnosis of orf or milker's nodules is usually based on clinical appearance and historical information
- Orf or milker's nodules may be confused with each other or with pyogenic granulomas, bacterial infections, or herpetic whitlow

When a biopsy is performed, histologic examination reveals acanthosis, papillary edema with vascular dilatation, and viral cytopathic effect with eosinophilic intranuclear inclusions.

Treatment

Key Points

- Orf and milker's nodules are self-limited conditions that resolve in 3–6 weeks
- Treatment is supportive in nature

Symptomatic care focuses upon moist dressings, local antiseptics, and finger immobilization. Secondary bacterial infection may occur and can be treated with topical or systemic antibiotics. Anecdotal response to topical imiquimod, resulting in rapid regression, has been reported. Rarely, large exophytic lesions may be surgically treated.

Hand, foot, and mouth (HFM) disease

Clinical presentation

Key Points

- HFM disease is a viral exanthem that most often affects young children
- Cutaneous findings include oral ulcerations and erythematous to gray papules and vesicles on the hands and feet

HFM disease is most often caused by coxsackie A16 virus and less often by enterovirus 71. Seasonal variation is noted, with cases being more common in summer and fall. Children, particularly those less than 4 years of age, are most often affected. After an incubation period of 3–7 days, the condition begins with a viral prodrome of malaise, fever, headache, abdominal pain, and even diarrhea. Anorexia and mouth soreness are common symptoms. Following this prodrome, painful ulcerations develop on the cheeks and lips, accompanied by small erythematous papules on the soles, palms, and ventral fingers and toes, or even the buttocks and perineum. These erythematous papules rapidly evolve into ovoid, gray vesicles (Figure 8-12). Aseptic meningitis can occur in up to 6% of cases caused by coxsackie A16.

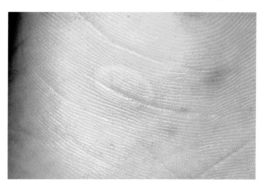

Figure 8-12 Hand, foot, and mouth disease

Diagnosis/differential diagnosis

Key Point

- HFM disease is diagnosed on clinical presentation and historical information

Treatment

Key Points

- Treatment for HFM disease is limited to supportive care
- Topical anesthetics may soothe painful oral ulcers
- Antipyretics and analgesics may help manage fever and arthralgias

Rubeola (Measles)

Clinical presentation

Key Points

- Measles is the classic example of a morbilliform viral exanthem of childhood
- Koplik's spots on the buccal mucosa are pathognomonic of measles
- A descending maculopapular eruption begins on day 4 or 5 after first symptoms and lasts for 5 days

Rubeola is caused by a single-stranded RNA virus of the Paramyxoviridae family. Even with the advent of an effective vaccine, measles still infects 50 million people annually and causes more than 1 million deaths in children. A prodrome of cough, coryza, and conjunctivitis follows a 7–14-day incubation period. Small blue-white spots with a surrounding red halo develop on the buccal mucosa (Koplik's spots) 2–3 days later. These are pathognomonic for measles. On day 4 or 5, the characteristic descending maculopapular eruption of measles begins, starting on the head, then spreading down the body. The rash worsens until day 7 or 8, and by day 10 it begins to clear. Complications of measles occur more commonly in developing countries and include dehydration, pneumonia, meningitis, and profound immunosuppression. A precipitous drop in vitamin A levels may lead to ocular complications.

Diagnosis/differential diagnosis

Key Points

- The diagnosis of measles is usually made by the clinical presentation and historical information
- Rubeola (measles) is sometimes confused with rubella (German measles)
  - The rash of measles lasts 5 days, whereas the rash of rubella lasts only 3 days
  - Rubella lacks Koplik's spots on the buccal mucosa
  - Rubella manifests postauricular and suboccipital lymphadenopathy

Treatment

Key Points

- Treatment for measles disease is limited to supportive care
- In malnourished patients, supplementation of vitamin A improves survival and decreases the risk of complications
- A combination live vaccine for measles, mumps, and rubella is widely utilized

The greatest medical advance against measles in the last 30 years was the development of a live attenuated vaccine. By 1991, 80% of the world's children were immunized by 1 year of age, and an estimated 1 million lives are saved annually through immunization. In the postvaccine era, the age of children sporadically affected by measles has increased in industrialized nations. This has led some to believe that effective immunity is lost with time, and some adults may be susceptible to the virus despite having had childhood vaccination.

BACTERIAL INFECTIONS

Impetigo contagiosa

Clinical presentation

Key Points

- Impetigo is a disease predominantly of young children
- The face is the most frequently affected site
- Both *Staphylococcus aureus* and *Streptococcus pyogenes* cause impetigo
- There are two clinical variants: classic or crusted and bullous impetigo
- Characteristic features of classic impetigo include a superficial plaque with a "honey-colored" crust

Impetigo most often presents in late summer or early fall. Patients may have one or multiple lesions, often from autoinoculation. The face is most often affected, particularly the perioral area. Classically, impetigo was caused by *Streptococcus pyogenes*, but recent evidence indicates that *Staphylococcus aureus* is actually the predominant cause of impetigo.

The initial lesion of classic, or crusted, impetigo is a transient, superficial, and fragile vesicle with surrounding erythema. As the lesion expands into a plaque, it develops a characteristic "honey-colored" crust (Figure 8-13). Systemic symptoms are uncommon. Streptococcal impetigo is not complicated by rheumatic fever, but may be associated with acute glomerulonephritis in 10–15% of cases. This glomerulonephritis is usually mild and complete recovery is the rule. Bullous impetigo (Figure 8-14) is always staphylococcal in etiology. It is most often associated with the group II, phage 71 form of *S. aureus*. The blisters are quite superficial and rupture easily. This bacterium produces an exfoliating toxin that inhibits keratinocyte adhesion. When present systemically, this same toxin causes staphylococcal scalded-skin syndrome (Ritter's disease). Lesions of impetigo heal without scarring.

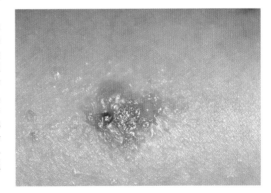

Figure 8-13 Impetigo

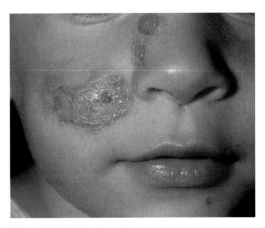

Figure 8-14 Bullous impetigo

Diagnosis/differential diagnosis

Key Points

- The diagnosis of impetigo is usually made on the clinical presentation and historical information
- Culture may confirm the diagnosis and provide antibiotic susceptibility information

A Gram stain from swabbed lesions may demonstrate Gram-positive cocci in chains (*Streptococcus*) or clusters (*Staphylococcus*); bacterial culture will confirm the identity of the organism and should be obtained if the diagnosis is unclear or if the condition fails to respond to initial antibacterial therapy. Partly because most impetigo is now caused by *S. aureus*, serologic testing for elevated ASO titers is positive in only 40% of cases. While the serum streptozyme levels are more often elevated in cases caused by streptococcus, this test is still less sensitive than culture. Rarely, pemphigus foliaceus, an autoimmune bullous disease that may occur on the face and neck of children, can be misdiagnosed as impetigo. Skin biopsy and possibly direct immunofluorescence studies should be obtained if impetigo fails to respond to an antibiotic.

Treatment

Key Points

- Most bacterial species that cause impetigo are resistant to penicillin and erythromycin
- Oral dicloxacillin and cephalexin are preferred first-line agents for treatment unless resistant bacteria are suspected or antibiotic susceptibility has been established
- Topical mupirocin and retapamulin can be used

One theoretical advantage of using oral medications to treat impetigo is eradication of bacteria in sites that are not clinically apparent. Also, topical treatment is more expensive than a 7-day course of either oral dicloxacillin or oral cephalexin. Still, provider or patient preference may be the final determinant in many situations.

Ecthyma

Clinical presentation

Key Points

- Ecthyma is most often a disease of teens and young adults
- Both *Staphylococcus* and *Streptococcus* can cause ecthyma
- Lesions often consist of eroded plaques or crusted ulcers on the extremities

Ecthyma is most common in teenagers and young adults. It was particularly common during the Vietnam conflict, during which it caused "jungle sores" on combat troops. Ecthyma is a more severe

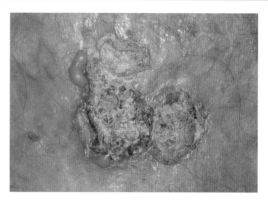

Figure 8-15 Ecthyma

form of impetigo in which there is full-thickness ulceration of the epidermis, with the formation of an overlying oyster shell-like crust (Figure 8-15). Patients may have lymphangitis, lymphadenopathy, or even a low-grade fever; all of which are uncommon in impetigo.

Diagnosis/differential diagnosis

Key Points

- The diagnosis of ecthyma is usually based on the clinical presentation and historical information
- Culture may be used to confirm the diagnosis and obtain antibiotic susceptibility

Treatment

Key Points

- Most bacterial species that cause ecthyma are resistant to penicillin and erythromycin
- Oral dicloxacillin and cephalexin are preferred first-line agents for treatment unless resistant bacteria are suspected or antibiotic susceptibility has been established
- Because the level of infection is fairly deep, topical medications such as mupirocin are not appropriate for treating ecthyma

Bacterial folliculitis

Clinical features

Key Points

- Folliculitis is an infection of the follicular unit; varied depths of infection cause a spectrum of related diseases:
  - Superficial folliculitis – small erythematous papules and fragile pustules located on the trunk, extremities, scalp, or face (Figure 8-16)
  - Furuncle/furnuculosis – more substantial infection of the hair follicle and the surrounding subcutis (referred by laypersons as a "boil")
  - Carbuncle/carbunculosis – the coalescence of several furuncles can form a subcutaneous abscess, which may be associated with systemic symptoms

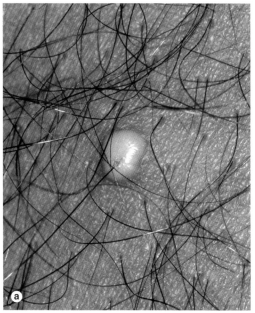

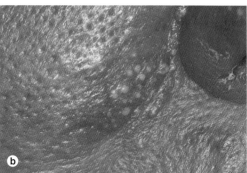

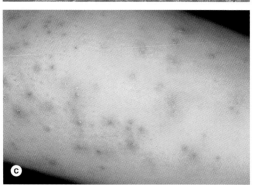

Figure 8-16 a, b, c Staphylococcal folliculitis

- The most common bacteria in these conditions is *Staphylococcus aureus*
- Painful and rapidly evolving lesions are suspicious for community-type methicillin-resistant *Staphylococcus aureus* (CA-MRSA) (Figure 8-17)
- Gram-negative bacteria may cause folliculitis in some cases, particularly in the anogenital region or in patients on chronic tetracycline therapy for acne

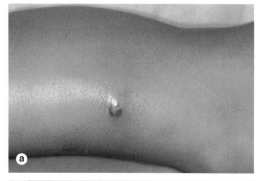

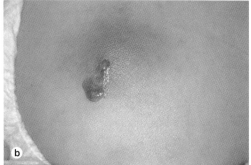

Figure 8-17 a Community-type methicillin-resistant *Staphylococcus aureus* (CA-MRSA) furuncle. **b** CA-MRSA abscess on thigh of an infant

- Up to 20% of patients with bacterial folliculitis may experience recurrent disease, and the rise of CA-MRSA contributes to this phenomenon
- Recreational folliculitis ("hot-tub folliculitis") is caused by transient infection with *Pseudomonas aeruginosa* from undertreated hot tubs or swimming pools.

Diagnosis/differential diagnosis

Key Points

- The diagnosis of bacterial folliculitis is based on the clinical presentation and historical information
- Culture of pustules may confirm the diagnosis and provide antibiotic susceptibility studies

Bacterial culture is the gold standard for diagnosis. It is important to obtain a culture in cases that are more severe, have not responded to treatment, or are located in the anogenital area, where Gram-negative infection is more common. The increasing prevalence of CA-MRSA has increased the importance of obtaining a culture. The differential diagnosis of bacterial folliculitis includes fungal folliculitis (Majocchi's granuloma), a condition discussed in the section on tinea, below.

Treatment

Oral azithromycin may be useful in penicillin-allergic patients. Gram-negative infections may be treated with levofloxacin or ciprofloxacin. Fortunately, many CA-MRSA have retained sensitivity to trimethoprim-sulfamethoxazole and the tetracycline family of drugs. If culture and antibiotic susceptibility testing have been performed, the results should guide selection of antimicrobials. Early lesions may require "ripening" with warm packs prior to drainage. Simple incision and drainage of fluctuant abscesses are generally adequate. Marsupialization or wicking is rarely necessary, but may be utilized in large or loculated lesions. Patients with carbuncles and systemic symptoms may require treatment with intravenous antibiotics.

Cellulitis and erysipelas

Clinical presentation

Cellulitis is caused by bacteria infecting the dermis and upper subcutis. Obesity, diabetes, and poor lymphatic drainage predispose patients to cellulitis. Patients with any of the above conditions, when coupled with tinea pedis, appear to be even more vulnerable to recurrent episodes of cellulitis, likely due to chronic fissuring in the feet from the tinea. Rarely, cellulitis may result from metastatic seeding of an organism from a distant site of infection, especially in immunocompromised individuals. This is particularly true of unusual forms of cellulitis due to *S. pneumoniae* or marine *Vibrio* species. Mortality with most forms of cellulitis is low (< 5%), but death may occur in neglected cases or when the infection is caused by highly virulent organisms, like *Pseudomonas aeruginosa*. Factors associated with an increased risk of death

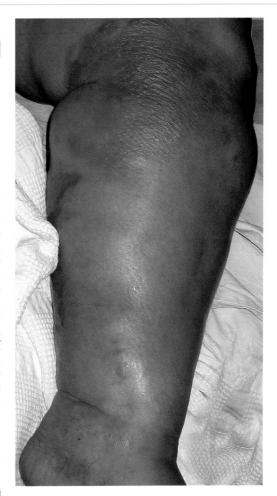

Figure 8-18 Cellulitis

include congestive heart failure, morbid obesity, hypoalbuminemia, or interconcurrent illness.

Erysipelas is a distinct subtype of cellulitis caused by *S. pyogenes*. It is characterized by sharp circumscription, bright red erythema ("fire red"), and brawny edema with a peau d'orange appearance (Figure 8-19). It is thought that the bright erythema and sharp circumscription occur because erysipelas involves a more superficial plane than does classic cellulitis. Erysipelas often involves the face or lower extremities. Regional lymphadenopathy is common with erysipelas, and systemic symptoms, including malaise, fever, and chills, may occur.

Diagnosis/differential diagnosis

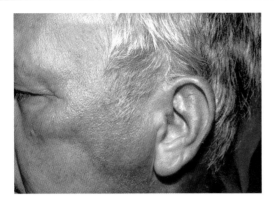

Figure 8-19 Erysipelas

Aspiration and culture at the edge of the erythematous area yield a positive result in only about 30% of cases; a negative study does not exclude the possibility of cellulitis. A complete blood count may be useful as an adjunctive test in questionable cases. Blood cultures should be routinely performed to exclude septicemia, which occurs in up to 2–10% of cases. The utility of a biopsy is limited as bacteria are infrequently identified and the histology is often nonspecific. Patients with tissue crepitus should be X-rayed to exclude the possibility of gas gangrene. As a general rule, bilateral involvement militates against infection, and favors other causes of edema and erythema, such as venous stasis dermatitis.

Treatment

Key Points

- Mild cases may be treated as an outpatient, but with close follow-up
- Oral cephalexin or dicloxacillin may be used as first-line agents unless resistant bacteria are suspected or antibiotic susceptibility has been established
- Treatment options in penicillin-allergic patients include clindamycin or vancomycin
- Ceftriaxone may be useful in the outpatient setting because it can be administered once daily
- Patients with erysipelas on the central face should be hospitalized and treated with intravenous antibiotics
- Strongly consider hospitalization and broad-spectrum intravenous antibiotics if the patient is diabetic or immunocompromised

Erysipelas involving the central face ("the danger-triangle area") has a significant risk of tracking into the cavernous sinus with resultant thrombosis, cranial nerve impairment, and death. Hospitalization is recommended for patients with this type of presentation. Selection of an antimicrobial may be based on the clinical response and results from culture and sensitivity testing.

Necrotizing fasciitis (NF)

Clinical presentation

Key Points

- NF is an insidious and deadly soft-tissue infection characterized by widespread tissue necrosis
- Clinically NF progresses rapidly and any delay in diagnosis may be fatal
- Early-warning signs include pain that is out of proportion to clinical findings

NF is an insidious soft-tissue infection characterized by widespread tissue necrosis. The majority of NF cases follow minor trauma, even bug bites, or less commonly, it may occur in surgical wounds. Immunocompromised patients, diabetics, alcoholics, or the obese are particularly predisposed to NF.

Three main subtypes of NF are recognized: type I (polymicrobial), type II (streptococcal, "flesh eating strep"), and type III (clostridial myonecrosis, "gas gangrene"). NF differs from classic cellulitis in that the infection spreads along a deeper plane between the subcutis and the fascia. Presumably, elaboration of unique bacterial enzymes and toxins facilitates this spread, and vascular occlusion, ischemia, and tissue necrosis result.

After an incubation period of 24–72 hours, the primary site demonstrates erythema and edema similar in appearance to classic cellulitis. However, pain is severe and exceeds that expected based on the cutaneous findings. Ultimately, the area develops a dusky-blue hue and serosanguineous bullae may be present; unfortunately, once these findings are noted, the opportunity for optimal intervention has largely passed. Systemic signs include high fever, prostration, tachycardia, mental confusion, obtundation, and, ultimately, hypotension and shock. Septicemia and metastatic abscesses may also occur. Mortality with NF has been as high as 50% in some series.

Diagnosis/differential diagnosis

Key Points

- NF is a true emergency that mandates early surgical consultation and evaluation
- A deep biopsy that includes the superficial fascia is required to confirm the diagnosis

A deep biopsy from the edge of a necrotic area is needed to make the diagnosis of NF. Histological examination reveals extensive thrombosis of the vasculature with resultant necrosis. Numerous bacteria are often seen, even with standard hematoxylin and eosin staining alone. Touch preparations may provide rapid presumptive evidence of the potential pathogen. Tissue biopsies should be submitted for both culture and histologic examination. Blood cultures, although often positive, are too delayed to be useful in making a rapid initial diagnosis. Soft-tissue X-rays may be useful to exclude gas-forming organisms.

Treatment

Key Points

- All patients with suspected NF should be immediately admitted to the hospital
- Intravenous access should be immediately established, as systemic toxicity with resultant hypotension may soon make future access difficult
- A surgeon and infectious disease specialist should be immediately consulted to assist with a biopsy and recommendations for empiric antibiotics, respectively
- Blood cultures should be obtained before administering antibiotics, unless the patient is unstable or a significant delay will ensue

NF is a surgical emergency and widespread debridement is the ultimate treatment of choice. When requesting consultation, it is important to impress upon the consultant the diagnostic suspicion and the concern that process could be potentially life-threatening; time is of the essence. If consultation with an infectious disease specialist is not available, intravenous antipseudomonal penicillin derivatives (ticarcillin/clavulanate, piperacillin/tazobactam, impipenem/cilastin, or meropenem) should be commenced. Vancomycin should be included if concern for MRSA exists. Hyperbaric oxygen may be used for anaerobic NF.

Syphilis

Clinical features

Key Points

- Syphilis is caused by the spirochete *Treponema pallidum*
- Infection with syphilis is commonly divided into the following stages:
  - Primary infection – chancre on exposed skin, usually from sexual contact
  - Secondary infection – systemic treponemia leads to widespread involvement of the skin, mucosa, and possibly the central nervous system
  - Latent infection – clinically inapparent infection in the viscera or central nervous system
  - Tertiary syphilis – tissue destruction and formation of gummas within the skin, mucosa, and viscera and severe central nervous system damage

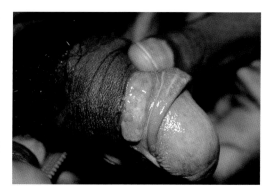

Figure 8-20 Syphilitic chancre

Clinical manifestations of syphilis may involve any organ system. In dermatology, however, we are primarily concerned with primary and secondary syphilis. After an incubation period of about 3 weeks, primary syphilis yields a chancre that is usually solitary, raised, and firm. The chancre is most often located upon the penis (Figure 8-20), vulva, or cervix, but it may be located in the oropharynx following oral sex or even on the hands or trunk. The chancre erodes to create an ulcer with rolled edges that is teeming with spirochetes and is highly infectious. The chancre heals with scarring over a period of 3–12 weeks.

Secondary syphilis is caused by systemic dissemination of the treponeme. Usually, but not always, the chancre has completely resolved by the time secondary disease develops. In the skin and mucosa, secondary syphilis may produce a variety of clinical manifestations. Most commonly, secondary syphilis presents with a papulosquamous rash on the trunk and extremities (Figure 8-21). The color of the rash in light-skinned individuals has been likened to "boiled ham" or "copper pennies." Involvement of the palms and soles is highly suggestive, but not diagnostic, of secondary syphilis. Other findings include mucous patches (also known as condyloma lata; Figure 8-22), split papules (at the corners of the mouth), or a non-scarring alopecia ("moth-eaten"). Lymphadenopathy is present in > 90% of cases.

Diagnosis/differential diagnosis

Key Points

- Primary syphilis is diagnosed by the clinical examination and performance of a screening rapid plasma reagin (RPR)/Venereal Disease Research Laboratory (VDRL) serology. Less commonly, dark-field examination on material from the chancre is used
- Secondary syphilis is diagnosed by clinical examination and performance of a screening RPR/VDRL, with confirmation using a treponeme-specific test such as fluorescent treponemal antibody absorption test (FTA-ABS)

- With appropriate treatment, RPR/VDRL titers decrease, but the FTA-ABS remains positive for life
- Patients with syphilis are often infected with HIV (as many as 40% in some studies); therefore, counseling and strong consideration of HIV-testing are encouraged
- HIV-positive patients with neurological symptoms, late latent syphilis or syphilus of an unknown duration should always receive a lumbar puncture with RPR/VDRL on spinal fluid to exclude neurosyphilis

Repeated studies indicate that many physicians do a poor job of diagnosing syphilis. In one retrospective study, upon presentation of a patient with the characteristic rash of secondary syphilis, only half of physicians entered such a suspicion into the medical record. The diagnosis of secondary syphilis can be made relatively easily with serologic screening tests (RPR/VDRL) and confirmed by more specific serologic tests (FTA-ABS) (Table 8-9); the critical step is considering the diagnosis. Occasionally a very high antibody response will render a screening exam falsely negative due to the prozone phenomenon, but most labs perform initial dilutions to eliminate this cause of error. Other diagnostic techniques include identification of the spirochete using a modified silver stain or special immunohistochemical techniques. Darkfield examination may be performed on primary or secondary lesions, although this is rarely done.

Treatment

Key Points

- Appropriate treatment for syphilis depends on the stage of disease and the patient's overall health
- *Treponema pallidum* remains exquisitely sensitive to penicillin G and most CDC-recommended treatment regimens utilize this antibiotic
- Doxycycline is the most widely used antibiotic for penicillin-allergic patients with primary or secondary uncomplicated syphilis

Treatment recommendations of syphilis consider both the stage of the disease and the overall health of the patient. The CDC issues annual guidelines for the treatment of primary and uncomplicated secondary syphilis (Table 8-10).

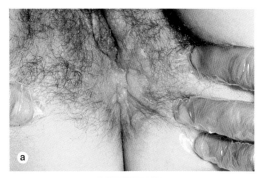

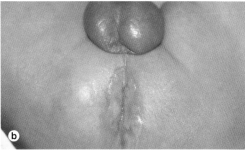

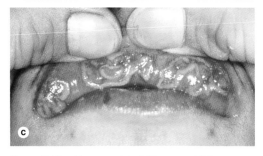

Figure 8-22 **a** Mucous patch. **b** Mucous patch in an infant. **c** Mucous patch (courtesy of Brooke Army Medical Center teaching file)

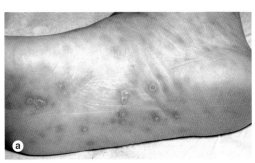

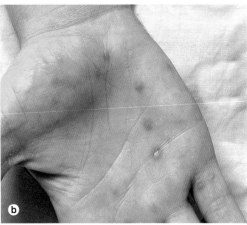

Figure 8-21 **a** Secondary syphilis. **b** Secondary syphilis in a human immunodeficiency virus-positive man

Table 8-9 Sensitivity of serological testing for syphilis in otherwise healthy individuals

	Key cutaneous manifestation	Test sensitivity	
		VDRL/RPR	FTA-ABS
Primary syphilis	Chancre	78–86%	76–84%
Secondary syphilis	Rash	~100%*	~100%*
Tertiary syphilis	Gumma	71–73%	94–96%

*Occasional false-negative results due to prozone phenomenon may be overcome by dilution prior to testing. Inexperienced laboratories may need to be reminded of this "pitfall," while experienced labs account for this automatically.
VDRL, Venereal Disease Research Laboratory; RPR, rapid plasma regain; FTA-ABS, fluorescent treponemal antibody absorption test.

Table 8-10 Summary of Centers for Disease Control and Prevention guidelines for treatment of primary and secondary syphilis in adults

| HIV-negative patient | Benzathine penicillin G 2.4 million units IM in a single dose
Doxycyline (penicillin-allergic) 100 mg PO bid × 14 days |
| --- | --- |
| HIV-positive patient | *Mandatory* lumbar puncture in secondary syphilis to exclude neurosyphilis
Benzathine penicillin G
2.4 million units IM as a single dose weekly × 3 weeks*
Doxycycline (penicillin-allergic) 100 mg PO bid × 14 days |

*Some experts recommend one-time-dosing, as per non-HIV-infected patients with syphilis but will retreat with three doses if follow-up RPR/VDRL testing in 3 months does not document a fourfold decrease in titers.
HIV, human immunodeficiency virus; IM, intramuscular; PO, orally; bid, twice a day;

Anthrax

Clinical features

Key Points

- Anthrax is a disease caused by the Gram-positive organism *Bacillus anthracis*
- Worldwide, anthrax remains a disease of significant morbidity and mortality
- 90% of all cases are limited to the skin
- Rare sporadic cases of anthrax (1 to 2 cases/year) occur in the United States, usually in those who come in contact with livestock
- During 2001, 22 cases were reported in the United States and all were in association with a bioterrorism plot propagated through the mail system

Anthrax is primarily a disease of domestic herbivores (cattle, sheep, horses, goats) and some wild animals. In humans, anthrax occurs in three forms: cutaneous, pulmonary, and gastrointestinal. More than 95% of all anthrax cases are cutaneous.

Cutaneous anthrax begins 1–14 days after inoculation as a painless pruritic papule resembling an insect bite. The head and neck region are most often involved. Lesions are often solitary, but may be multiple. The lesion enlarges rapidly, often with formation of a central vesicle, and with characteristic "brawny" edema. Edema may be extensive ("malignant edema") or it may extend over large areas. The vesicle then ulcerates, and a central black eschar reminiscent of a lump of coal develops. This central eschar may be surrounded by a "pearly wreath" of secondary vesicles. Systemic symptoms occur in 50% of cases. The lesions heal with scarring in 1–3 weeks. Approximately 20% of untreated cutaneous cases become systemic infections, often with disastrous consequences.

Diagnosis/differential diagnosis

Key Points

- Follow a recommended protocol for the evaluation of possible lesions of cutaneous anthrax
- Medical personnel are not considered at risk for pulmonary anthrax when evaluating skin lesions

The CDC and the American Academy of Dermatology have developed a protocol for use in the systemic evaluation of possible cases of cutaneous anthrax (Table 8-11).

Treatment

Key Points

- Ciprofloxacin is considered the treatment of choice until susceptibility studies are obtained (Table 8-12)
- Doxycycline represents an acceptable alternative medication
- Extensive cases require hospitalization and intravenous dosing of antibiotics

Table 8-11 Synopsis of recommendations for evaluation of possible anthrax

American Academy of Dermatology Bioterrorism Task Force cutaneous anthrax management algorithm	
Step 1	Notify the local health department to inform them of a patient with suspected anthrax and to obtain any additional instructions before performing diagnostic tests
	Take a picture of the lesion and record pertinent historical information
Step 2	Maintain universal precautions when evaluating patients with suspected cutaneous anthrax (a mask is not required)
Step 3	Swab exudates for Gram stain and culture
	If vesicles are present: soak two synthetic swabs in vesicular fluid
	If an eschar is present: lift the edge of the eschar and rotate two synthetic swabs beneath the eschar without dislodging it
	If only an ulcer is present: swab the base of the ulcer with two synthetic swabs moistened with sterile nonbacteriostatic saline
Step 4	Obtain a full-thickness 4-mm punch biopsy specimen and place in formalin for routine histopathology and polymerase chain reaction testing
	Obtain a second 4-mm sterile punch biopsy for culture and place the tissue in a sterile container with sterile nonbacteriostatic saline
Step 5	Draw one 5-mL tube of blood into a "red-topped" (serum separator) tube and transfer it to the laboratory for storage of serum at −70°C. Label the tube: "Anthrax serology. Store serum at −70°C for special pick-up"
Step 6	Draw one 5-mL tube of blood into a "purple-topped" tube (anticoagulated). This tube should be refrigerated and held for potential request by the Centers for Disease Control and Prevention for blood-based assays. Label this tube: "Anthrax blood-based assay. Store under refrigeration for special pick-up"
Step 7	Obtain blood cultures from febrile or hospitalized patients

Table 8-12 Treatment recommendations for cutaneous anthrax

Patient population	Initial oral therapy
Adults	**Ciprofloxacin** 500 mg PO bid × 60 days
	Doxycycline 100 mg PO bid × 60 days
Children	**Ciprofloxacin** 15 mg/kg PO bid × 60 days
	Doxycycline 100 mg PO bid (>45 kg) × 60 days 2.2 mg/kg PO bid (<45 kg)
Pregnant or nursing women	**Ciprofloxacin** 500 mg PO bid × 60 days (preferred)
	Doxycycline 100 mg PO bid × 60 days

PO, orally; bid, twice a day.

Although ciprofloxacin may cause arthropathy in children, and doxycycline may stain immature dental enamel, due to the risks involved with anthrax infection, such agents are considered necessary treatment for patients of all ages until susceptibilities are known. For penicillin-sensitive, nonweaponized strains of anthrax (either farm-acquired or susceptibility-proven strains), penicillin G may be used.

Erythema chronicum migrans (ECM)

Clinical features

Key Points

* ECM represents the cutaneous expression of Lyme disease
* ECM is present in up to 80% of patients with Lyme disease
* ECM typically develops in the first 4 weeks after infection

ECM (Figure 8-23), the cutaneous manifestation of Lyme disease, is a disorder caused by the spirochete, *Borrelia burgdorferi*. ECM develops 3–30 days after a bite by an infected tick. The *Ixodes* hard tick is the chief vector for Lyme disease, although the particular species involved varies from region to region (eastern United States – *I. scapularis*, western United States – *I. pacificus*). Ticks in all developmental stages are capable of transmitting the disease, but given their small size and mobility, nymphs are thought to cause most cases. Evidence suggests the tick must remain attached for *at least* 24–48 hours to transmit infection. Only one-third of patients recall the tick bite.

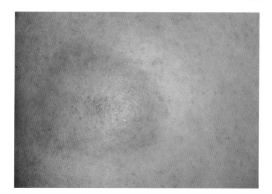

Figure 8-23 Erythema chronicum migrans

Table 8-13 Peroral treatment recommendations for acute Lyme disease

Patient population	Initial oral therapy
Adults	**Doxycycline** 100 mg PO bid × 30 days
	Cefuroxime* 500 mg PO bid × 30 days
Children	**Amoxicillin** 500–100 mg PO tid × 30 days
	Cefuroxime† 500 mg PO bid × 30 days
Pregnant or nursing women	**Amoxicillin** 500–100 mg PO tid × 30 days
	Cefuroxime* 500 mg PO bid × 30 days

*Only antibiotic with specific Food and Drug Administration approval for treatment of Lyme disease in adults.
†Experts who use cefuroxime in childhood Lyme disease dose as for adults.
PO, orally; bid, twice a day; tid, three times a day.

Diagnosis/differential diagnosis

Key Points

* A detailed exposure history is useful in evaluating for Lyme disease
* Histologic examination often demonstrates non-specific changes of arthropod assault such as eosinophils
* Silver-based stains (modified Steiner stain) demonstrate spirochetes in only one-half of cases
* False-negative serological testing for Lyme disease occurs most often in the first 6 weeks of infection, which correlates with the period when ECM is most apparent

Treatment

Key Points

* Routine antibacterial prophylaxis of patients with tick bites is controversial
* Early treatment of Lyme disease with doxycycline, amoxicillin, or cerfuroxime is highly successful (Table 8-13)

In two early randomized trials, investigators concluded that prophylactic treatment was not justified because of the cost, the potential side-effects, and the fact that early treatment prevented any long-term sequelae in patients from the control groups who did contract Lyme disease and did not receive prophylaxis. However, in a more recent study a single dose of 200 mg of doxycycline taken within 72 hours of a tick bite was shown to decrease the risk of developing Lyme disease. These studies were complicated by the fact that the tick must remain attached for > 24–48 hours to transmit infection. Early treatment of Lyme disease, during the period of ECM, is generally quite successful and prevents nearly all long-term sequelae. The management of disseminated disease or persistent disease is complex and consultation with specialists is advised.

Mycobacterium marinum

Clinical features

Key Points

* *Mycobacterium marinum* causes the most common type of atypical mycobacterial infection in the skin
* Infection with *M. marinum* is associated with exposure to contaminated water sources, hence the name "fish tank granuloma"

M. marinum is an atypical mycobacteria found in salt and fresh water (Table 8-14). Cutaneous infection in humans may follow inoculation of the skin or contamination of a pre-existing wound. The infection manifests as a localized granuloma consisting of a dermal plaque with minimal surrounding erythema. Less often, sporotrichoid spread with ascending lymphangitis may be observed. The upper extremity is involved in 90% of cases. Immunocompromised patients may have more extensive disease, including osteomyelitis and even disseminated infection, although this is rare because the organism grows optimally at a temperature of 25–32°C, rather than 37°C. *M. marinum* infection occurs worldwide in those with occupational or recreational exposure to fresh or salt water. The estimated annual incidence within the United States is 3 cases per 1 000 000 persons.

Table 8-14 Runyon classification of nontuberculous mycobacteria

Runyon group	Representative organisms
Group I (photochromogens)	*Mycobacterium kansasii, M. marinum, M. simiae*
Group II (scotochromogens)	*Mycobacterium scrofulaceum, M. gordonae, M. szulgai*
Group III (nonchromogens)	*Mycobacterium avium-intracellulare, M. xenopi, M. terrae*
Group IV (rapid-growing)	*Mycobacterium fortuitum, M. abscessus, M. chelonae*

Table 8-15 Systemic treatment recommendations for *Mycobacterium marinum* Infection limited to the skin

Medication	Dosage*
Minocycline	100 mg PO bid
Trimethoprim-sulfamethoxazole	One DS (160/800) tablet PO bid†
Rifampin	600 mg PO qd‡
Clarithromycin	500 mg PO bid

*For most medications, the duration of treatment is 4–6 weeks beyond the point of resolution.
†A duration as short as 10–14 days has been described for trimethoprim-sulfamethoxazole.
‡Rifampin has been described to be successful both as monotherapy and in combination with other agents.
PO, orally; bid, twice a day; DS, double-strength; qd, once a day.

Diagnosis/differential diagnosis

Key Points

* The diagnosis is suspected based on the clinical appearance and relevant historical information, including an exposure to contaminated water
* Tissue cultures held at a reduced temperature (32°C) may grow nonmotile acid-fast bacilli in 7–21 days
* Organisms are few in number and are not usually seen on histologic sections, even with performance of special stains for acid-fast bacilli

Treatment

Key Points

* Medical treatment usually involves prolonged courses of minocycline, trimethoprim-sulfamethoxazole, rifampin, or clarithromycin (Table 8-15)
* Antibiotics are usually dosed for a minimum of 4–6 weeks beyond resolution of the lesions
* Physiotherapy (heat packs) may be useful as an adjunctive treatment
* Debridement or excision may be utilized in certain cases

Colonized wounds

Clinical features

Key Points

* Any wound may become colonized with bacteria, but in dermatology, it is most frequent in chronic leg ulcers
* Antibiotics do not heal ulcers; they treat infections
* Infection usually manifests as:
  * New-onset wound pain
  * Deterioration of the wound bed with friable, dusky granulation tissue
  * Lack of granulation tissue
  * Development of a visible biofilm
  * Surrounding cellulitis
  * Constitutional symptoms

Simple colonized wounds have bacteria living in the tissues, but the presence of these microorganisms is not detrimental to healing.

Diagnosis/differential diagnosis

Key Points

* Colonization is distinguished from infection by an absence of inflammation and a lack of extension beyond the immediate area of the wound

Infection must be distinguished from colonization. Clinical signs of active infection include purulent drainage, edema, spreading erythema, lymphangitic streaking, or loss of granulation tissue with replacement by yellowed necrotic slough. Systemic antibiotic therapy is indicated in the case of wound infection. The only time to culture an ulcer is when infection is suspected; colonized wounds do not need to be cultured.

Treatment

* Heavy colonization is managed with wound debridement using an instrument such as a curette
* Antimicrobial dressings such as Acticoat, Actisorb silver, Aquacel AG, or Iodosorb may be used as adjuncts
* Topical or systemic antibiotics are not indicated for the treatment of colonization

Cutaneous diphtheria

Clinical presentation

Key Points

* Cutaneous diphtheria is unusual in the United States, but still commonly occurs in developing countries in tropical regions

- Lesions often begin as insect bites, which become infected with *Corynebacterium diphtheriae*
- Cutaneous diphtheria is characterized by shallow skin ulcers, possibly with a brown-gray membrane, that may occur anywhere on the body. They are usually chronic in nature
- Lesions are an important reservoir of infection and may cause respiratory or cutaneous infections in exposed persons
- Toxin production from the bacteria within the skin lesions is absorbed slowly and does not usually manifest as systemic toxicity

Diagnosis/differential diagnosis

Key Points

- The diagnosis is often suspected based on the clinical appearance coupled with a history of travel to an endemic area
- Swab culture specimens should be obtained from any chronic nonhealing skin ulcer in patients who have traveled to an endemic area
- Lesions of cutaneous diphtheria are often coinfected with *Staphylococcus aureus* and *Streptococcus pyogenes* and this may confound culture results

Treatment

Key Points

- Erythromycin (500 mg orally qid × 14 days) is the drug of choice for treating cutaneous diphtheria
- Vaccination and prophylaxis of contacts should be offered as exposed persons may develop oropharyngeal diphtheria, which can lead to death
- Following treatment, elimination of the organism should be documented by obtaining two successive cultures from the skin 24 hours apart

Erythrasma

Clinical presentation

Key Points

- Erythrasma is a superficial bacterial infection caused by *Corynebacterium minutissimum*
- Typically erythrasma presents as asymptomatic or mildly pruritic, slightly scaling, thin, erythematous to slightly brown plaques in the body folds
- The inguinal fold and medial thighs are most often affected

Erythrasma occurs primarily in adults, and it is decidedly more common in humid, tropical environments. The disease presents within the folds of the groin, pubic area, axillae, intergluteal folds, and inframammary areas. Clinically, it presents as thin, erythematous plaques that may become brown-red with a fine, wrinkled scale as they mature. Minimal pruritus is sometimes experienced, and systemic symptoms are absent.

Diagnosis/differential diagnosis

Key Points

- The diagnosis of erythrasma is based on the clinical presentation
- Examination using a Wood's lamp confirms the diagnosis, as the *Corynebacterium* fluoresce coral-red

Erythrasma is often confused for, and even mistakenly treated as, a dermatophyte infection. The diagnosis of erythrasma is established using a Wood's lamp that demonstrates characteristic coral-red fluorescence due to porphyrin production within the organism. However, these porphyrins are water-soluble, and may not be detected if the patient has just bathed. A biopsy is not usually necessary, but will demonstrate the organism within the stratum corneum. Bacterial cultures are not helpful, but a fungal culture will exclude tinea cruris.

Treatment

Key Points

- Topical erythromycin, topical clindamycin, topical benzoyl peroxide, topical imidazoles, Whitfield's ointment, and 20% aluminum chloride have all been described to be effective
- Oral erythromycin may be employed for those unable or unwilling to use topical medications

FUNGAL INFECTIONS

Tinea

Clinical presentation

Key Points

- Tinea infections are caused by superficial fungi that are capable of using keratin as an energy substrate
- Tinea infections are further subclassified based on the area of the body affected
- Tinea infections may be acquired from other humans (anthropophilic), from animals (zoophilic), or from the soil (geophilic)
- In general, infections that are acquired from animal or the soil cause the most inflammation, while those acquired from other humans result in the least inflammation
- Species from the genera *Epidermophyton*, *Microsporum*, and *Trichophyton* cause tinea infections in humans

- *Epidermophyton* often causes tinea pedis or tinea cruris; it does not involve the scalp
- *Microsporum* may infect a variety of areas; species fluoresce under Wood's lamp examination
- *Trichophyton* genus contains the most common species to infect humans (*T. rubrum*), and also the most common cause of tinea capitis (*T. tonsurans*)
- Most tinea infections are characterized by intensely pruritic, annular lesions with peripheral scale, central clearing, and variable inflammation
- Tinea involving hair-bearing skin may lead to alopecia
- Patients using immunosuppressive medications, including high-dose prednisone, are predisposed to extensive tinea infections

Tinea (Figure 8-24) is a Latin word meaning "gnawing worm or moth." Laypersons often refer to all forms of tinea as "ringworm," likely because of its tendency to form annular lesions. Traditionally, dermatologists have used Latin names to designate infections based upon the site of involvement. The most frequently encountered forms of tinea in dermatology include tinea pedis ("athlete's foot"), tinea capitis, tinea cruris ("jock itch"), and tinea corporis.

Prior misdiagnosis with mistaken treatment with topical steroids may alter the clinical appearance of tinea. While topical steroids initially lessen the inflammation and decrease pruritus, they also suppress the local immune response and act as "fertilizer" for the fungus. Under these conditions, the fungus may invade deeper into the follicular epithelium investing the hair shafts. This leads to a fungal folliculitis, often referred to as Majocchi's granuloma (Figure 8-25). Inflammatory kerion (Figure 8-26) in the scalp is also a form of fungal folliculitis.

Diagnosis/differential diagnosis

Key Points

- Tinea is often suspected because of clinical presentation and historical information
- A history of exposure to new pets or environments associated with tinea infections (health clubs, hotels, etc.) may be helpful
- Potassium hydroxide (KOH) preparation of scale from the edge of an annular lesion should reveal hyphal elements
- For tinea capitis, material for a KOH preparation may be obtained by vigorously rubbing the area with a moistened piece of gauze, swab, or even sterile toothbrush
- Fungal culture of scrapings is also useful, but results take several days to weeks to return

The diagnosis of tinea capitis is suspected based on the clinical features, with solicitation of a history of likely exposure being helpful. A KOH

preparation analyzed under a microscope has the advantage of immediate confirmation through the identification of fungal hyphae (Figure 8-27). Dissolving keratinocytes create an artifact known as "mosaic hypahe" (Figure 8-28). These polygonal structures must be differentiated from true hyphae. Fungal culture of tissue scrapings can confirm the diagnosis and provide species identification, but results are delayed a week or more.

Treatment

Key Points

- Limited tinea infections occurring on nonhair-bearing skin may be treated with topical antifungal medications (Table 8-16)
- Failure to use topical therapies for the prescribed duration is a leading cause of recurrence. Providing written instructions may enhance compliance
- Topical medications should be applied in a 2-cm radius beyond the visible border of the lesion
- When the distribution is extensive, the involved area is covered in terminal hair, or the patient has failed topical management, oral antifungal medications are indicated (Table 8-17)
- Oral griseofulvin remains the treatment of choice for tinea capitis in children, although oral terbinafine or oral azoles are being used more frequently.

Onychomycosis

Clinical features

Key Points

- Onychomycosis (Figure 8-29) includes all fungal infections of the fingernails or toenails
- Tinea unguium refers to a subset of nail infections caused exclusively by dermatophytes
- Not all thickened and yellowed fingernails or toenails are due to fungal infection, as similar changes are seen in psoriasis, lichen planus, lichen striatus, habit-tick deformity, repetitive trauma, and even aging itself
- In some studies, onychomycosis caused only about one-half of all nail dystrophy

Onychomycosis is a common condition, particularly with advancing age. Adults are 30 times more likely to have onychomycosis than are children. Dermatophyte infections cause one-half to two-thirds of cases. Nails are usually infected by the same fungal organisms involved in associated tinea pedis. Toenails are affected more often than are fingernails, and this likely reflects the high prevalence of tinea pedis. Typically, infected nails are asymptomatic, but occasionally they may become painful because of trauma, ingrowth, or severe dystrophy. Three clinical variants merit further discussion:

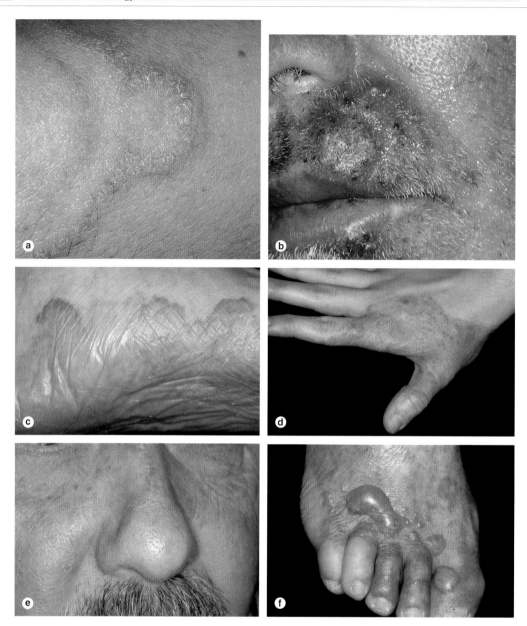

Figure 8-24 a Tinea. b Tinea barbae. c–e Tinea. f Bullous tinea with id reaction (autoeczematization)

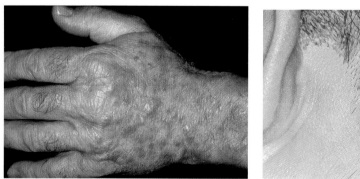

Figure 8-25 Majocchi's fungal folliculitis

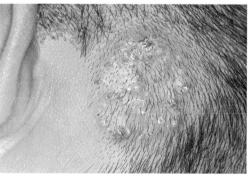

Figure 8-26 Kerion

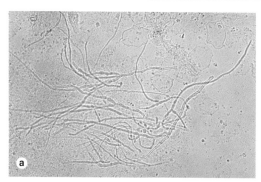

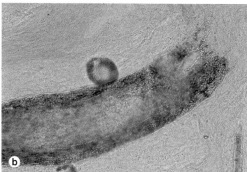

Figure 8-27 **a** Potassium hydroxide preparation of tinea. **b** Endothrix

1. Distal subungual onychomycosis – discoloration, thickening (onychogryphosis), and separation of the nail plate from the bed (onycholysis) that begins distally and progresses proximally
2. Proximal onychomycosis – an uncommon variant that begins near the matrix and is prevalent among immunocompromised patients (HIV/AIDS)
3. Superficial onychomycosis – an uncommon variant caused by superficial invasion of the nail with white opacities on the surface of the nail plate

Diagnosis/differential diagnosis

- Because nail dystrophy is not always caused by onychomycosis, the diagnosis *must* be confirmed prior to treatment
- Onychomycosis may be documented by identification of hyphae with KOH examination of subungual debris or by formal histologic examination of the involved nail plate using periodic acid–Schiff (PAS) stain
- Fungal culture of nail material and debris may also be utilized for diagnosis
- Histologic examination of nail clippings has been reported to have the highest sensitivity (> 90%), while fungal culture has the lowest sensitivity (~60%)
- A *representative* portion of the nail plate must be sampled for best results

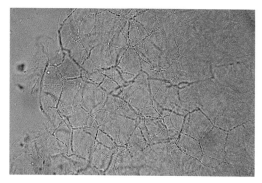

Figure 8-28 Epithelial cell outlines – so-called mosaic hyphae

Treatment

- Onychomycosis remains the superficial fungal infection that is most recalcitrant to treatment
- Medical therapy is relatively expensive and not without risk
- Infection of the fingernails is more socially stigmatizing and a lower threshold for treatment is often justified
- Patients with vascular insufficiency, diabetes, and/or recurrent cellulitis of the lower extremity likely benefit from treatment
- Enthusiasm for treatment must be balanced against long-term studies that have demonstrated recurrence rates of up to 50%
- Patients being considered for oral antifungal therapy should be questioned about liver disease, hepatitis, photosensitivity and a personal or family history of lupus

Only oral antifungal agents offer a reasonable rate of cure. Oral itraconazole and terbinafine have been widely utilized (Table 8-18). Recent meta-analyses have indicated that terbinafine is a superior treatment. Heart failure may complicate itraconazole therapy. Hepatotoxicity is a concern with both agents. Baseline liver function studies are recommended for patients anticipating a ≥ 6-week course of medication, or in any patient with a possible change in liver function. Routine testing during therapy is controversial, but is always indicated when there are clinical indications of liver toxicity. The estimated risk of fulminant hepatic necrosis is around 1:54 000 patients for terbinafine, and 1:500 000 patients for intraconazole. Topical treatment is inferior to oral management. Ciclopirox olamine lacquer has a reported 8% clinical cure rate, yet it remains an option for those with contraindications to oral medication, but who have a strong desire to treat. Nail avulsion remains an option. Alternative agents, including botanicals, bacterial extracts,

Table 8-16 Topical agents for treatment of limited tinea corporis, tinea cruris, and tinea pedis

Generic formulation	Form(s)	Dosing frequency	Treatment duration (weeks)		
			Corporis	Cruris	Pedis
Clotrimazole	1% cream, lotion, spray solution, solution	bid	4	2	Up to 8
Ketoconazole	1% and 2% cream	qd	2	2	6
Miconazole	2% cream, lotion, spray powder, spray solution	bid	2	2	4
Oxiconazole	1% cream, lotion	qd	2	2	4
Sulconazole	1% cream, solution	bid	3	3	4
Terbinafine	1% cream, spray solution, solution	qd to bid	1–4	1–4	1–2
Ciclopirox olamine	0.77% cream or lotion, solution	bid	2–4	2–4	2–4

bid, twice a day; qd, once a day.

Table 8-17 Systemic agents for treatment of tinea capitis or other extensive tinea infections

Medication	Dosage		Duration	
	Children	Adults	Tinea capitis	Extensive tinea elsewhere
Griseofulvin	20–25 mg/kg per day (micronized) 10–15 mg/kg per day (ultramicronized)	500–1000 mg qd (micronized) 250–500 mg qd (ultramicrosized)	6–8 weeks	4 weeks
Itraconazole	3–5 mg/kg per day	100 mg BID	4–6 weeks	2 weeks
Terbinafine	10–20 kg: 62.5 mg/day 20–40 kg: 125 mg/day >40 kg: 250 mg/day (adult dose)	250 md qd	4 weeks	2 weeks

qd, once a day; bid, twice a day.

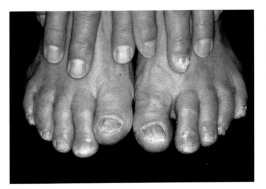

Figure 8-29 Onychomycosis

and various over-the-counter liniments deserve further study. Onychomycosis that is due to saprophytes is even more recalcitrant to treatment, and in this situation, treatment often fails.

Pityriasis versicolor

Clinical presentation

Key Points

- Pityriasis versicolor is the preferred term for a superficial infection of the epidermis caused by commensal yeast of the genus *Pityrosporum*
- Some authors use the genus *Malassezia* to refer to the pathogenic hyphal phase of this normal skin commensal
- Pityriasis versicolor is particularly common in young adults living in warm and humid climates
- Close inspection of the thin plaques of pityriasis versicolor reveals a fine, bran-like scale (Figure 8-30)

Pityriasis versicolor is a harmless and ubiquitous condition often seen in young adults in humid environments, particularly among those who exercise routinely. Multiple family members may be

Table 8-18 Systemic treatment recommendations for onychomycosis

| Medication | Area of the body involved | |
	Fingernails	Toenails
Terbinafine	250 mg qd × 6 weeks	250 mg qd × 12 weeks
Itraconazole	200 mg bid for 1 week of month × 2 months	200 mg bid for 1 week of month × 3 months

qd, once a day; bid, twice a day.

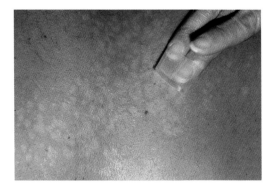

Figure 8-30 Tape collection of scale, tinea versicolor

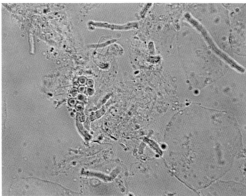

Figure 8-31 Tinea versicolor

affected, suggesting a possible familial disposition to overgrowth of this member of the normal skin flora. The yeast involved utilizes sebum as an energy source, and hence, the condition is more common on the superior trunk where sebum secretion is high. Most lesions are asymptomatic, although some patients will complain of pruritus. Azelaic acid derivatives secreted by the yeast interfere with melanin synthesis and packaging, resulting in patches of decreased pigmentation in affected skin. Tanning accentuates the color difference.

Diagnosis/differential diagnosis

Key Points

* The diagnosis of pityriasis versicolor is usually based on the clinical presentation and history
* Microscopic examination with KOH may be performed using a skin scraping, or alternatively, by touching the lesions with clear cellophane tape and then removing it ("tape stripping"; see Figure 8-30)
* Either KOH or methylene blue may be used to stain the specimen and identification of short hyphae and clusters of round yeast ("spaghetti and meat-balls") confirms the diagnosis (Figure 8-31)

The hypopigmentation macules of pityriasis versicolor can be confused with vitiligo. Unlike vitiligo, in which lesions are completely depigmented, lesions of pityriasis versicolor are only hypopigmented.

Pityriasis versicolor is distinguished from tinea by the lack of inflammation, the absence of central clearing, and the presence of yeast with short hyphae on KOH examination. Rarely, extensive cases of pityriasis versicolor have been confused with the islands of sparing in pityriasis rubra pilaris, but in this situation a KOH or biopsy allows for discrimination.

Treatment

Key Points

* A wide variety of treatments exist for pityriasis versicolor
* Patients with limited disease may be treated with the twice-daily application of a topical antifungal agent, such as an imidazole
* Patients may also be affordably treated with selenium sulfide 2.5% lotion (or over-the-counter 1% shampoo) applied to the skin for 10–30 minutes/day for 7–14 days or overnight once per month
* Topic zinc pyrithione and benzoyl peroxide bars have also been used
* Oral ketoconazole is an effective treatment for extensive pityriasis versicolor

There are nearly as many treatments for pityriasis versicolor as there are patients with the condition. Many medical regimens are effective in controlling the condition, but a "cure" is achieved in only 80–90% of cases. Recurrences are common and can be expected. Intermittent use of selenium sulfide or ketoconazole shampoo 2 or 3 times weekly may decrease the relapse rate by reducing the number of organisms colonizing the scalp; it can also be used as a body wash, but can be irritating for some patients.

Oral ketoconazole has historically been considered one of the most effective off-label treatments for extensive pityriasis versicolor. Ketoconazole 400 mg is taken as a single dose, followed in 90 minutes by physical activity to induce sweating. The sweat is allowed to dry and remain on the skin for 8 hours. Ketoconazole has a 1:50 000 risk of fulminant hepatic necrosis. Itraconazole (100 mg orally bid for 7–10 days) is also used, but is more expensive. Longer courses of therapy are needed because the drug is not delivered in eccrine sweat. Appropriate questioning regarding hepatitis or liver disease, although rare in the generally youthful population affected by pityrosporum versicolor, is essential prior to oral treatment.

Chromoblastomycosis (Chromomycosis)

Clinical presentation

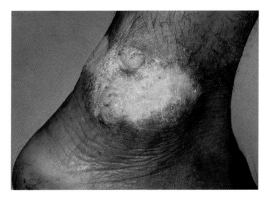

Figure 8-32 Chromomycosis

Key Points

- Chromoblastomycosis is a fungal infection by species of the genus *Cladosporium*, *Phialophora*, *Rhinocladiella*, or *Fonsecaea*
- These fungal species independently produce a melanin-based pigment, hence the name *chromoblastomycosis*
- Chromoblastomycosis is most often an infection of agricultural workers, particularly men, living in tropical and subtropical regions
- It is believed the fungus is introduced into the skin via traumatic implantation from splinters or other plant matter
- The lower leg and distal upper extremities are most often involved

Following implantation, an erythematous papule develops at the site of inoculation. Lesions of chromoblastomycosis progress slowly over many years to form a nodule or plaque (Figure 8-32). Chromoblastomycosis is often quite verrucous in appearance, and lesions spread laterally to involve contiguous healthy tissue. On the surface of the lesions, minute black dots may be observed, and are indicative of areas with a high number of pigmented fungal organisms. Purulent discharge is also a common feature.

Diagnosis/differential diagnosis

Key Points

- The diagnosis of chromoblastomycosis is made by biopsy, with histologic sections revealing pigmented, double-walled, refractile spores ("Medlar bodies" or "copper pennies") within the tissue

Histologic analysis of chromoblastomycosis often demonstrates significant pseudoepitheliomatous hyperplasia of the epidermis, and this correlates with the verrucous clinical appearance of the lesions. Pigmented fungal elements are often concentrated near neutrophilic abscesses within the acanthotic areas or in the underlying dermis.

Because the organisms produce melanin, they may often be located without special stains, but performance of a Fontana–Mason stain highlights melanin production within the spores.

Treatment

Key Points

- Chromoblastomycosis is best treated with a combination of surgical excision and prolonged courses of oral itraconoazole (200 mg orally bid)

Sporotrichosis

Clinical presentation

Key Points

- Sporotrichosis is an infection of the deep tissue caused by the dimorphic fungus *Sporothrix schenckii*
- *S. schenckii* is ubiquitous in the environment and most often infects farmers, gardeners, and horticulturists ("rose gardener's disease")
- Sporotrichosis classically spreads along ascending lymphatics; this pattern in other illness is called "sporotrichoid" spread

Following traumatic implantation, usually on the distal upper extremity, an erythematous papule develops within 1–10 weeks. Lymphangitic spread can lead to formation of secondary lesions that extend proximally along lines of lymphatic drainage. Fixed forms of disease may also result. Widespread dissemination of sporotrichosis may occur in immunosuppressed patients, particularly those with HIV/AIDS.

Diagnosis/differential diagnosis

Key Points

- The diagnosis of sporotrichosis is typically made by tissue culture
- *S. schenckii* grows rapidly, with most cultures yielding positive results within 1–2 weeks

While the clinical appearance and history may strongly suggest the diagnosis of sporotrichosis, tissue culture is the best diagnostic test. It is difficult to visualize the organism in histologic sections, even with special stains. The inability to visualize the organism in a biopsy does not exclude the diagnosis. Occasionally, cigar-shaped yeast or an extracellular asteroid body may be observed, but this is exceptional. Furthermore, the characteristic pattern of lymphangitic extension ("sporotrichoid spread") can occur in other diseases, including mycobacterial infections, cat-scratch disease, tularemia, nocardiosis, and leishmaniasis.

Treatment

Key Points

* Most cases of sporotrichosis are best treated with oral itraconoazole (100–200 mg orally bid × 3–6 months)
* Supersaturated solution of potassium iodide (SSKI) represents an older alternative treatment, but often produces significant gastrointestinal distress
* Disseminated cases are treated with intravenous amphotericin B

Histoplasmosis

Clinical presentation

Key Points

* Histoplasmosis refers to a broad category of fungal infections caused by the dimorphic fungus *Histoplasma capsulatum*
* *H. capsulatum* is found throughout the world, but is particularly prevalent in the Ohio, Missouri, and Mississippi river valleys
* Soil contaminated by bird droppings and bat guano is highly infectious

Exposure to histoplasmosis typically occurs by inhalation of aerosolized conidia. Most infected individuals are asymptomatic, but later may develop a small granuloma within the lungs. A minority of patients develop clinically evident disease. Typically, these patients are immunocompromised (HIV/AIDS) or have been exposed to large inocula (spelunkers in caves). Disseminated histoplasmosis may involve the reticular system, the bone marrow, the nervous system, or the skin. Cutaneous lesions are present in only about 10% of patients of all cases. Maculopapular eruptions, skin ulcerations, or oropharyngeal lesions may be observed.

Diagnosis/differential diagnosis

Key Points

* The easiest way to diagnose cutaneous involvement in disseminated histoplasmosis is with a skin biopsy for histologic assessment and culture
* Tissue specimens from lesions of histoplasmosis reveal small monomorphic yeast within macrophages
* Blood cultures are positive in 50–90% of patients with acute progressive disseminated histoplasmosis
* Serum *Histoplasma* antigen can also be useful for diagnosis

Mucosal and palatal lesions of histoplasmosis often resemble Kaposi's sarcoma, a neoplastic condition that, like histoplasmosis, often affects immunocompromised patients. The histopathology of cutaneous histoplasmosis is similar to that of cutaneous leishmaniasis; however, the yeast forms of histoplasmosis are smaller and lack a kinetoplast common to amastigotes of leishmaniasis.

Treatment

Key Points

* The finding of cutaneous histoplasmosis is presumptive evidence of systemic involvement, including the bone marrow and reticuloendothelial system, and consultation with infectious disease experts is strongly recommended
* Patients with disseminated histoplasmosis are treated with intravenous liposomal amphotericin B, followed by oral itraconazole as a maintenance medication

North American blastomycosis

Clinical presentation

Key Points

* North American blastomycosis (Gilchrist's disease) is an unusual fungal infection caused by the dimorphic fungus *Blastomyces dermatitidis*
* *B. dermatitidis* is particularly prevalent in the southeastern United States and the Great Lakes region
* North American blastomycosis has been associated with exposure to beaver dams and is a common fungal infection of dogs

Exposure to *B. dermatitidis* occurs through inhalation of aerosolized conidia. While the infection may begin in the lungs, blastomycosis disseminates widely in about 50% of cases. Those with immunocompromised states or chronic health issues may be predisposed to dissemination. The skin is the most common extrapulmonary site of infection, with involvement in 20–40% of disseminated cases. Other common sites of involvement include the bones (10–25%), prostate and genitourinary organs (5–15%), and the central nervous system (~5%).

In cutaneous blastomycosis, nonspecific lesions usually develop upon the face, neck, and extremities. Early in the course of disease, the lesions may exist as papules or pustules. Later lesions may be verrucous in appearance, and ultimately scarring may develop.

Clinical presentation

Key Points

- Histologic examination of blastomycosis reveals yeasts of 8–20 μm in diameter, with broad-based buds and doubly refractile walls
- Culture may confirm the diagnosis and is particularly useful when microscopic examination fails to reveal budding yeast forms

The finding of broad-based yeast forms in tissue sections may allow an experienced pathologist to distinguish blastomycosis from other yeast infections, particularly *Cryptococcus*, which exhibits narrow-based budding. However, budding may be missed depending upon the plane of section and, for this reason, tissue culture may be needed to clarify the diagnosis.

Treatment

Key Points

- Patients with severe blastomycosis, including central nervous system involvement, should be treated with high-dose intravenous amphotericin B
- Oral itraconazole (200 mg orally bid) is the drug of choice for mild to moderate disease
- Prolonged treatment may be necessary in patients with fungal osteomyelitis

Cryptococcosis

Clinical presentation

Key Points

- Cryptococcosis is a fungal infection caused by the encapsulated yeast, *Cryptococcus neoformans*
- In the United States, cryptococcus is associated with pigeon excrement
- Cryptococcosis is almost always a systemic infection that begins in the lungs before disseminating widely; however, the skin is affected in only about 10% of cases

Four serotypes of cryptococcus exist: serotypes A and D (*C. neoformans var. neoformans*), and serotypes B and C (*C. neoformans var. gattii*). Serotypes A and D are most common in the United States, and are the types associated with pigeon excrement. Worldwide, serotype A causes most cryptococcal infections in immunocompromised patients, particularly those infected with HIV.

Diagnosis/differential diagnosis

Key Points

- Serologic studies are the most expedient test to diagnose systemic cryptococcosis
- Tissue biopsy of cutaneous cryptococcosis reveals one of two general histological patterns:
  - A pauci-inflammatory mucoid form
  - A granulomatous inflammatory form
- Visualized yeast appears pleomorphic with a surrounding halo, which represents the remnants of the mucoid capsule

The mucoid capsule common to *Cryptococcus* species stains with mucicarmine, while the fungal wall itself highlights with PAS staining. Cutaneous lesions of cryptococcosis in HIV/AIDS patients can resemble molluscum, another disease common in this population. A cryptococcosis variant that mimics cellulitis is also well described in immunocompromised patients.

Treatment

Key Points

- Because cryptococcosis is a systemic infection, consultation with an infectious disease expert is recommended
- A lumbar puncture is indicated to rule out central nervous system disease in all patients, even in the absence of symptoms
- Intravenous amphotericin B, chronic therapy with fluconazole, and even therapeutic lumbar puncture may be utilized in treatment

Coccidioidomycosis

Key Points

- Endemic to the desert southwest and San Joaquin valley
- Histology demonstrates large granular spores with a refractile wall
- Never attempt to culture in the office, as culture plates will develop easily aerosolized arthrospores that are highly infectious

Coccidioidomycosis (Figure 8-33) is caused by the dimorphic fungus, *Coccidioides immitis*. Infections are particularly associated with the Sonoran desert region. Valley fever is typically a self-limited infection, but some ethnic groups, including Blacks, Hispanics, and Filipinos, are more prone to dissemination. Skin lesions are usually the result of dissemination from a pulmonary focus. Skin testing and complement fixation titers may be of benefit in establishing the diagnosis and guiding therapy. Those with disseminated disease may require treatment with fluconazole, oral itraconazole, or intravenous amphotericin B.

Hyalohyphomycosis (Aspergillosis and fusariosis)

Key Points

- Important causes of fungal sepsis in immuno-compromised hosts
- Often presents with crusted eschars, as the vasculotropic fungus leads to vessel obstruction and damage with resultant tissue necrosis
- Histology demonstrates thin-walled, narrow hyphae with bubbly cytoplasm

Hyalohyphomycosis is seen in patients with neutropenia. Voriconazole is currently the drug of choice for disseminated aspergillosis.

Phaeohyphomycosis

Key Points

- Important causes of invasive skin infection (Figure 8-34) and fungal sepsis in immunocompromised hosts
- Presents with localized "cysts" and tinea nigra (Figure 8-35) in immunocompetent hosts
- Histology demonstrates thick-walled, septate hyphae with bubbly cytoplasm

Itraconazole has been used most often, but antifungal therapy is unreliable.

Mucormycosis

Key Points

- Diabetic patients, particularly those in ketoacidosis, are particularly susceptible
- Presentation often involves the central face with edema and tissue necrosis
- Histology demonstrates thick-walled, broad, red, hollow hyphae

Mucormycosis refers to infection with any zygomycete. *Rhizopus* is the most common organism, but various species of *Rhizomucor*, *Absidia*, and *Mucor* have been implicated. Treatment is primarily surgical, although posaconazole shows some activity.

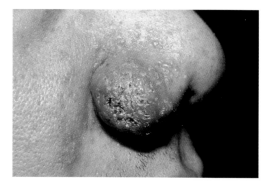

Figure 8-33 Coccidioidomycosis (courtesy of Dr. Larry Anderson)

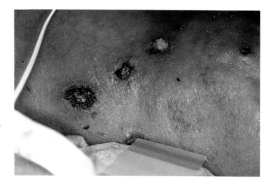

Figure 8-34 Phaeohyphomycosis

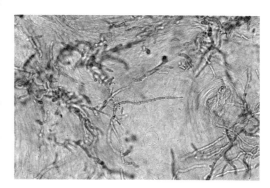

Figure 8-35 Tinea nigra, potassium hydroxide preparation

Further reading

DiCaudo DJ. Coccidioidomycosis: a review and update. J Am Acad Dermatol 2006;55:929–942.

Elston DM. Community-acquired methicillin-resistant *Staphylococcus aureus*. J Am Acad Dermatol 2007;56:1–16.

Gabillot-Carre M, Roujeau JC. Acute bacterial skin infections and cellulitis. Curr Opin Infect Dis 2007;20:118–123.

Hankin A, Everett WW. Are antibiotics necessary after incision and drainage of a cutaneous abscess? Ann Emerg Med 2007;50:49–51.

Hay RJ. *Fusarium* infections of the skin. Curr Opin Infect Dis 2007;20:115–117.

Hirschmann JV. Antimicrobial therapy for skin infections. Cutis 2007;79(Suppl):26–36.

Johnson RP, Xia Y, Cho S, et al. *Mycobacterium marinum* infection: a case report and review of the literature. Cutis 2007;79:33–36.

Jones S, Kress D. Treatment of molluscum contagiosum and herpes simplex virus cutaneous infections. Cutis 2007;79(Suppl):11–17.

Kravitz SR, McGuire JB, Sharma S. The treatment of diabetic foot ulcers: reviewing the literature and a surgical algorithm. Adv Skin Wound Care 2007;20:227–237.

Sims CR, Ostrosky-Zeichner L. Contemporary treatment and outcomes of zygomycosis in a non-oncologic tertiary care center. Arch Med Res 2007;38:90–93.

Dermatologic conditions of pregnancy

9

Lisa C. Edsall and Julia R. Nunley

Introduction

A variety of dermatologic conditions occur during pregnancy, many of which are the result of immunologic, hormonal, and metabolic changes unique to gestation. Whereas pregnancy-induced physiologic changes affect almost all pregnant women, a subset of inflammatory pruritic disorders specifically classified as the dermatoses of pregnancy are less common. Other conditions have been incorrectly attributed to pregnancy; these are actually primary cutaneous diseases that may be influenced by the pregnant milieu. Although this chapter will outline all of these alterations, the dermatoses of pregnancy will be highlighted because of potential maternal and fetal risk.

PHYSIOLOGIC SKIN CHANGES DURING PREGNANCY

Key Points

- Affect most pregnancies
- Hyperpigmentation is most common
- Many reverse postpartum
- No adverse fetal outcomes
- Biopsy of a suspicious mole should not be delayed because of pregnancy

Pregnancy-induced physiologic skin changes, outlined in Box 9-1, include a wide array of pigmentary, vascular, glandular, and miscellaneous alterations that occur in nearly every pregnancy. Precise physiologic mechanisms remain speculative because of the multitude and variable fluctuation of hormones throughout pregnancy. Since most resolve postpartum, there is little need for study or treatment.

Pigmentary changes

Hyperpigmentation occurs in 90% of pregnancies. Theoretically, placental lipids stimulate melanin production by upregulating tyrosinase activity. Areolae are uniformly involved, whereas other sites are variably so (Table 9-1; Figure 9-1). Darkening develops within the first trimester and fades after childbirth. However, pigment-prone areas such as the areolae, nipples, and genitalia may not return to their prepregnancy color. Pigmentary demarcation lines (lines of Voigt or Futcher; Figure 9-2) may also become more evident in pregnancy.

Melasma affects 50–75% of pregnant women, most commonly in a centrofacial distribution (Figure 9-3). Pregnancy is only one of the factors associated with melasma (Box 9-2). The high prevalence of melasma in both pregnant and nonpregnant women on oral contraceptives supports a pathogenic role for estrogens. Treatment should be delayed until after delivery since the color may fade spontaneously and the safety of hypopigmenting agents in pregnancy has not been established.

Vascular and hematologic changes

Several hormones, including an adrenocorticotropic hormone-like substance, human chorionic gonadotropin, luteinizing hormone-releasing hormone, and thyrotropin-releasing hormone most likely contribute to the production of the pregnancy-associated vascular changes. These hormones induce blood volume expansion, increase intravascular pressure, and stimulate vessel proliferation, causing the conditions outlined in Table 9-2.

Neoplasms

A variety of neoplasms, most of which are benign, can develop or proliferate during pregnancy (Box 9-3). Pyogenic granulomas (Figure 9-4) are the most common, appearing in up to 27% of women between the second and fifth months of pregnancy. Believed to be a result of hormonally induced capillary proliferation, pyogenic granulomas often regress spontaneously postpartum. Treatment during pregnancy may be needed because of bleeding and pain.

BOX 9-1

Physiologic skin changes in pregnancy

Pigmentary changes
    Hyperpigmentation
    Melasma
Vascular and hematologic changes
    Varicosities
    Palmar erythema
    Spider angiomas
    Purpura
    Cutis marmorata
    Edema
    Unilateral nevoid telangiectasia
Cutaneous neoplasms
Striae distensae
Glandular activity
    Eccrine
    Apocrine
    Sebaceous
Hair changes
Nail changes
Mucosal changes
    Gingivitis and periodontitis
    Vascular changes

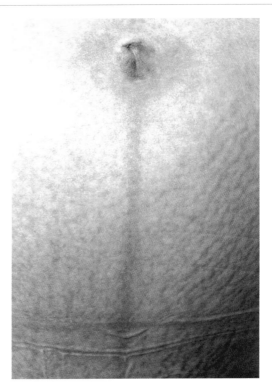

Figure 9-1 Darkening of the linea alba occurs in approximately one-third of pregnant women

Table 9-1 Prevalence of pregnancy-induced hyperpigmentation

Sites	Prevalence (%)
Areolae	100
Genitalia	49
Linea alba	35
Generalized hypermelanosis	32
Neck	20
Axillae	4.7
Scar pigmentation	4
Darkening of freckles	1.5
Pigmentary demarcation lines (Voigt or Futcher lines)	Rare reports

Some patients describe the abrupt development of numerous dermatofibromas and molluscum gravidarum (skin tags). Vascular tumors are less common. Hemangiomas, hemangioendotheliomas, and glomangiomas are reported in approximately 5% of pregnancies, appearing as subcutaneous nodules during the second or

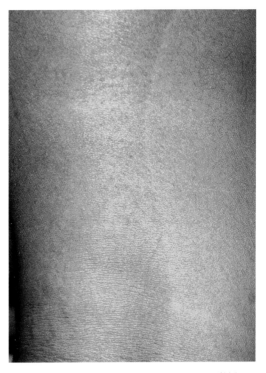

Figure 9-2 Pigmentary demarcation lines (lines of Voigt or Futcher) can be more evident during pregnancy

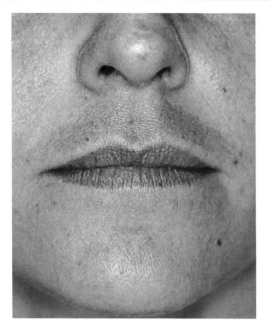

Figure 9-3 Melasma appears as patchy hyperpigmentation, most commonly in a centrofacial distribution

---

BOX 9-2

Factors associated with the development of melasma

Ultraviolet B therapy

Sunlight/lack of sunscreen use

Hormonal contraception methods

Hormone replacement

Increased parity

Family history

Skin phototype III to VI

Dark eye and hair color

Increased freckling tendency

Pregnancy

BOX 9-3

Neoplasms associated with pregnancy

Pyogenic granuloma

Molluscum fibrosum gravidarum

Dermatofibromas

Eruptive collagenomas

Hemangiomas

Hemangioendotheliomas

Anetoderma of Jadassohn

Desmoid tumors

Glomus tumors

Neurofibromas

Leiomyomas

Keloids

Dermatofibrosarcoma protuberans

---

third trimesters. They may increase in size until delivery.

The influence of pregnancy on melanocytic lesions remains controversial. Beliefs that nevi were more likely to become malignant and that a melanoma developing during pregnancy had a worse prognosis were based entirely on case reports and uncontrolled studies. Although there are reports of histological atypia developing in nevi during pregnancy, most of the recent information suggests that pregnancy neither impacts major changes in nevi, nor affects the prognosis of melanoma. However, in the past, erroneous interpretation that color and size changes were physiologic may have delayed the diagnosis of melanoma, allowing progression to a greater stage. Current data suggest that melanoma prognosis is not affected by pregnancy; prognosis is based, as in nongravid women, on the stage of disease at time of diagnosis. It is now recommended that the exact same standards for excising nevi be applied to all patients regardless of pregnancy. Biopsy of a changing or atypical-appearing nevus should never be delayed because of pregnancy.

Patients with melanoma often seek advice about future pregnancy and contraceptive choices. No evidence consistently links estrogen or other hormones to melanoma, therefore neither subsequent pregnancy nor hormonal contraceptives are contraindicated. It is not necessary to delay subsequent pregnancy following excision of a thin, early-stage melanoma; however, a delay of 2–3 years would be reasonable in a patient with high risk for recurrence, since most recurrences occur within this time frame.

Striae

Striae distensae may be the most prominent and concerning cutaneous consequence of pregnancy (Figure 9-5). Linear, violaceous, atrophic bands develop most commonly on the abdomen and proximal extremities beginning at the end of the second trimester. Occurring in close to 90% of Caucasian women, striae are unusual in Asian or African American women. Development is influenced by numerous factors (Box 9-4). Although bland emollients are strongly recommended to pregnant women, pre-emptive therapy has not been definitively shown to prevent the formation of striae. Unfortunately postpartum treatment

Table 9-2 Vascular and hematologic changes associated with pregnancy

Condition	Prevalence	Clinical appearance	Location	Comments	Treatment
Varicosities	Affects 40% of pregnancies Presents late in first trimester	Swollen, congested vessels	Lower extremities, rectum, vulva, vagina, and vestibule	10% risk of thrombosis	Leg elevation, Trendelenburg or lateral decubitus sleeping position Typically regresses postpartum
Palmar erythema	Affects 66% of Caucasians and 35% of African-Americans Presents in second month of pregnancy but incidence increases until delivery	Diffuse mottled erythema	Uniform involvement of thenar/hypothenar eminences with sparing of digits	If persists postpartum, evaluate for other causes	Generally resolves within 1–7 weeks postpartum
Spider angiomas	Affects 66% of Caucasians and 10% of African-Americans Presents in first to second trimesters	Central arteriole with radiating vessels and surrounding erythema	Upper chest, arms, hands, face, neck	If persist postpartum, evaluate for liver disease	Spontaneous resolution within 3 months postpartum; 10% may persist
Purpura/ petechiae	Prevalence unknown Presents in second half of pregnancy	Small purpuric macules or papules	Most commonly on lower extremities	If persist postpartum, evaluate for vasculitis	Postpartum resolution
Cutis marmorata	Prevalence unknown Appears any time during pregnancy	Mottled bluish, reticulated discoloration	Most commonly on lower extremities	Common after cold exposure Rare venous occlusion leading to phlegmasia alba dolens and phlegmasia cerulean dolens	Postpartum resolution
Edema	Lower-extremity edema in 70% of pregnancies; eyelid edema in 50% Appears during the third trimester	Nonpitting and pitting edema	Lower extremities, eyelids, and hands	Must exclude cardiac, nephrogenic, hepatic and pre-eclamptic edema	Leg elevation Reduction in salt intake Diuretic use is controversial; may be used in severe cases for short periods Postpartum resolution
Unilateral nevoid telangiectasia	Rare Appears any time during pregnancy	Patches of superficial, blanchable telangiectasia in a unilateral linear distribution	Most commonly affects cervical dermatomes (C3–C7)	May appear for first time in later pregnancies	Postpartum resolution May recur with subsequent pregnancies or hormone therapy

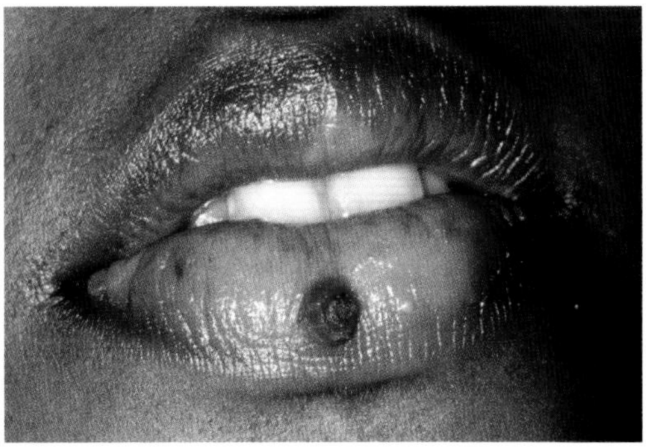

Figure 9-4 Pyogenic granulomas occur commonly in pregnancy and may affect the oral mucosa

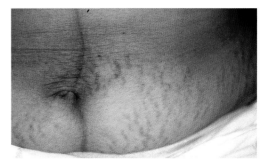

Figure 9-5 Stretch marks (striae) are most common in patients with excessive or rapid weight gain

also has limited benefits; options include topical tretinoin or laser.

Glandular activity

Alterations in glandular activity are well documented throughout pregnancy. Apocrine activity decreases whereas both eccrine and sebaceous gland activities increase. Affected conditions are listed in Table 9-3. Although acne typically correlates with sebaceous gland activity, its course is entirely unpredictable during pregnancy. Treatment options are limited due to unacceptable fetal risk from most oral medications and the lack of information regarding fetal risk of topical treatments (Table 9-4).

Hair changes

Pregnancy-associated hair changes, summarized in Table 9-5, are primarily a result of hormonal effects on the hair cycle. Theoretically, estrogen increases the proportion of the anagen-to-telogen ratio. Prolongation of anagen results in hair retention, causing thicker, more luxurious hair during pregnancy. The abrupt postpartum decrease in estrogen drops this ratio back to normal, shifting these recruited hairs back to telogen. Hair shedding (telogen effluvium) begins 2–3 months after delivery and typically lasts 1–5 months, although it may continue up to 1 year. This "normalization" of the hair cycle may overshoot and hair loss may exceed that which was retained. However, complete regrowth generally occurs within 15 months. Incomplete hair growth may be due to an underlying female-pattern alopecia.

Pregnancy can also trigger hirsutism and patterned hair loss. Excessive hair growth is most common on the face, although the limbs and back may also be affected. Frontoparietal recession and even diffuse thinning can develop late in pregnancy. Both conditions are attributed to

BOX 9-4

Factors affecting the development of striae

Caucasian heritage

Degree of abdominal distension during pregnancy

Younger age

Excessive or rapid maternal weight gain

Family history

Hormonal changes (estradiols, adrenocorticosteroids, relaxin)

Table 9-3 Pregnancy-induced glandular effects

Gland	Activity	Associated conditions
Eccrine	Increased	Hyperhidrosis
		Miliaria
Apocrine	Decreased	Improvement in Fox–Fordyce disease
		Improvement in hidradenitis suppurativa
Sebaceous	Increased	Hypertrophy of areolar sebaceous glands (Montgomery tubercles)
		Variable effect on acne

hormonal fluctuations since hair growth typically normalizes after delivery.

Nail changes

The rate of nail growth typically increases early in pregnancy then slows postpartum. Other reported nail changes are listed in Box 9-5. Longitudinal melanonychia that appears during pregnancy and fades spontaneously postpartum may be another manifestation of hyperpigmentaion. Persistence of nail changes postpartum should trigger an investigation of other diseases such as psoriasis, lichen planus, and fungal infections.

Table 9-4 Medications commonly prescribed by dermatologists

Medication	Food and Drug Administration pregnancy prescribing category*	Special considerations
Topical acne preparations		
Azelaic acid	B	
Benzoyl peroxide	C	May be systemically absorbed
		Minor risk can not be excluded
Clindamycin	B	
Erythromycin	B	
Metronidazole	B	
Adapalene	C	It is not known if adapalene crosses the placenta
Tazarotene	X	Pregnancy testing indicated before initial prescription
Tretinoin	C	Possible retinoic acid embryopathy congenital malformations associated with first-trimester use
Anesthetics		
Lidocaine	B	No contraindications with limited use
Lidocaine with epinephrine	B	No contraindications with limited use
Lidocaine with prilocaine	B	Less data available than above anesthetics
Antibiotics – oral		
Azithromycin	B	Avoid in first trimester; possible associations with congenital malformations
		No adverse fetal effects reported during second- and third-trimester use
Cephalexin	B	Possible risk of congenital malformations during first-trimester use of cephalosporins
Clindamycin	Oral: B	No adverse fetal effects reported to date
	Topical: B	
Erythromycin	Oral: B	Oral form in early pregnancy may be associated with fetal cardiovascular defects
	Topical: B	Avoid estolate salt of erythromycin since use has been associated with maternal hepatotoxicity
Fluoroquinolones	C	
Penicillins	C	
Sulfonamides	C	
Tetracyclines	D	Fetal dental anomalies when used during second and third trimester
		Possible risk of decreased fetal bone growth and maternal liver toxicity
Antibiotics – topical		
Bacitracin	C	No adverse fetal effects reported to date
		No large studies conducted
Mupirocin	B	No adverse fetal effects reported to date
		No larger studies conducted
Neomycin	Unrated	No adverse fetal effects reported to date
Polymyxin B	B	No adverse fetal effects reported to date
Silver sulfadiazine	B	Theoretical risk of kernicterus and hemorrhage in infant with glucose-6-phosphate dehydrogenase deficiency
Topical sulfur	C	

Table 9-4 Medications commonly prescribed by dermatologists—cont'd

Medication	Food and Drug Administration pregnancy prescribing category*	Special considerations
Antifungals		
Clotrimazole	B	
Fluconazole	C	Single or low dose, risk is unlikely
		Continuous daily dose of >400 mg/day may be teratogenic
Griseofulvin	C	Possible association with congenital malformations and fetal death
Ketoconazole	C	No adverse fetal effects reported to date with topical use
		Oral form should be avoided in first trimester as it may impair progesterone secretion and implantation
Miconazole	C	Reported to cause toxicity in animal studies
Naftifine	B	No adverse fetal effects reported to date with topical use
Nystatin	C	No adverse fetal effects reported to date with topical use
Selenium sulfide	C	
Terbinafine	B	No adverse human fetal affects reported to date with topical or oral use
Antihistamines		Avoidance of antihistamines during the last 2 weeks of pregnancy is advised for presumed risk of retrolental fibroplasia
Cetirizine	B	
Chlorpheniramine	B	May be oral antihistamine of choice during pregnancy
Cyproheptadine	B	Human data limited
Diphenhydramine	B	May be antihistamine of choice for parenteral use during pregnancy
Doxepin	Oral: C	
	Topical: B	
Fexofenadine	C	
Hydroxyzine	C	Per manufacturer, early trimester use is contraindicated secondary to lack of clinical data
Loratadine	B	Avoid first-trimester use
Antiscabietics and antipediculocides		
Ivermectin	C	No adverse human fetal effects reported to date
		Teratogenic in high doses in animal studies
Lindane	B	Possible association with hypospadia
Permethrin	B	No adverse fetal effects reported to date
Antivirals		
Acyclovir	Topical: B	No adverse human fetal affects reported with topical or oral use
	Oral: B	May reduce mortality of disseminated viral infection
		Best studied antiviral
Famciclovir	B	Causes benign tumors in animal studies
		No adverse human fetal effects reported to date
Valacyclovir	B	No adverse human fetal effects reported to date
Corticosteroids		
Prednisone	C	First-trimester use may result in orofacial clefts
		Fetal immunosuppression if high dose given throughout pregnancy

Continued

Table 9-4 Medications commonly prescribed by dermatologists—cont'd

Medication	Food and Drug Administration pregnancy prescribing category*	Special considerations
Topical corticosteroids	C	Limited use not thought to be of significant risk to fetus
		Excessive use during pregnancy theoretically associated with low birth weight
Immunomodulators and immunosuppressants		
Adalimumab	B	No adverse human fetal affects reported to date
		A pregnancy directory has been established
Azathioprine	D	May cause fetal immunosuppression and intrauterine growth retardation
		May interfere with intrauterine contraceptive device
Cyclosporine	C	Poses a risk for intrauterine growth retardation
Etanercept	B	No adverse human fetal affects reported to date
		A pregnancy directory has been established
Imiquimod	B	Suprapharmacologic doses in animals have been associated with low birth weight
Infliximab	B	No adverse human fetal affects reported to date
		A pregnancy directory has been established
Mycophenolate mofetil	C	Fetal structural defects reported in animal studies
		Caution advised for use during pregnancy
Pimecrolimus	C	No adverse human fetal affects reported to date with topical use
		Although scientific data is insufficient, a Public Health Advisory has been issued regarding a potential risk of lymphoma after topical use
Tacrolimus	Topical: C Oral: C	No adverse human fetal effects reported to date with topical use
		Although scientific data are insufficient, a Public Health Advisory has been issued regarding a potential risk of lymphoma after topical use
		Oral use has been associated with an increase in fetal toxicity and teratogenicity in animal studies
		Oral use may be associated with human fetal growth retardation, prematurity, renal toxicity, and hyperkalemia
Miscellaneous drugs/therapies		
Calcipotriene	C	Skeletal abnormalities shown in animal studies
		Approximately 6% systemic absorption when applied to psoriatic plaques
		A pregnancy directory has been established
Coal tar	C	Known carcinogen and mutagen
		Topical use associated with systemic uptake
		No human studies
Cholestyramine	B	May reduce vitamin K absorption
Dapsone	C	Has been successfully used in pregnant patients with leprosy and dermatitis herpetiformis
		May worsen maternal anemia
		Theoretic risk of neonatal kernicterus or methemoglobinemia when used during last month of pregnancy
Hydroquinones	C	No human studies

Table 9-4 Medications commonly prescribed by dermatologists—cont'd

Medication	Food and Drug Administration pregnancy prescribing category*	Special considerations
Hydroxychloroquine	C	Because it has a prolonged half-life, discontinuation when pregnant will not eliminate fetal exposure
		Flair of systemic lupus after discontinuation may adversely affect pregnancy
Isotretinoin	X	Avoid conception for at least 1 month after discontinuation
Menthol	Unrated	
Ultraviolet B	Unrated	No adverse human fetal affects reported with use during pregnancy
		Maternal hyperthermia increases the risk of fetal neural tube defects
Permethrin	B	
Pramoxine	C	
Psoralen and ultraviolet A	C	Psoralen is a potential teratogen, although risk of adverse human fetal effects is unknown
		Maternal hyperthermia increases the risk of fetal neural tube defects
Ursodeoxycholic acid	B	May decrease premature labor, fetal distress, and mortality

*See Table 9-9 for explanation of Food and Drug Administration pregnancy prescribing category definitions.

Table 9-5 Hair changes due to pregnancy

Condition	Clinical presentation	Resolution	Comments	Treatment
Hirsutism	Occurs early in pregnancy with increased hair on upper lips, cheeks, chin, and mid suprapubic area	Typically regresses by 6 months postpartum	Favors women with dark, thick hair	Shaving, electrolysis, laser
Telogen effluvium	Occurs 1–5 months postpartum with diffuse hair loss and thinning	Regrowth is generally noted within 15 months postpartum	Incomplete regrowth may unmask female-pattern alopecia	Evaluate for other causes of alopecia if persistent postpartum
Androgenetic alopecia	Occurs in third trimester with frontoparietal recession and diffuse thinning	Regrowth is generally noted within 15 months postpartum	May be due to pregnancy hormone-induced inhibition of gonadotropic activity	Evaluate for other causes of alopecia if persistent postpartum

BOX 9-5

Nail changes associated with pregnancy

Transverse grooving (Beau's lines)

Brittle nails

Distal onycholysis

Subungual hyperkeratosis

Longitudinal melanonychia

Mucosal changes

Mucous membrane changes, also very common during pregnancy, are outlined in Table 9-6.

DERMATOSES OF PREGNANCY

Pruritus is common in pregnancy, affecting 17% of all pregnancies due to a myriad of conditions (Table 9-7). Although one of the dermatoses of pregnancy should always be considered, other nonpregnancy-related conditions must first be excluded.

The dermatoses of pregnancy are a group of unrelated, pregnancy-associated disorders that share the common clinical presentation of severe pruritus. Some are merely uncomfortable conditions for the mother, whereas others may adversely affect maternal and fetal outcomes. The paucity of diagnostic laboratory tests and specific

Table 9-6 Mucous membrane changes associated with pregnancy

Condition	Timing	Clinical findings	Pathogenesis	Comments
Gingivitis	First trimester	Enlargement, darkening, and swelling in up to 80% of women	Heightened gingival reactivity to local irritants Pre-existing periodontal disease	2% of patients develop epulis gravidarum on gingiva (histologically indistinguishable from pyogenic granuloma)
Periodontitis	Throughout pregnancy	Dental decay and gum regression	Progesterone-induced inhibition of matrix metalloproteinases Altered salivary composition	Potentially a risk factor for premature rupture of membranes and preterm delivery
Goodell sign	First weeks of pregnancy	Cervical bluish discoloration	Increased vascularity and venous congestion	Early sign of pregnancy
Jacquemier–Chadwick sign	First weeks of pregnancy	Vestibular erythema	Increased vascularity and venous congestion	Early sign of pregnancy

Table 9-7 Pregnancy-associated pruritic disorders

Condition	Frequency
Eczematous eruptions of pregnancy	50%
Atopic dermatitis	
Prurigo of pregnancy (1%)	
Pruritic folliculitis (<1%)	
Pruritic urticarial papules and plaques of pregnancy	22%
Pemphigoid gestationis	4%
Cholestasis of pregnancy	3%
Other	21%
Scabies	
Pediculosis	
Infection	
Neurodermatitis	
Drug eruption	
Contact dermatitis	
Urticaria	
Acne	
Pityrosporum folliculitis	
Psoriasis	

histologic features has made definitive diagnosis and classification of these disorders difficult. As a result, each entity has several names (Table 9-8), complicating the literature. More recent reviews have grouped these entities into four categories, which have been adopted for this chapter. Practical details regarding diagnosis and treatment are summarized in Figure 9-6 and Table 9-8. Pregnancy prescribing guidelines should be consulted before selecting any medication.

Eczematous eruptions of pregnancy

Key Points

- Account for up to 50% of all cases of pregnancy-associated pruritus
- Up to 70% of individuals have an elevated immunoglobulin (Ig) E; up to 90% have a personal or family history of atopy
- Frequently the first occurrence of an eczematous eruption
- No adverse fetal outcome

Recent studies indicate that this is a group of conditions including atopic dermatitis, prurigo of pregnancy, and pruritic folliculitis. These account for nearly one-half of pregnancy-associated pruritic disorders.

Clinical presentation

Although all patients present with papules and excoriations, anatomic sites may vary accordingly. Atopic dermatitis tends to favor flexural sites whereas prurigo of pregnancy appears more commonly on extensor surfaces. Typically, pruritic folliculitis begins on the trunk as follicular-based papules or pustules and may spread centrifugally to involve the extremities. For 80% of patients, this is their first occurrence of an eczematous eruption.

Diagnosis

The multitude of names associated with this condition reflects the difficulty in making the diagnosis. Although not pathognomonic, an elevated IgE can be found in 70% of cases. Intrahepatic cholestasis of pregnancy (ICP) must be excluded.

Pathogenesis

Since these conditions have considerable histological and clinical overlap, a common pathogenesis is suspected. Atopy may be the common

Table 9-8 Dermatoses of pregnancy

	Eczematous eruptions of pregnancy (EEP)	Pruritic urticarial papules and plaques of pregnancy (PUPPP)	Pemphigoid gestationis (PG)	Intrahepatic cholestasis of pregnancy (ICP)
Incidence	1:10 pregnancies	1:160 to 1:300 pregnancies	1:10,000–1:50,000 pregnancies	Wide geographic variability; reported 1:10 to 1:10,000 pregnancies
Other terminology	Atopic dermatitis Prurigo of pregnancy Pruritic folliculitis	Polymorphic eruption of pregnancy Toxic erythema of pregnancy Late-onset prurigo of pregnancy Toxemic rash of pregnancy	Herpes gestationis	Obstetric cholestasis
Theoretical pathogenesis	Pregnancy-induced alteration in the TH1/TH2 cytokine balance to favor a TH2 response	Antigenic stimulation by fetal DNA within maternal skin Physical stress from skin stretching may alter fibroblast activity and connective tissue homeostasis	Aberrant MHC class II placental molecules homologous to BPAG2 stimulate maternal antibody production Immune complex deposition in BMZ with complement activation Increased frequency of HLA-DR3 (60–80%) and HLA-DR4 (52–53%)	Hormonal inhibition of hepatic uptake and protein transport of bile acids, resulting in increased circulating bile acids Increased frequency of HLA-A31, B8 haplotypes
Associations	Family history Personal or family history of atopy >90% meet the clinical criteria for atopic dermatitis according to Hanifin and Rajka	Primiparous women Multiple gestation	Hydatidiform moles Choriocarcinoma Graves disease (11%) Alopecia areata Ulcerative colitis Vitiligo Antithyroid antibodies Hashimoto's thyroiditis Pernicious anemia	Family history Multiple gestation Geographic location (10–14% of pregnancies in Chile; 1.5% in Sweden; 0.02% in USA)
Onset	Any time during pregnancy	Late third trimester or postpartum	Second to third trimester Postpartum flares in 75% of cases (up to 18 months after delivery) Exacerbations triggered by oral contraceptives	Third trimester
Clinical findings	Atopic dermatitis: affects flexural areas Pruritic folliculitis: follicular-based papules or pustules primarily on trunk Prurigo of pregnancy: pruritic papules and nodules, mostly on extremities	Urticarial plaques beginning within striae of abdomen and thighs Periumbilical sparing Rare involvement of palms, soles, or face May have vesicles but no bullae Erythema multiforme-like lesions noted in 20% of cases	Begins as urticarial plaques within the periumbilical area Progression to a generalized bullous eruption Spares the face, mucous membranes, palms, and soles	No primary eruption Skin lesions (excoriations) due to scratching Jaundice in severe cases (<20%)

Continued

Table 9-8 Dermatoses of pregnancy—cont'd

	Eczematous eruptions of pregnancy (EEP)	Pruritic urticarial papules and plaques of pregnancy (PUPPP)	Pemphigoid gestationis (PG)	Intrahepatic cholestasis of pregnancy (ICP)
Laboratory findings	Elevated serum immunoglobulin E in 70% of cases	Decreased serum cortisol inconsistently reported at onset	Biopsy: Subepidermal split with a primarily eosinophilic inflammatory infiltrate DIF: Linear C3 (± IgG) at BMZ IIF: Low-titer IgG variably reported	Increased total serum bile acids (cholic acid, deoxycholic acid, chenodeoxycholic acid) Variably increased conjugated bilirubin, alkaline phosphatase, lipids and hepatic transaminases
Prognosis	No maternal or fetal risk reported	No maternal or fetal risk reported	Small-for-gestational-age newborns Prematurity Neonatal lesions (10%) No reported increase in fetal or maternal mortality	Stillbirth (3.5–15%) Prematurity Maternal postpartum hemorrhage Fetal intracranial hemorrhage
Treatment options*	Emollients Topical antipruritics Topical corticosteroids	Emollients Topical antipruritics Topical corticosteroids Oral corticosteroids	Topical corticosteroids Oral corticosteroids **Postpartum** Cyclophosphamide Pyridoxine Gold Methotrexate Plasmapheresis Chemical oophorectomy Ritrodine IVIg Tetracyclines	Delivery at 38 weeks Rest, low-fat diet Emollients Topical antipruritics Ursodeoxycholic acid Cholestyramine Vitamin K Phenobarbital UVB phototherapy Prolonged oral corticosteroids

MHC, major histocompatibility complex; BPAG2, bullous pemphigoid antigen 2; BMZ, basement membrane zone; HLA, human leukocyte antigens; DIF, direct immunofluorescence; IgG, immunoglobulin G; IIF, indirect immunofluorescence; IVIG, intravenous immunoglobulin; UVB, ultraviolet B light.
*Refer to Tables 9-8 and 9-9 summarizing Food and Drug Administration pregnancy prescribing categories and treatments.

denominator as over 90% have a personal or family history of atopy.

Treatment

Lesions tend to resolve spontaneously within weeks to months postpartum. Treatment is geared toward symptomatic relief with topical emollients, steroids, and antipruritic agents, as well as oral antihistamines.

Controversies

There are no associated maternal or fetal risks in these conditions, although some earlier studies reported low fetal birth weight for patients with pruritic folliculitis. Topical immunomodulators should probably be avoided due to the recent controversy regarding their use.

Pruritic urticarial papules and plaques of pregnancy

Key Points

- Consists of urticarial and polycyclic papules and plaques
- Spares the umbilicus
- May have scattered vesicles, but no bullae
- No adverse fetal outcome

Pruritic urticarial papules and plaques of pregnancy (PUPPP) is the next most common dermatosis

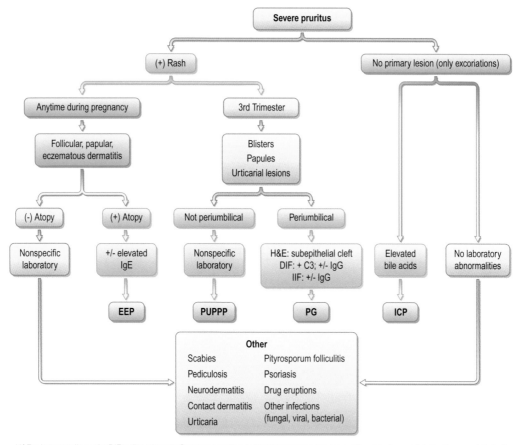

H&E = hematoxylin-eosin; DIF = direct immunofluorescence; III = indirect immunofluorescence; C3 = complement 3; IgG = immunoglobulin G;
IgE = immunoglobulin E; EEP = eczematous eruptions of pregnancy; PUPPP = pruritic urticarial papules and plaques of pregnancy;
PG = pemphigoid gestationis; ICP = intrahepatic cholestasis of pregnancy

Figure 9-6 Diagnostic algorithm for pruritic dermatoses in pregnancy

of pregnancy, generally affecting primiparous or multiple-gestation pregnancies.

Clinical presentation

This eruption consists primarily of urticarial, polycyclic, or targetoid lesions that classically begin within the striae of the abdomen or thighs late in pregnancy (Figure 9-7). Although it may spread down the extremities, the face, palms, and soles are generally spared. Fine vesicles may develop over the surface of the plaques, but frank bullae are not seen. Pruritus is quite severe at onset, but typically lessens after the first week.

Diagnosis

This disorder remains difficult to diagnose as a result of its varied clinical presentations and its lack of specific laboratory, genetic, or histological findings. Periumbilical sparing and lack of bullae help to differentiate PUPPP from pemphigoid gestationis (PG) clinically; histologic features are also dissimilar.

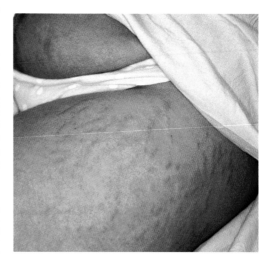

Figure 9-7 Urticarial lesions of pruritic urticarial papules and plaques of pregnancy (PUPPP) typically begin in the striae of the abdomen or thighs

Pathogenesis

No immunologic or human leukocyte antigen (HLA) associations have been found, although the discovery of fetal DNA within maternal skin has triggered speculation by some investigators that PUPPP may be a hypersensitivity reaction. Its association with rapid weight gain and multiple births suggests that abdominal wall stretching may also be a pathogenic factor. A role for pregnancy-associated hormones has also been suggested.

Treatment

Treatment is geared toward symptomatic relief and includes topical antipruritics, steroids, and oral antihistamines. Systemic steroids may be needed in severe cases.

Controversies

Although topical steroid use later in pregnancy poses low fetal risk, frequent or excessive use may worsen the striae associated with pregnancy.

Pemphigoid gestationis

Key Points

- Only dermatosis of pregnancy with well-defined pathogenesis
- Consists of urticarial plaques that eventually develop into bullae
- Begins in the periumbilical area
- May recur with hormonal contraceptive methods
- Mothers are at increased risk for autoimmune disorders, most commonly Graves disease
- 2–10 % of neonates with transient rash; may be small-for-gestational-age

Of the listed dermatoses of pregnancy, only PG has a well-defined pathogenesis.

Clinical presentation

The onset of PG is generally abrupt and may be associated with fever and malaise. Lesions characteristically involve the periumbilical area and spare the face, mucous membranes, palms, and soles. Early lesions consist of intensely pruritic, urticarial papules and plaques; as the eruption progresses, bullae form within these areas (Figure 9-8). Although PG flares at delivery in 75% of cases, it typically resolves quickly thereafter. However, blistering may continue for an additional 2–3 months and rarely up to a year in some patients. Recurrences have been reported with menses, the use of oral contraceptives, and in subsequent pregnancies. Curiously, outbreaks may "skip" pregnancies 8% of the time. Recurrent disease is frequently more severe. Rare cases of PG have reportedly progressed to bullous pemphigoid.

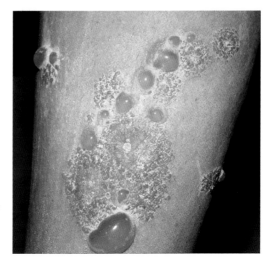

Figure 9-8 Pemphigoid gestationis (courtesy of Martha McCullough, MD)

Diagnosis

Diagnosis is often delayed because early lesions may mimic those of PUPPP. Biopsy demonstrating a subepithelial cleft with linear deposition of C3 by direct immunofluorescence confirms the diagnosis. IgG is variably found within the lesion or in circulation by indirect immunofluorescence.

Pathogenesis

Studies indicate that PG is the result of a circulating IgG antibody that targets bullous pemphigoid antigen 2 (BPAG2) in the epidermis. Speculatively, aberrant major histocompatibility complex (MHC) class II placental structure(s) share homology with BPAG2. Production of a circulating maternal autoantibody to these placental antigens subsequently results in cutaneous blisters. As placental tissue is derived predominantly from a paternal origin, PG hypothetically may be under paternal influence. Maternal immunogenetic predisposition is suspected since 50% of patients have the presence of both HLA-DR3 and HLA-DR4.

Treatment

Treatment typically requires systemic corticosteroids, although mild cases may respond to topical therapy. Severe cases may benefit from plasmapheresis. A variety of other agents have been used for this condition (see Table 9-8); most are utilized postpartum because of fetal risk.

Controversies

Small-for-gestational-age infants and preterm delivery have been reported in patients with PG and may result from placental insufficiency associated with the maternal immunological reaction to placental antigens. There appears to be no increased risk in spontaneous abortions or stillbirths, although 2–10% of newborns may develop a transient rash.

Patients should be advised that use of hormonal contraception may trigger PG. Patients are also at risk for the development of a variety of other autoimmune diseases, most commonly Graves disease.

Intrahepatic cholestasis of pregnancy

Key Points

- Severe itching with no primary skin lesions
- Associated with elevated bile acids
- A significant number of patients have hepatitis C
- Most likely dermatosis of pregnancy to be associated with adverse maternal and fetal outcomes, including maternal postpartum hemorrhage, intracranial fetal hemorrhage, and stillbirth

Of all the dermatoses of pregnancy, ICP is most likely to be linked with adverse maternal and fetal outcomes. Premature labor and meconium staining occur in up to 45% of cases. Stillbirth is reported in 3.5–15% cases. Due to impaired absorption, vitamin K deficiency may result in postpartum maternal hemorrhage and fetal intracranial hemorrhage.

Clinical presentation

ICP typically presents late in pregnancy. Severe pruritus begins on the palms and soles, but may become generalized. There are no primary lesions, although widespread excoriations may be present; only 20–60% of patients develop clinical jaundice, usually within a month of the onset of pruritus. An occasional patient may complain of right upper quadrant discomfort.

Diagnosis

Many patients develop an increase in serum bile acid levels, conjugated bilirubin, alkaline phosphatase, hepatic transaminases, and lipids, although laboratory testing may be normal. In some cases aspartate aminotransaminase may be increased fourfold. Liver ultrasound is normal, and skin biopsy is nondiagnostic.

Pathogenesis

ICP may be a consequence of maternal estrogens interfering with hepatic bile acid secretion affected by genetic, environmental, and hormonal factors. Its prevalence varies widely in accordance with geographic location, affecting 10% of pregnancies in Chile, 1.5% in Sweden, yet only 0.2% in the United States. Uncommon in Asians or African Americans, ICP affects primarily Caucasians. Fifty percent of patients have a positive family history and specific HLA subtypes may be more susceptible. Twin pregnancies tend to increase the risk of ICP, as may maternal coinfection; hepatitis C infection has been reported in up to 16% of patients and frequently there is a history of a preceding urinary tract infection.

Treatment

Delivery is usually induced at 38 weeks of gestation to reduce maternal and fetal complications. Intramuscular vitamin K should be considered to decrease the risk of hemorrhage. Pruritus generally resolves within 24–48 hours after delivery. Associated jaundice and laboratory abnormalities return to normal 2–4 weeks postpartum.

Treating the pruritus before delivery is problematic. Emollients, topical steroids and antipruritics, and oral antihistamines are rarely effective. Bile acid binders such as cholestyramine should be used cautiously, as they may worsen an existing vitamin K deficiency. Although not approved by the Food and Drug Administration (FDA) for ICP, ursodeoxycholic acid at a dose of 15 mg/kg per day is probably the treatment of choice for the highly symptomatic patient if immediate delivery is not an option. Its use has been shown to reduce premature labor, fetal distress, and demise.

Controversies

Persistence in laboratory abnormalities several months postpartum should trigger an investigation for other liver diseases.

OTHER CONDITIONS AFFECTED BY PREGNANCY

Key Points

- Pregnancy can accelerate progression to acquired immunodeficiency syndrome (AIDS) in human immunodeficiency virus (HIV)-infected women
- Pregnancy's effect on psoriasis is highly variable
- Impetigo herpetiformis (Figure 9-9) is a form of pustular psoriasis developing de novo in pregnancy; it may be associated with hypocalcemia, placental insufficiency, and stillbirth

Other dermatological conditions may also be affected by pregnancy. Acne and eczema are discussed above. Condyloma or verruca may proliferate. Cutaneous stigmata of AIDS, including recalcitrant orovulvar candidiasis and seborrheic dermatitis, may develop in HIV-infected women since pregnancy tends to accelerate the progression to AIDS. Identification of these individuals is important because the fetus is at risk for intrauterine growth retardation and prematurity and initiation of antiretroviral therapy may minimize maternal and fetal complications. Although interesting, these conditions are beyond the scope of

Table 9-9 US Food and Drug Administration pregnancy prescribing category definitions

A	Controlled studies in women fail to demonstrate a risk to the fetus in the first trimester
	No evidence of a risk in later trimesters
	Possibility of fetal harm appears remote
B	Animal reproduction studies have not demonstrated a fetal risk but there are no controlled studies in pregnant women
	Animal reproduction studies have shown adverse effect other than a decrease in fertility not confirmed in controlled studies in women in the first trimester, with no evidence of a risk in later trimesters
C	Studies in animals have revealed adverse effects on the fetus (teratogenic or embryocidal or other) and there are no controlled studies in women
	Studies in women and animals may not be available
	Drugs should be only given if the potential benefit justifies the potential risk to the fetus
D	There is positive evidence of human fetal risk
	Benefits from use in pregnant women may be acceptable despite the risk (e.g., for life-threatening situations or serious disease with no safer alternative)
X	Studies in animals or human beings have demonstrated fetal abnormalities
	There is evidence of fetal risk based on human experience
	The risk of the use of the drug in pregnant women clearly outweighs any possible benefit
	The drug is contraindicated in women who are or may become pregnant

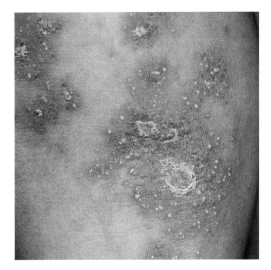

Figure 9-9 Impetigo herpetiformis (courtesy of Karen Warschaw, MD)

Table 9-10 Medications to avoid during pregnancy

Drug	Food and Drug Administration pregnancy prescribing category
Acitretin	X
Aspirin	D
Azathioprine	D
Bleomycin	D
Colchicine	D
Cyclophosphamide	D
Estrogens	X
Etretinate	X
Finasteride	X
Fluorouracil	X
Flutamide	X
Griseofulvin	C
Hydroxyurea	D
Isotretinoin	X
Methotrexate	X
Penicillamine	D
Potassium iodide	D
Stanozolol	X
Tazarotene	X
Tetracyclines	D
Thalidomide	X

*See Table 9-9 for explanation of Food and Drug Administration pregnancy prescribing category definitions.

this chapter. The remainder of this discussion will focus on psoriasis during pregnancy.

Pregnancy's effect on psoriasis is highly variable. A recent compilation of studies found that psoriasis improved in twice as many pregnant patients compared to the number in whom it worsened. However, close to half of the patients experienced no subjective change in their disease.

Pustular psoriasis, referred to as impetigo herpetiformis when developing de novo during pregnancy, deserves special attention since it may result in placental insufficiency and stillbirth. Development of pustule-studded erythematous plaques in a flexural distribution is most common, with relative sparing of the hands, feet, and face. Constitutional symptoms such as malaise, fever, delirium, diarrhea, and vomiting may be present. Potential abnormal laboratory findings include an elevated white blood cell count and sedimentation rate as well as hypocalcemia, which may induce tetany. Remittance postpartum is common, as is recurrence with subsequent pregnancies. Treatment typically requires systemic steroids, although future treatment regimens may include the biologic agents. Pregnancy prescribing guidelines should always be consulted.

MEDICATIONS IN PREGNANCY

A recent survey indicates that greater than 80% of women use at least two medications during their pregnancy. Potential fetal risk of a medication must always be considered. Table 9-4 outlines the FDA pregnancy prescribing categories for medications commonly prescribed by dermatologists; it also highlights other pertinent information. Table 9-10 lists medications that should be avoided during pregnancy. A conservative approach to prescribing medications during pregnancy and lactation is suggested.

Further references

Al-Fares SI, Jones SV, Black MM. The specific dermatoses of pregnancy: a re-appraisal. J Eur Acad Dermatol Venereol 2001;15:197–206.

Ambros-Rudolph CM, Mullegger RR, Vaughan-Jones SA, et al. The specific dermatoses of pregnancy revisited and reclassified: results of a retrospective two-center study on 505 pregnant patients. J Am Acad Dermatol 2006;54:395–404.

Briggs GG, Freeman RK, Yaffe SJ. Drugs in Pregnancy and Lactation, 5th edn. Baltimore, MD: Williams & Wilkins, 1998.

Dahdah MJ, Kibbi AG. Less well-defined dermatoses of pregnancy. Clin Dermatol 2006;24:118–121.

Driscoll MS, Grant-Kels JM. Nevi and melanoma in pregnancy. Dermatol Clin 2006;24:199–204.

Elling SV, Powell FC. Physiological changes in the skin during pregnancy. Clin Dermatol 1997;15:35–43.

Grin CM, Driscoll MS, Grant-Kels JM. The relationship of pregnancy, hormones, and melanoma. Semin Cutan Med Surg 1998;17:167–171.

Kroumpouzos G, Cohen LM. Specific dermatoses of pregnancy: an evidence-based systematic review. Am J Obstet Gynecol 2003;188:1083–1092.

Leachman SA, Reed BR. The use of dermatologic drugs in pregnancy and lactation. Dermatol Clin 2006;24:167–197.

MacKie RM. Pregnancy and exogenous hormones in patients with cutaneous malignant melanoma. Curr Opin Oncol 1999;11:129–131.

Martin AG, Leal-Khouri S. Physiologic skin changes associated with pregnancy. Int J Dermatol 1992;31:375–378.

McDonald JA. Cholestasis of pregnancy. J Gastroenterol Hepatol 1999;14:515–518.

Muallem MM, Rubeiz NG. Physiological and biological skin changes in pregnancy. Clin Dermatol 2006;24:80–83.

Murray JC. Pregnancy and the skin. Dermatol Clin 1990;8:327–334.

Muzaffar F, Hussain I, Haroon TS. Physiologic skin changes during pregnancy: a study of 140 cases. Int J Dermatol 1998;37:429–431.

Nichols AA. Cholestasis of pregnancy: a review of the evidence. J Perinat Neonatal Nurs 2005;19:217–225.

Nussbaum R, Benedetto AV. Cosmetic aspects of pregnancy. Clin Dermatol 2006;24:133–141.

Oumeish OY, Al-Fouzan AW. Miscellaneous diseases affected by pregnancy. Clin Dermatol 2006;24:113–117.

Poupon R. Intrahepatic cholestasis of pregnancy: from bedside to bench to bedside. Liver Int 2005;25:467–468.

Shornick JK. Dermatoses of pregnancy. Semin Cutan Med Surg 1998;17:172–181.

Teplitzky S, Sabates B, Yu K, et al. Melanoma during pregnancy: a case report and review of the literature. J La State Med Soc 1998;150:539–543.

Vaughan Jones SA, Hern S, Nelson-Piercy C, et al. A prospective study of 200 women with dermatoses of pregnancy correlating clinical findings with hormonal and immunopathological profiles. Br J Dermatol 1999;141:71–81.

Diseases of the mouth and oral mucosa

Katy Burris, Geeta K. Patel
and Eve J. Lowenstein

Introduction

Disorders of the oral cavity may present as a primary problem or as a manifestation of systemic disease. This chapter provides an overview of oral mucosa and lip diseases. Diseases of particular interest are covered in the text, while specifics of most conditions are included in the tables.

Developmental/embryologic and other benign, idiopathic oral disorders

Key Points

- Most developmental and embryologic disorders are benign and require no treatment. They are important to recognize, however, since they must be distinguished from more significant conditions. They are summarized in Table 10-1
- Geographic tongue is most often sporadic, but may be associated with pustular psoriasis, Reiter's syndrome, atopic dermatitis, pityriasis rubra pilaris, or human immunodeficiency virus (HIV) infection
- Fissured tongue is a common isolated finding, but may be associated with psoriasis, developmental anomalies, Melkersson–Rosenthal and Down syndromes
- Black tongue is often associated with a history of coffee or tea drinking, antibiotic use, or tobacco use

Genetic disorders

Key Points

- Peutz–Jeghers syndrome presents with mucocutaneous lentigines at birth and is associated with a 15-fold increased risk of developing intestinal cancer
- Lipoid proteinosis presents with a hoarse cry and hyaline papules on the lid margin
- Acanthosis nigricans can involve mucosal surfaces

Several genetic diseases are associated with disorders of the oral mucosa (Table 10-2).

Peutz–Jeghers syndrome is a genodermatosis that can be diagnosed at birth or during early childhood. Mucocutaneous lentigines are typically present at birth and tend to fade with age. However, oral mucosal maculae persist as a marker. This paraneoplastic syndrome is associated with a 15-fold increased risk of developing intestinal cancer.

Lipoid proteinosis, another rare genodermatosis, classically presents in infancy with a hoarse cry from laryngeal infiltration. The disease typically follows a slowly progressive, yet often benign, course.

White sponge nevus is an uncommon inherited condition with asymptomatic, white patches on the bilateral buccal mucosa. It appears at birth or early childhood, rarely later. Once present, the lesions remain stable throughout life, although they may become more pronounced during pregnancy.

Hereditary gingival fibromatosis is characterized by a slowly progressive, benign enlargement of the oral gingival tissues. The gingival enlargement may occur as an isolated finding or may be associated with hypertrichosis and epilepsy. Mental retardation, hearing loss, and supernumerary teeth are more variable findings. The clinical differential includes drug-induced gingival fibromatosis secondary to pregnancy or drugs (dilantin, cyclosporin A or nifedipine).

Acanthosis nigricans is a relatively common skin condition that rarely involves the oral mucosa. Oral acanthosis, unlike its cutaneous component, is often not pigmented. Cutaneous acanthosis nigricans is associated with many diseases and conditions; however, rapidly appearing acanthosis nigricans often presages malignancy, most commonly gastric (in up to 60%).

Infections

Key Points

- The best test for herpes simplex virus (HSV) is viral culture. Direct fluorescent antibody is also a good test
- Actinomycosis (lumpy jaw) usually occurs following oral surgery

Table 10-1 Developmental and embryologic entities

Condition	Etiology	Clinical features	Treatments	Complications
Torus palatinus/torus mandibularis (Figure 10-1)	Familial, heritable bony growth	Common asymptomatic, heritable, developmental exostoses on the hard palate or floor of mouth. Most common among the Asian and Inuit. Appears after puberty, more common in females	None; benign	Affects denture design
Fordyce spots	Ectopic/heterotopic sebaceous glands	Cream-yellow dots along the vermilion and oral mucosa. Appear in childhood and increase during puberty and adulthood. 80–90% of adults affected	None; benign	None
Cleft lip/palate	Incomplete embryonic fusion of facial growth processes; May be sporadic, familial (20%) or syndromic	The most common congenital craniofacial anomaly (1:1000 births). Clefting may be incomplete or complete, unilateral or bilateral, true cleft or pseudocleft. Bifid uvula may be seen with cleft palate	Prevention: risk reduction with folate supplementation early in pregnancy. Treatment is surgical	Difficulty with speech and swallowing
Geographic tongue/benign migratory glossitis (Figure 10-2)	Unknown; physiologic variant, familial or sporadic	Patterned patches on the dorsum tongue that change within hours. Common (2% prevalence). Female > male	None needed; Zinc 200 mg tid for 3 months	Occasional soreness, may be found with fissuring
Fissured tongue/ plicated tongue (Figure 10-3)	Unknown; normal anatomic variant	Asymptomatic deep furrows in tongue of 5% population, increasing prevalence with age	None	None
Hairy tongue/black tongue (Figure 10-4)	Elongation and defective desquamation of filiform papillae	Usually a black discoloration of dorsum tongue. Male > female; increased prevalence with increased age	Brush the tongue with a toothbrush or tongue scraper	None
Median rhomboid glossitis (Figure 10-5)	Etiology unknown; Candida implicated. Defective formation of filiform papillae	Red, atrophic patch in the posterior midline dorsal tongue, usually < 2 cm and anterior to the circumvallate papillae. Male > female	None	None
Linea alba	Phylogenetic remnant of embryologic fusion	Slightly raised white line on cheek at level of dental occlusion	None	None
Epstein's pearls	Embryologic developmental defect resulting in gingival keratin cysts	Small superficial white papules on midline palate, maxillary and mandibular gingiva. Found in newborns; these resolve spontaneously in the first months of life	None	None

tid, three times a day.

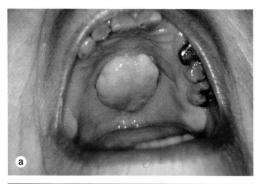

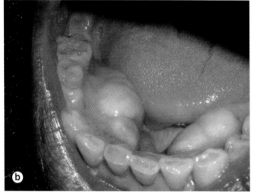

Figure 10-1 a Torus palatinus. **b** Torus mandibularis

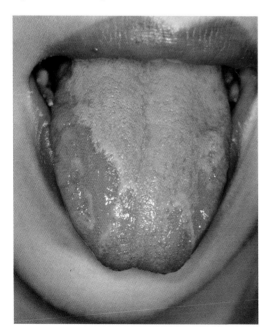

Figure 10-2 Geographic tongue

- Focal epithelial hyperplasia, also known as Heck's disease, is a rare benign, verrucous disorder caused by human papillomavirus (HPV) types 13 and 32
- Oral manifestations of syphilis include chancres, "split papules," mucous patches, and granulomatous lesions

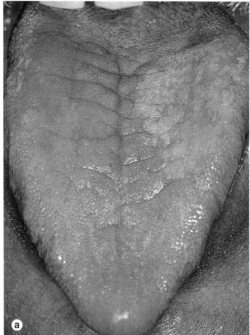

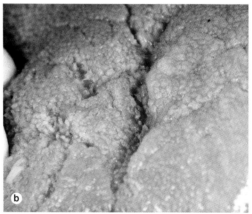

Figure 10-3 a Fissured geographic tongue in pustular psoriasis flare. **b** Tongue fissure

- Acute necrotizing ulcerative gingivitis (ANUG) can progress very rapidly
- Cancrum oris (noma) occurs in severely malnourished children
- Yaws, also a disease of developing countries, is a contagious, nonvenereal treponeme that mainly affects children younger than 15 years
- HIV infection may first manifest with oral disease. A high prevalence of oral candidiasis, melanotic pigmentation, xerostomia, and periodontitis has been reported
- Hand, foot, and mouth disease is caused by epidemic infections with coxsackievirus A16 or enterovirus 71
- Oral hairy leukoplakia (OHL) is an opportunistic Epstein–Barr virus infection predominantly seen in younger HIV patients

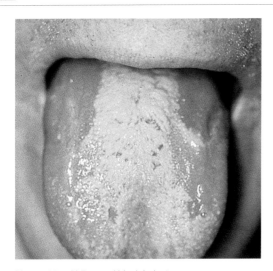

Figure 10-4 Yellow and black hairy tongue

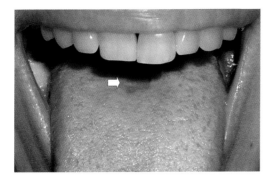

Figure 10-5 Median rhomboid glossitis

Many infections affect the oral mucosa (Table 10-3). For HSV, the diagnostic gold standard is viral culture, with a sensitivity of 75%. This test also distinguishes between HSV-1 and HSV-2 with >90% sensitivity. Where available, direct fluorescent antibody tests obtained from intact vesicles also provide rapid diagnostic confirmation. Serologies offer variable sensitivity of 50–90% in adults with antibodies to HSV and are clinically less useful. Treatment with oral antiviral drugs decreases the duration and pain of recurrent episodes by approximately 1 day; however, they do not eradicate the viral infection. The majority of patients with recurrent HSV-1 oral lesions shed viral DNA. Shedding primarily occurs before and after the appearance of the lesions, but can be asymptomatic.

Actinomycosis usually occurs following oral surgery, and is most common in patients with poor oral hygiene. A preliminary diagnosis can be confirmed by finding sulfur granules on microscopic examination of the discharge.

HPV infection of the oral mucosa is thought to occur primarily via sexual transmission. Non-cancer-causing HPV types 6 and 11 have been isolated from the nares, mouth, and larynx. HPV has been implicated as a risk factor in head and neck cancers.

Focal epithelial hyperplasia, also known as Heck's disease, is a rare benign, verrucous disorder of the oral mucosa that is caused by HPV types 13 and 32. Found in Native Americans and other ethnic predisposed groups, it affects children and young adults, girls more than boys. The clinical course varies; some cases persist for years, and others resolve spontaneously. Treatments include interferon-beta, surgery, cryosurgery, or laser excision.

The incidence of syphilis has declined over the last 30 years. Oral manifestations of syphilis can occur at all stages of disease, beginning with the primary chancre, which can appear in the mouth 21–28 days after exposure, and heals spontaneously within 3–6 weeks. After hematogenous spread, secondary syphilis may cause "split papules" at the corners of the mouth or syphilitic perleche, grey oval patches on the palate, buccal mucosa or tongue, erosions with flattened papillae on the tongue, or condyloma lata lesions. A gumma of tertiary syphilis is a destructive granulomatous lesion. Hutchinson teeth (widely spaced incisors with large notches) and "mulberry molars" are characteristic of congenital syphilis. The nontreponemal tests, Venereal Disease Research Laboratory (VDRL) and rapid plasma reagin (RPR), are used as screening methods. Treponemal tests, including the fluorescent treponemal antibody absorption (FTA-ABS) and microhemagglutination test for antibodies to *Treponema pallidum*, confirm the diagnosis. Dark-field microscopy of oral lesions is of limited value because of the presence of nonpathogenic spirochetes in the normal oral flora.

Oral candidiasis can be seen in the context of several risk factors, including HIV infection, diabetes, use of antibiotics, inhaled steroids, and smoking.

ANUG can progress very rapidly and have severe complications. If an abscess is present, needle drainage and culture is the most accurate method of diagnosis. Pantomography may reveal the full extent of advanced periodontitis or the presence of single or multiple abscesses. Ultrasonography, radionuclide scanning, computed tomography, and magnetic resonance imaging are also useful for the localization of deep infections of the head and neck.

Cancrum oris (noma) occurs in severely malnourished children living in underdeveloped countries. Risk factors include poor hygiene, immunodeficiency, measles, scarlet fever, tuberculosis, and malignancy. Treatment is directed at eradication of underlying organism and salvage of remaining tissue.

Yaws, also a disease of developing countries, is a contagious, nonvenereal treponeme that mainly affects children younger than 15 years. The disease

Table 10-2 Genetic disorders

Syndrome	Inheritance	Clinical features	Treatment	Differential diagnosis	Other features
Peutz–Jeghers syndrome/periorificial lentiginosis (Figure 10-6)	Autosomal dominant, 40% spontaneous mutations; STK11/LKB1 proto-oncogene; (a serine threonine kinase)	Lentigines on lips and mucosal surfaces, also acral, genital, and perineal	Ruby, potassium titanyl phosphate (KTP) or CO_2 lasers for cosmesis	Laugier–Hunziker syndrome; Bannayan–Ruvalcaba–Riley syndrome; Cronkhite–Canada syndrome	Benign intestinal hamartomas, a paraneoplastic syndrome (ovarian, breast, and pancreatic carcinoma, rarely adenocarcinoma within polyps)
Cowden's syndrome/multiple hamartoma syndrome	Autosomal dominant; PTEN (tyrosine phosphatase) tumor suppressor	Oral papillomas on lips, tongue, gums, and palate, coalesce to cobblestone appearance; facial tricholemmomas and acral keratoses	CO_2 laser ablation for lesions; surveillance for malignancy (paraneoplastic); prophylactic mastectomy option	Muir–Torre syndrome; multiple endocrine neoplasia IIb; lipoid proteinosis; tuberous sclerosis	A paraneoplastic syndrome (breast and thyroid), ovarian cysts, colonic polyps
Focal dermal hypoplasia/Goltz syndrome	X-linked dominant	Papillomatous growths of mucosa lip pits; gingival hyperplasia; hemihypoplasia of tongue and hypo/oligodontia, Blaschkoid poikilodermatous plaques; fat herniation; aplasia cutis congenita; skin hyper/hypopigmentation	Cosmetic cryotherapy, curettage, or photodynamic therapy for growths	Incontinentia pigmenti; nevus lipomatosus superficialis; Rothmund–Thomson syndrome	Lobster claw deformity, mental retardation; craniofacial, ocular, dental, and musculoskeletal abnormalities
Keratosis follicularis/Darier's disease	Autosomal dominant; SERCA2 (Ca^{2+}-ATPase (ATP2A2)	Mucosal cobblestone papules on palatal and alveolar mucosa; infrequent oral involvement; halitosis	Long-term systemic retinoids; topical retinoids; antibacterial soap; nonalcohol mouthwash	Hailey–Hailey disease; Grovers disease	Greasy papules and plaques in a seborrheic distribution; acral acrokeratosis; verruciformis of Hopf with punctuate pits; nails with longitudinal red and white streaks, distal notching
Lipoid proteinosis/Urbach Wiethe disease/hyalinosis cutis et mucosae	Autosomal recessive; extracellular matrix protein 1 gene (ECM1)	Progressive development of yellow papules, plaques, and nodules of skin, lips, and oral mucosa; thickened, indurated tongue; decreased motility, xerostomia and recurrent parotitis; dental anomalies	CO_2 laser of skin papules	Cowden's syndrome; pseudoxanthoma elasticum; xanthomas	Pockmarks and indurated plaques of face, axillae and extremities; eyelid "string of pearls" appearance; patchy alopecia, hoarseness, dysphagia; central nervous system calcification (bean-shaped in suprasellar area) and seizures

Continued

Table 10-2 Genetic disorders—cont'd

Syndrome	Inheritance	Clinical features	Treatment	Differential diagnosis	Other features
Cyclic neutropenia	Autosomal dominant; elastase-2 gene	Oral ulcers (gingival and mucosal) with fever, anorexia, pharyngitis. Usually onset first year of life with decreased severity with time; however, adult-onset form exists	Granulocyte colony-stimulating factor (1–5 µg/kg) during episodes; antibacterial mouthwash; aggressive dental care	Kostmann syndrome	Recurrent neutropenia in a 21-day cycle presenting with recurrent fever, malaise, headaches
White sponge nevus (Figure 10-7)	Autosomal dominant; keratin 4 or 13 gene	Asymptomatic symmetric plaques on the buccal mucosa, tongue, labial mucosa, alveolar ridges, and floor of the mouth	Oral tetracycline rinse	Pachyonychia congenita; Darier–White disease; pseudomembranous candidiasis	Genitorectal mucosal involvement can be observed
Gingival fibromatosis	Autosomal dominant; growth hormone–releasing factor deficiency	Pebbled gingival interdental papillae, late dental eruption	Surgical gingivectomy, improved oral hygiene	Squamous cell carcinoma	Generalized hypertrichosis, epilepsy, and mental retardation
Acanthosis nigricans	Autosomal dominant or sporadic	Skin flexures and mucosal lesions	Topical or oral retinoids, keratolytic agents	Addison's disease; hemochromatosis; pellagra; Gougerot–Carteaud syndrome	Nongenetic form is more common and is associated with obesity, diabetes, and autoimmune disease; may be drug-related or a marker of paraneoplastic disease

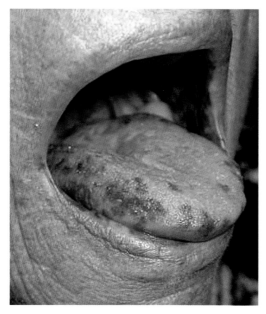

Figure 10-6 Peutz–Jeghers syndrome (courtesy of Dr Benjamin Fisher, Israel)

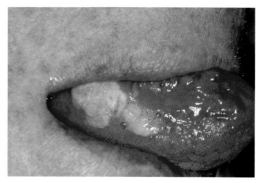

Figure 10-7 Oral white sponge nevus

BOX 10-1

Human immunodeficiency virus (HIV)-associated mucosal diseases

Candidiasis

Melanotic pigmentation (especially with highly active antiretroviral therapy (HAART))

Xerostomia

Periodontitis

Oral hairy leukoplakia (OHL)

Kaposi's sarcoma (Figure 10-10)

Non-Hodgkin lymphoma

Acute necrotizing ulcerative gingivitis (ANUG)

Human papillomavirus-associated papillomas

Salivary gland disease

---

tends to occur in warm, humid, tropical areas of Africa, Asia, and South America, and among poor rural populations where there is overcrowding and poor hygiene. Goundou refers to nasal bone involvement by yaws.

Orofacial tuberculosis is caused by primary autoinoculation of the mucosa or secondarily on mucosa/skin adjacent to an active draining internal tuberculosis infection.

HIV infection may first manifest with oral disease. A high prevalence of oral candidiasis, melanotic pigmentation, xerostomia, and periodontitis has been reported in HIV (Box 10-1). Oral hairy leukoplakia (OHL), Kaposi's sarcoma (KS), non-Hodgkin lymphoma (NHL), and ANUG are less prevalent oral markers for HIV. With the advent of highly active antiretroviral therapy (HAART), the prevalence of *Candida*, OHL, and periodontitis has decreased in adults, but not in children. HAART is associated with an increased prevalence of melanotic pigmentation, HPV-associated papillomas, and salivary gland disease.

Hand, foot, and mouth disease is a contagious infection usually caused by epidemic infections with coxsackievirus A16 or enterovirus 71. Primarily observed in children under 10 years of age, it is characterized by erosive stomatitis and an acral, vesicular eruption. Usually a benign infection, it can be rarely complicated by meningoencephalitis and myocarditis. Treatment is symptomatic. Children are infectious while blisters are present, but fecal viral shedding may persist for weeks after infection.

OHL is an opportunistic Epstein–Barr virus infection predominantly seen in younger HIV

patients. It responds to HAART therapy. It has also been associated with Behçet's disease and ulcerative colitis. Treatments for oral infectious diseases are listed in Table 10-4.

Allergic/toxic/drug

Key Points

- Urticaria and angioedema may involve the oral mucosa
- Hereditary angioedema does not present with urticaria
- Erythema multiforme (EM) affects the mouth in 25% of cases
- Lichen planus and lichenoid contact dermatitis occur in the mouth

Allergic, toxic, and drug-induced reactions affecting the oral mucosa range from very mild and self-limiting to life-threatening, particularly if left untreated. In most cases, treatment involves removal of the offending agent and supportive, symptomatic care (Table 10-5).

Table 10-3 Infectious diseases involving the mouth

Disease	Causative organism	Clinical presentation	Diagnostic tests	Serious complications
Herpes simplex virus (HSV) (Figure 10-8)	HSV-1 > HSV-2	Primary infection much more severe than subsequent infections. Painful prodrome followed by the development of erythematous papules that rapidly develop into tiny, thin-walled, intraepidermal vesicles	Culture (gold standard – sensitivity of 75%; distinguishes between HSV-1 and HSV-2 with >90% sensitivity;) polymerase chain reaction; serologies; clinical judgment; Tzanck smear; DFA	Bacterial and fungal superinfection; HSV encephalitis; visceral infections; aseptic meningitis
Actinomycosis/"lumpy jaw"	Actinomyces species	Follows oral surgery; also seen in patients with poor oral hygiene. Cervicofacial infection is the most common presentation (50–70%). Erythema and swelling of perimandibular skin, followed by ulceration	Culture is gold standard; histology (sulfur granules may be seen)	Spread to cranium, brain, and blood; fistula development
Human papillomavirus (HPV)	HPV	Benign oral verrucous lesions	Polymerase chain reaction; histology	Squamous cell cancer of the head and neck (tonsillar and oropharyngeal)
Focal epithelial hyperplasia/Heck's disease	Rare; caused by HPV 13 or 32	Increased prevalence in native Americans and other ethnically predisposed groups; affects children and young adults, girls more than boys. Asymptomatic diffuse pink-white papules and confluent plaques on the lips, buccal mucosa, and lateral tongue. The clinical course is variable, with some cases persisting for years and others resolving spontaneously.	Clinical presentation; histology	Anogenital mucosa may be affected, other skin involvement rare; malignant transformation rare
Syphilis	Treponema pallidum	Oral lesions of primary syphilis: chancre (single, painless ulcer) – appears 18–21 days after exposure and heals spontaneously within 3–6 weeks. Secondary syphilis (secondary to hematogenous spread): split papules, syphilitic perleche, grey oral patches on palate/buccal mucosa/tongue, erosions with flattened papillae on the tongue, and condyloma lata. Tertiary syphilis: gummas (destructive granulomatous lesions) Congenital syphilis: Hutchinson's teeth (widely spaced incisors with large notches), mulberry molars	RPR/VDRL; FTA-ABS; immunofluorescence staining	Cardiovascular syphilis, neurosyphilis (progression to secondary and tertiary disease), skeletal degeneration of maxilla/mandible

Table 10-3 Infectious diseases involving the mouth—cont'd

Disease	Causative organism	Clinical presentation	Diagnostic tests	Serious complications
Gonorrhea	*Neisseria gonorrhoeae*	Sexually acquired oral disease is uncommon. Slight erythema to severe ulceration with a pseudomembranous coating and discharge	Culture; gram stain	Meningitis, endocarditis
Candidiasis	*Candida* species (*C. albicans* most common)	Risk factors include human immunodeficiency virus (HIV), diabetes, the use of antibiotics, inhaled steroids and smoking. Perleche: fissure and inflammation of angle of the lips (Figure 10-9) Oropharyngeal candidiasis: Painful mouth and pharynx, white plaques, red plaques	Culture; wet mount or potassium hydroxide smears	Resistance to therapy; severe pain may limit oral intake, causing wasting and malnutrition
Acute necrotizing ulcerative gingivitis (ANUG)/Vincent's angina	*Prevotella intermedia*, alpha-hemolytic streptococci, *Actinomyces* species, spirochetes	Sudden onset of gingival pain, eroded appearance, necrosis of the interdental gingivae, pseudomembrane formation, halitosis, and dysageusia	Clinical presentation; needle drainage with culture is the most accurate method of diagnosis; ultrasonography, radionuclide scanning, computed tomography and magnetic resonance imaging (to diagnose periodontitis or the presence of single or multiple abscesses)	Hematogenous spread, osteomyelitis, disfiguring facial ulceration
Cancrum oris (noma)	Fusiform bacilli	Affects severely malnourished children in underdeveloped countries. Risk factors include poor hygiene, immunodeficiency, measles, scarlet fever, tuberculosis, and malignancy. Mucosal inflammation and ulcers progress to rapid tissue destruction	Clinical + culture of likely organism	Deformity of soft tissue and bone, loss of teeth
Leishmaniasis	*Leishmania* "New World" species (*L. mexicana, L. amazonensis, L. donovani, L. chagasi, and others*)	Initial cutaneous lesion typically heals spontaneously. Years later, oral and respiratory mucosal involvement may occur, with destruction of the nose, mouth, oropharynx, and trachea	Polymerase chain reaction; serology; biopsy and culture	Death may occur from respiratory compromise and malnutrition

Continued

Table 10-3 Infectious diseases involving the mouth—cont'd

Disease	Causative organism	Clinical presentation	Diagnostic tests	Serious complications
Yaws	*Treponema pertenue*	Usually in patients younger than 15 years in rural, overcrowded areas of Africa, Asia, and South America. Primary lesion ("mother yaw") develops at the site of inoculation after 3-week incubation, resolves spontaneously after 3–6 months. Secondary lesions may occur near primary lesions or elsewhere; goundou refers to nasal involvement.	Usually diagnosed clinically; may use serologies	Irreversible tissue damage
Orofacial tuberculosis (TB)	*Mycobacterium tuberculosis*	Rare presentation usually secondary to extension of internal disease or sometimes autoinoculation; a painful indurated ulcer on the gingiva, lips, and buccal mucosa	Ziehl–Neelsen stain for acid-fast bacilli; culture of lesion	Systemic TB, pulmonary TB
Blastomycosis	*Blastomyces dermatitidis*	Verrucous or ulcerated lesions with raised irregular borders, crusting and purulent drainage (endemic in south-central, south-eastern, and mid-western United States)	Culture; chemiluminescent DNA probes	Pulmonary disease, neurological involvement
Hand, foot, and mouth disease	*Coxsackie viruses, especially A16, enterovirus 71*	Primarily affects children. Erythematous macules develop into 2–3-mm ulcers involving palate, buccal mucosa, gingiva, and tongue. Lesions are very painful and make eating difficult. Acral vesicles	Clinical; viral culture	Meningitis, encephalitis, myocarditis
Oral hairy leukoplakia	*Epstein–Barr virus*	Associated with younger HIV patients and patients with Behçet's disease or ulcerative colitis; painless, changing white plaque along the lateral borders of the tongue. "Hairy" appearance relatively uncommon despite name. Responds to highly active antiretroval therapy (HAART) in HIV patients	Clinical; polymerase chain reaction for Epstein–Barr virus; biopsy (generally to rule out other causes)	Superinfection with *Candida*

DFA, direct fluorescent antibody; RPR, rapid plasma reagin; VDRL, Venereal Disease Research Laboratory; FTA-ABS, fluorescent treponemal antibody absorption test.

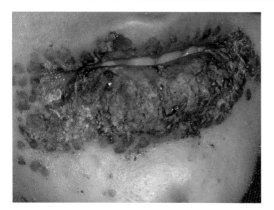

Figure 10-8 Herpes simplex

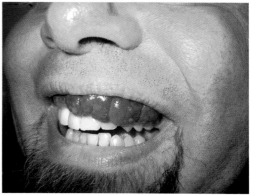

Figure 10-10 Kaposi's sarcoma (courtesy of Dr Naana Boakye, SUNY Health Science Center at Brooklyn)

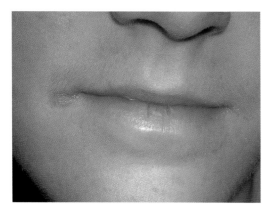

Figure 10-9 Perleche

Urticaria and angioedema can affect the oral mucosa in an allergic reaction. Drugs that commonly induce these reactions include penicillin, sulfur-containing drugs, and salicylic acid, among others. If lesions last longer than 36 hours, they should be biopsied to rule out urticarial vasculitis. Other indications for biopsy include presence of petechiae, fever, arthralgia, and elevated erythrocyte sedimentation rate. Low levels of C4, C1q, and C1 esterase inhibitor (C1-INH) may be associated with hereditary angioedema.

EM involves mucosal surfaces in about 25% of cases. It is usually mild and typically involves the oral cavity. There may be a recent or concomitant history of recurrent HSV infection, although this is not always symptomatic.. Mucosae are always involved in Stevens–Johnson syndrome/toxic epidermal necrolysis (SJS/TEN; Figure 10-11) and it is generally more severe than that of EM. Necrotic sloughing and crusting of the lips are characteristic of SJS/TEN, with the main differential diagnosis being paraneoplastic pemphigus.

A fixed drug eruption typically appears within hours of exposure to a drug and recurs in exactly the same location upon rechallenge. Common offenders include aspirin, barbiturates, methaqualone, phenylbutazone, phenolphthalein, sulfonamides, tetracyclines, and trimethoprim-sulfamethoxazole.

Cheilitis can be a consequence of lip licking and contact dermatitis and is the most common side-effect of isotretinoin therapy (Figure 10-12). The severity of isotretinoin-induced cheilitis is dose-dependent, and it can be managed with topical emollients, use of lower dosage of isotretinoin, and anecdotally, vitamin E supplementation (1200 units/day).

Oral lichenoid eruptions may be associated with allergic contact dermatitis to metals or chemicals in dental restorations. Lesions are typically found adjacent to the dental work. Patch testing should be done before replacing dental work, which is both expensive and not universally helpful. Metal allergens identified include mercury, gold, beryllium, nickel, ticonium, cobalt, palladium, chrome, platinum, zinc, and manganese. Oral lichenoid drug reactions typically affect the skin, rather than mucosa. The most common culprit drugs include angiotensin-converting enzyme inhibitors, nonsteroidal anti-inflammatory drugs (NSAIDS), antihypertensives, diuretics, and oral hypoglycemic agents.

Hyperpigmentation of the tongue is a side-effect of antiretroviral medications such as zidovudine and the tenofovir/emtricitabine combination. It is seen at a higher rate in dark-skinned as compared to light-skinned individuals. The pigmentation may be localized or diffuse. The diagnostic differential includes benign melanosis, melanocytic dysplasia, and KS, which rarely affects the tongue. Two-thirds of oral melanomas arise from oral melanotic macules and, therefore, these lesions warrant attention.

Autoimmune/rheumatologic

Key Points

- Aphthous stomatitis presents with gray painful ulcers on a red base
- A variety of systemic diseases present with oral lesions

Table 10-4 Treatments for infectious oral diseases

Disease	Treatment	Adult dosage	Pediatric dosage	Pregnancy category
HSV labialis recurrent infection	Acyclovir	200–400 mg PO five times daily for 5 days	Severe infections in immunocompromised children: 10 mg/kg per day IV q8 hours for 7 days	B
	Valacyclovir	2000 mg PO q12 hours for 1 day	>12 years old: same as adult	B
		1500 mg PO single dose within 6 hours of symptoms		
Actinomycosis	Penicillin G (drug of choice)	12–24 million u/day IV infusion or in divided dose q4 hours for 1–2 weeks, then PO for 6–12 months	200 000–400 000 U/kg per day IV infusion or in divided doses q4 hours for 1–2 weeks, then switch to PO for 6–12 months	B
	Penicillin VK	500 mg PO q6 hours for 6–12 months	25–50 mg/kg per day PO in divided doses q6 hours for 6–12 months	B
	Doxycycline	100 mg PO/IV q12 hours	>8 years: 1 mg/kg PO/IV q12 hours; not to exceed 200 mg/day	D
	Clindamycin	600 mg IV q8 hours, or 150–300 mg PO q8 hours	8–20 mg/kg per day as hydrochloride or 8–25 mg/kg per day as palmitate PO divided tid/qid *or* 20–40 mg/kg per day IV divided tid/qid	B
Syphilis and yaws	Benzathine penicillin G	Primary or secondary syphilis: 2.4 million U IM in a single dose	Primary or secondary syphilis: 50 000 U/kg IM single dose; not to exceed 2.4 million units	B
Gonorrhea	Ceftriaxone (drug of choice)	125–250 mg IM once	<45 kg 125 mg IM once; >45 kg, same as adult	B
	Ciprofloxacin	500 mg PO	n/a	B
Candidiasis	Fluconazole	Esophageal/oral/pharyngeal: 200 mg on day one, then 100 mg per day PO/IV for 7–14 days	6 mg/kg day one, then 3 mg/kg/day PO/IV for 7-14 days. Children <2 weeks old should be treated with same dose, but given every 72 hours.	C
	Itraconazole	200 mg/day PO/IV for 7–14 days	n/a	C
Acute necrotizing ulcerative gingivitis	Penicillin VK (drug of choice)	500 mg PO qid for 10 days	<12 years: 25–50 mg/kg per day PO divided q6–8 hours; not to exceed 3 g/day; >12 years: same as adults	C
	Minocycline microspheres	Insert a unit-dose cartridge into base of periodontal pocket	n/a	D
Leishmaniasis	Sodium stibogluconate	20 mg/kg/day IV for 28 days	Same as adults	C
Blastomycosis	Itraconazole	200–400 mg/day PO with food	5–7 mg/kg per day PO once daily or divided q12 hours	C
	Ketoconazole	400–800 mg/day PO	n/a	C

HSV, herpes simplex virus; PO, orally; IV, intravenously; IM, intramuscularly; qid, four times a day; tid, three times a day.

Table 10-5 Allergic, toxic, and drug-induced disease of the mouth

Disease	Etiology	Clinical presentation	Diagnosis	Differential diagnosis	Complications
Urticaria/ angioedema	Caused most often by drugs (penicillin, sulfur- containing drugs, and salicylic acid, and others) in adults, and by infections in children	Urticaria: red papules/patches with associated pruritus Angioedema: massive swelling of lips, mild if any pruritus; <72 hours' duration	Clinical; subtle histopathology findings; low C4, C1q, and C1-INH levels in hereditary angioedema	Urticarial vasculitis (especially with lesions lasting >24 hours)	Anaphylaxis and death
Erythema multiforme	Herpes simplex virus most common, drugs, or infections less common	Sudden, rapidly progressive, symmetrical lesions. Characteristic concentric targetoid lesions	Clinical judgment; biopsy for confirmation		Rare secondary bacterial infections/ sepsis
Stevens– Johnson syndrome (SJS)/ toxic epidermal necrolysis (TEN) (Fig 10-11)	Drugs; rarely malignancy or infection	Vesiculobullous lesions; eroded or crusted lips and mucosa. More extensive and severe mucous membrane involvement in TEN than SJS	Clinical	Paraneoplastic pemphigus	Esophageal strictures, ocular scarring, respiratory failure, sepsis, high-output cardiac failure, death
Fixed drug eruption	Allergy; unknown mechanism; common offending drugs include aspirin, barbiturates, methaqualone, phenylbutazone, phenolphthalein, sulfonamides, tetracyclines, and trimethoprim-sulfamethoxisole	Single or multiple, round, sharply demarcated, dusky plaques, recur in same site after re-exposure to inciting drug	History and clinical		Risk of generalized bullous eruptions
Cheilitis/ stomatitis	Lip licking Isotretinoin Contact dermatitis (i.e., cinnamon)	Dryness, dysesthesia, fissuring, erythema, burning	Clinical judgment; history		Bacterial or yeast superinfection, dyschromia
Lichenoid amalgam reaction	Allergy to metals (mercury most commonly) in dental fillings	Reticulate, lacy, plaque-like, or erosive lichenoid changes near amalgam dental fillings	History of dental work; patch testing helpful (allergens identified include mercury, gold, beryllium, nickel, ticonium, cobalt, palladium, chrome, platinum, zinc, and manganese)	Lichen planus Lichenoid drug reaction (common culprit drugs include ACE inhibitors, NSAIDs, antihypertensives, diuretics, and oral hypoglycemic agents)	None
Chemical burn	Aspirin or other low-pH compound	White patches with subsequent desquamation, mainly affecting buccal mucosa	History of aspirin placement in mouth for local pain relief		None

Continued

Table 10-5 Allergic, toxic, and drug-induced disease of the mouth—cont'd

Disease	Etiology	Clinical presentation	Diagnosis	Differential diagnosis	Complications
Tongue pigmentation due to antiretroviral therapy	Hypermelanocytosis as side-effect of medication (especially zidovudine and tenofovir/emtricitabine	Diffuse oral pigmentation and hyperpigmentation of the tongue	Clinical; medication history	Benign melanosis; melanocytic dysplasia; Kaposi sarcoma (which rarely affects the tongue); melanoma; Addison's disease	None

ACE, angiotensin-converting enzyme; NSAIDs, nonsteroidal anti-inflammatory drugs.

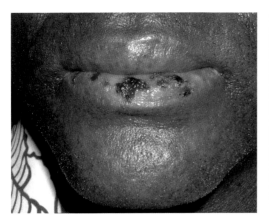

Figure 10-11 Stevens–Johnson syndrome

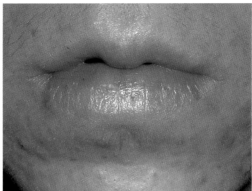

Figure 10-12 Isotretinoin cheilitis

Several rheumatologic diseases affect the mouth (Table 10-6). Recurrent aphthous stomatitis (RAS) is very common, especially in higher socioeconomic classes. RAS has three subtypes, which are outlined in Table 10-7.

Wegener granulomatosis affects the oral cavity in 6–13% of cases, but is rarely the primary sign of the disease. The antineutrophil cytoplasmic antibody c-ANCA has 96% sensitivity in active disease, 41% sensitivity in remission.

Pyostomatitis vegetans is a rare disorder that is a highly specific marker for inflammatory bowel disease, especially ulcerative colitis. Oral disease may be present without skin involvement, but rarely without intestinal involvement. Lesions may reflect intestinal disease activity. The skin lesions are annular pustular lesions. In most cases, bowel disease precedes the onset of oral lesions by months to years.

Oral lichen planus is often associated with cutaneous involvement. Erosive lesions have a predilection to scar and form strictures in up to 90% of patients. Esophageal involvement, although rare, can lead to severe complications, such as stenosis. The vulvovaginal–gingival syndrome is a rare and severe subgroup of lichen planus, with human leukocyte antigen linkage implicated.

Nutritional disorders

Key Point

- Nutritional disorders may present with bleeding gums, glossitis, cheilitis, and angular stomatitis

Nutritional deficiencies (Table 10-8) are rare in developed countries, but can be seen in the elderly and from medication, alcoholism, eating disorders, gastrointestinal surgery, and genodermatoses.

Idiopathic pyridoxine deficiency is rare, but risk increases with age, in pregnancy, malnutrition, and with the use of certain drugs (isoniazid, pyrazinamide, d-penicillamine, and hydralazine).

Vitamin C deficiency (scurvy) is now relatively rare and occurs primarily among the poor, elderly, and alcoholics who consume < 10 mg/day of vitamin C. Scurvy generally occurs at levels less than 0.1 mg/dL. Serious complications are generally not seen until the late stages of the disease.

Folate and vitamin B_{12} deficiency are most common in the elderly. Peripheral vibratory sensation is frequently abnormal in B_{12} deficiency. Complete blood count will reveal macrocytic anemia in both deficiencies. Other informative labs include serum B_{12}. Serum methylmalonic acid and total

Table 10-6 Autoimmune and rheumatological oral disease

Syndrome	Clinical features	Diagnosis	Treatment	Differential diagnosis	Other findings
Systemic lupus erythematosus (SLE), discoid lupus erythematosus	Erythema, atrophy, depigmentation; oral ulcers (SLE), scarring, leukoplakia, and telangiectasias	Biopsy; serologies	Topical or intralesional steroids	Malignant leukoplakia; lichen planus; Sjögren's syndrome	Photosensitivity "butterfly" rash, neurological, joint pain, alopecia, thrombophlebitis, cytopenias, hypertension, pleurisy, pericarditis, and renal disease
Sjögren's disease	Sicca syndrome; xerostomia; smooth tongue with atrophy of the filiform papillae; angular chelitis; dental decay; episodic or chronic parotid enlargement	Clinical diagnostic criteria: ocular, oral, Schirmer's test, histopathology and serologies; Ro(SS-A) and La(SS-B) antibodies	Oral hygiene; topical antibiotics; antifungals; pilocarpine; artificial saliva	Xerostomia secondary to drugs (antihypertensives, diuretics); radiation	Keratoconjunctivitis sicca, arthralgia, Raynaud's phenomenon, fatigue, atrophic gastritis, and constipation
Pemphigus vulgaris and paraneoplastic pemphigus (PNP)	Painful crusted erosions of the mouth	Skin or mucosal biopsy with direct or indirect immunofluorescence; serologies (enzyme-linked immunosorbent assay (ELISA) test)	Systemic prednisone ± mycophenolate mofetil, intravenous immunoglobulin, azathioprine, cyclophosphamide; resection of tumor in PNP	Cicatricial pemphigoid; Stevens–Johnson syndrome; bullous lupus	Generalized Nikolsky-positive bullous eruption
Recurrent aphthous stomatitis (RAS)/Mikulicz's aphthae	Minor, major, and herpetiform (see Table 10-7)	Clinical presentation, biopsy	Amlexanox 5% paste qid; silver nitrate; topical/intralesional steroids, oral vitamin B_{12}, zinc supplementation; tetracycline rinses; chlorhexidine mouthwash 0.12% bid; 50 mg penicillin G troches; for severe disease: levamisole or thalidomide	Recurrent oral herpes simplex virus; herpangina; hand, foot, and mouth disease; vitamin deficiency	
Behçet's syndrome	Nonscarring painful ulcers 2–10 mm in diameter, with a yellow necrotic base. May appear singly or in crops; persist for 1–2 weeks	Clinical presentation; biopsy	Tetracycline swish and spit qid or topical corticosteroids; lidocaine gel (2%); sucralfate suspension; 5% amlexanox; systemic steroids; methotrexate; azathioprine; cyclosporine; thalidomide	Aphthous stomatitis, herpes simplex, lupus erythematosus	Uveitis and cutaneous lesions, erythema nodosum, neutrophilic pustular folliculitis. Also arthritis, gastrointestinal and neurological symptoms

Continued

Table 10-6 Autoimmune and rheumatological oral disease—cont'd

Syndrome	Clinical features	Diagnosis	Treatment	Differential diagnosis	Other findings
Wegener's granulomatosis	Aphthae, cheilitis, cobblestone plaques, mucosal tags, dysgeusia, "strawberry gingival hyperplasia"	Clinical findings; biopsy; c-ANCA test (96% sensitivity in active disease, 41% sensitivity in remission)	Systemic steroids or cyclophosphamide	SLE, leishmaniasis, relapsing polychondritis	Sinusitis, rhinorrhea, other respiratory involvement, renal, arthralgia, ocular disease
Oral Crohn's	Diffuse gingival or mucosal swelling; cobblestoning; aphthous ulcers; mucosal tags; and angular cheilitis	Clinical findings; biopsy; elevated C-reactive protein; erythrocyte sedimentation rate, and low albumin	Systemic steroids; topical steroids; lidocaine	Miescher cheilitis; Melkersson–Rosenthal	Oral lesions may either precede or follow intestinal symptoms
Pyostomatitis vegetans	Painful pustules, erosions, and vegetations of mucosal lips and gingiva; "snail track" chronic appearance; lesions may reflect intestinal disease activity; skin lesions are annular pustular lesions. In most cases, bowel disease precedes oral lesions by months to years	Direct and indirect immunofluorescence	Topical and oral prednisolone; dapsone; topical tacrolimus; infliximab; methotrexate	Oral herpes simplex virus, syphilis, Crohn's disease, Behçet's disease	Usually a marker for inflammatory bowel diseases, particularly ulcerative colitis.
Oral lichen planus (Figure 10-13)	Reticular, erythematous or erosive lesions (ulcerated or bullous) – have a tendency to scar and form strictures in 90%, xerostomia, dysaguesia	Biopsy; clinical findings	Treat if symptomatic; topical steroids, systemic retinoids	Lichenoid drug/contact eruption; graft-versus-host disease; lichenoid dysplasia	Generalized rash and pruritus, nail abnormalities, hair loss (lichen planopilaris); genital ulcers; esophageal stenosis in severe cases

qid, four times a day; bid, twice a day; c-ANCA, antineutrophil cytoplasmic antibody.

Table 10-7 Clinical subtypes of recurrent aphthous stomatitis (RAS)

Minor aphthae (most common form, 80% of RAS)	Painful, small (< 1 cm) round ulcers with a gray membrane surrounded by erythema that heal without scarring
Major aphthae	Larger (> 1 cm) deeper painful ulcers that heal slowly and usually scar, often accompanied by fever and malaise
Herpetiform aphthae	Multiple, grouped 1–2-mm ulcers, which can coalesce; heal in 7–30 days, sometimes with scarring

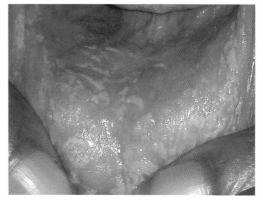

Figure 10-13 Oral lichen planus

homocysteine levels are sensitive indicators of vitamin B_{12} deficiency, whereas red blood cell folate is the best measure of metabolically active folate.

Fatigue, palpitations, lightheadedness, hair loss, and lack of energy are common in iron deficiency. A blood smear reveals hypochromic microcytic anemia. Total ferritin may be low, and the total iron-binding capacity (TIBC) will be elevated. Screening colonoscopy is indicated for adults > 50 years old to rule out iron deficiency from an intestinal malignancy.

Perioral erythematous patches and plaques of dry, scaly, eczematous skin are seen in zinc deficiency. Causes of zinc deficiency include exclusive breastfeeding of infants, malabsorption due to cystic fibrosis or small-bowel resection, abnormal metabolism of essential fatty acids, and kwashiorkor, among others. Acrodermatitis enteropathica is an autosomal-recessive disorder which causes inhibition of zinc uptake in intestinal cells, leading to periorificial and acral dermatitis, alopecia, and diarrhea.

Acquired diseases

Key Points

- History and physical exam are adequate for the diagnosis of most acquired oral lesions
- Biopsy should be considered for clinically nondiagnostic lesions

Acquired oral conditions tend to develop later in life and may be self-induced or a sign of additional underlying illness (Table 10-9).

Venous lakes are harmless vascular lesions that are common in adults over 50. A history of chronic sun exposure is the main risk factor. The typical presentation is an asymptomatic, soft, compressible, blue-purple papule that measures up to 1 cm in size. Elective therapies include surgical ablation/excision, laser, or cryosurgery. Malignancy

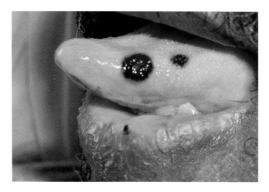

Figure 10-14 Tongue purpura secondary to minor trauma in hospitalized patient with coagulopathy

should be ruled out with biopsy if the clinical exam is not definitive.

Primary systemic amyloidosis presents with macroglossia in 19% of cases. Amyloidosis localized in the tongue, lips, rhinopharynx, and larynx is most common, although there are reports of palatal involvement. Other skin lesions include petechiae, ecchymoses, and waxy papules, nodules, or plaques around the eyelids, neck, and anogenital area. Usually associated with myeloma, the prognosis for primary systemic amyloidosis is poor. Dialysis-related amyloidosis of the tongue has been reported.

Glossodynia is thought to have a wide range of possible etiologies, including hematological diseases, vitamin deficiencies, dental work, hormonal factors, infections, and psychological disorders (neuroses, depression, or phobias). Typically, the oral mucosa is normal in most patients. Therapy is treatment of the underlying cause, and involves antidepressants, vitamin B supplementation, and transcutaneous electrical nerve stimulation.

Cheilitis granulomatosa may or may not be a monosymptomatic form of Melkersson–Rosenthal syndrome. Episodic swelling of lips is observed in this condition, and 20–40% of patients develop a

Table 10-8 Nutritional deficiencies

Endocrine/nutritional disease	Clinical presentation	Diagnosis	Causes	Associated findings
Vitamin B$_2$ (riboflavin) deficiency/oro-oculogenital syndrome	Angular stomatitis, cheilitis, glossitis (magenta tongue) and seborrheic dermatitis (especially peri-nasal),scrotal and vulvar dermatitis	Clinical findings		Increased corneal vascularity, neurological damage
Vitamin B$_3$ (niacin) deficiency/pellagra	Burning mouth (earliest symptom), tongue red, swollen, and smooth due to atrophic papillae. Patchy loss of epithelium; gingiva may bleed and appear raw	Low niacin levels		Secondary infection, malaise, diarrhea, dementia, death
Vitamin B$_6$ (pyridoxine) deficiency	Increased incidence with advanced age, pregnancy, malnutrition, and with the use of certain drugs (isoniazid, pyrazinamide, d-penicillamine, and hydralazine); "scalding" pain, erythema, ulceration, and cheilitis	Decreased pyridoxal 5'-phosphate (active form)		Cheilitis may be unresponsive to replacement treatment
Vitamin C deficiency (scurvy)	Seen in the poor, elderly, and alcoholics who consume <10 mg/day of vitamin C. Gingivitis, petechiae, ecchymoses, and perifollicular hemorrhages; corkscrew hairs	Plasma or leukocyte vitamin C level (generally occurs at levels less than 0.1 mg/dL)		Jaundice, oliguria, neuropathy, skeletal, fracture/ changes, fever and convulsions
Folate/vitamin B$_{12}$ deficiency	Tongue erythema, shiny and smooth	Serum B$_{12}$; red blood cell folate; complete blood count/ mean cell volume		B$_{12}$: neurological impairment Folate: birth defects
Iron deficiency	Angular cheilitis, atrophic glossitis, and generalized mucosal atrophy	Ferritin; total iron-binding capacity; complete blood count/mean cell volume		Pallor, lethargy, palpitations, lightheadedness, hypochromic microcytic anemia, alopecia; may be secondary to an intestinal malignancy
Zinc deficiency	Perioral erythematous patches and plaques, hypogeusia, inflammation, poor wound healing	Low plasma zinc levels	Genetic (see Table 10-2); exclusive breastfeeding; malabsorption due to cystic fibrosis or small-bowel resection; abnormal metabolism of essential fatty acids; kwashiorkor	Infection of poorly healing wounds

Table 10-9 Acquired oral diseases

Disease	Etiology	Clinical presentation	Diagnosis	Complications	Treatment
Oral purpura (Figure 10-14)	Bleeding into the skin or mucosa due to trauma, vascular disorder, amyloidosis, hematologic disorders, infectious mononucleosis, rubella, human immunodeficiency virus (HIV), and other rare diseases, such as Chédiak–Higashi syndrome, and Wiskott–Aldrich syndrome	May present with petechiae, ecchymoses or bullae (angina bullosa haemorrhagica), the latter being most frequent among the elderly	Clinical findings; may require work-up for hemostatic function, thrombocytopenia, infections, or nutrient deficiencies	Depends on underlying etiology	
Venous lake	Dilation of venules (vascular ectasia); may be partially related to chronic sun exposure	Dark blue to purple compressible papules up to 1 cm, typically on vermilion of lower lip. Much more frequent in males over age 50	Diascopy; dermoscopy; biopsy; clinical findings	Rule out melanoma and pigmented basal cell neoplasm	Surgical ablation, excision, laser, cryotherapy
Aphthous stomatitis (canker sores)	Unknown, likely to be multifactorial; 10–25% of the population; more common in females	Recurrent, self-healing ulcers with pseudomembrane, usually affecting nonkeratinized mucosa (inside the lips, buccal mucosa, or tongue)	Complete history of recurrent self-healing ulcers at regular intervals	None	
Amyloid/macroglossia	Production of amyloid fibrils by myeloma	Mucocutaneous rubbery papules (tongue, lips, rhinopharynx, larynx, palate; eyelids; neck, anogenital), petechiae, and ecchymoses, macroglossia (the presenting sign of amyloidosis in 19% of patients)	Biopsy of involved tissue; clinical correlation	Dysphagia, dysarthria; associated with myeloma; sialysis-related amyloid of the tongue has also been reported	
Strawberry tongue	Unknown etiology; seen in Kawasaki's, scarlet fever, and toxic shock syndrome	Intense erythema and swelling of papillae on the surface of the tongue, which is covered by a whitish coat	Clinical findings	Related to systemic disease associated with Kawasaki disease, toxic shock syndrome, and scarlet fever	
Glossodynia (burning-mouth syndrome)	Increasing evidence for an underlying sensory neuropathy; females > males, especially postmenopausal women; wide range of possible etiologies, including hematological diseases, vitamin deficiencies, dental work, hormonal factors, infections, and psychological disorders (neuroses, depression, or phobias)	Burning or tingling on the lips, tongue, or entire mouth; usually no visual signs. Pain typically increases over the course of the day	History; clinical judgment	None	Treatment of the underlying cause (antidepressants, vitamin B supplements, transcutaneous electrical nerve stimulation)

Continued

Table 10-9 Acquired oral diseases—cont'd

Disease	Etiology	Clinical presentation	Diagnosis	Complications	Treatment
Angular cheilitis	Fungal, bacterial, and viral infections; nutritional deficiency (especially B vitamins)	Deep cracks and fissures of corners of mouth; may bleed and form a crust	Clinical findings; history; culture	None	Treat underlying condition
Cheilitis glandularis	Unknown; thought to be a reaction chronic irritation (actinic damage, trauma, atopy, infection, and tobacco)	Progressive enlargement of the lower lip, eversion, and induration, mucopurulent exudates, salivary gland dilation. Patients may describe a burning or raw sensation. Male predominance in fourth to seventh decades	Clinical; biopsy to rule out other granulomatous diseases; bacterial/fungal culture	Increased risk of squamous cell carcinoma	
Cheilitis granulomatosa	Unknown; may be monosymptomatic variant of MRS	Onset in early childhood or adolescence. Nontender, episodic (over months to years; may increase in duration over time) swelling of one or both lips; upper lip is most commonly involved, followed by lower lip, then cheeks. Fissured tongue in 20–40%. Rarely, forehead, eyelid, chin, and vulvar involvement have been reported.	Clinical findings Biopsy and culture to rule out other causes (sarcoidosis, Crohn's disease)	None	Nonsteroidal anti-inflammatory drugs and steroids, anticholinergic drugs, and surgical procedures. Botulinum toxin injection into the lacrimal gland has been reported
Melkersson–Rosenthal syndrome (MRS)	Unknown	Triad: lingua plicata (furrowed tongue), chronic labial swelling, and facial nerve palsy. The classic triad is infrequent, with monosymptomatic variants more frequently observed	Clinical findings	May recur intermittently, or may not resolve completely	

Table 10-9 Acquired oral diseases—cont'd

Disease	Etiology	Clinical presentation	Diagnosis	Complications	Treatment
Morsicatio buccarum et labiorum	Chronic, low-grade, mechanical irritation by the teeth (may be a fixed neurosis)	More common in young adults. Lesions are distinct, focal, and translucent to opaque white asymptomatic patches, sharply delineated borders. 2:1 female-to-male ratio	Clinical exam; history	None	Lesions heal with reduction of friction
Tobacco-related changes	Smoking and chewing tobacco	Stained or discolored teeth, halitosis, hairy tongue, "smoker's palate," "smoker's melanosis," "smoker's lip"	Clinical; history	Tobacco increases the risk of oral cancer (squamous cell carcinoma is most common), gingivitis and acute necrotizing ulcerative gingivitis	
Xerostomia (dry mouth)	Anxiety, drugs (anticholinergic tricyclics, phenothiazides, antihypertensive drugs, antihistamines, cytotoxic drugs, retinoids, lithium, opioids, and protease inhibitors), salivary gland diseases (Sjögren's syndrome, sarcoidosis, HIV), systemic disease (graft-versus-host disease, hepatitis C), dehydration, irradiation	Difficulty with speech, swallowing, altered taste, mastication, and suppurative sialadenitis	Clinical; serologies (SS-A and SS-B antibodies); sialometry; salivary gland biopsy; sialography	Candidiasis Dental caries	Avoid exacerbating medications, alcohol, and smoking. Salivation may be stimulated by chewing sugar-free gum and the use of salivary substitutes or sialogogues such as pyridostigmine.
Halitosis	Secondary to volatile sulfur compounds generated by bacteria. Risk factors include poor oral hygiene, dental infections and sepsis, ulcers, xerostomia, starvation, smoking, drugs, diabetic ketosis, nasal foreign body, hepatic or renal failure, psychiatric disease, and advanced age	Bad breath, sour/bitter taste, yellow film on tongue, white tonsillar nodules; normal finding on awakening	Clinical	Depends on underlying cause	Good oral hygiene (brush teeth and tongue, floss and mouthwash), regular meals, avoiding smoking and certain foods (garlic, onions); chewing gum or breath fresheners

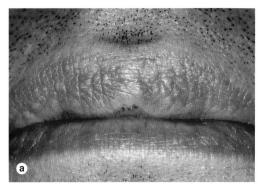

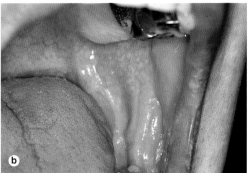

Figure 10-15 a Fordyce spots on the lips. **b** Fordyce spots on the buccal mucosa

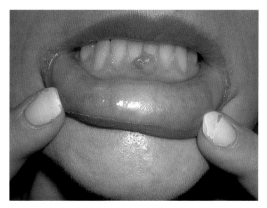

Figure 10-16 Pyogenic granuloma

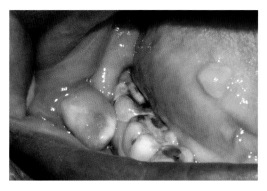

Figure 10-17 Granular cell tumor

fissured tongue. Recurrences may last from months to years and increase in duration. Facial swelling may persist and increase, potentially becoming permanent after recurrent episodes. Melkersson–Rosenthal syndrome tends to begin in childhood or early adolescence. Rarely, forehead, eyelid, chin, and vulvar involvement have been reported. Sarcoidosis and Crohn's disease are in the differential diagnosis. The therapeutic approach mainly consists of NSAIDS and steroids, anticholinergic drugs, and surgical procedures. Botulinum toxin injection into the lacrimal gland is the most recent therapeutic option.

Melkersson–Rosenthal syndrome is a rare neurological disorder characterized by the triad of recurrent orofacial swelling, relapsing facial paralysis, and fissured tongue. The classic triad is infrequent, with monosymptomatic variants more frequently observed. Morsicatio buccarum et labiorum is a frictional keratosis found in young adults. Cheek or lip biting may be observed as a fixed neurosis. Diagnosis can be confirmed by biopsy, and lesions heal spontaneously.

Xerostomia is a common disorder that affects many people. It may result from anxiety, dehydration, and iatrogenic causes, including drugs (anticholinergic tricyclics, phenothiazines, antihypertensive drugs, antihistamines, cytotoxic drugs, retinoids, lithium, opioids, and protease inhibitors), irradiation, and graft-versus-host disease. Salivary gland diseases, such as Sjögren's syndrome,

sarcoidosis, HIV, and hepatitis C can also cause dry mouth. Treatment includes avoiding exacerbating medications, alcohol, and smoking. Salivation may be stimulated by chewing sugar-free gum and the use of salivary substitutes or sialogogues such as pyridostigmine.

Halitosis ("bad breath") is a relatively common complaint among adults. Halitosis results from bacterially generated volatile sulfur compounds. Its prevalence increases with age. Halitosis is normal upon waking, but can become a more persistent and pathologic problem, affecting taste. Treatment includes good oral hygiene (brush teeth and tongue, floss and mouthwash), regular meals, avoiding smoking and certain foods (garlic, onions), chewing gum or breath fresheners. Halitosis may also be a sign of chronic dental infection, gastrointestinal *Helicobacter pylori* infection, or ANUG and must be evaluated for such causes.

Neoplastic disease

Key Points

- Leukoplakia may be premalignant
- Erythroplakia is usually malignant
- Plummer–Vinson syndrome presents with a triad of dysphagia, iron-deficiency anemia, and esophageal webs

- Oral submucous fibrosis is a premalignant condition observed among betel nut/areca nut chewers
- Squamous carcinoma can present as an ulcer, red or white lesion, lump, or fissure

Neoplasms of the oral mucosa may be benign, premalignant, or malignant (Table 10-10).

Pyogenic granulomas are benign vascular growths that occur more commonly in women, during pregnancy (1% incidence), with poor oral hygiene or a history of oral trauma.

Oral papillomas are verrucous lesions usually associated with benign HPV 6 or 11, although premalignant viral subtypes and potential have been reported.

Leukoplakia, white patchy mucosal changes found in 1–4% of the population, has a 100-fold increased rate of cancer development when compared with baseline normal population. In western populations, a 4–5% 10-year malignant transformation rate has been reported. The floor of mouth is at highest risk for neoplasia, whereas palatal lesions have a relatively low risk. Lesions homogeneous in appearance are less likely to transform (5%) than are speckled lesions (30%). Erythroplakia, red mucosal patches, has a higher rate of carcinoma development than does leukoplakia, and generally warrants removal.

Plummer–Vinson syndrome is a very rare, idiopathic disorder with a classical triad of dysphagia, iron-deficiency anemia, and esophageal webs. Most patients are white, middle-aged (40–70 years old) women. The dysphagia involving solid foods is usually painless, intermittent, or progressive, and may be associated with weight loss. Symptoms of anemia (weakness, pallor, fatigue, tachycardia) may dominate the clinical picture. Glossitis, angular cheilitis, koilonychias, splenomegaly, and thyromegaly may also be observed. The syndrome is associated with development of squamous cell carcinoma (SCC) of the pharynx and esophagus, and thus malignancy surveillance is crucial, as are iron supplementation and mechanical dilation of the esophageal lumen.

Oral submucous fibrosis is an idiopathic condition observed among betel nut/areca nut chewers in India. The condition involves a chronic insidious atrophy and fibrosis of the tongue and oral mucosa, with ensuing premalignant changes. A dose-dependent relationship between the areca nut (which is independent of tobacco) and the development of the condition has been demonstrated. The diagnosis is clinical and is confirmed by biopsy.

Oral cancer has a 2:1 prevalence ratio in males:females and is most prevalent in the > 40-year age group. In the oral cavity, 90% of malignancies are SCC, 8% are adenocarcinomas (salivary gland), and 2% are sarcomas. These tumors appear on the lower lip (30%), tongue (20%), floor of mouth (15%), mandibular alveolus (15%), buccal mucosa (10%), and maxillary alveolus and palate (10%). Implicated etiologic factors include social habits (tobacco, alcohol, areca nut/betel nut), infections (bacterial: tertiary syphilis; fungal: *Candida* leukoplakia; and viral: HSV, HPV, and HIV), extrinsic factors (ultraviolet radiation, poor oral hygiene, and ill-fitting dentures), and intrinsic factors (genetics, such as dyskeratosis congenita, Paterson–Kelly sideropenic dysphagia syndrome), nutritional deficiencies (iron: Plummer–Vinson syndrome; folate: vitamin B_{12}), and drug or HIV-induced immunosuppression. Chronic wounds secondary to inflammatory/autoimmune diseases such as lichen planus, oral lichenoid dysplasia, and discoid lupus erythematosus also predispose to the development of SCC. Chronic immunosuppression in combination with fair skin and sun damage/actinic cheilitis predispose to development of SCC of the lip. Tobacco is commonly regarded as the most influential factor, especially with verrucous carcinoma and leukoplakia. Pipe and cigar smoking can cause intraoral keratosis; unfiltered cigarettes cause lip carcinoma; and snuff dipping typically results in carcinoma of the buccal sulcus, where it is habitually positioned.

Oral SCC is most prevalent in the developing world. SCC can present as an ulcer, red or white lesion, lump, or fissure. Diagnosis is confirmed by biopsy. Verrucous carcinoma, usually a slow-growing exophytic mass, is a low-grade SCC in the elderly.

Premalignant changes of actinic cheilitis can be treated topically with diclofenac, 5-fluorouracil, imiquimod, and retinoids. Other destructive modalities include topical trichloracetic acid, cryotherapy, curettage, and carbon dioxide laser therapy. Treatments for SCC include surgery, radiotherapy, and chemotherapy most frequently. Systemic retinoids and chemotherapy are also useful in advanced or metastatic disease. SCC prognosis based upon tumor, node, metastasis (TNM) clinical staging, with stage 1 through 4 offering 5-year survivals of 85, 65, 40, and 10%, respectively.

Kaposi's sarcoma (KS) is a human herpesvirus 8-associated neoplasm, usually found in HIV patients, rarely in transplant and other iatrogenically immunosuppressed patients. Lesions are most often found on the palate or oropharynx. Clinical lesions and viral load have been reported to respond to HIV therapy or decreased immunosuppression in transplant patients.

Oral malignant melanoma is a rare disease. It is most commonly found on the maxillary arch of the palate (80%), but also on the gingiva. Oral mucosal melanoma represents about 8% of total melanomas in Asians and 20% in blacks. Often diagnosed at a late stage of disease, these lesions are associated with a poor prognosis.

Table 10-10 Neoplastic disorders of the mouth

Disease	Clinical presentation	Treatment	Complications
Fordyce spots (Figure 10-15) (ectopic sebaceous glands)	Yellow papules on lips or buccal mucosa	None	None
Papilloma	Verrucous papule or nodule	Excision; laser; cryotherapy	
Pyogenic granuloma (lobular capillary hemangioma) (Figure 10-16)	More common in pregnancy and women. May be secondary to trauma. Soft, painless rubbery red-to-purple nodule, decreases in vascularity with time. Anterior maxillary gingiva most frequently affected site	Biopsy	Always benign, but be sure to exclude other tumors
Oral leukoplakia/ erythroplakia/oral lichenoid dysplasia	Found in 1–4% of the population; asymptomatic, white/red, sharply defined elevated patch or plaque that cannot be rubbed off	Biopsy; surgical/destructive removal; discontinue alcohol use and smoking	Oral cancer (100-fold increased rate of cancer development compared with baseline normal population; in western populations, a 4–5% 10-year malignant transformation rate has been reported)
			Floor of the mouth is at highest risk for neoplasia
			Lesions homogeneous in appearance are less likely to transform (5%) than speckled lesions (30%)
Erythroplakia	Red mucosal patches	Excision	Oral cancer (more common than in leukoplakia)
Leukokeratosis nicotina palate ("smoker's palate")	Appears as a diffuse, uniform, white keratosis on the hard palate; multiple red, umbilicated papules due to inflamed salivary glands	Cessation of smoking; biopsy if lesion involves soft palate	Premalignant potential
Squamous cell carcinoma	Red or white patch, plaque, or ulcer of the oral mucosa. Location frequency: lateral tongue > floor of mouth > lower vermilion lip border > alveolar ridge	Excisional biopsy; Mohs micrographic surgery; adjunctive chemotherapy and radiation if lymphatic spread has occurred; systemic retinoids	Metastasis and death
Basal cell carcinoma	Rarely occurs in the oral cavity; most commonly on lip. Pearly telangiectatic nodule or patch; may ulcerate and bleed	Excisional biopsy; Mohs micrographic surgery; adjunctive radiation and chemotherapy if advanced	Rare metastasis and bone involvement
Granular cell tumor (Figure 10-17)	Painless orange to yellowish firm nodules< 2 cm in size; most commonly on the tongue	Surgical excision	Risks of simple excision (infection, bleeding, etc); tend not to recur
Kaposi sarcoma (Figure 10-10)	Violaceous patches, plaques or nodules associated with HIV or other causes of immunosuppression (i.e., transplant patients); intraoral is most common location on body with prevalence: palate > lips > tongue	Various treatments: surgical excision; low-dose radiation; intralesional chemotherapy; sclerosing agents; resolves with highly active antiretroviral therapy (HAART) or reduction of immunosuppression	Systemic involvement

Table 10-10 Neoplastic disorders of the mouth—cont'd

Disease	Clinical presentation	Treatment	Complications
Salivary gland tumor	Small, mobile, slow-growing, painless mass, usually in the parotid region. Spares seventh cranial nerve, even when large	Complete surgical excision	Metastasis
Leukemia/leukemia cutis	Varied presentations: Gingival hypertrophy, petechiae, ulcers, and ecchymoses	Treat underlying leukemia	Bacterial superinfection
Melanoma	Brown/black lesion/ulcer; most commonly found on the maxillary arch of the palate (80%), but also on the gingival	Surgical, other adjunctive therapies	Metastasis and death

HIV, human immunodeficiency virus.

Further reading

Cawson RA, Odell EW. Essentials of Oral Pathology and Oral Medicine, 7th edn. London: Churchill Livingstone, 2002.

Dimitroulis G, Avery BS. Oral Cancer: A Synopsis of Pathology and Management. Oxford: Reed, 1998.

Eisen D. The clinical manifestations and treatment of oral lichen planus. Dermatol Clin 2003;21:79–89.

Ficarra G, Cicchi P, Amorosi A, et al. Oral Crohn's disease and pyostomatitis vegetans. Oral Surg Oral Med Oral Pathol Oral Radiol Endod 1993; 75:220–224.

Hand JL, Rogers RS. Oral manifestations of genodermatoses. Dermatol Clin 2003;23:183–194.

Hildebrand C, Burgdorf WHC, Lautenschlager S. Cowden syndrome: diagnostic skin signs. Dermatology 2001;202:362–366.

Mahoney EJ. Sjögren's disease. Otolaryngol Clin North Am 2003;36:733–745.

Messadi DV, Mirowski GW. White lesions of the oral cavity. Dermatol Clin 2003;21:63–78.

Regezi J, Sciubba J, Pogrel MA. Atlas of Oral and Maxillofacial Pathology. Philadelphia: WB Saunders, 2000.

Witman PM, Rogers RS. Pediatric oral medicine. Dermatol Clin 2003;21:157–170.

Wolff K, Johnson RA, Suurmond D. Fitzpatrick's Color Atlas and Synopsis of Clinical Dermatology, 5th edn. New York: McGraw Hill, 2005.

Spongiotic disorders

Sharon E. Jacob and Juan P. Jaimes

Introduction

Several diseases fall under the umbrella category of "eczematous dermatoses" because of their similar clinical and histological presentations. Eczema, from the Greek word meaning to "boil over," is synonymous with dermatitis. A common unifying characteristic of this group of dermatoses is spongiotic inflammation of the epidermis, which histologically consists of exocytosis of lymphocytes and intracellular edema. This chapter differentiates and delineates these dermatoses (Box 11-1 and Table 11-1) and offers a guide to diagnosis and treatment (see overview in Table 11-11, later).

Allergic contact dermatitis (ACD)

Clinical presentation

Key Points

- Eczematous and edematous, scaly pruritic plaques, which may be accentuated by papules and vesicles
- History and geographic distribution are important clues to the causal allergen

Allergic contact dermatitis (ACD) (Figure 11-1) is the inflammatory state that results from a T-cell-mediated, type IV delayed-type hypersensitivity (DTH) reaction to a percutaneously-exposed allergen. This type of allergic reaction is characterized by erythema, edema, and, in severe cases, papulovesicles, usually in the distribution of contact with the instigating allergen. The presentation may vary, however, because of inherent differences in the area of epidermis involved, the potency of the allergen, and the chronicity of the disease. This dermatosis may be divided into subacute, acute, and chronic subtypes. The subacute presentation is likely to demonstrate macular erythema and scaling. On the other hand, the acute form typically exhibits erythema, edema, and papulovesicles. One distinguishing feature of acute ACD, which

helps differentiate it from irritant contact dermatitis (ICD) and patch-stage mycosis fungoides, is its intense pruritus. However, when the dermatitis becomes chronic, the clinical picture of lichenified, fissured plaques predominates, and differentiation between ICD and ACD may not be possible.

In general, primary lesions arise in the distribution of allergen contact on the skin, providing a very important diagnostic clue as to the identity of the instigating allergen. Although not all allergens "obey the rules," location of the dermatitis is a chief factor in the diagnostic algorithm. Site-specific clinical presentations and high-probability allergens are grouped in Table 11-2.

ACD presents in all age groups, although it is less common in the first few months and after the sixth decade of life. It is generally thought that the low incidence of ACD in infants and the elderly results from a lack of exposure and failure to respond immunologically in the former, and to a decline in the immune response (senesce) in the latter. Although ACD in children was once believed to be very rare, new evidence suggests

---

BOX 11-1

Differential diagnoses of eczematous diseases

1. Allergic contact dermatitis (ACD)
2. Asteatotic dermatitis
3. Atopic dermatitis (fundamentally a pathologic itch, but secondary spongiotic change common)
4. Autosensitization reaction
5. Dyshidrotic eczema
6. Irritant contact dermatitis (ICD)
7. Mycosis fungoides (patch to plaque stage)
8. Nummular dermatitis
9. Psoriasis vulgaris
10. Seborrheic dermatitis
11. Venous stasis dermatitis

Table 11-1 Overview of spongiotic disorders

Differential diagnosis	Differences in clinical presentation	Histopathology	Differentiating tests
Irritant contact dermatitis	Burning, and stinging exceed itching Rapid presentation of disease (hours) compared to allergic contact dermatitis (days) Macular erythema, hyperkeratosis	Superficial ballooning Neutrophilic infiltrates and necrosis Separation of the dermoepidermal junction can be observed, resulting in vesicles or bullae	Patch testing Biopsy findings variable (depending on the irritant); some irritants produce superficial necrosis of the epidermis with neutrophils
Allergic contact dermatitis	Pruritic eczematous, scaly edematous plaques accentuated by papulovesicles	Vesiculation and spongiosis with an ordered pattern Presence of mild exocytosis of lymphocytes Eosinophilic dermal infiltrate Superficial dermal edema	Patch testing
Nummular dermatitis	Coin-shaped, well-demarcated plaques with scale and vesicles Usually first observed on the extremities Intense pruritus Koebner phenomenon observed	Spongiosis in a disorganized pattern Occasional neutrophils in the dermal infiltrate Occasional neutrophils in the epidermis	
Seborrheic dermatitis	Erythematous or pink papulosquamous greasy plaques Presents on skin surfaces containing large numbers of sebaceous glands such as the face, scalp, chest, back, and flexural areas	Variable spongiosis Scale crust and spongiosis may localize to follicular ostia	
Atopic dermatitis	Acute: Eczematous, honey-crusted scaly plaques, marked by excoriation Chronic: Lichenified, scaly, fissured plaques	Vessels are prominent in the papillary dermis Presence of eosinophil major basic protein and eosinophils around vessels Secondary spongiosis or lichenification with dermal angiofibroplasia and compact hyperkeratosis	Clinical history
Pompholyx	Distribution of the lesions is bilateral and symmetrical Vesicular eruptions of palms and soles Presence of pruritus, burning, and prickling sensations	Vesicle formation with peripheral displacement of acrosyringia Usually more sharply defined than allergic contact dermatitis of palms and soles	
Stasis dermatitis	Pruritic, erythematous, shiny, and scaly plaques located in medial lower legs Excoriations and lichenification are often observed as well as brown puncta, purpura, hemosiderosis, and/or patches of white atrophy	Dermal hemosiderin Mild spongiosis Nodular proliferation of vessels in the superficial dermis Extravasation of erythrocytes	

Table 11-1 Overview of spongiotic disorders—Cont'd

Differential diagnosis	Differences in clinical presentation	Histopathology	Differentiating tests
Autoeczematization	Eczematous, poorly defined patches of vesiculation History of chronic dermatitis patch with new widespread, less defined patches	Variable spongiosis Edema of papillary dermis and activated lymphocytes often present	
Mycosis fungoides	Poorly demarcated, atrophic scaly pink patches and plaques Torso predominance	Little spongiosis Pautrier microabscesses Atypical lymphocytes in epidermis surrounded by white halo "(lump of coal on a pillow)" Papillary dermal fibrosis Lymphocytes often line up at dermal–epidermal junction	Biopsy
Psoriasis	Sharply demarcated papulosquamous plaques with no vesiculation Scalp, retroauricular area, elbows, knees, genitalia, nails Predominance to areas of trauma (koebnerization) Pustules may be acutely present, particularly on the palms and soles Concomitant arthritis	Regular acanthosis Thinning of suprapapillary plate Alternating neutrophils and parakeratosis in stratum corneum	Biopsy

Adapted from Weedon D. Skin Pathology, 2nd edn. New York: Churchill Livingstone, 2002.

that as many as 20% of the pediatric population are affected. In all, 20–65% of children referred to patch-testing centers have been found to have positive reactions.

In 2004, 9.2 million patients visited dermatologists in the United States for evaluation of ACD, making it the third most common reason for visits in outpatient dermatology. Because of its chronicity and relentless nature, it has a high impact on morbidity and health care costs.

The North American Contact Dermatitis Group regularly reports their patch test study data and identifies their top allergens. In the most recently reported data set (between 2001 and 2002), nickel was the allergen most frequently identified, followed by neomycin and balsam of Peru (Table 11-3).

Diagnostic tests

The epicutaneous patch test is the *gold standard* for diagnosing ACD (Figure 11-2). There are two commercially available patch test *screening* tools in the United States with Food and Drug Administration indications: the 29-chamber thin-layer rapid-use epicutaneous panel (T.R.U.E Test™) and the Hermal/Trolab 20-allergen standard test.

Beyond this, more comprehensive testing may be performed in which allergens are specifically selected for the patient based on the history and clinical distribution of the dermatosis.

Per standardized procedure protocol, the screening chemical substances in chambers are placed in contact with clinically unaffected skin on the back (and sometimes inner arm) for 48 hours. After the initial 48-hour application period, the patches are removed, marked, and evaluated. Reactions are graded on a scale of 0–3+ (Table 11-4). Irritant reactions may also be seen at this reading. A delayed reading between 72 and 120 hours postapplication is strongly recommended to identify late-appearing DTH reactions; however, this is not always done. Reactions to several allergens, including bacitracin and corticosteroids, are frequently delayed. Studies suggest that up to one-third of reactions are missed because of failure to perform a delayed reading.

If patch testing detects any allergies, it is important to establish the likely relevance of these allergies to the patient's dermatitis. In some cases, the relevance is clear, particularly if there was known exposure to a particular chemical that elicited the rash, and the same reaction is confirmed by testing. However, in other situations, the relevance is unclear. Some allergens, such as thimerosal, are frequently positive on testing, but are rarely relevant to most dermatoses. This is particularly important when occupational, or potentially legal, issues are involved with the purported allergy. If the suspect products are nontoxic and noncaustic, direct testing can, in many cases, be performed with specific products, such as personal care products. A repeat open-application test can also confirm allergies to some products. Several reference texts provide information about patch testing with nonstandardized products, and it is strongly recommended that these be consulted, or that the patient be referred to a center that performs regular patch testing, if patch testing with nonstandardized allergens is desired.

Pathogenesis

Key Points

- ACD is a delayed-type (type IV) T-cell mediated hypersensitivity reaction
- Two phases of the reaction: sensitization (induction) and elicitation (challenge)

ACD is the clinical outcome of an aberrant T-cell-mediated immunity. In the susceptible person, the process is initiated when small, electrophilic haptens (< 500 Da) penetrate the epidermis and covalently bind to keratinocytes. One exception

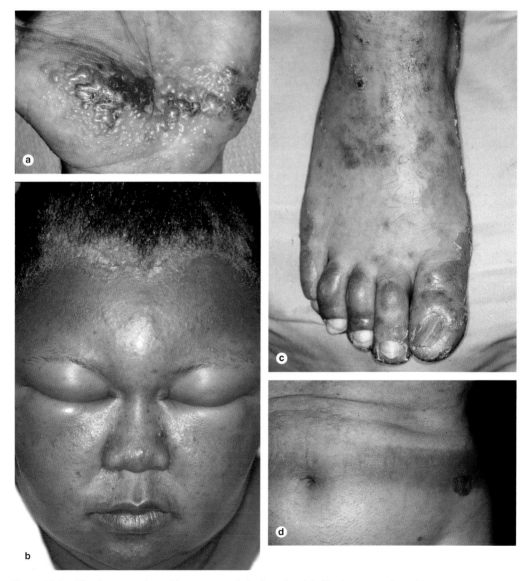

Figure 11-1 **a** Allergic contact dermatitis to neoprene in keyboard pad. **b** Allergic contact dermatitis to paraphenylenediamene. **c** Allergic contact shoe dermatitis. **d** Bleached rubber dermatitis.

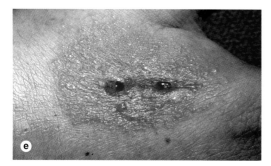

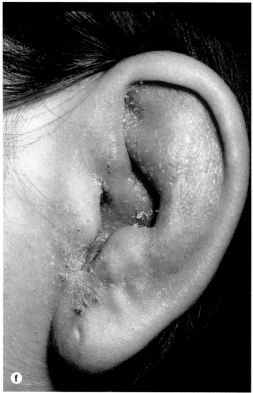

Figure 11-1, cont'd e Allergic contact dermatitis to bacitracin. **f** Allergic contact dermatitis to neomycin in an otic suspension

Table 11-2 Algorithm for suspecting allergens

Location	Regional suspects	Likely allergens
Scalp, hairline	Hair dyes, styling products	Hair dye (paraphenylenediamine, PPD)
Face	Cosmetics and airborne allergens	Preservatives: formaldehyde-releasing products (quaternium-15, diazolidinyl urea), fragrances, paraben mix
Eyelids	Nail polish, eye makeup, contact lens solutions, airborne allergens	Formaldehyde, FRP, gold, PPD, fragrances, cyanoacrylates
Lips	Foods, lip balm, nail polish, toothpaste	Balsam of Peru, lanolin derivatives, parabens, surfactants (cocamidopropyl-betaine; CAPB)
Ears	Jewelry, eardrops	Nickel, neomycin, corticosteroids
Preauricular region	Hair dye, styling products	PPD
Post-auricular region	Shampoo, conditioner, soap	FRP, fragrances, CAPB
Neck	Hair products, jewelry, perfumes	Nickel, fragrance mix, PPD, balsam of Peru
Axilla	Deodorant, clothing	Fragrance mix, formaldehyde, resins
Trunk	Clothing, zippers, buttons	Formaldehyde resins, dyes, nickel, balsam of Peru
Hands	Gloves and occupational contacts	Rubber additives (thiuram, black rubber mix), formaldehydes, CAPB
Feet	Shoes	*Para*-tertiary butylphenol formaldehyde resin, formaldehyde, antibiotics, potassium dichromate

Adapted from de Groot A. Allergic contact dermatitis. In: Marks R, ed. Eczema. London: Martin Dunitz, 1992:104–125.

is metals, which form a complex similar to that formed by cobalt in vitamin B_{12}. The keratinocyte-hapten interaction forms a neoallergen, which is then captured by Langerhans cells. Through a complex immunologic function, the Langerhans cell carries the allergen to the lymph node, where it presents the allergen to naive T-helper cells. If production of major histocompatibility (MHC) I class-restricted CD8+ T cells (suppressor cells) occurs, immunologic tolerance to the allergen develops. However, if production of MHC II class-restricted CD4+ T cells (effector cells) results, the patient becomes sensitized to the allergen. The sensitization process can take as little as 10–14 days with a potent allergen or as long as 21 days with a lesser allergenic substance.

Upon subsequent exposure to this same antigen, activated clonal T cells proliferate and cytotoxic T cells migrate to the site of original antigen contact. This may be likened to a bee which surveys the garden (skin) and then returns to the hive (lymph node of cloning) to perpetuate the information to the next set of bees. With each subsequent contact of the allergen to sensitized skin, a proinflammatory cytokine cascade is released, causing the clinical picture of ACD within 48–120 hours.

Table 11-3 Top North American Contact Dermatitis Group allergens 2001–2002

Order	Substance	Number of tests	Positive reactions (%)
1	Nickel sulfate (2.5%)	4901	16.7
2	Neomycin (20%)	4904	11.6
3	Balsam of Peru (25%)	4910	11.6
4	Fragrance mix (8%)	4896	10.4
5	Thimerosal (0.1%)	4899	10.2
6	Sodium gold thiosulfate (0.5%)	4900	10.2
7	Quaternium-15 (2%)	4910	9.3
8	Formaldehyde (1% aqs)	4909	8.4
9	Bacitracin (20%)	4900	7.9
10	Cobalt chloride (1%)	4899	7.4
11	Methyldibromoglutaronitrile/ phenoxyethanol	4897	5.8

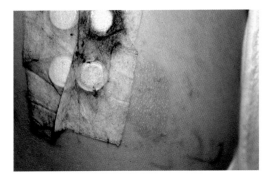

Figure 11-2 Positive patch test reaction to nickel

Table 11-4 North American Contact Dermatitis Group scoring system

Score	Clinical characteristics
0	Negative
?	Macular erythema
1+	Erythema, infiltration, possible papules
2+	Erythema, infiltration, papules, vesicles
3+	Intense erythema, infiltration, coalescing vesicles, crusting with ulceration
IR	Irritant

Data from Marks JG, Belsito DV, DeLeo VA, et al. North American Contact Dermatitis Group standard tray patch test results (1992–1994). Am J Contact Dermatis 1995;6:160–165, and Marks JG, Belsito DV, DeLeo VA, et al. North American Contact Dermatitis Group patch test results for the detection of delayed-type hypersensitivity to topical allergens. J Am Acad Dermatol 1998;38:911–918.

Treatment

The primary step in management of ACD is the identification of the culprit allergen(s). The second step is avoidance of exposure to the allergen and any cross-reactive substances. Patients should be educated as to likely sources of exposure to their relevant allergens, and an alternative product substitution list should be offered to them. Treatment consists of topical corticosteroids or topical immunomodulators. When there is widespread involvement, either by acute or chronic ACD, use of systemic immunomodulating medications may be considered. Treatments used may include oral corticosteroids, oral tacrolimus, cyclosporine, and mycophenolate mofetil. A summary of treatments available for ACD is given in Table 11-5.

Asteatotic dermatitis (Eczema craquelé)

Clinical presentation

Key Points

- Crackled parchment-like patches with notable absence of edema and vesiculation
- Very pruritic
- Hallmark: anterior shin predominance, usually limited to lower extremities in aged persons

This pruritic dermatitis is most commonly located in the lower extremities of elderly individuals, but may present in other parts of the body as well. The affected areas appear dry, with fine scales and cracks that can coalesce in a perpendicular fashion, resembling cracks in porcelain (Figure 11-3) or cement. The diagnosis is based on the

Table 11-5 Allergic contact dermatitis treatment

Treatment	Schedule
Topical corticosteroids	Select appropriate potency by clinical assessment with once- or twice-daily applications
Immunomodulators	Topical tacrolimus 0.1% ointment twice daily
Systemic corticosteroids	Prednisone 1 mg/kg per day for several days with a 2-week taper

Table 11-6 Treatments available for asteatotic dermatitis

Treatment	Schedule
12% ammonium lactate containing-lotions	Applied daily
Topical steroids (class III–IV)	Once or twice daily

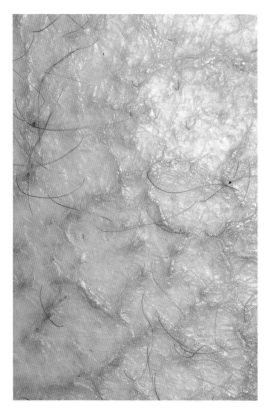

Figure 11-3 Eczema craquelé

clinical presentation and the history. It is most commonly associated with vigorous cleaning and rubbing, hot baths, and a history of xerosis.

Pathogenesis

It is thought to occur more commonly in the elderly population in the setting of xerosis, secondary to a decrease in sebaceous and sweat gland activity, in addition to epidermal water loss in the barrier. Frequent bathing with soap, especially during the winter, is a common factor in the elderly. Fundamentally, most asteatotic eczema represents a barrier defect. Spongiotic change is secondary. Some cases represent mild forms of nummular eczema.

Treatment

Gentle cleaning with emollients and lukewarm water is recommended. Topical corticosteroids can be considered if there is an inflammatory component. In addition, 12% ammonium lactate lotion may help soften dry skin, but patients should be cautioned that it occasionally stings and irritates fissured areas. Topical steroids (class III–IV) are recommended for severe cases. A summary of treatments available for asteatotic dermatitis is given in Table 11-6.

Atopic dermatitis (AD)

Clinical presentation

Key Points

- Acute: eczematous, honey crusted scaly plaques, marked by excoriation
- Chronic: lichenified, scaly, fissured plaques
- Pruritus is extremely common
- Facial and extensor involvement in infants
- Flexural lichenification in adults and children

AD is a chronic, pruritic disease that can occur at any age, but is most common in early childhood. The remitting and flaring course of this condition may be exacerbated by social, environmental, and biological triggers. There is a history of allergic rhinitis or asthma in up to 50% of patients with AD, and in 75%, there is a family history of atopy. Notably, AD appears to resolve during early adolescence in over half of the cases.

AD (Figure 11-4) is considered to be part of the inflammatory (type I) hypersensitivity triad that includes allergic rhinitis and bronchial asthma. It may have a variety of clinical features. A summary of differential diagnoses and their clinical presentation is given in Table 11-7.

Diagnostic tests

Key Points

- Prick testing for immunoglobulin (Ig) E-mediated allergies
- Radioallergosorbent test (RAST) for associated IgE-mediated allergies
- IgE levels > 1000 ng/mL and increased blood eosinophils support diagnosis

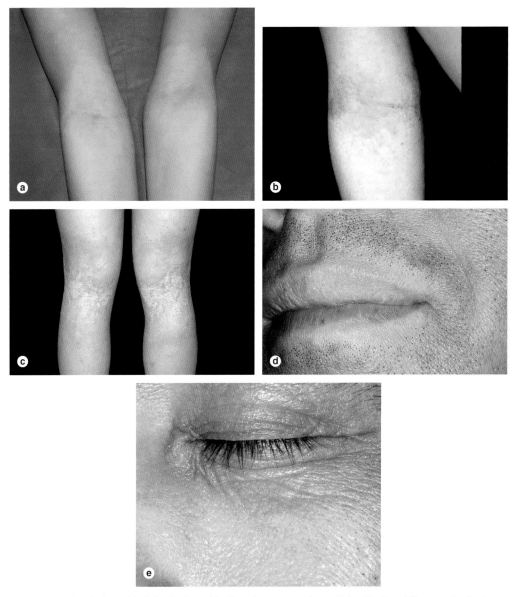

Figure 11-4 a Atopic dermatitis. **b** Atopic dermatitis, flexural eczema. **c** Flexural lichenification. **d** Circumoral pallor in atopic dermatitis. **e** Dennie Morgan folds

Although the tests mentioned above might be helpful, in order to diagnose AD the criteria in Table 11-8, and in Table 11-9 for infants, have to be met.

Pathogenesis

- Inherited reduction or loss of the epidermal barrier protein filaggrin is a major predisposing factor for AD
- Due in part to genetic susceptibility, immune dysfunction, and epidermal barrier dysfunction.
- Associated with increased serum IgE levels, eosinophilia, increased basophil spontaneous histamine release, and expansion of interleukin (IL)-4 and IL-5-secreting TH2-type cells

AD is in part due to genetic susceptibility, immune dysfunction, and epidermal barrier dysfunction. AD is associated with increased serum IgE production. It is thought that AD is in part related to a defect in filaggrin.

Treatment

The mainstay of treatment is to control the inflammation by avoiding triggers (excessive washing, contact with irritating substances, and certain foods) and restoring the epidermal barrier with emollients. In addition, topical steroids, immunomodulators, and antihistamines may be needed. As clinically appropriate, measures may be needed to control secondary infections, particularly those

Table 11-7 Clinical presentation and differential diagnosis of atopic dermatitis

Age	Clinical presentation	Differential diagnosis
Infantile	Pruritus	Seborrheic dermatitis
	Erythema of the cheeks, spreading rapidly to other parts of the body, such as scalp, neck, forehead, and legs	Immunodeficiency
		Psoriasis
	Perioral sparing	
	Moist, crusted lesions are often observed	
	Secondary infection is common	
Childhood	Pruritus	Scabies
	Drier lesions, less exudative and more papular	Tinea corporis
	Located classically in antecubital and popliteal fossae, flexor wrists, face, and neck	Perioral dermatitis
		Nummular dermatitis
		Contact dermatitis
		Molluscum dermatitis
		Mycosis fungoides
Adult	Flexural involvement	
	Lesions are coalescent papules that form lichenified scaly plaques which can be erythematous or hyperpigmented	
	Typical features of childhood atopic dermatitis may resolve, leaving only "sensitive skin" and/or hand dermatitis	

Adapted from Krol A, Krafchik B. The differential diagnosis of atopic dermatitis in childhood. Dermatol Ther 2006;19:73–82.

from *Staphylococcus aureus*. A summary of treatments available for AD is given in Table 11-10.

Autosensitization reaction (Id reaction)

Clinical presentation

Key Points

- Eczematous, poorly defined patches of vesicles
- History of chronic dermatitis with new, widespread, less well-defined patches

The autosensitization reaction (id reaction) is a secondary dermatitis that results from a distant dermatitis occurring elsewhere in the body. This autoeczematization usually develops 1 week to several weeks after the original lesion arises. The most common presentation of these "initial" lesions is on the lower extremities, in the form of chronic eczema or venous stasis dermatitis. On clinical presentation, symmetrical, pruritic, erythematous papulovesicular plaques may appear in a variety of different body locations. Diagnosing this eczematous condition can be challenging, as it is a diagnosis of exclusion.

Pathogenesis

The pathogenesis is largely unknown; however, it is thought that cytokines produced in the initial lesion circulate in the bloodstream and cause sensitization in distant skin regions. An increased number of activated T cells, as well as an elevated ratio of T-helper cells to T-suppressor cells, has been observed, providing a rationale for this purported cytokine effect.

Treatment

Key Points

- Identify the primary lesion; in particular, look for chronic eczema on the lower legs
- Treat the "primary" lesion
- Topical and/or systemic corticosteroids may be needed, depending on the intensity of the widespread dermatitis

Dyshidrotic eczema

Clinical presentation

Key Points

- Recurrent vesicular eruption of the palms and soles
- Presence of pruritus, burning, and prickling sensations

Dyshidrotic eczema (Figure 11-5) has also been called *episodic vesiculobullous eczema of the palms and soles, hand and foot eczema,* and *pompholyx.* There has been some controversy as to whether dyshidrotic eczema and pompholyx are the same disease or represent different entities. The

Table 11-8 Diagnostic criteria for atopic dermatitis

Major features	Minor features
1. Pruritus	Cataracts
2. Typical morphology and distribution • Flexural lichenification in adults • Facial and extensor involvement in infants and children	Cheilitis
	Conjunctivitis – recurrent
	Eczema – perifollicular accentuation
	Facial pallor/facial erythema
	Food intolerance
3. Chronic or chronically relapsing dermatitis	Hand dermatitis – nonallergic, irritant
4. Personal or family history of atopy (asthma, allergic rhinitis, atopic dermatitis)	Ichthyosis
	Serum immunoglobulin E elevated
	Immediate type 1 skin test reactivity
	Cutaneous infections
	Infraorbital fold (Dennie–Morgan lines)
	Itching when sweating
	Keratoconus
	Keratosis pilaris
	Nipple dermatitis
	Orbital darkening
	Palmar hyperlinearity
	Pityriasis alba
	White dermographism
	Wool intolerance
	Xerosis

Three or more from major and minor criteria are necessary to confirm the diagnosis.
Adapted from Habif T. Clinical Dermatology: A Color Guide to Diagnosis and Therapy, 4th edn, Philadelphia: Mosby, 2004.

Table 11-9 Diagnostic criteria for atopic dermatitis, modified for young infants

Major features	Minor features
Pruritus	Xerosis/ichthyosis/hyperlinear palms
Family history of atopy (asthma, allergic rhinitis, atopic dermatitis)	Perifollicular accentuation
	Postauricular fissures
Facial and extensor involvement	Chronic scalp scaling

Three or more from major and minor criteria are necessary to confirm the diagnosis.
Adapted from Odom R, James W, Berger T. Andrews' Diseases of the Skin: Clinical Dermatology, 9th edn. Philadelphia: WB Saunders, 2000.

Table 11-10 Treatments available for atopic dermatitis

Treatment	Schedule
Topical corticosteroids	Potency and structural class selection will depend on clinical judgment
	Hydrocortisone ointment 1 or 2.5%
	Triamcinolone acetonide ointment 0.1% (limit use in children from 7 to 21 days)
	Hydrocortisone valerate ointment 0.2%
Immunomod-ulators	Topical tacrolimus, 0.03% ointment (children) and 0.1% (adults)
Systemic corticosteroids	Prednisone in varied doses
Antibiotics	Cephalexin 250–500 mg qid
	Cefadroxil 500 mg bid
	Dicloxacillin 250 mg qid
Antihistamines	Hydroxyzine 25–75 mg qhs
Emollients	10% urea in a hydrophilic cream
	Various emollient preparations
	Petrolatum
	1% hydrocortisone in 10% urea
	Crude coal tar 1–5% in white petrolatum

qid, four times a day; bid, twice a day; qhs, at bedtime.

characteristic finding of dyshidrosis is vesicles on the palms and soles, which are often preceded by pruritic, burning, and prickling sensations. The distribution of the lesions is typically bilateral and symmetrical. Notably, the eruption may last 2–3 weeks and it resolves without scarring. Recurrence at various intervals is commonplace. Keratolysis exfoliativa (Figure 11-6) presents with oval fine white scaling areas that evolve from subclinical spongiotic vesicles. It generally represents a mild form of dyshidrotic eczema. Tinea can present with a similar appearance.

Diagnostic tests

Key Points

- Clinical history
- Rule out an associated dermatosis, particularly ACD

An important aspect in the evaluation and treatment of dyshidrosis is identifying concomitant dermatoses (Table 11-11).

Pathogenesis

Key Points

- Unknown etiology
- May be related to stress, atopy, and allergens (topical and ingested). Although the etiology of this eczematous disease is unknown, higher relative risks are seen in association with stress, atopy, and ingested or topical allergens. Tinea pedis may contribute to dyshidrotic eczema in the form of an id reaction

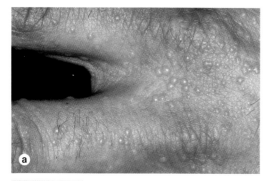

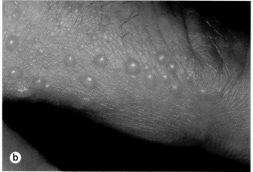

Figure 11-5 a Dyshidrotic vesicular dermatitis.
b Dyshidrotic eczema

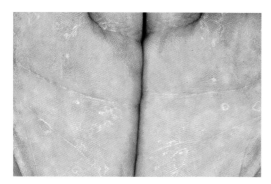

Figure 11-6 Keratolysis exfoliativa

Table 11-11 Differential diagnosis of dyshidrosis

Differential diagnosis	Differentiating tests
Allergic contact dermatitis	Patch test
Pustular psoriasis, tinea, atopic dermatitis, rarely mycosis fungoides	Biopsy

Treatment

The treatment options for dyshidrotic eczema are listed in Table 11-12. It is important to note that, although this vesicular process can resolve without treatment, relapse is common.

Table 11-12 Medical treatment of dyshidrosis

Treatment*	Schedule
Topical corticosteroids	Mometasone furoate 0.1% ointment bid
Immunomodulators	Tacrolimus (FK506) 0.1% ointment bid
Systemic steroids	Oral prednisone
	Intramuscular triamcinolone
Cyclosporine	2.5–4 mg/kg daily, divided dose
	Monitoring:
	Baseline blood pressure, BUN/Cr, Mg
	Recheck in 2 weeks, then monthly
Methotrexate	2.5–25 mg weekly
	Monitoring:
	Baseline: CBC, AST/ALT, BUN, creatinine, serologies for hepatitis B and C
	Recheck labs (except for hepatitis serologies) weekly for 4 weeks, then monthly, and with any subsequent elevation in dose
Mycophenolate mofetil	6–40 mg/kg daily, divided dose
	Monitoring:
	Baseline: CBC, chemistries, AST/ALT
	Recheck CBC weekly for 4 weeks, then monthly and with dose elevation
Phototherapy	Ultraviolet A-1 (40 J/cm^2) five times a week for 3 weeks

*Warshaw E, Lee G, Storrs FJ. Hand dermatitis: a review of clinical features, therapeutic options, and long-term outcomes. Am J Contact Dermatis 2003;14:119–137.
bid, twice daily; BUN, blood urea nitrogen; CBC, complete blood count; AST, aspartate aminotransferase; ALT, alanine aminotransferase.

Irritant contact dermatitis

Clinical presentation

Key Points

- Nonimmunologic
- No previous exposure is needed, although repeated exposure to weak irritants such as soap may precipitate onset of dermatitis
- Sharply demarcated macular erythema, hyperkeratosis, and fissuring
- Burning sensation more common than itch
- Therapy is directed at barrier repair, hand protection, and avoidance of wet work
- Corticosteroids of limited benefit

About 80% of all cases of contact dermatitis cases are ICD (Figure 11-7). Distinguishing between chronic ACD and ICD can be very challenging, from both clinical and histopathological standpoints. ICD can occur in an immunologically naïve person with no previous exposure. ICD usually results when a strong or irritating chemical contacts the relatively weak epidermis. Repeated exposures to even weak irritants, such as soaps, can cause a reaction. Lesions usually appear as macular erythema with scale and, in severe cases, the skin may fissure. Burning and soreness are more common than is pruritus. Symptoms may begin immediately upon exposure, or may take up to 48 hours to develop. Mild irritants may produce a spongiotic dermatitis that mimics ACD. It is notable that most ICD reactions begin to resolve within 96 hours.

Diagnosis

Key Points

- ICD is usually a diagnosis of exclusion. Often ICD is diagnosed after patch testing fails to identify a relevant allergy
- If patch testing with sodium lauryl sulfate (SLS) is positive, macular, erythematous skin reactions are more likely to be irritant than allergic in nature

Recently, the SLS test has been used in patch testing as a way of differentiating between allergic and irritant reactions. If SLS reacts during patch testing, it is likely that macular, erythematous reactions to patch test samples have an irritant etiology. On the other hand, if the skin does not react to SLS, it is likely that these reactions to allergens during patch testing are allergic in etiology. Although the SLS can be helpful, it is very important to keep in mind that it is impossible to correlate results with every possible irritant. The clinical presentation and the exposure history to the suspect irritant should play an important and complementary role in the diagnosis of ACD versus ICD. Hand eczema (Figure 11-8) may be multifactorial. Patients often have an atopic background. Irritants play an important role. ACD may play a role and can only be assessed by means of patch testing. Some cases of hand dermatitis represent psoriasis (Figure 11-9). Napkin dermatitis in infants (Figure 11-10) shares many features in common with hand eczema.

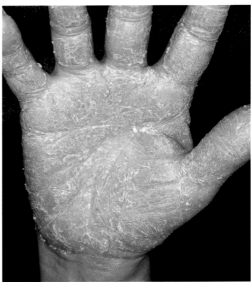

Figure 11-8 Hand eczema

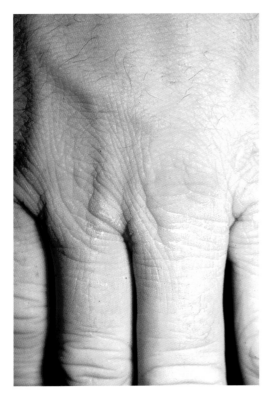

Figure 11-7 Irritant dermatitis

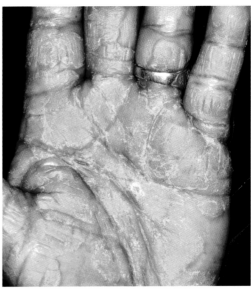

Figure 11-9 Psoriasis

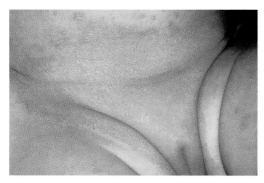

Figure 11-10 Napkin dermatitis

There is often an atopic background. Irritants play a role, and some patients later develop psoriasis.

Pathogenesis

Key Points

- Nonimmunologic
- Direct toxic effect of chemical on keratinocytes

Irritation can result from chronic exposure to friction, wet work, frequent use of soaps and detergents, exposure to organic or alkaline solvents, exposure to an environment with low humidity, or chronic exposure to saliva (lip smacking), urine, or feces.

Treatment

The mainstay of treatment is to identify and avoid irritants. Any contributory environmental conditions such as "wet work" should be sought and, when possible, changed. Furthermore, measures taken to ensure skin barrier integrity (i.e., decreased hand washing with soaps and increased emollient use) may be beneficial. The use of corticosteroids in ICD is controversial. Barrier creams, especially those containing dimethicone, may be of benefit.

Mycosis fungoides (Patch to plaque stage)

Clinical presentation

Key Points

- A form of T-cell lymphoma that first manifests in the skin
- Poorly demarcated, atrophic scaly pink patches and plaques
- Torso predominance

The incidence of cutaneous T-cell lymphoma (CTCL) is 0.5 per 100 000. Males are affected more than females with a ratio (male-to-female) of 1.6:1 to 2:1. Mycosis fungoides is the most common presentation of CTCL, with over 50%

of the cases. Initial clinical presentations include nonspecific eczema, chronic dermatitis, and psoriasis-like plaques that respond poorly to treatment with topical steroids and emollients. In most cases, the diagnosis is made in an adult who has a chronic history of eczema or nonspecific dermatitis. The lesions tend to increase in size and number over time. It is a difficult disease to diagnose, because in its early stages, biopsies may not be diagnostic. The disease may progress from patch to plaque or tumor stage.

Diagnosis

Key Point

- See the algorithm for diagnosis of early mycosis fungoides presented in Table 11-13

Pathogenesis

Key Point

- T-cell proliferation that first appears in the skin

Treatment

Key Point

- See Chapter 14

Nummular dermatitis

Clinical presentation

Key Points

- Coin-shaped, well-demarcated plaques with scale and tiny vesicles
- Variably exudative
- Legs, dorsal hands, extensor surfaces
- Intensely pruritic
- Koebner phenomenon may be observed
- Worsens during the winter, due to less humidity in the air, increasing skin dryness

Nummular dermatitis (Figure 11-11) predominantly affects older individuals, but, unlike other types of eczema such as asteotic dermatitis, it may also occur in younger populations. This dermatitis is characterized by coin-shaped, well-demarcated erythematous plaques with fine scale. In severe cases, small vesicles may also be seen. The disease typically begins with a single (herald-type) plaque or a few lesions on one of the extremities. Irregular patches of eczema may also occur (Figure 11-12). Children with nummular dermatitis may also develop patches of pityriasis alba (Figure 11-13). This represents mild eczema.

It is important that this entity should not be mistaken for Bowen's disease, which can be distinguished with a biopsy (Table 11-14). Without treatment and within a few months, more lesions

Table 11-13 Algorithm for diagnosis of early mycosis fungoides

	Basic	Additional
Clinical		
2 points for basic criteria plus two additional criteria	Persistent and/or progressive patches and/or thin plaques	Nonsun-exposed location
		Size/shape variation
1 point for basic criteria plus one additional criterion		Poikiloderma
Histopathologic		
2 points for basic criteria plus two additional criteria	Superficial lymphoid infiltrate	Epidermotropism without spongiosis
		Lymphoid atypia
1 point for basic criteria plus one additional criterion		
Molecular biological		
1 point for clonality	Clonal T-cell receptor gene rearrangement	
Immunopathologic		
1 point for one or more criteria	<50% CD2+, CD3+, and/or CD5+ T cells	
	<10% CD7+ T cells	
	Epidermal/dermal discordance of CD2, CD3, CD5, or CD7	

Adapted from Pimpinelli N, et al. Defining early mycosis fungoides. J Am Acad Dermatol 2005;53:1053-1063. A total of 4 points from all the above categories is required for diagnosis of mycosis fungoides.

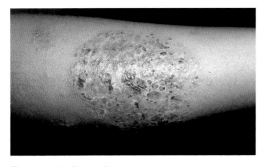

Figure 11-11 Nummular eczema

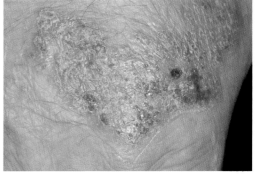

Figure 11-12 Eczema

may develop to involve all four extremities and then, the trunk. Characteristically, small "satellite" lesions may coalesce with the coin-shaped lesions, and expand into larger plaques. Nummular dermatitis is commonly seen in patients with a history of dry skin or eczema.

Diagnostic tests

Key Point

- Biopsy

Pathogenesis

Key Point

- Unknown

Treatment

It is very important to preserve and restore the skin barrier with moisturizers and emollients. An inflammatory component warrants use of topical corticosteroids. In nonresponsive cases, or if the lesions worsen with treatment, allergy to the topical treatment may be considered, necessitating a switch to an alternate class. In severe cases, intralesional or systemic therapy may be warranted (antihistamines and immunosuppressive agents). If the skin becomes secondarily infected, antibiotics with appropriate sensitivities should be used. A list of treatments for nummular eczema is given in Table 11-15.

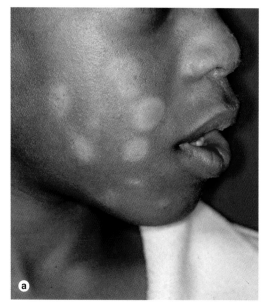

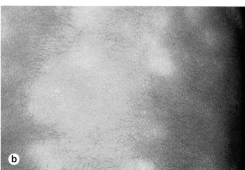

Figure 11-13 a Pityriasis alba. **b** Pityriasis alba and follicular eczema

Table 11-15 Treatments for nummular eczema

Treatment	Schedule
Topical corticosteroids	Potent or superpotent creams or ointments bid
Intralesional steroids	
Systemic steroids	Intramuscular triamcinolone acetonide 40 mg
	Oral prednisone in a tapering dose, starting at 40–60 mg daily
Antihistamines	Hydroxyzine 25 mg tid
Emollient creams	Continuous

bid, twice daily; tid, three times daily.

Table 11-14 Differential diagnosis of nummular dermatitis

Differential diagnosis	Differences in clinical presentation (compared to nummular dermatitis)	Differentiating tests
Psoriasis	Thicker lesions	Biopsy
	Less pruritus	
Bowen's disease	Single lesions	Biopsy
	Often not nummular	
	Slower development	
Tinea corporis	More rapid development	Skin scraping for potassium hydroxide examination
	More inflammatory	
	Scale may be more prominent at periphery	

Adapted from Marks R. Eczema in the elderly. In: Marks R, ed. Eczema. London: Martin Dunitz, 1992: 178–181, 182–183.

Psoriasis vulgaris (See Chapter 12)

Clinical presentation

Key Points

- Sharply demarcated, papulosquamous plaques without vesicles
- Common areas of involvement include the scalp, retroauricular area, elbows, knees, genitalia, gluteal cleft, and nails
- Predominance in areas of trauma (koebnerization)
- Pustules may be acutely present, particularly on the palms and soles
- Concomitant arthritis is common

Psoriasis is a common chronic and recurrent inflammation of the skin that affects 2–3% of the United States population. The lesions are well-demarcated, pink to violaceous plaques with overlying silvery gray/white scale. Nails are often involved, and findings include nail pits, oil spots, onycholysis, hyperkeratosis, and deformities.

Psoriasis vulgaris (chronic plaque) is the most common presentation; however, the other morphologic variants include guttate, erythroderma, and pustular (von Zumbusch) psoriasis.

Diagnostic tests

Clinical presentation

Key Point

- Biopsy is helpful, but is of limited value on the palms and soles, where confusion with spongiotic dermatitis is most likely

Seborrheic dermatitis

Clinical presentation

Key Points

- Erythematous to pink papulosquamous greasy papules and plaques
- Affects hair-bearing regions, flexural areas, and nasolabial folds, likely because of increased number of sebaceous glands

This inflammatory dermatosis is characterized by greasy, scaly papules and plaques on skin that contains large numbers of sebaceous glands, including the face (Figure 11-14), scalp, chest, back, and flexural areas. Seborrheic dermatitis is particularly common in patients with human immunodeficiency virus (HIV) and Parkinson's disease. During periods of stress or sleep deprivation, there is also an increase in the number of flares. Nutritional deficiencies to riboflavin, pyridoxine, niacin, and zinc have also been reported to cause a seborrheic dermatitis-like clinical presentation.

Diagnostic tests

Key Point

- Biopsy is helpful and will show spongiosis with parakeratosis at the lips of follicles

Pathogenesis

Key Points

Thought to be due to a combination of:
- *Malassezia furfur*, or its yeast form, *Pityrosporum ovale*
- Sebaceous lipids
- Individual sensitivity

Treatment

See Table 11-16.

Controversies

Some authors question the active role of *M. furfur* or its yeast form *P. ovale* in the pathogenesis of seborrhea. Furthermore, the role of sebaceous glands and sebum is also under investigation because of the preponderance of the distribution in the areas of numerous sebaceous glands.

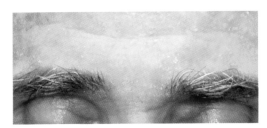

Figure 11-14 Seborrheic dermatitis

Table 11-16 Treatment of seborrheic dermatitis

Treatment	Schedule
Shampoos	Ketaconazole 2% applied twice a week
	Selenium sulfide 2.5% applied two to three times per week
	Tar shampoos applied two to three times per week
	Zinc pyrithione, applied two to three times per week
Topical corticosteroids	Group V through VII
Antifungal creams	Ketoconazole 2% cream applied daily
	Ciclopirox olamine cream or gel, applied daily

Adapted from Odom R, James W, Berger T. Andrews' Diseases of the Skin: Clinical Dermatology, 9th edn. Philadelphia: WB Saunders, 2000.

Stasis dermatitis

Clinical presentation

Key Points

- Papulosquamous plaques with dyschromia
- Shins and medial surfaces of lower legs are affected
- Concomitant venous varicosities

Stasis dermatitis is thought to be preceded by pitting edema in the medial aspect of the lower leg rostrally to the medial malleolus. Later in the course of disease, the medial lower third of the lower leg may become erythematous and indurated with resultant hair loss and scale. Excoriations and lichenification often develop as a consequence of intense pruritus. Brown puncta, purpura, hemosiderosis, and/or patches of white atrophy are also observed as the disease progresses.

Diagnostic tests

Key Points

- Diagnosis is based on the clinical presentation and history
- In particular, any history of venous thrombosis, prior injury to the affected limb, or prior treatment of varicose veins should be reviewed
- Vascular evalution of the lower extremities – both venous and, when indicated, arterial sides – should be done

Pathogenesis

Key Points

- Venous insufficiency underlies the condition
- Rubbing and scratching worsen the condition and make the skin changes chronic
- Increased sensitization to allergens can result in an ACD

Table 11-17 Treatment for stasis dermatitis

Treatment	Schedule
Topical steroids	Watch for development of atrophy with corticosteroids stronger than 1% hydrocortisone
Emollients	
Compression with stockings and wraps	
Leg elevation	

Affected skin is very sensitive and susceptible to the development of eczematous reactions from topical medications. In severe cases in which leg ulcers develop, patients frequently become sensitized to topical allergens such as neomycin sulfate, lanolin (Amerchol), alcohols, *Myroxylon pereirae* (balsam of Peru), colophony, fragrance mix, propylene glycol, parabens mix, corticosteroids, thiuram mix, and nickel sulfate. Autosensitization reactions may also be observed in stasis dermatitis.

Treatment

Compression is the key to the treatment of venous insufficiency. Since topical medication allergy could worsen stasis dermatitis, careful selection of medications with low sensitizing potential is encouraged. Table 11-17 has a list of available treatments.

Further reading

Abel EA, Wood GS, Hoppe RT. Mycosis fungoides: clinical and histologic features, staging, evaluation, and approach to treatment. CA Cancer J Clin 1993;43:93–115.

Belsito DV. The diagnostic evaluation, treatment, and prevention of allergic contact dermatitis in the new millennium. J Allergy Clin Immunol 2000;105:409–420.

Bickers DR, Lim HW, Margolis D, et al. The burden of skin diseases: 2004. A joint project of the American Academy of Dermatology Association and the Society for Investigative Dermatology. J Am Acad Dermatol 2006;55:490–500.

Boguniewicz M, Leung DY. 10. Atopic dermatitis. J Allergy Clin Immunol 2006;117(Suppl):S475–S480.

DeAngelis YM, Gemmer CM, Kaczvinsky JR, et.al. Three etiologic facets of dandruff and seborrheic dermatitis: Malassezia fungi, sebaceous lipids, and individual sensitivity. J Invest Dermatol Symp Proc 2005;10:295–297.

de Groot A. Allergic contact dermatitis. In: Marks R, ed. Eczema. London: Martin Dunitz, 1992:104–125.

Gupta AK, Bluhm R. Seborrheic dermatitis. J Eur Acad Dermatol Venereol 2004;18:13–26.

Jacob SE, Steel T. Allergic contact dermatitis, early recognition and diagnosis of important allergens. Dermatol Nurs 2006;18:433–439, 446.

Krol A, Krafchik B. The differential diagnosis of atopic dermatitis in childhood. Dermatol Ther 2006;19:73–82.

Mark BJ, Slavin RG. Allergic contact dermatitis. Med Clin North Am 2006;90:169–185.

Marks R. The pathology and pathogenesis of the eczematous reaction. In: Marks R, ed. Eczema London: Martin Dunitz, 1992:21–33.

McGirt LY, Beck LA. Innate immune defects in atopic dermatitis. J Allergy Clin Immunol 2006;118:202–208.

Norman RA. Xerosis and pruritus in the elderly: recognition and management. Dermatol Ther 2003;16:254–259.

Odom R, James W, Berger T. Andrews' Diseases of The Skin: Clinical Dermatology, 9th edn. Philadelphia: WB Saunders, 2000:52, 70, 74–76, 82, 83–84, 216–218, 244–245.

Palmer CN, Irvine AD, Terron-Kwiatkowski A, et al. Common loss-of-function variants of the epidermal barrier protein filaggrin are a major predisposing factor for atopic dermatitis. Nat Genet 2006;38:441–446.

Pratt MD, Belsito DV, DeLeo VA, et al. North American Contact Dermatitis Group patch-test results, 2001–2002 study period. Dermatitis 2004;15:176–183.

Rietschel RL. Clues to an accurate diagnosis of contact dermatitis. Dermatol Ther 2004;7: 224–223.

Smith CH, Barker JN. Psoriasis and its management. Br Med J 2006;333:380–384.

Warshaw EM. Therapeutic options for chronic hand dermatitis. Dermatol Ther 2004;17:240–250.

Willemze R. Cutaneous T-cell lymphoma: epidemiology, etiology, and classification. Leuk Lymphoma 2003;44(Suppl 3):S49–S54.

Papulosquamous disorders **12**

Melvin W. Chiu

Psoriasis

Clinical presentation

Key Points

- Plaque type is the most common variant
- Plaque psoriasis presents with erythematous plaques and an adherent silvery scale
- Psoriasis can also affect the nails and joints

Psoriasis (Figure 12-1) affects approximately 2% of the population. It can present at any age, but it occurs most commonly in the third and sixth decades. There is a significant genetic component, and patients frequently have a family history of psoriasis. There are four main variants: plaque-type, guttate, pustular, and erythrodermic psoriasis (Table 12-1). Plaque-type psoriasis, the most common variant, is characterized by well-demarcated, erythematous plaques with an adherent, silver to white-colored scale. When the adherent scales are removed, pinpoint bleeding on the skin may be seen (Auspitz's sign). Plaques may have surrounding hypopigmentation called Woronoff's ring; this can be spontaneous or arise from treatment. Plaques are most prevalent on the scalp, extensor surfaces of the extremities, and the periumbilical and sacral trunk; they rarely occur on the face, or on intertriginous areas of the body (inverse psoriasis). Lesions may arise at sites of trauma, termed the Koebner phenomenon. Plaques may be pruritic, but are often asymptomatic.

Guttate psoriasis is the second most common variant. It occurs more commonly in young adults, and it presents with multiple small "drop-shaped" erythematous scaly plaques diffusely on the body, most frequently on the trunk. This variant of psoriasis is often preceded by streptococcal infections, especially pharyngitis.

Pustular psoriasis is characterized by superficial pustules. These pustules may be localized on the palms and soles, as in palmoplantar pustulosis, or they may be generalized (Von Zumbusch). This generalized variant may be accompanied by fever

and malaise. When it occurs during pregnancy, it is called impetigo herpetiformis. The final variant of psoriasis is the erythrodermic variant, which is characterized by diffuse erythroderma with fine scaling.

Other clinical findings found in psoriasis include mucosal and nail changes. The dorsal tongue may exhibit geographic, annular white patches. Psoriatic nail changes include "oil spots," nail pitting, distal onycholysis, and accumulation of subungual debris. Severe nail dystrophy resulting from severe pustular psoriasis is termed acrodermatitis of Hallopeau.

Thirty percent or more of psoriasis patients may also have associated inflammatory arthritis. Psoriatic arthritis most commonly presents as an asymmetric oligoarthritis affecting the distal or proximal interphalangeal joints. However, psoriatic arthritis may also present as isolated monoarthritis, sacroiliitis, arthritis mutilans, or enthesitis. In addition, psoriasis patients appear to be at an increased risk for developing obesity, diabetes mellitus, hyperlipidemia, hypertension, and cardiovascular disease.

Diagnosis

Key Points

- Psoriasis is primarily diagnosed by clinical findings
- Skin biopsy may be useful in atypical cases

The diagnosis of psoriasis is usually based on clinical findings. Evidence supporting the diagnosis includes typical morphology and anatomic location of the skin lesions, presence of nail lesions or arthritis, and a positive family history of psoriasis. If lesions appear atypical, a skin biopsy may be useful in establishing a diagnosis.

Histologic findings in psoriasis include hyperkeratosis, parakeratosis, collections of neutrophils in the stratum corneum (Munro's microabscesses), hypogranulosis, regular acanthosis, spongiform collections of neutrophils in the epidermis (spongiform pustules of Kogoj), thinned suprapapillary plates, vascular ectasia in the papillary dermis, and superficial perivascular lymphocytic infiltrate.

Differential diagnosis

- The differential diagnosis of psoriasis varies according to the psoriasis variant

The differential diagnosis of psoriasis depends on the clinical psoriasis morphology. The differential diagnosis for plaque-type and guttate-type psoriasis includes other papulosquamous dermatoses such as nummular dermatitis, pityriasis rosea, mycosis fungoides, parapsoriasis, Reiter's disease (Figure 12-2), secondary syphilis, and pityriasis rubra pilaris (PRP). The differential diagnosis for pustular psoriasis includes acute generalized exanthematous pustulosis, subcorneal pustular dermatosis, and acute folliculitis. The differential diagnosis for erythrodermic psoriasis includes mycosis fungoides or its leukemic variant Sézary's syndrome, atopic dermatitis, seborrheic dermatitis, drug eruption, or PRP. Geographic tongue is similar to psoriasis histologically and may accompany flares of psoriasis (Figure 12-3).

Pathogenesis

Key Points

- Once thought to be a disease of epidermal hyperproliferation, psoriasis is now understood to be a T-cell-mediated inflammatory disease
- Genetic factors have a role in the etiology of psoriasis

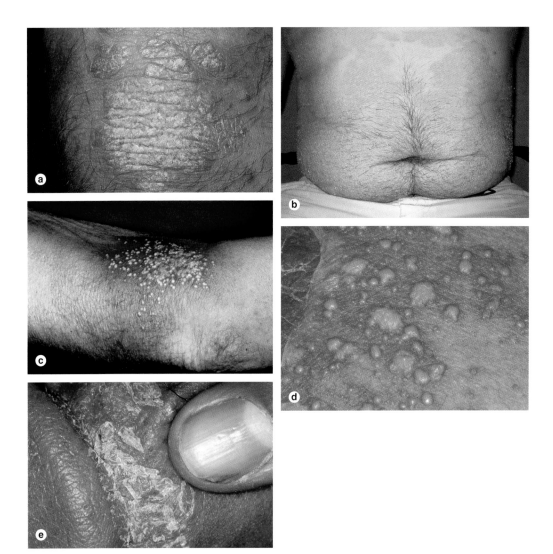

Figure 12-1 a, b Psoriasis. c, d Pustular psoriasis. e Penile psoriasis

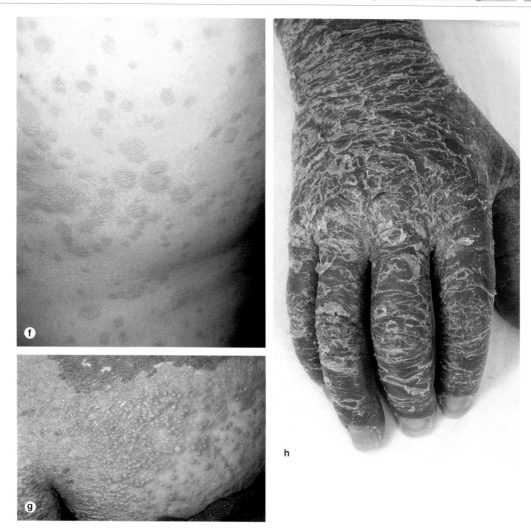

Figure 12-1, cont'd f Guttate psoriasis. g Generalized pustular psoriasis. h Erythrodermic psoriasis

Table 12-1 Clinical types of psoriasis

Type of psoriasis	Comments
Plaque	Most common type
Guttate	Often preceded by streptococcal infection
Pustular	May be localized or diffuse (von Zumbusch)
Erythrodermic	Diffuse erythema and scaling
Inverse	In the skin folds

- Psoriasis can be exacerbated by trauma, diminished sunlight, increased stress, and certain medications

Psoriasis is thought to result from an elaborate interplay between the epidermis and both the innate and adaptive immune system. Resident skin dendritic cells interact with T cells, which in turn interact with keratinocytes to produce the clinical phenotype of psoriasis. T cells in psoriasis are predominantly of the TH1 and cytotoxic CD8+ variety, with some having the newly described TH17 phenotype. Cytokines involved in the pathogenesis of psoriasis include interleukin-1 (IL-1), IL-6, IL-8, IL-12, IL-17, IL-20, IL-22, IL-23, interferon-gamma (IFN-γ), and tumor necrosis factor alpha (TNF-α). The importance of T cells and these TH1 and TH17 cytokines in the pathogenesis of psoriasis can be demonstrated in the clinical improvement seen in patients treated with specific T-cell inhibitors and antagonists of IL-12, IL-23, or TNF-α.

Genetic factors seem to play a role in psoriasis pathogenesis as well. Different psoriasis susceptibility genes have been identified, including *PSORS1*, which may represent human leukocyte antigen (HLA) markers like HLA-Cw6. Several other susceptibility loci have been identified (*PSORS2–8*), further exemplifying the potential polygenic nature of the disease. In addition, patients with

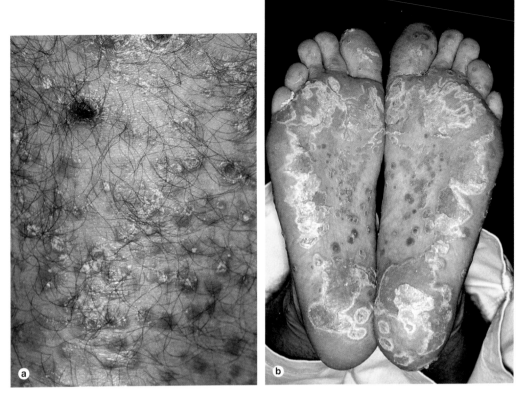

Figure 12-2 **a** Reiter's syndrome guttate lesions. **b** keratoderma blenorrhagicum

polymorphisms in IL-12B or the IL-23 receptor were recently found to have an increased likelihood of having psoriasis.

Psoriasis can be exacerbated by various environmental stimuli such as trauma (Koebner phenomenon), diminished exposure to sunlight, or stress. In addition, psoriasis can be triggered by or exacerbated by certain medications, including lithium, interferon, antimalarials, and beta-blockers. Pustular psoriasis sometimes erupts after treatment with systemic steroids.

Treatment

Key Points

- Topical treatments for psoriasis include topical steroids, topical retinoids, topical vitamin D analogs, topical keratolytics, topical tar products, and phototherapy
- Systemic treatments for psoriasis include oral retinoids, immunosuppressive agents, and "biologics"
- Systemic steroids should not be used for the treatment of psoriasis because of the risk of disease flare upon discontinuation of the steroids

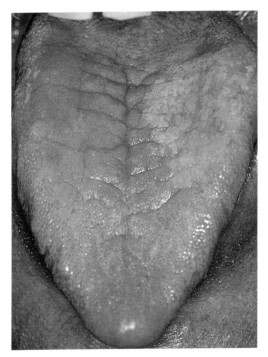

Figure 12-3 Fissured geographic tongue in pustular flare of psoriasis

Topical treatments include corticosteroids, retinoids such as tazarotene, vitamin D analogs such as calcipotriene, keratolytics like salicylic acid, and tar products such as anthralin (Table 12-2). Topical therapies are an excellent treatment option for limited disease, but are not practical when the disease is more widespread. Topical steroids are very effective and are the mainstay of topical psoriasis treatment. Long-term side-effects of their use include skin atrophy, telangiectasia formation, striae distensae, or even adrenal suppression, especially when used under occlusion or when ultrapotent corticosteroids are used. Use of systemic steroids should be avoided in psoriasis as discontinuation of the steroid can result in a disease flare or a change in morphology to a more inflammatory variant such as pustular or erythrodermic psoriasis.

Several nonsteroidal topical therapies can be used in conjunction with, or in lieu of, topical steroids. Tazarotene, a topical retinoid, has been shown to be useful as monotherapy or in combination with topical steroids or systemic phototherapy in the treatment of plaque psoriasis. The most common side-effect of tazarotene is skin irritation. Tazarotene is also teratogenic. Calcipotriene is a vitamin D analog that is used as monotherapy and in combination with topical steroids. The main adverse effects of calcipotriene are skin irritation and the potential for hypercalcemia at very high doses (it is recommended to use no more than 100 grams of calcipotriene per week). Salicylic acid, a topical keratolytic agent, may help decrease scale; its main potential adverse effect is systemic salicylate toxicity, which usually occurs with higher concentration formulations of salicylic acid and use over very large body surface areas. Symptoms of salicylate toxicity include dizziness, tinnitus, gastrointestinal complaints, psychiatric complaints, and hypoglycemia. Tar-based topical therapies such as anthralin are effective for psoriasis, but because of skin irritation and staining, are used infrequently.

Systemic treatments for psoriasis can be broadly categorized into nonimmunosuppressive and immunosuppressive therapies (Table 12-3). Nonimmunosuppressive therapies include ultraviolet (UV) phototherapy and acitretin. Immunosuppressive therapies for psoriasis include medications such as methotrexate and cyclosporine, and newer "biologic" agents, including etanercept, adalimumab, infliximab, efalizumab, and alefacept.

Effective types of UV phototherapy include psoralen plus UVA (PUVA) photochemotherapy, broadband UVB (BBUVB), and narrowband UVB (NBUVB). Different modes of delivering the UV light have been used, including whole-body units, hand-and-foot units, excimer laser, and directed monochromatic NBUVB light sources. UV phototherapy may act by inhibiting Langerhans cells and decreasing the cutaneous

immune hyperactivity associated with psoriasis. The adverse effects of UV phototherapy include phototoxicity and an elevated risk for skin cancer (both nonmelanoma and melanoma), especially with PUVA.

Acitretin is a systemic retinoid that is moderately efficacious for the treatment of plaque psoriasis. Its efficacy may be improved if used in conjunction with UV phototherapy. Acitretin is particularly effective in the treatment of pustular and erythrodermic psoriasis. Cutaneous adverse effects include alopecia, cheilitis, and asteatotic dermatitis. Other side-effects include hyperlipidemia, transaminitis, and hyperostosis. Acitretin is teratogenic and should be avoided in women with

Table 12-2 Topical psoriasis treatments

Medication	Adverse effect(s)
Steroids	Skin atrophy, telangiectasia. striae distensae, adrenal suppression
Tazarotene	Skin irritation, teratogenic
Calcipotriene	Skin irritation, hypercalcemia
Salicylic acid	Salicylate toxicity
Tar	Skin irritation, staining of clothes/linens

Table 12-3 Systemic psoriasis treatments

Medication	Mechanism of action	Adverse effect(s)
Ultraviolet light	Potentially decreases Langerhans cells	Phototoxicity Skin cancer
Acitretin	Unknown	Alopecia Cheilitis Asteatosis Hyperlipidemia Liver toxicity Hyperostosis Teratogenic
Methotrexate	Inhibits dihydrofolate reductase	Pancytopenia Gastrointestinal upset Liver toxicity Alopecia Teratogenic
Cyclosporine	Inhibits T cells	Hypertension Renal toxicity Electrolyte abnormalities Hypertriglyceridemia

child-bearing potential. In addition, concomitant alcohol consumption catalyzes the esterification of acitretin to etretinate, which can remain in the body for up to 3 years after a single dose.

Methotrexate is a systemic antimetabolite used in the treatment of psoriasis and psoriatic arthritis. Methotrexate inhibits the immune system via inhibition of dihydrofolate reductase, decreasing the inflammatory component associated with psoriasis. Methotrexate can be administered intramuscularly, intravenously, subcutaneously, or orally. It is usually dosed weekly, and potential adverse effects include bone marrow toxicity, gastrointestinal upset, hepatotoxicity and teratogenicity. Interval liver biopsies are generally recommended in psoriatic patients receiving long-term methotrexate.

Cyclosporine is an immunosuppressive molecule effective in the treatment of psoriasis. It selectively inhibits T cells and has a rapid onset of action; because of this, it may be particularly useful in the management of pustular flares. Potential side-effects include hypertension, renal toxicity, and increased risk for malignancy. Given these potential toxicities, it is generally advised that patients use cyclosporine for no longer than 1 year.

Recently, the development of newer systemic medications termed "biologics" has ushered in a new era of psoriasis therapy. These bioengineered molecules target specific inflammatory mediators of the immune system. Inhibition of the inflammatory cytokine TNF-α with targeted biologic agents has proven to be effective against both psoriasis and psoriatic arthritis. There are currently three anti-TNF-α molecules approved by the Food and Drug Administration for the treatment of psoriasis and psoriatic arthritis in the United States: etanercept, adalimumab, and infliximab (Table 12-4). Etanercept is a fusion protein made of the Fc fragment of immunoglobulin (Ig) G_1 and two TNF-α receptors. Adalimumab is a human monoclonal antibody targeted against TNF-α, and infliximab is a human–mouse chimeric monoclonal antibody targeted against TNF-α.

Major risks associated with use of TNF-α inhibitors include an increased risk of malignancy or infection. Reactivation of latent tuberculosis has been seen, and all patients should be screened for latent tuberculosis infection prior to beginning immunosuppressive medications such as TNF-α inhibitors. Other potential side-effects of TNF-α inhibitors include injection site reactions, exacerbation or triggering of congestive heart failure, demyelinating disorders, lupus-like syndromes, and, paradoxically, new onset or exacerbation of pre-existing psoriasis (Table 12-5).

Other biologic therapies are targeted against T cells. Efalizumab is a human monoclonal antibody directed against the CD11a subunit of LFA-1 on T cells. Its main potential adverse effects include injection reactions, psoriasis flares while on or upon discontinuing the medication, and rare thrombocytopenia. Alefacept is a fusion protein made of the Fc fragment of IgG_1 and LFA3, which binds to memory T cells. The main potential adverse effect of alefacept is a reversible decrease in CD4+ T cells during therapy. Because of this, it is not recommended that human immunodeficiency virus (HIV)-positive psoriasis patients be treated with alefacept.

Table 12-4 Biologics for psoriasis/psoriatic arthritis

Medication	Type/target	Food and Drug Administration indication
Etanercept	Fusion protein (Fc + TNF-alpha receptors)	Psoriasis + PsA
Adalimumab	Human monoclonal Ab against TNF-alpha	Psoriasis and PsA
Infliximab	Mouse-human chimeric monoclonal Ab against TNF-alpha	Psoriasis + PsA
Efalizumab	Human monoclonal Ab against CD11a subunit of LFA-1	Psoriasis
Alefacept	Fusion protein (Fc + LFA3)	Psoriasis

TNF, tumor necrosis factor; PsA, psoriatic arthritis; Ab, antibody; LFA-1, leukocyte function-associated antigen-1.

Table 12-5 Biologics for psoriasis/psoriatic arthritis – adverse effects

Medication	Adverse effects
Etanercept	Increased risk of malignancy/infection (including tuberculosis)
	Injection site reactions
	Worsening congestive heart failure
	Demyelinating disorders
	Lupus-like syndrome
	Psoriasis flares
Adalimumab	Same as etanercept
Infliximab	Same as etanercept
Efalizumab	Thrombocytopenia, injection reactions, psoriasis flares
Alefacept	Decrease in CD4+ T cells

Pityriasis rubra pilaris

Clinical presentation

Key Points

- Seen during childhood or at 40–60 years of age
- Coalescing erythematous to slightly orange plaques with islands of sparing
- Palmoplantar keratoderma
- May evolve into erythroderma

PRP (Figure 12-4) can be familial or acquired. If familial, most cases appear to be autosomal-dominant with variable penetrance. The incidence is bimodal, with peaks occurring during childhood and at 40–60 years of age. PRP can be classified into six types (Table 12-6).

PRP presents with coalescing erythematous to slightly orange scaly macules and follicular hyperkeratotic papules, often starting on the head, scalp, neck, and trunk. Palms and soles are frequently hyperkeratotic, appearing like "carnuba wax," and the eruption may evolve into erythroderma and exfoliative dermatitis. Rare oral involvement has been reported. Patients may have rheumatologic findings such as arthritis or dermatomyositis (so-called Wong's dermatomyositis). Exacerbation by UV light has also been reported, as have rare associations with underlying malignancy.

Diagnosis

Key Points

- Characteristic clinical findings include erythematous or orange patches and plaques with islands of sparing, follicular hyperkeratosis, and palmoplantar keratoderma
- Diagnosis is usually based on clinical findings; if uncertain, biopsy may help clarify the diagnosis

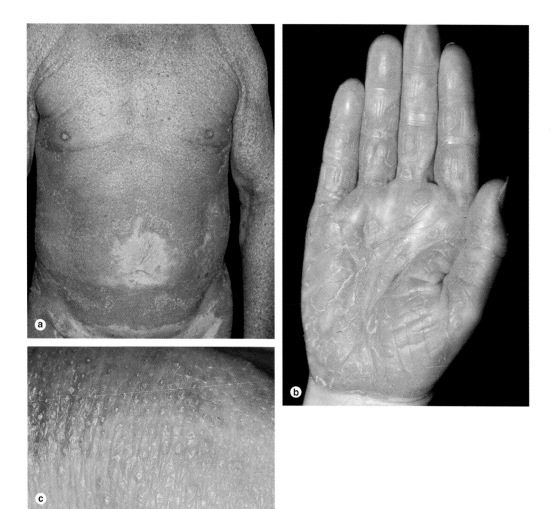

Figure 12-4 Pityriasis rubra pilaris **a** Islands of sparing. **b** Palmar keratoderma. **c** Follicular hyperkeratosis

Differential diagnosis

- PRP may resemble other papulosquamous diseases (Figure 12-5)

Other conditions that may present with similar clinical findings include psoriasis, mycosis fungoides, atopic dermatitis, seborrheic dermatitis, drug eruption, and Wong-type dermatomyositis. Histologic findings distinguish these conditions from PRP.

Laboratory testing

- Skin biopsy may help distinguish PRP from similar conditions (Table 12-7)

PRP may show both horizontally and vertically oriented alternating ortho- and parakeratosis, hypergranulosis, follicular plugging with perifollicular parakeratosis, psoriasiform epidermal hyperplasia, thickened suprapapillary plates, widened rete ridges, variable acantholytic dyskeratosis, and a superficial perivascular lymphocytic infiltrate.

Pathogenesis

- Familial cases have an unidentified genetic basis, but the pathogenesis of PRP is currently unknown

The pathogenesis of PRP is currently not known. Genetic factors seem apparent in familial cases, but a culprit gene has yet to be identified. Reports of streptococcal infections preceding juvenile PRP suggest that bacterial superantigens may play a role in pathogenesis.

Treatment

- Oral retinoids with or without UV phototherapy are the mainstay of therapy
- Second-line therapies include methotrexate, cyclosporine, TNF-α inhibitors, and extracorporeal photochemotherapy

Juvenile PRP may spontaneously resolve after 1–2 years. Generalized type III PRP sometimes improves to become circumscribed type IV PRP. However, juvenile PRP can persist into adulthood in some cases. Adult cases tend to remit spontaneously in 1–3 years, but familial types may persist throughout life.

First-line therapy for PRP involves oral retinoids (Box 12-1). Retinoids in combination with UV phototherapy have also been successful, although UV radiation has been reported to exacerbate PRP in some cases. Second-line treatments include methotrexate, cyclosporine, TNF-α inhibitors, and extracorporeal photochemotherapy. HIV-associated PRP may best be treated with a combination of oral retinoid and antiretroviral therapy.

Controversies

- PRP may be associated with internal malignancy

Some authors have reported an association between PRP and internal malignancy. PRP can precede, occur concurrently with, or follow the diagnosis of malignancy. Some authors suggest that atypical PRP may be more likely to be paraneoplastic. Since both PRP and malignancies are more common in older persons, the association may be coincidental.

Table 12-6 Classification of pityriasis rubra pilaris	
Type	**Comments**
I. Adult, classic	Most common type
II. Adult, atypical	More resistant to therapy
III. Juvenile, classic	Similar to type I, most common type seen in children
IV. Juvenile, circumscribed	Localized to knees and elbows
V. Juvenile, atypical	Ichthyosiform
VI. HIV-associated	Often associated with acne conglobata and more often recalcitrant to therapy. Also known as HIV-associated follicular syndrome

HIV, human immunodeficiency virus.

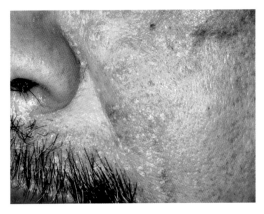

Figure 12-5 Seborrheic dermatitis

Table 12-7 Distinguishing pityriasis rubra pilaris from other conditions

Disease	Clinical findings	Histologic findings
Pityriasis rubra pilaris	Follicular papules, confluent erythematous scaly plaques with islands of sparing, palmoplantar keratoderma	Alternating ortho- and parakeratosis, perifollicular parakeratosis, follicular plugging, hypergranulosis, psoriasiform epidermal hyperplasia
Psoriasis	Erythematous plaques with silver scale on extensor surfaces, nail pitting, and oil spots	Parakeratosis, hypogranulosis, Munro's microabscesses (neutrophil collections in the stratum corneum), regular acanthosis, spongiform pustules of Kogoj (neutrophil collections in the epidermis), thinning of the suprapapillary plates, dilation of dermal papillary vasculature
Mycosis fungoides	Erythematous patches or plaques with fine scale on trunk, buttocks, proximal extremities	Pautrier's microabscesses (collections of atypical lymphocytes in the epidermis), epidermotropic atypical lymphocytes, acanthosis, lichenoid infiltrate of atypical lymphocytes
Atopic dermatitis	Erythematous, scaly, lichenified plaques on flexor surfaces	Parakeratosis, variable spongiosis, exocytosis, superficial perivascular lymphohistiocytic infiltrate
Seborrheic dermatitis	Erythematous scaly patches on scalp, face, chest, back	Perifollicular parakeratotic scale crust, spongiosis, superficial perivascular lymphohistiocytic infiltrate
Drug eruption	Diffuse, coalescing erythematous papules	Superficial and deep perivascular lymphohistiocytic infiltrate with eosinophils
Wong-type dermatomyositis	Erythematous, follicular hyperkeratotic papules over the dorsal hands ± keratoderma in the setting of dermatomyositis	Follicular hyperkeratosis and interface dermatitis with arrector pilorum myositis

BOX 12-1

Treatment options for pityriasis rubra pilaris

Retinoids ± ultraviolet phototherapy

Methotrexate

Cyclosporine

Tumor necrosis factor-α inhibitors

Extracorporeal photochemotherapy

Reiter's disease

Clinical presentation

Key Points

- Triad of arthritis, conjunctivitis, and urethritis
- Cutaneous findings include psoriasiform dermatitis, keratoderma blenorrhagicum, and balanitis circinata

Reiter's disease, also known as Reiter's syndrome or reactive arthritis, is a seronegative spondyloarthropathy comprised of the triad of arthritis, conjunctivitis, and urethritis. Not all components of the triad are present in all Reiter's disease patients. The arthritis usually involves more than one joint, tends to be asymmetric, and often occurs on the lower extremities. Dactylitis, sacroiliitis, and enthesitis may also be seen. Ocular signs include unilateral or sometimes bilateral conjunctivitis, anterior uveitis, posterior uveitis, keratitis, cataract, and glaucoma. Urethritis may present with dysuria and urethral discharge or may be completely asymptomatic. Mucocutaneous findings include psoriasiform dermatitis, keratoderma blenorrhagicum, balanitis circinata, and mucosal ulcerations. Keratoderma blenorrhagicum is characterized by thick, yellow plaques on the plantar surface of the feet. Balanitis circinata are shallow ulcers at the meatus and glans penis that can evolve into crusted plaques.

Diagnosis

Key Point

- Characteristic clinical triad of arthritis, conjunctivitis, and urethritis with classic cutaneous findings

Reiter's syndrome is usually diagnosed based on clinical findings of arthritis, conjunctivitis, urethritis, and typical cutaneous findings such as psoriasiform plaques, keratoderma blenorrhagicum, and balanitis circinata.

Differential diagnosis

Key Point

- Differential diagnoses include psoriasiform dermatoses

Other papulosquamous conditions, such as psoriasis, PRP, and mycosis fungoides, can mimic the psoriasiform plaques of Reiter's disease. Lesions resembling balanitis circinata may be seen in psoriasis, seborrheic dermatitis, mycosis fungoides, PRP, contact dermatitis, Zoon's balanitis, Bowen's disease, and extramammary Paget's disease. Scaling on the soles resembling keratoderma blenorrhagicum may be seen in psoriasis, palmoplantar pustulosis, contact dermatitis, chronic palmoplantar eczema, atopic dermatitis, or other palmoplantar keratodermas.

Pathogenesis

Key Points

- Often follows gastrointestinal or genitourinary infection
- May occur after intravesicular bacille Calmette–Guérin (BCG) infusion

Reiter's disease is thought to be a reactive process following certain gastrointestinal or genitourinary infections. Causative infections include *Chlamydia*, *Ureaplasma*, *Salmonella*, *Shigella*, *Campylobacter*, *Yersinia*, *Clostridium*, *Streptococcus*, *Mycoplasma*, *Cyclospora*, and traveler's diarrhea. Symptoms of Reiter's disease usually follow the infectious episode by 1–3 weeks.

Reiter's disease has also been reported to occur in 0.5% of patients after intravesicular infusion of BCG for bladder carcinoma.

Men are affected more than women, and a disproportionately high number of patients have the HLA-B27 antigen. Peak incidence occurs from 15 to 35 years of age.

DNA of genitourinary pathogens *Chlamydia trachomatis* and *Ureaplasma urealyticum*, as well as DNA from enteric pathogens *Salmonella*, *Shigella*, and *Campylobacter*, has been isolated from the synovial fluid of Reiter's disease patients.

Treatment

Key Points

- Any underlying infections should be treated
- Systemic treatments include NSAIDs, sulfasalazine, methotrexate, azathioprine, and TNF-α inhibitors

First line treatment for Reiter's disease includes nonsteroidal anti-inflammatory drugs (NSAIDs) such as indomethacin and doxycycline to treat any potential *Chlamydia* infection. Persistent disease can be treated with sulfasalazine, methotrexate, or azathioprine. Recently, TNF-α inhibitors have been reported to improve Reiter's disease. Large joint effusions can be treated with intra-articular steroid injections. Patients with unexplained reactive arthritis should be evaluated for HIV.

The treatment of ocular Reiter's disease consists of topical corticosteroid and/or antibiotic eyedrops. BCG-induced Reiter's disease can be treated with NSAIDs or systemic steroids, sometimes in combination with isoniazid.

Acquired immunodeficiency syndrome (AIDS)-related Reiter's disease has been reported to improve with a combination of NSAIDs, antiretroviral therapy, and acitretin.

Controversies

Key Point

- The name "Reiter's syndrome" has fallen out of favor. The term "reactive arthritis" is used more commonly

Reiter's syndrome is named after German physician Hans Reiter. There is controversy surrounding the eponym, partly because Dr. Reiter may not have been the first to describe the condition, but mostly because Dr. Reiter was a high-ranking Nazi physician who, during World War II, authorized unethical experiments on concentration camp prisoners. Many now recommend that Reiter's syndrome be called reactive arthritis.

Parapsoriasis

Clinical presentation

Key Points

- Two variants: small plaque (< 5 cm in diameter) or large plaque (≥ 5 cm in diameter)
- Presents with erythematous scaly patches on the trunk and proximal extremities
- Large plaque parapsoriasis (LPP) and some small plaque parapsoriasis (SPP) are early forms of mycosis fungoides

Parapsoriasis consists of persistent, asymptomatic, or slightly pruritic erythematous patches that favor the trunk and proximal extremities. Parapsoriasis is split into two categories: SPP and LPP. SPP consists of lesions less then 5 cm in diameter, whereas LPP consists of lesions ≥ 5 cm in diameter. Digitate dermatosis is a variant of SPP that presents with orange to pink finger-shaped or oval patches on the trunk and extremities (Figure 12-6).

Diagnosis

Key Points

- Parapsoriasis shows nonspecific histologic findings
- T-cell gene rearrangement studies are not usually helpful

The diagnosis of parapsoriasis is based on characteristic clinical findings. Histologic findings are not diagnostic. Parapsoriasis shows nonspecific changes which include parakeratosis, spongiosis, and variable interface lymphocytic infiltrate. T-cell gene rearrangement studies are not typically helpful in diagnosis as both parapsoriasis and mycosis fungoides can show monoclonal T-cell populations. Digitate dermatosis rarely if ever progresses to mycosis fungoides, but most other forms of parapsoriasis represent early mycosis fungoides.

Differential diagnosis

Key Point

- The main diagnostic considerations include mycosis fungoides, psoriasis, atopic dermatitis, nummular dermatitis, and pityriasis rosea

The differential diagnosis for parapsoriasis includes other papulosquamous dermatoses such as mycosis fungoides, psoriasis, atopic dermatitis, nummular dermatitis, and pityriasis rosea.

Pathogenesis

Key Point

- Parapsoriasis is thought to be an early cutaneous lymphoproliferative condition similar to pityriasis lichenoides or lymphomatoid papulosis

The etiology of parapsoriasis remains unclear, but most authors consider it to be an early cutaneous lymphoproliferative condition similar to pityriasis lichenoides or lymphomatoid papulosis. T-cell clonality has been detected in lesions of both SPP and LPP. Infectious etiologies have been sought, but none have been found to date.

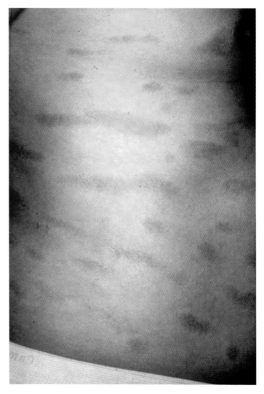

Figure 12-6 Digitate dermatosis

Treatment

Key Point

- Treatment of parapsoriasis involves topical corticosteroids and phototherapy

Parapsoriasis has been shown to respond to topical corticosteroids, NBUVB, PUVA, 308-nm excimer laser, and balneotherapy.

Controversies

Key Point

- Parapsoriasis may be an early form of mycosis fungoides

Currently, the relationship between parapsoriasis and mycosis fungoides is somewhat controversial. Many authors contend that parapsoriasis is a member of a group of clonal potentially premalignant lymphoproliferative cutaneous disorders which also include pityriasis lichenoides and lymphomatoid papulosis. LPP has been shown to exhibit monoclonality and classically been thought to develop eventually into mycosis fungoides in up to 46% of cases, but there is now evidence that some cases of SPP also displays monoclonality and may have the ability to evolve into mycosis fungoides.

Classic digitate dermatosis rarely, if ever, evolves into lymphoma. Patients with LPP may also have a predisposition to developing other lymphoproliferative conditions, such as CD30+ cutaneous T-cell lymphoma.

Pityriasis rosea

Clinical presentation

Key Points

- Pityriasis rosea usually occurs in children or young adults
- The hallmark of pityriasis rosea is a "herald patch" followed by a secondary eruption of smaller scaly patches in a "Christmas-tree" distribution
- Atypical variants exist

Pityriasis rosea (Figure 12-7) occurs in 0.68 per 100 dermatologic patients. The peak incidence occurs in patients aged 10–35 years old, and there is a slight female predominance. Patients classically present with a 2–10-cm oval patch with a collarette of scale called a "herald patch." In fair-skinned individuals, the lesion is often salmon-colored, but in darker-skinned patients the lesion is usually hyperpigmented. This "herald patch" is usually followed in 7–14 days by a secondary eruption of smaller scaly patches that mimic the herald patch in color and morphology, but differ in size. These 5–10-mm secondary lesions are often numerous and situated along Langer's lines on the trunk in a "Christmas-tree" distribution. The eruption is either asymptomatic or variably pruritic.

Atypical presentations of pityriasis rosea include vesicular, purpuric, papular, localized, and erythema multiforme-like.

The differential diagnosis includes secondary syphilis, tinea corporis, nummular eczema, guttate psoriasis, and viral exanthem.

Histopathologic findings are nonspecific. Skin biopsies show slight epidermal acanthosis and

spongiosis with mounds of parakeratosis. The dermis shows a superficial perivascular infiltrate composed predominantly of lymphocytes and histiocytes, and variable numbers of extravasated erythrocytes.

Diagnosis

Key Point

- Diagnosis is based on the clinical finding of a herald patch and the characteristic secondary eruption

Diagnosis is based on clinical findings; histopathologic findings are usually nonspecific.

Differential diagnosis

Key Point

- Differential diagnosis includes other papulosquamous dermatoses

The differential diagnosis of pityriasis rosea includes secondary syphilis, nummular dermatitis, psoriasis, parapsoriasis, and mycosis fungoides.

Pathogenesis

Key Points

- Pityriasis rosea may be caused by an as-yet undetermined virus, but definitive proof is lacking
- Pityriasis rosea can be caused by certain medications

A great deal of circumstantial evidence exists to suggest an infectious etiology for pityriasis rosea, but definitive evidence for a causative link is lacking. Temporal clustering of cases suggests an infectious etiology. Virus-like particles have been seen in keratinocytes in electron microscopic analyses of pityriasis rosea lesions; however, the exact nature of these particles remains to be elucidated. The association of pityriasis rosea with human herpesvirus-6 (HHV6) or HHV7 is controversial. Some reports have linked pityriasis rosea to HHV-6 and HHV-7, while others have failed to find an association. Pityriasis rosea has also been potentially linked to enterovirus.

Pityriasis rosea-like eruptions have been associated with different medications (Box 12-2).

Treatment

Key Points

- Pityriasis rosea usually resolves spontaneously
- Topical steroids may help control symptomatic pruritus
- Oral erythromycin, oral acyclovir, and UVB phototherapy have been reported to improve pityriasis rosea

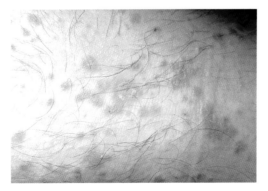

Figure 12-7 Pityriasis rosea

Barth WF, Segal K. Reactive arthritis (Reiter's syndrome). Am Fam Physician 1999; 60:499–503, 507.

Berlau J, Junker U, Groh A, et al. In situ hybridisation and direct fluorescence antibodies for the detection of *Chlamydia trachomatis* in synovial tissue from patients with reactive arthritis. J Clin Pathol 1998;51:803–806.

Chan H, Liu FT, Naguwa S. A review of pityriasis rubra pilaris and rheumatologic associations. Clin Dev Immunol 2004;11:57–60.

Chuh A, Chan H, Zawar V. Pityriasis rosea – evidence for and against an infectious aetiology. Epidemiol Infect 2004;132:381–390.

Dicken CH. Treatment of classic pityriasis rubra pilaris. J Am Acad Dermatol 1994;31:997–999.

Drago F, Vecchio F, Rebora A. Use of high-dose acyclovir in pityriasis rosea. J Am Acad Dermatol 2006;54:82–85.

Gonzalez LM, Allen R, Janniger CK, et al. Pityriasis rosea: an important papulosquamous disorder. Int J Dermatol 2005;44:757–764.

Kikuchi A, Naka W, Harada T, et al. Parapsoriasis en plaques: its potential for progression to malignant lymphoma. J Am Acad Dermatol 1993;29:419–422.

Lowes MA, Bowcock AM, Krueger JG. Pathogenesis and therapy of psoriasis. Nature 2007;445:866–873.

Lu DW, Katz KA. Declining use of the eponym "Reiter's syndrome" in the medical literature, 1998–2003. J Am Acad Dermatol 2005;53:720–723.

Magro CM, Crowson AN. The clinical and histomorphological features of pityriasis rubra pilaris. A comparative analysis with psoriasis. J Cutan Pathol 1997;24:416–424.

Mueller KK, Yeager JK. Clinical considerations in digitate dermatosis. Int J Dermatol 1997;36:767–768.

Myers WA, Gottlieb AB, Mease P. Psoriasis and psoriatic arthritis: clinical features and disease mechanisms. Clin Dermatol 2006;24:438–447.

Neimann AL, Shin DB, Wang X, et al. Prevalence of cardiovascular risk factors in patients with psoriasis. J Am Acad Dermatol 2006;55:829–835.

Sharma PK, Yadav TP, Gautam RK, et al. Erythromycin in pityriasis rosea: A double-blind, placebo-controlled clinical trial. J Am Acad Dermatol 2000;42:241–244.

Simon M, Flaig MJ, Kind P, et al. Large plaque parapsoriasis: clinical and genotypic correlations. J Cutan Pathol 2000;27:57–60.

Vakeva L, Sarna S, Vaalasti A, et al. A retrospective study of the probability of the evolution of parapsoriasis en plaques into mycosis fungoides. Acta Dermatol Venereol 2005;85:318–323.

BOX 12-2

Drugs that can cause a pityriasis rubra-like eruption

Angiotensin-converting enzyme inhibitors

Angiotensin receptor blockers

Bismuth

Hydrochlorothiazide

Ketotifen

Acetylsalicylic acid

Omeprazole

Allopurinol

Imatinib

Terbinafine

Isotretinoin

The eruption frequently spontaneously resolves within 8 weeks. Symptomatic control of pruritus may be attempted by using topical corticosteroids. Erythromycin appears effective for the treatment of pityriasis rosea, with complete response reported in 73% versus none with placebo. Azithromycin, however, has been shown to be ineffective. Antiviral medications, specifically acyclovir, and UVB phototherapy have shown some efficacy in the treatment of pityriasis rosea. UVB phototherapy generally shows little response until erythema is achieved, but a single erythemogenic dose of UVB will commonly result in widespread desquamation, with rapid resolution of the itch and subsequent healing of the eruption. BBUVB and natural sunlight may be superior to NBUVB in the treatment of pityriasis rosea

Controversies

Key Point

- No infectious etiology of pityriasis rosea has been definitively proven

The etiology of pityriasis rosea remains unclear. Certainly data from immunohistochemical and polymerase chain reaction studies suggest a possible infectious etiology, but definitive evidence is still lacking.

Further reading

Arndt KA, Paul BS, Stern RS, et al. Treatment of pityriasis rosea with UV radiation. Arch Dermatol 1983;119:381–382.

Atzori L, Pinna AL, Ferreli C, et al. Pityriasis rosea-like adverse reaction: review of the literature and experience of an Italian drug-surveillance center. Dermatol Online J 2006;12:1.

Lichenoid dermatoses **13**

Christopher B. Skvarka
and Christine J. Ko

The lichenoid/interface dermatoses share a pink to violaceous color and histologic features of vacuolar change, epidermal basal cell damage, and/or a band-like infiltrate. This chapter highlights the unique features of each major lichenoid dermatosis (Box 13-1), along with illustrating basic pathogenesis and treatment options.

Lichen planus

Clinical presentation

> **Key Points**
>
> - Inflammatory disorder that affects skin, scalp, mucous membranes, and nails
> - Hepatitis C is more prevalent in patients with lichen planus than in controls
> - Atypical presentations are more likely to be associated with hepatitis C

Skin findings

- Pruritic, purple, polygonal, flat-topped papules with a fine reticulated network of white lines (Wickham's striae) corresponding to areas of periadnexal hypergranulosis
- Lesions koebnerize and are commonly found on the flexor wrists, forearms, dorsal hands, lower legs, presacral area, neck, and glans penis
- In children, the pattern is often linear/zosteriform and mucosal involvement is uncommon

Scalp findings

- Lichen planopilaris (LPP), the follicular variant of lichen planus, causes scarring alopecia
- Anagen hairs release on the hair-pull test in active lesions. This can be helpful to monitor disease activity and response to treatment
- LPP shares the typical histopathological and immunohistochemical features of lichen planus

Mucous membranes

- Up to 60% of patients with lichen planus on the skin have mucous membrane involvement

---

BOX 13-1

Lichenoid/interface dermatoses

Lichen planus (Figure 13-1)

Lichen nitidus (Figure 13-2)

Lichen striatus (Figure 13-3)

Lichen sclerosus et atrophicus (Figure 13-4)

Pityriasis lichenoides

Lichenoid contact

Lichenoid purpura

Porokeratosis

Erythema dyschromicum perstans

Graft-versus-host disease

Eruption of lymphocyte recovery

Acquired immunodeficiency syndrome (AIDS) interface dermatitis

Late secondary syphilis

Mycosis fungoides

Lichenoid drug eruption

Fixed drug reaction

Erythema multiforme

Lupus erythematosus

Dermatomyositis

Perniosis

Paraneoplastic pemphigus

- Six morphologic forms of oral lichen planus have been described: atrophic, reticular, papular, plaque, erosive, and bullous
- The most common pattern reported is reticular

Nails

- Nail changes are found in 5–10% of patients with lichen planus

- Trachyonychia, or twenty-nail dystrophy, is a form of lichen planus that, especially in children, may spare other cutaneous surfaces

Approximately 20 clinical variants of lichen planus have been described. Many of these distinct variants are summarized in Tables 13-1 through 13-3. This disease has no racial predilection and is uncommon in children. Two-thirds of patients with lichen planus present between the ages of 30 and 60 years old. Fewer than 2–3% of all cases are reported in patients less than 20 years old. Familial clustering of lichen planus is seen in 1.5–10.7% of reported cases.

Pruritus is common in patients with early lesions of lichen planus. Pruritus generally worsens with increased body surface area involvement, with the exception of hypertrophic lichen planus of the shins. This variant may be localized, yet extremely pruritic. Typically, the pruritus in lichen planus leads to rubbing, rather than scratching. The duration of the disease varies for each patient. Hypertrophic, nail, or oral lichen planus tend to run prolonged courses.

Diagnosis

Key Points

- Clinical features are often diagnostic
- Histologically, lichen planus is the prototypical lichenoid dermatitis

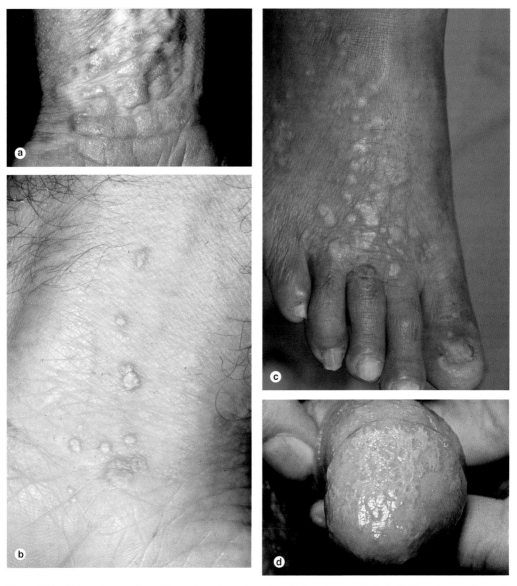

Figure 13-1 **a** Lichen planus on the wrist **b** purple, polygonal papules **c** Lichen planus on the foot. **d** Lichen planus on the penis.

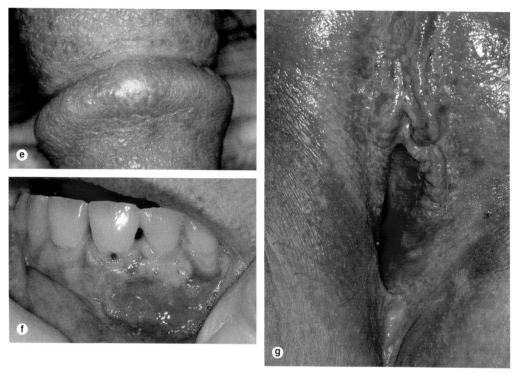

Figure 13-1, cont'd e Lichen planus. f Erosive oral lichen planus. g Vulvar lichen planus

Histological features include hyperkeratosis without parakeratosis, hypergranulosis, acanthosis, a "saw-tooth" pattern of the rete ridges, a high-hugging band-like infiltrate composed of lymphocytes, and apoptotic keratinocytes, referred to as Civatte bodies.

Clumps of IgM, IgA, or C3 are present and correspond to the Civatte bodies on direct immunofluorescence.

Differential diagnosis is given in Box 13-2.

Pathogenesis

Key Points

- Likely involves an autoimmune reaction against antigens on lesional keratinocytes
- Medications may induce or exacerbate lichen planus (Box 13-3)

The pathogenesis of lichen planus is not fully understood. Current evidence suggests that the damage to the basal cells of the epidermis results from primed T cells that recognize antigens on the surface of the keratinocytes. Viruses, contact allergens, and medications (see Chapter 23 for more information) have been implicated as inciting agents in the development of lichen planus.

Particular focus has been paid to the hepatitis C virus (HCV). The oral form of lichen planus is more commonly implicated as a manifestation of HCV infection. HCV RNA was detected in 93%

of oral lichen planus specimens from patients with diagnosed lichen planus and known HCV infection. Different prevalences of HCV infection among lichen planus patients are reported from different geographic regions. In countries such as Japan with high rates of HCV infection, anti-HCV antibodies have been demonstrated in up to 62% of patients with oral lichen planus. Similar studies from the United Kingdom, in which the prevalence of hepatitis C is lower, found no anti-HCV antibodies in patients with oral lichen planus.

Several factors likely influence the development of lichen planus in HCV-infected patients. An Italian study noted a significant association of oral lichen planus and HCV infection with the major histocompatibility complex (MHC) allele human leukocyte antigen (HLA)-DR6. Possibly, cytotoxic T cells become primed to recognize antigens on the surface of keratinocytes after the presentation of exogenous antigens in genetically susceptible individuals.

Analysis of the role of the MHC antigens in the pathogenesis of lichen planus has been unclear and contradictory at times. Different antigens have been described in diverse populations and include HLA-B8, HLA-B27, HLA-Bw57, HLA-DR1, HLA-DR6, and HLA-DR9.

Contact allergy to amalgam (mercury) dental fillings, gold, and copper has also received attention in the development of oral lichenoid

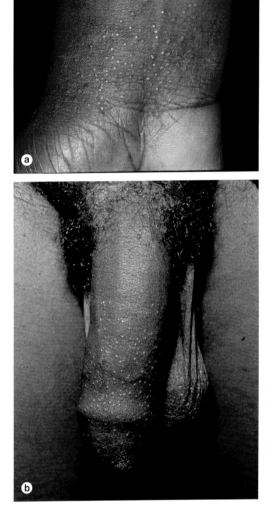

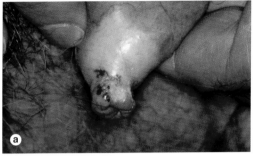

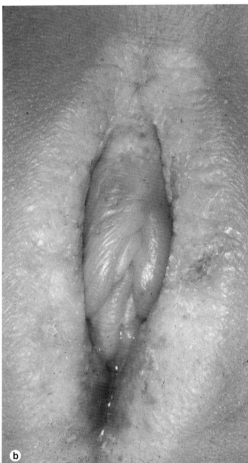

Figure 13-2 a Lichen nitidus. b Lichen nitidus of the penis

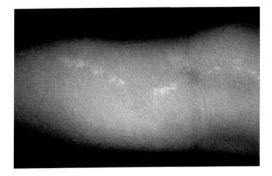

Figure 13-3 Lichen striatus

Figure 13-4 a Lichen sclerosus. b Vulvar lichen sclerosus

eruptions and cutaneous lichen planus. The contributory role of dental products to the development of oral lichen planus remains a subject of debate. While some patients with identified allergies to dental metals have improved after removal of the implicated dental work, it remains unclear whether the metals in some way caused the lichen planus, or if the contact allergy is a secondary phenomenon. Systemic medications are also associated with lichen planus (see Box 13-3). A lichen planus-like eruption has occurred in up to 32% of patients receiving gold treatments.

Tumor necrosis factor-α (TNF-α) has also been implicated in the development of lichen planus. TNF-α levels have been found to be elevated in patients with lichen planus versus controls. Medications that inhibit TNF-α such as

Table 13-1 Variants of lichen planus (LP) involving the skin

	Summary
Actinic LP	
Clinical presentation	Annular red-brown to dark brown plaques surrounded by hypopigmentation
Site of predilection	Sun-exposed areas (face, dorsal hands, forearms, and neck)
Special comments	More common in patients of Middle Eastern descent; frequently improves in the winter
	Ashy dermatosis is closely related, but tends to occur in Hispanic patients
Acute LP	
Clinical presentation	Rapid onset of lesions, sometimes progress from a red to black color
Site of predilection	Disseminated
Special comments	May resolve in 3–6 months
Annular LP	
Clinical presentation	Annular lesions
Site of predilection	Penis, scrotum, and vermilion lips; also intertriginous sites such as the axilla and groin
Atrophic LP	
Clinical presentation	Centrally depressed atrophic lesions
Site of predilection	Lower leg
Special comments	Resembles porokeratosis
Annular atrophic lichen planus (AALP)	
Clinical presentation	Purple papules that enlarge with an atrophic center
Site of predilection	Involves the same sites as regular lichen planus
Special comments	The atrophy is reported to be a consequence of inflammatory elastolysis
Bullous LP	
Clinical presentation	Bullous
Site of predilection	Lower extremity
Special comments	Bullous lichen planus can arise in pre-existing lesions of LP secondary to severe basal damage and dermal edema. Histologically, this vesicular lesion corresponds to an enlarged Max–Joseph space
LP pemphigoides	
Clinical presentation	Bullous
Site of predilection	Diffuse distribution, but bullae tend to be located on the limbs
Special comments	Bullae arising in skin uninvolved with lichen planus; circulating IgG autoantibodies recognize the epitope (MCW-4) within the C-terminal NC16A domain of the 180 kDa BP antigen (BPAG2, type XVII collagen). Biopsied lesions demonstrate linear deposits of IgG and C3 along the basement membrane
Hypertrophic lichen planus	
Clinical presentation	Hyperkeratotic plaques
Site of predilection	Anterior shins
Special comments	The lesions are pruritic and have a chronic course secondary to repetitive rubbing. Histologically, changes of lichen simplex are evident. Squamous cell carcinoma is more frequently reported in patients with hypertrophic lichen planus than in those with normal cutaneous lichen planus
Keratosis lichenoides chronica	
Clinical presentation	Intersecting linear lesions form "Chinese characters". Associated seborrheic dermatitis-like scaling plaques
Site of predilection	Extremities (papules and nodules), head and neck (scaling)
Special comments	Biopsy reveals hyper- and parakeratosis, hypergranulosis, vacuolar change, and perivascular and periappendageal infiltrates

Table 13-1 Variants of lichen planus (LP) involving the skin—Cont'd

	Summary
Linear LP	
Clinical presentation	Lichenoid, purple papules following Blaschko's lines
Site of predilection	Extremities, trunk, head, and neck
Special comments	Presumably due to postzygotic mutations; now more commonly reported in adults than children
LP-lupus erythematosus overlap syndrome	
Clinical presentation	Chronic plaques with central atrophic hypopigmentation with a purple border
Site of predilection	Extremities
Special comments	Histologic and immunofluorescence examinations share features of both lichen planus and lupus. Patients often have elevated antinuclear antibody titers and other serologies indicative of lupus
LP pigmentosus	
Clinical presentation	Slate gray to brown-black macules and papules in a reticulated pattern
Site of predilection	Appear on the face, neck, and flexor folds; oral lesions also occur
Special comments	Overlap with LP actinicus, and often histologically indistinguishable from erythema dyschromicum perstans; more common in the Indian and Hispanic populations
Ulcerative (Erosive) LP	
Clinical presentation	Erosions, ulcers
Site of predilection	Palms and soles; mucous membranes
Special comments	Associated with onychoatrophy; an increased risk of malignant transformation (0.4–5.6% of cases) has been reported with ulcerative LP of the mucous membranes
Vulvovaginal gingival syndrome	
Clinical presentation	Erosive or desquamative lesions
Site of predilection	Vulva, vagina, and gingiva
Special comments	Significant morbidity may be associated with HLA-DRB1

Ig, immunoglobulin; HLA, human leukocyte antigen.

thalidomide as well as the biologic alefacept have been reported to be successful in the treatment of lichen planus. The implications for these findings need further clarification.

Treatment

Key Points

- Includes topical, intralesional, systemic corticosteroids, and topical calcineurin inhibitors
- Resistant cases may require acitretin, psoralen with ultraviolet A, or cyclosporine
- Oral and erosive genital lichen planus may be particularly difficult to treat

Therapy for lichen planus is often difficult and disappointing. The Food and Drug Administration has not approved any specific therapy for lichen planus. Controlled studies with large numbers of patients are rare and challenging to perform without a standardized method for evaluating the severity of the disease. Reports from large series note spontaneous remission in 64–68% of cases after 1 year. Recurrence rates have not been studied in a large series of patients.

The initial treatment for lichen planus includes topical and intralesional corticosteroids. Hypertrophic lichen planus can be treated with high-potency corticosteroids under occlusion or intralesional corticosteroids. Although systemic corticosteroids are effective, relapses frequently occur after discontinuing the medication. When corticosteroids do not provide adequate or safe therapy, other options include acitretin, hydroxychloroquine, photochemotherapy, metronidazole, and cyclosporine. Topical calcineurin inhibitors can be helpful in some cases, but have mostly been used to treat mucosal disease.

The treatment of mucosal lichen planus is especially challenging. In addition to the above therapies, many topical therapies – topical corticosteroids, topical tretinoin, and cyclosporine swish and spit – have been used with variable success. Oral cyclosporine is expensive. Some patients have refrigerated and reused the swish and spit solution, coining the term "recyclosporine."

Table 13-2 Variants of lichen planus (LP) involving the scalp

	Summary
Lichen planopilaris (LPP)	
Clinical presentation	Follicular keratotic papules, tufted hairs, perifollicular erythema, and scarring alopecia
Special comments	More common in females
Frontal fibrosing alopecia (FFA)	
Clinical presentation	Scarring alopecia characterized by selective hair loss
Site of predilection	Frontoparietal region and eyebrows
Special comments	It is primarily observed in postmenopausal women
Graham–Little syndrome	LPP with follicular papules on the trunk and extremities

Table 13-3 Variants of lichen planus (LP) involving the mucous membranes

	Summary
Reticular	
Clinical presentation	White lacy striae
Special comments	Most common variant seen by dermatologists
Erosive	
Clinical presentation	Irregular erosions that may have a yellow or white exudate
Special comments	Usually the most symptomatic
Atrophic	
Clinical presentation	Red patches with white striae on the edge
Special comments	Frequently involves the gingiva
Papular	
Clinical presentation	Pinpoint white papules
Plaque	
Clinical presentation	Slightly elevated plaques that are homogenously white
Bullous	
Clinical presentation	Small vesicles/bullae
Special comments	Rare

BOX 13-2

The clinical differential diagnosis of lichen planus

Skin

Lichenoid drug reaction

Secondary syphilis

Lichen nitidus

Lichen striatus

Erythema dyschromicum perstans

Guttate psoriasis

Pityriasis rosea

Scalp

Lupus erythematosus

Pseudopelade of Brocq

Folliculitis decalvans

Mucous membrane

Benign leukoplakia

Malignant leukoplakia

Lupus erythematosus

Mucous patches of syphilis

Aphthous stomatitis

Normal bite line

Candidiasis

Blistering disorders (pemphigus, pemphigoid)

BOX 13-3

Medications that induce or exacerbate lichen planus

Gold

Antimalarials

Beta-blockers

Penicillamine

Thiazides

Furosemide

Spironolactone

Angiotensin-converting enzyme (ACE) inhibitors

Calcium-channel blockers

Nonsteroidal anti-inflammatory medications

Tetracycline

Triamcinolone in Orabase is indicated for intraoral use; however, its gritty vehicle is considered unpalatable by some users. High-potency topical corticosteroid gels, such as fluocinonide gel, are used off-label with some benefit. Recently, the off-label use of the topical calcineurin inhibitors tacrolimus and pimecrolimus has been reported as an effective alternative for controlling oral and vulvovaginal lichen planus. Additional research is vital for future therapy in patients with mucosal and generalized lichen planus.

A summary of the treatments available for lichen planus is given in Table 13-4. Reports supporting their use are often anecdotal.

Controversy

Key Point

- An up to 10% incidence of oral lichen planus degenerating into oral squamous cell carcinoma has been reported. The percentage has varied and all estimates likely reflect a strong reporting bias. The actual risk is likely to be far lower

Controversy exists: does oral lichen planus have an inherent risk of developing squamous cell carcinoma or do other external factors cause this risk?

Close surveillance for the development of malignancy in lesions of oral lichen planus is recommended by many authors. While increased rates of malignant degeneration are reported, oral lichen planus has not been established as a premalignant condition. Two recent studies found rates of 1.5% and 0.8% of oral squamous cell carcinoma in patients with oral lichen planus. Confounding factors included smoking and systemic immunosuppression.

External risk factors that may influence the development of squamous cell carcinoma in a patient with oral lichen planus include smoking, alcohol abuse, oral candidiasis, poor nutrition, and the use of systemic immunosuppressants for lichen planus. It is possible that the synergistic effect between the chronic inflammation of lichen planus and these external risk factors may lead to the increased incidence of malignancy.

Lichen striatus

Clinical presentation

Key Points

- Uncommon, self-limited, linear dermatosis primarily in children
- Flat-topped tan to pink, scaly papules with an interrupted linear pattern that follows Blaschko's lines

Lichen striatus primarily affects children between the ages of 4 months and 15 years. Adults are rarely affected. The female to male ratio is 2–3:1. There is rarely a positive family history for the disease.

Case series consistently identify the arms and legs as the most common sites of involvement. The head is infrequently involved. Both the left and right sides of the body are equally affected, and, rarely, bilateral lesions or multiple streaks develop. Lesions occasionally resolve with hypo- or hyperpigmentation that can persist for years.

Table 13-4 Treatments available for lichen planus

Treatment	Schedule
Topical corticosteroids	
Intralesional corticosteroids	
Systemic corticosteroids	Prednisone 30–60 mg PO qd
Topical tretinoin	
Topical cyclosporine	
Topical tacrolimus 0.1% ointment	
Topical pimecrolimus 1% cream	
Acitretin*	30 mg PO qd
PUVA/UVB/UVA1/bath PUVA	
Cyclosporine	1–6 mg/kg PO qd
Dapsone	200 mg PO qd[†]
Alefacept[‡]	15 mg^2/week × 12 weeks
Mycophenolate mofetil[§]	1 g PO bid
Thalidomide	150 mg PO qd
Metronidazole	250 mg PO tid/500 mg PO bid
Hydroxychloroquine	200–400 mg PO qd × 6 months
Azathioprine	50 mg bid PO × 3-7 months
Cyclophosphamide	50–100 mg PO qd
Griseofulvin[¶]	Griseofulvin FP 125 mg PO bid × 3–6 months
Methotrexate	10–15 mg/week
Enoxaparin**	3 mg subcutaneously once weekly × 4–6 weeks

PO, orally, qd, once daily; PUVA, psoralen ultraviolet A; bid, twice daily; tid, three times daily

*In a double-blind placebo-controlled study, treatment with acitretin for 8 weeks demonstrated significant improvement or remission versus placebo.
[†]Two-thirds healed after 4 months, 19% with partial response.
[‡]Two patients with recalcitrant generalized lichen planus.
[§]Benefit in 3 patients.
[¶]The authors have had little success with griseofulvin.
**In a recent report, 6 patients had no response.

Nail changes are rare, but onychodystrophy does occur. Reported nail changes include nail pitting; longitudinal ridging, splitting, and fissuring; striate leukonychia; onycholysis; and nail bed hyperkeratosis. Lichen striatus of the nail can occur without skin involvement and should be suspected when changes affect only the medial or lateral nail. Nail changes regress spontaneously after an average of 23 months.

Pruritus is the most common symptom reported in up to one-third of patients with lichen striatus. Symptomatic patients are more likely to have a history of atopy.

Traditionally, cases of lichen striatus cluster in the spring and summer months. This has led authors to propose a viral etiology for the disease.

Diagnosis

Key Points

* Primarily a clinical diagnosis made when characteristic lesions follow Blaschko's lines in children
* Skin biopsy is rarely needed, but can help clarify diagnosis

Helpful clues on light microscopy include a lichenoid or dense perivascular inflammatory infiltrate composed of lymphocytes and histiocytes in the upper dermis. The infiltrate may also surround the eccrine glands or hair follicles deeper in the dermis. Spongiosis and dyskeratosis are occasionally found in the epidermis. As opposed to lichen planus, direct immunofluorescence is negative in lichen striatus.

The differential diagnosis of linear lesions that follow Blaschko's lines is found in Box 13-4.

Pathogenesis

Key Point

* Loss of immune tolerance to an embryonically abnormal clone of epidermal cells has been suggested

Blaschko's lines represent the path and direction of growth followed by cutaneous cells during embryonic development. It is thought that a somatic mutation occurring after fertilization might create a peculiar clone of cells in one of the Blaschko's lines. After years of immune tolerance to this clone, an inciting event likely induces the immune system to recognize the clone as foreign. On histopathology, CD8+ T lymphocytes are found surrounding dyskeratotic keratinocytes and activated Langerhans cells in the epidermis, supporting this autoimmune hypothesis.

The inciting event has been proposed to be a virus, given the seasonal clustering of cases. Lichen striatus has been reported to occur after a flu-like illnesses, tonsillitis, application of retinoic acid lotion, sunburn, hepatitis B virus, and bacille Calmette–Guérin (BCG) vaccination. However, most patients do not report an inciting event.

Though disputed by recent reports, atopic disease (personal and family history of atopy) may be more frequent in patients with lichen striatus. It has been proposed that altered immunity in atopic patients allows for the loss of tolerance after a viral infection.

BOX 13-4

Differential diagnosis of raised lesions that follow Blaschko's lines

Linear psoriasis

Linear lichen planus

Lichen striatus

Inflammatory linear verrucous epidermal nevus (ILVEN)

Linear porokeratosis

Linear chronic graft-versus-host disease

Linear lichen nitidus

Linear lupus erythematosus

Linear fixed drug eruption

Linear Darier's disease

Incontinentia pigmenti

Treatment

Key Points

* Lichen striatus spontaneously resolves, with a mean duration of 6–9 months
* Symptomatic treatment is usually sufficient

Relapses have been reported. Topical corticosteroids do not affect the duration of the disease, but can be used for the treatment of pruritus. Other reported therapies include salicylic acid and coal tar. Anecdotal response to tacrolimus ointment has been reported.

Lichen nitidus

Clinical presentation

Key Points

* Multiple, firm, discrete, 1–2-mm, flat papules with a shiny surface
* Papules display the Koebner phenomenon
* Found on the upper extremities, chest, abdomen, and glans penis
* Asymptomatic with a spontaneous remission
* Actinic lichen nitidus is a photodistributed variant of lichen nitidus

Lichen nitidus is an uncommon inflammatory dermatosis found primarily in school-aged children and young adults. No obvious racial or sex predilection exists. The papules can be flesh-colored, hypopigmented, pink, or purple, depending on skin color of the individual. They tend to be grouped in circinate arrays, but linear groups occur and disseminated lesions may occur on the penis, especially in dark-skinned individuals. As in lichen planus, the isomorphic phenomenon of Koebner occurs in lichen nitidus and is a hallmark for the disease. This accounts for the linear arrays of lesions. Unlike lichen planus, lichen nitidus is usually asymptomatic. There are rare reports of familial lichen nitidus. Generalized lichen nitidus has also been described. Lichen nitidus can involve the nails, causing linear ridges and pits. Rarely, lichen nitidus can affect the palms, soles, and mucous membranes.

Actinic lichen nitidus (also called summertime actinic lichenoid eruption) is characterized by multiple, shiny, pinhead-sized papules that erupt in sun-exposed areas. This entity has been described in children and adult patients and is clustered in the subtropical regions, especially the Middle East and India. Seasonal recurrences are common with re-exposure to the sun.

Diagnosis

Key Points

* Characteristic clinical presentation
* Biopsy is also characteristic with elongated rete ridges cupping an infiltrate of lymphocytes and histiocytes

Histopathologically, lichen nitidus is a unique example of a lichenoid infiltrate. This disease is characterized by a focal, closely packed infiltrate of lymphocytes, histiocytes, and giant cells in the papillary dermis. The width of these cells spans one to two dermal papillae. At the periphery of this collection or "ball" of cells, the rete ridges elongate and extend downward around it. This is referred to as the pathognomonic "ball and claw" formation. The overlying epidermis is often atrophic and contains parakeratosis. Biopsy specimens of lichen nitidus are negative on immunofluorescence evaluation. Thus, lichen nitidus differs from lichen planus histologically by the ball-in-claw morphology, presence of histiocytes, and lack of cytoid bodies. The differential diagnosis of lichen nitidus is given in Box 13-5.

Pathogenesis

Key Point

* The cause of lichen nitidus is unknown

Authors have speculated about alterations in the immune system's recognition of epidermal cell antigens, as likely occurs in lichen planus. However, the population of cells in lichen nitidus is different on immunohistochemical evaluation when compared to lichen planus. Lichen nitidus is mediated by a diverse population of helper, nonhelper, and activated T lymphocytes; macrophages; and giant cells. Lichen planus lacks the number of macrophages and giant cells seen in lichen nitidus.

Often, systemic associations can be useful in evaluating the pathogenesis of a rare disease. See Box 13-6 for the associations with lichen nitidus.

Treatment

Key Point

* Treatment is generally not required for lichen nitidus – it has a tendency towards spontaneous remission and is asymptomatic for many patients

Therapy with mid- to high-potency topical corticosteroids and topical dinitrochlorobenzene has been reported to accelerate clearance. Systemic therapies reported to be effective include systemic corticosteroids, antihistamines, acitretin, low-dose cyclosporine, antituberculosis agents (isoniazid 300 mg orally daily for 6 months), itraconazole, psoralen with ultraviolet A, narrowband ultraviolet B, and sun exposure. Sun avoidance is important for patients with actinic lichen nitidus.

Controversy

Key Point

* Some argue that lichen nitidus is a variant of lichen planus

---

BOX 13-5

Differential diagnosis of lichen nitidus

Lichen planus

Keratosis pilaris

Papular eczema

Lichen amyloidosis

Pityriasis rubra pilaris

Papular mucinosis

Phrynoderma

BOX 13-6

Systemic associations with lichen nitidus

Amenorrhea

Crohn's disease

Human immunodeficiency virus infection

Atopic dermatitis

Hepatitis B vaccination

Some authors describe lichen nitidus as a form of lichen planus. Patients can have both diseases simultaneously; others have developed lichen nitidus after the diagnosis of lichen planus. Both of these diseases demonstrate the Koebner phenomenon and have a lichenoid infiltrate on histopathology. A photodistributed version of both also exists.

Clinically, differences between these two disorders are found. Lichen planus demonstrates Wickham's striae and is commonly pruritic (two features usually absent in lichen nitidus). The two diseases have different distributions, as lichen planus more commonly affects the nails and oral mucosa. Histologically, important differences also exist. Lichen nitidus often has parakeratosis; inflammation with lymphocytes, macrophages, and giant cells; and lacks immunofluorescent deposits. In contrast, lichen planus lacks parakeratosis, has prominent hypergranulosis, has a primarily lymphocytic infiltrate, and contains Civatte bodies (cytoid bodies) that stain with immunoglobulin (Ig) M, IgA, or C3.

Immunohistochemical studies have tried to differentiate the population of lymphocytes in each disorder. Some studies favor the involvement of CD4+ T lymphocytes more than CD8+ lymphocytes in lichen nitidus and vice versa for lichen planus. Studies are contradictory at times and further research is needed for clarification.

Benign lichenoid keratosis (BLK, lichen planus-like keratosis)

Clinical presentation

Key Points

* A red to purple to brown macule, papule, or plaque that can mimic basal cell carcinoma clinically
* The most common location is the trunk

First described in 1966 as a solitary variant of lichen planus, BLKs are common lesions found on the trunk and upper extremities of adults after the fifth and seventh decades. The female-to-male ratio is 3:1. The average size of a BLK is 5.5 mm.

Diagnosis

Key Point

* BLKs resemble lichen planus on histopathology, but are more likely to demonstrate parakeratosis (Table 13-5)

The BLK is often submitted as a basal cell carcinoma, seborrheic keratosis, or actinic keratosis. Histologically, the differential diagnosis includes lichen planus, lichenoid drug eruption, lichenoid acral lupus erythematosus, lichenoid graft-versus-host disease, inflamed seborrheic keratosis, halo nevus, and lichenoid regression of melanoma.

Pathogenesis

Key Points

* Likely the inflammatory involution of a pre-existing lentigo or lichenoid actinic keratosis
* Unknown triggering event

Treatment

Key Points

* A diagnosis of BLK is reassuring
* Cryotherapy can be used to hasten clearance

Erythema dyschromicum perstans

Clinical presentation

Key Points

* Multiple ash-gray, hyperpigmented macules on the trunk, proximal extremities, neck, and face
* Early active lesions have a red raised border that spreads centrifugally
* Generally asymptomatic, although lesions may be pruritic

Erythema dyschromicum perstans, also described as "ashy dermatosis," is an uncommon dermatosis first reported in patients from Latin America.

Cases have been described from the age of 2 years through adult life. However, the majority are found in patients under the age of 30. Conflicting reports exist concerning the sex

Table 13-5 Comparison between benign lichenoid keratosis and lichen planus

Features shared by benign lichenoid keratosis and lichen planus	Features that may be seen with benign lichenoid keratosis, but are not seen in lichen planus
Hyperkeratosis	Epidermal parakeratosis
Hypergranulosis	Flanking features of a lentigo
Epidermal acanthosis	Inclusion of eosinophils and plasma cells
Necrotic basal keratinocytes	
High-hugging infiltrate composed of lymphocytes	

predilection. The disease is primarily reported in Latin America and India.

Diagnosis

Key Points

- A lichenoid reaction pattern may be found
- No histopathologic change is pathognomonic
- The differential diagnosis is listed in Box 13-7

Suspicious clinical lesions are often biopsied. Biopsies taken from the active border demonstrate a prominent high-hugging lymphocytic infiltrate with pigment incontinence and basal layer vacuolation. Colloid bodies are detected and label with IgG or IgM by direct immunofluorescence. Prominent features of developed lesions include a superficial perivascular infiltrate and melanophagocytosis. The disease may represent a variant of lichen planus.

Pathogenesis

Key Point

- Unknown etiology

An abnormality in cell-mediated immunity with alterations of adhesion and activation molecules on basal keratinocytes has been proposed. Three observations of erythema dyschromicum perstans and human immunodeficiency virus (HIV) infection support the idea of an altered immune status. Box 13-8 lists other associations seen.

On immunopathological investigation, similar patterns of MHC class II antigen expression on keratinocytes, staining of Langerhans cells, and infiltration of T lymphocytes are seen in both erythema dyschromicum perstans and lichen planus.

Treatment

Key Points

- Various treatment modalities have been reported
- Treatment is often disappointing

Treatment with topical hydroquinone, steroids, or tretinoin is often inadequate. Laser therapy offers potential. The use of antibiotics, vitamins, isoniazid, and chloroquine has not been beneficial. Griseofulvin has been reported to induce remission, but the lesions recur after discontinuing this medication. Clofazimine (100 mg daily for 3 months) and dapsone (100 mg daily for 6–8 weeks) have been reported to be effective.

Lichen sclerosus

Clinical presentation

Key Points

- Chronic inflammatory dermatosis with a predilection for the anogenital region in women, men, and children
- Characterized by white, atrophic, or indurated papules that coalesce into porcelain-white plaques
- Extragenital lichen sclerosis occurs in up to 10–20% of patients and is more common in women

Malignancy occurs in some women with genital lichen sclerosus, but quoted figures up to 4–5% reflect a strong reporting bias. The actual risk is likely far lower.

Lichen sclerosus has been reported in patients ranging from 6 months old to late adulthood. The mean age of onset is the fifth and sixth decade.

BOX 13-7

Differential diagnosis of erythema dyschromicum perstans

Fixed drug eruption

Lichen planus pigmentosus

Postinflammatory hyperpigmentation

Pityriasis rosea

Drug-induced hyperpigmentation

Hyperpigmentation due to heavy metals

Addison's disease

Late pinta

Tinea versicolor

BOX 13-8

Associations reported with erythema dyschromicum perstans

Ammonium nitrate ingestion

Whipworm infestation

Human immunodeficiency virus infection

Chlorothalonil (a fungicide used on banana plantations) allergy

Cobalt allergy in plumbers

Orally administered X-ray contrast material

Bronchial carcinoma

Lichen planus and lichen planopilaris

Endocrinopathies

Hepatitis C

Most patients are Caucasian, but other ethnic groups are also affected. The prevalence of the disorder is estimated to be between 1:300 and 1:1000. The female-to-male ratio is 10:1 to 6:1. Familial cases of lichen sclerosus occur.

Up to 15% of cases of lichen sclerosus are in children. The prevalence of vulval lichen sclerosus in children is 1:900, with an average age at diagnosis of 7 years.

In women, atrophic pink to white plaques are found on the vulva, perineum, and perianal skin. The mucous membranes, commonly the vaginal mucosa, may be involved. A "figure-of-eight" configuration is common with disease involvement extending from the clitoris to the anus. Erosions and fissures are common. In addition to the white plaques, hemorrhagic bullae and ecchymosis may form and resolve with hyperpigmentation. Follicular plugging and scarring can be seen. Women may experience pruritus, irritation, dyspareunia, dysuria, bleeding, and painful skin fissures. Up to 9% of women are asymptomatic.

Lichen sclerosus in men primarily affects the glans penis or foreskin. In this location, it has been called balanitis xerotica obliterans. Presenting signs and symptoms include urinary obstruction, phimosis, painful erection, and decreased penile sensitivity. Young boys commonly present with phimosis.

The most common symptoms in prepubertal girls are pruritus and soreness. The clinical features of lichen sclerosus, particularly vulvar ecchymoses, may be mistaken for sexual abuse. Spontaneous remissions have been reported with the onset of puberty.

Extragenital lesions affect the head, neck, and torso, particularly under the breasts. Lesions are atrophic, hyper- to hypopigmented macules that are usually asymptomatic. Extragenital lesions are not associated with malignancy.

Complications of lichen sclerosus are listed in Box 13-9. Squamous cell carcinoma and verrucous carcinoma are the most common malignancies, but basal cell carcinoma and melanoma have been reported.

Diagnosis

Key Points

* Clinical features are often diagnostic, but histopathological changes are characteristic
* Histologic features include epidermal atrophy with homogenization, hyalinization, and sclerosis of the papillary dermis
* The differential diagnosis is listed in Box 13-10

Other histological features include compact orthohyperkeratosis, vacuolar degeneration of the basal layer, and a dense lymphocytic infiltrate underneath the basement membrane in early lesions. This interface dermatitis may be sparse in developed lesions.

Pathogenesis

Key Points

* Associated with autoimmune disorders and HLA class II antigen DQ7
* Autoantibodies to extracellular matrix protein 1 (ECM 1) have been implicated

The cause of lichen sclerosus is not fully understood. Some 20–40% of patients with lichen sclerosus have an associated autoimmune disease. Box 13-11 lists the most commonly associated autoimmune disorders.

This association led researchers to investigate the role of autoantibodies in the etiology of lichen sclerosus. Autoantibodies to ECM 1 are commonly found in patients with lichen sclerosus (74% of patients with lichen sclerosus versus 7% of controls). Although it has not been established whether the antibodies to ECM 1 are a cause or epiphenomenon, this association

BOX 13-9

Complications of lichen sclerosus

Malignancy

Secondary infection with candidiasis

Introital narrowing

Pseudocysts of the clitoris

Sexual dysfunction

Vulvodynia

Penile dysesthesia

Meatal stenosis

Phimosis

BOX 13-10

The differential diagnosis of lichen sclerosus

Erosive lichen planus

Morphea/scleroderma

Candidiasis

Child sexual abuse

Vulvar eczema

Herpes simplex infection

Blistering disorders (pemphigus and pemphigoid)

Squamous cell carcinoma in situ

Autoimmune disorders commonly associated with lichen sclerosus

Alopecia areata

Vitiligo

Thyroid disease

Pernicious anemia

Cicatricial pemphigoid

illustrates an interesting connection. The glycoprotein, ECM 1, is mutated in lipoid proteinosis, a disease that shares many features histologically with lichen sclerosus. ECM 1 binds to proteoglycans in the dermis, helps to aid in epidermal differentiation, and is involved in angiogenesis. Disruption of these functions likely leads to the dermal hyalinization, epidermal atrophy, and ecchymosis seen in lichen sclerosus.

Studies have investigated *Borrelia burgdorferi* as a cause of lichen sclerosus. No consistent association has been demonstrated in North America, although it has been associated with some cases in Europe. Geographic variations in the strains of *Borrelia* species may account for these conflicting reports.

Authors have suggested that the development of lichen sclerosus may be due to a loss of androgen sensitivity. Studies have shown a loss of androgen receptor nuclear antigen staining in lesional genital skin compared with controls. Although a higher percentage of lichen sclerosus occurs most commonly in premenarchal and postmenopausal women, no protective effect from estrogen has been clearly demonstrated. Further investigation is needed into many of the above associations.

Treatment

Key Points

- The treatment of choice is ultrapotent topical steroids
- Surgical management may be required for postinflammatory scarring
- Surveillance is needed to screen patients for malignancy

The treatment of choice for lichen sclerosus in male or female adults and children is ultrapotent topical steroids such as clobetasol 0.05% ointment. The ointment form is preferred over creams, which usually contain alcohols and can sting. Ultrapotent corticosteroids decrease pruritus, improve the clinical appearance of the white plaques, and can reverse phimosis.

Topical progesterone has been reported to be effective, whereas topical testosterone is no more effective than emollient. Resistant cases may require treatment with a topical steroid in combination with a topical or systemic retinoid. See Table 13-6 for a full list of therapies and dosing regimens.

Given the association of autoimmune disorders, laboratory screening can be offered for thyroid disease, diabetes, and anemia. Surgical management has traditionally been utilized for malignancies that arise. Surgery should be performed carefully, as the procedure can create new lesions through koebnerization.

Controversies

Key Points

- There may be overlap between lichen sclerosus and morphea, both clinically and histologically
- Certain histologic features may allow for a diagnosis of lichen sclerosus to be favored

There are cases that clinically and histologically are difficult to classify as either morphea or lichen sclerosus. Histologic features that favor lichen sclerosus include loss of elastic fibers in the papillary dermis, vacuolar change at the dermoepidermal junction, presence of a lymphoid band, and absence of sclerosis in the reticular dermis and subcutaneous fat.

Table 13-6 Treatment of lichen sclerosus

Treatment	Schedule
Clobetasol 0.05% ointment	Daily for 2 weeks, followed by application on Saturday and Sunday only
Topical progesterone	qod alternating therapy with topical corticosteroids
Tretinoin 0.025% cream	q day, five days a week × 1 year
Acitretin	30 mg PO q day × 16 weeks*
Carbon dioxide laser	One session – Sharplan 1020 5–6 W with continuous discharge mode
Stanozolol	2 mg PO q day
Cryotherapy	
Ultraviolet A1 phototherapy	4 times a week × 10 weeks
Photodynamic therapy with 5-aminolevulinic acid	1–3 cycles of 5-aminolevuline acid with 80 J/cm² at an irradiance of 40–70 mW/cm²

qod, every other day; q, every; PO, orally.
*Randomized, placebo-controlled, double-bind study of 78 women

PITYRIASIS LICHENOIDES ET VARIOLIFORMIS ACUTA AND PITYRIASIS LICHENOIDIES CHRONICA

Pityriasis lichenoides is a rare inflammatory dermatosis of unknown etiology. The disease commonly affects children and young adults with equal sex ratios. The mean age of onset is 7.5 years. No racial or geographic predilection exists. Pityriasis lichenoides occurs on a spectrum with acute and chronic variants: pityriasis lichenoides et varioliformis acuta (PLEVA) and pityriasis lichenoides chronica (PLC), respectively. Some patients have lesions of both PLEVA and PLC simultaneously. As classic presentations of PLEVA, PLC, and the febrile variant of pityriasis lichenoides differ, the clinical presentations and diagnosis for each will be addressed separately below. The pathogenesis and treatment sections will address the spectrum of the disease as a whole.

Pityriasis lichenoides et varioliformis acuta

Clinical presentation

> **Key Points**
>
> - Characteristic crops of asymptomatic pink to red papulovesicles that usually resolve in weeks to months
> - Vesicles are often hemorrhagic or necrotic and may resemble chicken pox
> - Lesions are characteristically found in different stages
> - Predilection for the proximal and flexor extremities and anterior trunk, sparing the face, palms, soles, and mucous membranes
> - PLEVA may transition into PLC

PLEVA is also known as Mucha–Habermann disease. The lesions occasionally itch and resolve with scarring and postinflammatory dyspigmentation. Occasionally, patients report a low-grade fever, malaise, or headache and can have lymphadenopathy.

Diagnosis

> **Key Points**
>
> - Histologic features include a vacuolar interface dermatitis with a lymphocyte in nearly every vacuole, keratinocyte necrosis, a superficial and deep wedge-shaped perivascular lymphocytic infiltrate, neutrophils within dermal vessels, an overlying compact corneum with neutrophils, extravasation of red blood cells,

and transepidermal elimination of red blood cells
- The apex of the wedge-shaped infiltrate points toward the deep dermis with the base in the papillary dermis
- The differential diagnosis is listed in Box 13-12

Febrile ulceronecrotic Mucha–Habermann disease

Clinical presentation

> **Key Points**
>
> - A fulminant type of PLEVA, known as febrile ulceronecrotic Mucha-Habermann disease (FUMHD), in children
> - Diffuse, large necrotic papules, coalescent ulcerations, and high-grade fever
> - Several cases have been fatal

Diagnosis

> **Key Points**
>
> - Changes of leukocytoclastic vasculitis are seen in addition to the changes of PLEVA

Pityriasis lichenoides chronica

Clinical presentation

> **Key Points**
>
> - Recurrent crops of red-brown papules with adherent scale that resolve with postinflammatory pigmentary changes
> - A prolonged course that may last up to 1 year with exacerbations and remissions

---

BOX 13-12

The differential diagnosis of pityriasis lichenoides et varioliformis acuta

Lymphomatoid papulosis

Varicella

Small vessel vasculitis

Erythema multiforme

Arthropod reaction (papular urticaria)

Viral exanthem

Gianotti–Crosti syndrome

Drug eruption

Dermatitis herpetiformis

Folliculitis

Diagnosis

Key Points

- Histologic features include parakeratosis, a compact corneum, vacuolar interface dermatitis with a lymphocyte in almost every vacuole, and extravasated erythrocytes
- The cellular infiltrate in PLC is less dense than that of PLEVA

The differential diagnosis is listed in Box 13-13. Lymphomatoid papulosis may present in a similar fashion to pityriasis lichenoides. Lymphomatoid papulosis (considered by some authors to be in the spectrum of pityriasis lichenoides) progresses to mycosis fungoides in 10–20% of cases and is distinguished on histology by atypical CD30-positive lymphocytes.

Pathogenesis

Key Points

- Exact etiology of pityriasis lichenoides is unknown.
- PLEVA demonstrates a predominance of CD8+ cells, whereas PLC has a predominance of CD4+ cells
- Clonal T-cell rearrangements have been documented in adults and children with pityriasis lichenoides
- No clear infectious agent, although toxoplasmosis, Epstein–Barr virus, cytomegalovirus, parvovirus, HIV, and adenovirus have been implicated

Activated T cells and macrophages are found in both PLEVA and PLC, and immunohistochemical analyses have shown similar patterns in both entities. Clonal populations of T cells have been demonstrated in PLEVA, PLC, and FUMHD. Recently, a T-cell receptor gene rearrangement study demonstrated a dominant clonal population of T cells in 57% of patients with PLEVA and 8% of patients with PLC. The clonal population in PLEVA may arise from a subset of cells as a result of an altered immune response or as a

true lymphoproliferative disorder. Rare cases of lymphoma arising in patients with pityriasis lichenoides have been reported.

The presence of IgM and C3 in dermal vessels of patients with PLEVA suggests that immune complex deposition may play a role. Infectious agents have been proposed as the cause of the immune complex deposition and altered immune response.

Elevated levels of TNF-α have been found in FUMHD.

Treatment

Key Points

- Includes topical corticosteroids, oral antibiotics, psoralen with ultraviolet A and ultraviolet B phototherapy, and low-dose methotrexate
- Both tetracycline and erythromycin induce remission, likely secondary to their anti-inflammatory effects
- In children, erythromycin and ultraviolet B have been used

Tacrolimus has been shown to be efficacious for treatment of PLEVA and PLC in a few cases. Methotrexate may be beneficial when other therapies fail and in particular may be needed for the FUMHD. Prednisolone in doses greater than 1 mg/kg per day have also been used for FUMHD. Table 13-7 lists the treatments available for pityriasis lichenoides.

Table 13-7 Treatment for pityriasis lichenoides

Treatment	Schedule
Tacrolimus 0.03%/0.1% ointment	bid application × 4–6 weeks
Erythromycin	30–50 mg/kg per day × 8 weeks
Tetracycline	2 g/day
Ultraviolet B	3–5 times weekly with an average of 29 treatments for clearance; 4–8-week courses
Psoralen ultraviolet A	Three times weekly
Methotrexate	7.5–20 mg PO q week
Prednisolone in FUMHD	Greater than 1 mg/kg per day

bid, twice daily; PO, orally; q, every; FUMHD, febrile ulceronecrotic Mucha-Habermann disease.

Further reading

Arizaga AT, Gaughan MD, Bang RH. Generalized lichen nitidus. Clin Exp Dermatol 2002;27: 115–117.

Boyd AS, Neldner KH. Lichen planus. J Am Acad Dermatol 1991;25:593–619.

Combemale P, Faisant M, Guennoc B, et al. Erythema dyschromicum perstans: report of a new case and critical review of the literature. J Dermatol 1998;25:747–753.

Cribier B, Frances C, Chosidow O. Treatment of lichen planus. An evidence-based medicine analysis of efficacy. Arch Dermatol 1998;134:1521–1530.

Dalziel KL, Millard PR, Wojnarowska F. The treatment of vulval lichen sclerosus with a very potent topical steroid (clobetasol propionate 0.05%) cream. Br J Dermatol 1991;124:461–464.

Gelmetti C, Rigoni C, Alessi E, et al. Pityriasis lichenoides in children: a long-term follow-up of eighty-nine cases. J Am Acad Dermatol 1990;23:473–478.

Glorioso S, Jackson SC, Kopel AJ, et al. Actinic lichen nitidus in 3 African American patients. J Am Acad Dermatol 2006;54(Suppl):S48–S49.

Handa S, Sahoo B. Childhood lichen planus: a study of 87 cases. Int J Dermatol 2002;41:423–427.

Helmbold P, Gaisbauer G, Fiedler E, et al. Self-limited variant of febrile ulceronecrotic Mucha–Habermann disease with polyclonal T-cell receptor rearrangement. J Am Acad Dermatol 2006;54:1113–1115.

Kato N. Familial lichen nitidus. Clin Exp Dermatol 1995;20:336–338.

Loening-Baucke V. Lichen sclerosus et atrophicus in children. Am J Dis Children 1991;145:1058–1061.

Lumpkin LR, Helwig EB. Solitary lichen planus. Arch Dermatol 1966;93:54–55.

Meffert JJ, Davis BM, Grimwood RE. Lichen sclerosus. J Am Acad Dermatol 1995;32:393–416.

Morgan MB, Stevens GL, Switlyk S. Benign lichenoid keratosis: a clinical and pathologic reappraisal of 1040 cases. Am J Dermatopathol 2005;27: 387–392.

Nagao Y, Sata M. Hepatitis C virus and lichen planus. J Gastroenterol Hepatol 2004;19:1101–1113.

Patel DG, Kihiczak G, Schwartz RA, et al. Pityriasis lichenoides. Cutis 2000;65:17–23.

Patrizi A, Neri I, Fiorentini C, et al. Lichen striatus: clinical and laboratory features of 115 children. Pediatr Dermatol 2004;21:197–204.

Shapiro L, Ackerman AB. Solitary lichen planus-like keratosis. Dermatologica 1966;132:386–392.

Taniguchi Abagge K, Parolin Marinoni L, Giraldi S, et al. Lichen striatus: description of 89 cases in children. Pediatr Dermatol 2004;21:440–443.

Tilly JJ, Drolet BA, Esterly NB. Lichenoid eruptions in children. J Am Acad Dermatol 2004;51:606–624.

Cutaneous malignancies

14

Elizabeth Satter

Cutaneous carcinomas are the most common malignancies seen in humans. Basal cell carcinomas (BCCs) and squamous cell carcinomas (SCCs) are extremely common, and are expected to increase in frequency with the aging demographics of our population. Although less common, the cutaneous carcinomas that have the greatest mortality include melanomas and Merkel cell carcinomas. The following chapter will review cutaneous malignancies as well as soft-tissue tumors, lymphomas, and metastases that are frequently encountered in dermatology.

SUBTYPES OF SQUAMOUS CELL CARCINOMA

SCC is composed of a multitude of histological variants including a precursor lesion (actinic keratosis: AK), an in-situ variant (Bowen's disease), as well as multiple invasive variants. These include adenoid (acantholytic or pseudoglandular), adenosquamous, pseudovascular, desmoplastic, spindle cell, clear cell, signet-ring type, papillary, follicular, pigmented, verrucous carcinoma, Marjolin's ulcer, and keratoacanthoma (KA). Similar to melanoma, greater depth of invasion may portend a worse prognosis; however, some histologic variants may also have a more aggressive behavior, including SCC arising in Bowen's disease, adenosquamous carcinoma, desmoplastic SCC, and SCC arising in Marjolin's ulcers. Furthermore, SCC occurring in certain locations, particularly the lip, ear, and genital region, may have greater metastatic potential, such as rapidly growing SCC occurring in immunosuppressed patients. On the contrary, some SCCs, such as verrucous carcinoma and KA, may be locally aggressive, but have a lower metastatic potential.

Actinic (Solar) keratosis

Key Points

- Typically present with a hard keratotic surface with erythematous base
- Precancerous – may give rise to invasive SCC
- Destruction via cryotherapy, photodynamic therapy (PDT), or topical therapy

Clinical presentation

AK (Figure 14-1) is a precancerous epidermal neoplasm with the potential to develop into SCC. Clinically, AKs appear as 1–10-mm skin-colored to erythematous to brown, ill-defined, rough, scaly papules or plaques. They are often easier to feel than to see, making palpation a key element of the physical examination. Lesions may be solitary, numerous, or confluent. Often there is surrounding evidence of sun damage such as solar elastosis and lentigines. Eighty percent occur on sun-exposed areas, including the face, dorsum of hands and arms, neck, and upper torso. Most are asymptomatic, but AKs can be pruritic or tender. Predictable risk factors include ultraviolet (UV) exposure, age, male sex, immunosuppression (organ transplant recipients), and genetic syndromes (including xeroderma pigmentosum and albinism). Up to 25% regress spontaneously, while approximately 1 in 1000 develop into SCC within 1 year. Metastases from SCC arising in AKs are uncommon.

Several AK variants exist. The *hypertrophic AK* (HAK) is thicker with significant scale. It is most common on the dorsal hands and arms. Cutaneous horns may develop on HAKs, and biopsy is often needed to distinguish from SCC. The *superficial pigmented AK* (SPAK) is an uncommon variant that is characterized by size greater than 1.5 cm, brown to black pigmentation, a verrucous or smooth surface, and lateral growth. These are found most often on the

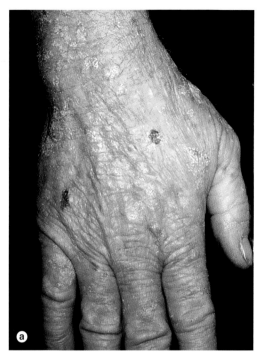

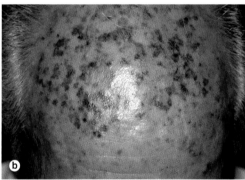

Figure 14-1 a Actinic keratosis. b Pigmented actinic keratosis

face and may be confused with lentigo maligna. *Lichenoid AKs* clinically mimic BCC with their pink, pearly appearance. These occur most frequently on the extremities and upper torso and histologically have a dense band of lymphocytic infiltrate at the papillary dermis. *Proliferative AKs* have ill-defined borders, are often larger than 1 cm, and have higher rates of recurrence following cryotherapy. *Actinic cheilitis* presents on the vermilion border with diffuse dryness or scaling. Because SCC of the lip has a higher rate of metastasis than do SCCs located elsewhere, these lesions must be carefully evaluated and aggressively treated.

Diagnosis

Diagnosis can be made clinically by the experienced observer, but histopathologic evaluation may be needed to rule out SCC.

Differential diagnosis

AKs can mimic SCC, seborrheic keratoses, Bowen's disease, discoid lupus erythematosus, and superficial BCC.

Pathogenesis

Prolonged exposure to UV radiation, especially UVB, causes cumulative damage to keratinocyte DNA. When mutations are not repaired or are repaired with errors, abnormal replication and epidermal cell hyperplasia cause neoplastic growth. AKs are common in Caucasians with fair skin, and those individuals with a history of significant sunlight exposure are at highest risk. It has been shown that AKs may regress with decreased UV exposure and that recent exposure is especially important in the development of new AKs. It is not possible to predict which AKs will regress and which will undergo malignant transformation.

Histological Features

Any thick or indurated AK should be biopsied to rule out SCC. Other poor prognostic signs include large size, ulceration, bleeding, rapid growth, and recurrence following treatment. Biopsy demonstrates partial-thickness dysplasia with atypical keratinocytes limited to the epidermis and an inflammatory response at the dermis. Lesions on the lips should be carefully evaluated and there should be a lower threshold for biopsy because of the increased rate of metastasis compared to nonmucosal SCCs.

Treatment

Treatment of AKs should be considered to prevent progression to SCC. Decreasing sun exposure, wearing protective clothing, and use of sunscreen all help prevent the formation of new AKs, and allows some existing lesions to heal. Treatment can be lesion-directed or field-directed, depending on the number of lesions present. Lesion-directed cryotherapy with liquid nitrogen is the treatment of choice for isolated AKs or for thick, hypertrophic AKs. Lesions can be removed surgically with curettage and electrodesiccation, but scarring may result.

When numerous lesions are present, topical application of 5-fluorouracil (5-FU) (0.5–5%) is effective. 5-FU blocks the enzyme thymidylate synthase and inhibits DNA synthesis. Little reaction occurs on normal skin; however, clinical and subclinical AKs become inflamed, crusted, and eroded. Treatment requires several weeks and may be repeated every 1–2 years in susceptible populations. 5-FU is less effective for treating hypertrophic AKs and another method should be considered for these lesions. Imiquimod, a topical immune response modifier, is also effective in the treatment of AKs. Local reactions to imiquimod tend to be milder than those seen with 5-FU, but prolonged use can cause frank erosions in the area of application.

In patients with extensive photodamage, subclinical AKs should be suspected, and field-directed treatment considered. High-risk patients, including those with xeroderma pigmentosum and chronically immunosuppressed organ transplant recipients, benefit from a combination of oral and topical retinoids for prophylaxis. Long-term use is required, as lesions again develop upon discontinuation of medicine. Other treatments include PDT and skin resurfacing with chemical peels or dermabrasion.

Pharmaceuticals

- 5-FU
- Imiquimod
- Topical diclofenac
- Oral and topical retinoids

Prognosis

Hyperkeratotic AKs respond better when treated or pretreated with cryotherapy. Head-to-head comparisons of the field-directed drugs are not available, but individual drug studies have shown complete clearance in 30–50% of cases (Table 14-1).

Controversies

Although AKs are referred to as "precancerous" lesions in this text, some believe that all AKs are intraepithelial SCCs and should therefore be redefined as true malignant neoplasms. It has been suggested that a grading system be developed to describe the continuum from AK to SCC (KIN system), similar to that of female cervical intraepithelial neoplasia (CIN). However, not all AKs become SCCs and approximately 40% of SCCs develop de novo, making the utility of such a system questionable.

Squamous cell carcinoma in situ (Bowen's disease)

Clinical presentation

Key Points

- Clinically the lesions appear as slow-growing, solitary, sharply demarcated, erythematous plaques with superficial scale; Figure 14-2
- Multiple lesions may be seen
- Although most lesions occur in sun-exposed skin, they may occur in sun-protected areas, such as the penis and the subungual region
- Velvety penile lesions are referred to as erythroplasia of Queyrat

Differential diagnosis

- Inflammatory dermatoses such as eczema, psoriasis, or seborrheic keratosis, as well as Paget's disease and superficial BCC

Pathogenesis

UV light exposure plays a role in lesions associated with actinic damage, but lesions on the penis, anogenital, region or subungual lesions are often associated with human papillomavirus (HPV) infection. Arsenic may act as an initiator/promotor contributing to the development of Bowen's disease.

Histological features

- Full-thickness epidermal atypia with loss of polarity

Keratinocytes may be markedly enlarged and pleomorphic, often with bizarre mitoses, or may simply be crowded with an architecture likened to a "wind-blown" appearance (i.e., the keratinocytes fail to maintain an orderly progression of maturation). Bowen's disease, in contrast to actinic keratoses, often spares the basal layer of the epidermis. The squamous atypia often involves the hair follicle, occasionally sparing eccrine ostia. The overlying stratum corneum shows confluent parakeratosis. Histological variants include clear cell, pagetoid, pigmented, and clonal (Borst–Jadassohn) types.

Treatment

- Topical therapies similar to treatment of AK such as 5-FU (Efudex and Carac), imiquimod (Aldara) and PDT, electrodesiccation and curettage, primary excision, and Mohs micrographic surgery

Prognosis

- Approximately 5–26% of cases ultimately become invasive, and up to 13–33% of these cases develop metastases

Controversies

The association of Bowen's disease with internal malignancies has been a subject of debate for many years. Initially it was claimed that 25% of patients with Bowen's disease occurring in non-actinically damaged skin developed other malignancies; however, subsequent studies have failed to substantiate this finding. However, 42% of patient's with Bowen's disease will develop other premalignant or malignant cutaneous lesions within 7 years of diagnosis.

Table 14-1 Actinic keratoses (AK): treatment methods and outcomes[†]

Name of topical medication or type of destruction	Cryotherapy	Electrodesiccation and curettage	Photodynamic therapy	Chemical or laser peel, or dermabrasion	5-fluorouracil	Imiquimod	Diclofenac	Colchicine (Not available in US)	Retinoids Off label use
Indication	One or a few lesions	One or a few lesions	Multiple AKs, diffuse actinic damage	Multiple AKs, diffuse actinic damage	Multiple AKs, diffuse actinic damage	Multiple AKs, diffuse actinic damage	Multiple AKs, diffuse actinic damage	Multiple AKs, diffuse actinic damage	Multiple AKs, diffuse actinic damage
Mechanism of action	Physical Destruction	Physical Destruction	Aminolevulinic acid (ALA) absorbed by damaged cells and is photoactivated with blue or red light resulting in cell apoptosis	Physical destruction of both the normal and damaged epidermis	Inhibition of thymidylate synthase results in reduced DNA synthesis and cell death	A toll-like receptor agonist that eventuates in increased production of inflammatory cytokines and apoptosis of damaged cells	Inhibits cyclooxygenase and decreases the downstream byproducts of arachidonic acid metabolism	Disrupts tubulin and arrests microtubule formation leading to mitotic arrest	Local antiproliferative and differentiating inducer
Dosing	One or two freeze thaw cycles in a single setting	1–3 cycles of curettage followed by electrodesiccation in a single setting	Topical application of ALA followed 4–14 later by red or blue light in a single setting	Treatment occurs in a single setting	Various Protocols: QD to BID application for 2–4 weeks until ulceration occurs	Various Protocols: 3 to 7 times a week for 4–16 weeks depending on inflammatory response	BID for 8–12 weeks	BID for 10 days	BID for 24 weeks
Side effects	Hypopigmentation Scarring (rare)	Need for anesthesia Hypopigmentation Scarring	Pain Hypopigmentation Scarring (rare)	Need for anesthesia Hypopigmentation Infection Scarring (rare)	Irritation Inflammation Allergic contact dermatitis Ulceration	Irritation Inflammation Ulceration Can worsen psoriasis or eczema, local vitiligo (rare), Flu-like symptoms	Irritation Inflammation Dry skin	Irritation Inflammation Ulceration	Irritation Inflammation
% of patients with complete clearance of lesions*	67–99%	Similar to 5-FU	69–93%	75% reduction in visible lesions	26.3–47.5%	45–82%	33–81%	70–87%	56% complete regression one small study, but most studies show 50–84% reduction in number of lesions

*The approximate clearance rate depends upon the thickness of the AKs and either the freeze-thaw cycle duration, or the duration of the topical therapy and patient compliance with treatment.
BID, twice daily; QD, once daily
[†]Biopsy and histopathological evaluation to rule out squamous cell carcinoma if necessary, especially if thick, indurated lesion or with ulceration, bleeding, large size, rapid growth, or recurrence.

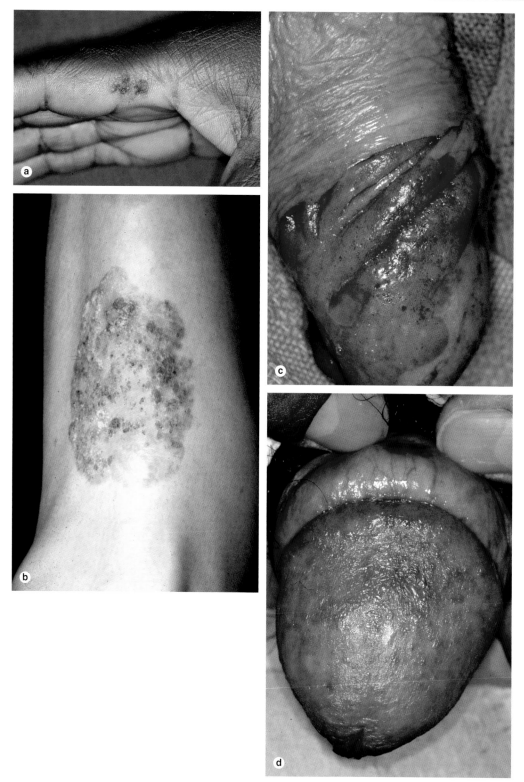

Figure 14-2 a Pigmented Bowen's disease. **b–d** Bowen's disease

Squamous cell carcinoma

Clinical presentation

Key Points

- The lesions typically occur in the same distribution as AKs, but additionally can occur in the anogenital or mucosal regions, subungual areas, within chronic ulcers or scars, at the site of radiation exposure, and on the palms and soles
- Typically presents as a slow-growing erythematous papule, nodule, or plaque that may be smooth, keratotic, eroded, or ulcerated (Figure 14-3)

Differential diagnosis

- Adnexal neoplasms, deep fungal infection amelanotic melanoma

Pathogenesis

Key Points

- UV exposure plays a significant role in the development of SCC. Specifically, UVB causes a signature mutation in the DNA where cytosine is exchanged for thymine. Once this mutation has occurred in the p53 suppressor gene located on chromosome 17p, its regulatory effects on cell growth and proliferation are lost and oncogenesis is possible
- Approximately 90% of SCCs are associated with a mutated p53 suppressor gene
- Additional factors involved in the pathogenesis include exposure to psoralen with ultraviolet A (PUVA), ionizing radiation, arsenic, HPV, and cigarette smoking
- Patients with certain genetic syndromes (epidermodysplasia verruciformis, xeroderma pigmentosa, oculocutaneous albinism, and dystrophic epidermolysis bullosa) as well as

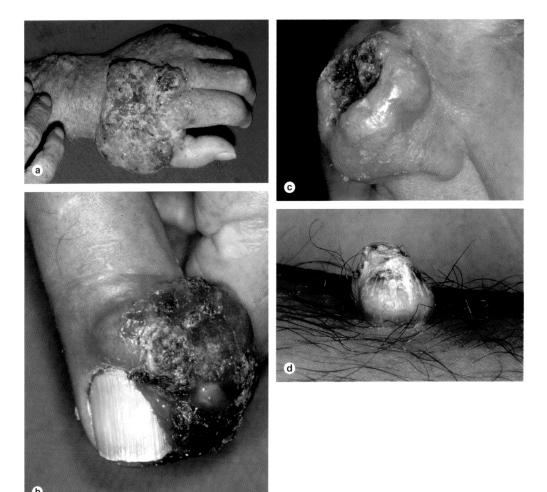

Figure 14-3 a–c Squamous cell carcinoma. d Cutaneous horn with underlying squamous cell carcinoma

immunosuppression, most commonly from organ transplantation, have a higher incidence of developing SCC

Histological features

Conventional SCC arises from the epidermis and consists of a downward proliferation of atypical keratinocytes that irregularly extend into the dermis in an infiltrative fashion. The keratinocytes are enlarged with abundant ground-glass eosinophilic cytoplasm. The nuclei are pleomorphic and hyperchromatic and mitotic figures are frequently encountered. The keratinocytes display individual cell dyskeratosis and form keratin pearls (dyskeratotic keratinocyte that centrally encases anucleated keratin in a concentric fashion). SCCs can be graded based upon the degree of differentiation, Broder's classification, with grade I representing well-differentiated lesions and grade IV being the least differentiated. There are multiple histological variants of SCC, some of which have different clinical presentations as well as prognoses. The most common are Marjolin's ulcer, verrucous carcinoma, and KA and they will be discussed separately.

Treatment

Shallow lesions in low-risk sites can be treated with electrodesiccation and curettage; however, if the fat is breached, excision must be performed with primary excision providing histologic margin assessment, Mohs micrographic surgery, and radiation therapy as a primary treatment or adjuvant therapy in high-risk tumors.

Prognosis

For SCC arising in AK, the recurrence rate if completely excised and metastatic rate are approximately 1–2%. Tumors that have evidence of

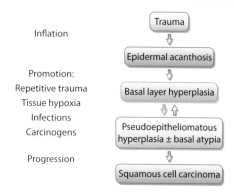

Figure 14-4 Trauma and co-carcinogen theory

perineural invasion have a higher risk of recurrence. Tumors that arise in high-risk locations (lip, ear, genital region), show evidence of vascular invasion, have recurred, are associated with chronic ulcers or scars, or are deeper than 6 mm have a higher metastatic potential (Table 14-2).

Marjolin's Ulcer

Clinical presentation

Key Points

- Presents as a slow-growing exophytic verrucous nodule, can be painful, and is often associated with a mixed infection
- Often arises with burn scars, but can occur in other chronically injured or diseased skin such as sinus tracts associated with osteomyelitis, scars of chronic cutaneous lupus or dystrophic epidermolysis bullosa, and radiation sites
- Affected patients are usually younger than those who develop conventional SCCs
- Tumors are most often located on the extremities
- Rate of malignant transformation of chronically wounded tissues is approximately 0.3–0.7%

Differential diagnosis

- Pseudoepitheliomatous hyperplasia associated with an underlying infection, verrucous carcinoma and keratoacanthoma.

Pathogenesis

Although the exact pathogenesis for malignant transformation is unknown it is hypothesized that repetitive trauma, tissue hypoxia, toxic metabolites and inflammatory mediators that accumulate from chronic infections and/or other carcinogens contribute to unregulated growth, unchecked tumor surveillance, and a persistent growth activated phenotype of the epithelium undergoing regeneration. (Figure 14–4)

Table 14-2 Clinical and histologic features of high-risk squamous cell carcinomas	
Clinical features	**Histologic features**
Size > 2 cm	Depth of invasion > 4 mm
Rapid growth	Breslow level IV or V
Recurrent tumors	Poorly differentiated (Broders 3 or 4)
Immunosuppression, including transplant recipients	Perineural invasion
Genetic abnormalities	Vascular or lymphatic invasion
Etiology: scars, chronic ulceration, radiation	
Anatomic location: ear, lip, mucosa, genitalia	

Histological features

The tumor has the appearance of a well-differentiated SCC, consisting of an atypical proliferation of keratinocytes that extend into the dermis and frequently invades muscle, nerve, and bone. The amount of cytological atypia varies. There is individual cell dyskeratosis, formation of keratin pearls, and frequent mitoses.

Treatment

- Wide excision, sometimes requiring amputation

Prognosis

- Typically more locally aggressive with a higher rate of recurrence (11–50%) and metastasis (20–54%), with the highest rates seen in lesions from the lower extremities

Controversies

The pathogenesis for malignant transformation is controversial, with proposed mechanisms including accumulation of toxic metabolites and inflammatory mediator from chronic infections contributing to unregulated growth, unchecked tumor surveillance, and persistent growth activated phenotype of the epithelium undergoing regeneration.

Verrucous carcinoma (Also known as oral florid papillomatosis, giant condyloma of Buschke and Löwenstein, and carcinoma cuniculatum)

Clinical presentation

- Presents as a slow-growing verrucous fungating mass in the oral, genital, or plantar surface, often with multiple burrow-like openings

Differential diagnosis

- Verrucae, condyloma, and pseudoepitheliomatous hyperplasia (Table 14-3)

Pathogenesis

- Some lesions are associated with HPV infections; others may occur as a result of chronic trauma/maceration or infection, as is seen in scar carcinoma

Histological features

The growth is typically endoexophytic with marked epidermal acanthosis and papillomatosis. There is often overlying hyperkeratosis and parakeratosis which often results in keratin-filled sinus tracks. The base of the lesion is broad with bulbous pushing advancing borders that extend into the deep dermis or subcutaneous tissues. The cytology of the keratinocytes is bland with minimal atypia and few mitoses.

Treatment

- Complete surgical excision

Prognosis

Locally aggressive and deeply invasive, but rarely metastatic except in the case of hybrid tumors, which are verrucous carcinomas that show focal areas that are less differentiated and invasive.

Controversies

Although some studies have suggested that radiation should be avoided due to risk of anaplastic transformation, others have failed to replicate this finding.

Keratoacanthoma

Key Points

- Crateriform neoplasms that grow rapidly
- Often demonstrate explosive growth after biopsy
- Capable of spontaneous involution and often respond to intralesional 5-FU or methotrexate

Clinical presentation

KAs (Figure 14-5) are epithelial neoplasms characterized by rapid growth (4–6 weeks), histologic similarity to conventional SCC, and spontaneous involution. They appear as solitary, round nodules with a central keratotic plug on sun-exposed areas of middle age and older persons, with a peak age of 60 years. They typically occur on hair-bearing skin, but may present anywhere, including mucosal surfaces. The lesion progresses rapidly through three clinical stages: proliferation, maturation, and resolution. The entire process usually occurs within 6 months. Multiple KAs can develop in an autosomal-dominant, inherited familial form (Ferguson–Smith) in which patients acquire lesions in adolescence and early adulthood. Generalized eruptive KAs of Gryzbowski appear as hundreds of keratotic follicular papules occurring all over the body. KAs are also found along with other visceral malignancies in the autosomal-dominant Muir–Torre syndrome, which is associated with a defect in a mismatch DNA repair gene.

Diagnosis

- KA morphology and growth pattern are distinctive

Table 14.3 Clinical and histopathological features of well-differentiated squamous cell carcinomas as compared to pseudoepitheliomatous hyperplasia

	Pseudoepitheliomatous hyperplasia	Keratoacanthoma	Verrucous carcinoma	Scar carcimoma
Clinical features				
Solitary, fungating lesion	Usually a solitary plaque, but can be multiple sites	Usually solitary with rapid onset but can be multiple	Solitary, slowly enlarging	Solitary, can be ulcerative or exophytic
Location	Various	Solitary lesions in actinically exposed; multiple anywhere	Oral, genital, plantar foot	Extremities most common
Concurrent dermal inflammation	Mixed inflammatory cells, often with associated fungi, bacteria or viruses	Mixed infiltrate with increased number of eosinophils	Mixed inflammation, can be associated with HPV infection	Yes; mixed ± associated infection
Pain	Depends on etiology	Occasionally	Yes	Yes
Enlargement of lymph nodes	Yes: reactive nodes	Usually not	Yes, but more often reactive	Yes, often metastasis
Histological features				
Endophytic proliferation of squamous cells	Irregular acanthosis mostly adnexal	Exoendophytic cratiform, follicular centered	Exoendoendophytic with pushing bulbous margins	Often endophytic with infiltrative margins
Epidermal projections extend into lower dermis	No	Not beyond level of sweat glands	Yes	Yes
Extend into lower dermis				
Disruption of basement membrane	No	Occasionally, focally disrupted	Occasionally, focally disrupted	Yes, but may occur only focally
Cytologic atypia	No	Slight	Minimal	Varies
Mitosis	Few superficial	Yes, mostly superficial	Few superficial	Yes
Atypical mitosis	No	Few	No	Yes
Dyskeratosis	No	Varies, superficial	No	Yes
Individual cell necrosis	No	No	No	Varies
Squamous eddies	Yes	Varies	Varies	Varies
Keratin pearls	No	Varies	No	Yes
Invasion of bone or muscle	No	Yes, especially subungual	Varies	Varies
Perineural invasion	No	Varies	Varies	Varies
Metastases	No	Rare	None, but up to 10% in hybrid tumors	20–54%
Recurrence	None: withdrawal of stimuli	Up to 8%	18–50%	11–50%

HPV, human papillomavirus.

- Crateriform lesion with glassy atypia, elastic trapping, neutrophil microabscesses, and eosinophils in stroma. Acantholysis is absent

Differential diagnosis

A KA may be impossible to differentiate from SCC, even by histopathologic evaluation. The diagnosis is based more on architectural features than on cytologic changes. KA is favored by the presence of a symmetrical lesion with a central keratin core and lack of acantholysis. Common warts and molluscum contagiosum are also in the clinical differential.

Laboratory testing

Biopsy to rule out SCC may be necessary; however, even with histopathological evaluation, it is difficult to differentiate between the two. KAs demonstrate well-differentiated squamous epithelium with only mild pleomorphism.

Pathogenesis

Wart viruses, UV radiation, and chemical carcinogens have been implicated in the development of KAs. HPV has been identified in lesions by polymerase chain reaction in several studies; however, others have failed to find a link. Genetic factors and immunosuppression also play a role. Regression is thought to be mediated by the immune system.

Treatment

Because KAs may cause significant inflammation, growth, and tissue destruction, observation is generally not recommended despite their tendency to involute spontaneously. Prompt surgical excision is recommended for a solitary KA when possible (Table 14-4). Partial shave biopsy does not allow for definitive diagnosis, but smaller lesions may be treated with deep excisional shave and curettage. Cryosurgery can be successful, especially with small, early lesions. Partial punch biopsies should be avoided because evaluation of the entire tumor is necessary; punch excisions are acceptable. Excision with adequate margins and histopathological evaluation is often the treatment of choice. KAs are radiosensitive and low-dose radiotherapy may be used to treat large or anatomically difficult-to-remove lesions. Medical treatment is reserved for cases in which surgical intervention is not possible, including lesions that are large in size and present in a difficult location, or in patients with comorbidities that make surgery undesirable. Systemic retinoids with close follow-up may be used in these cases or in patients with multiple familial or generalized eruptive forms. Intralesional chemotherapy with 5-FU or methotrexate or topical imiquimod and 5-FU have been used with success. If a patient has a family history significant for KAs and/or visceral malignancies, Muir–Torre syndrome should be considered.

Lesions recur 4–8% of the time after surgical excision. Data comparing the effectiveness of cryosurgery, intralesional chemotherapy, and oral retinoids are not available. However, all have been reported to have good success rates.

Controversies

Although some consider KAs to be a benign cutaneous tumor, others consider them to be a variant of SCC ("well-differentiated SCC with KA features"); some even suggest renaming them "keratocarcinomas."

Basal cell carcinoma

Clinical presentation

Key Points

* Often presents as a pearly erythematous papule with a rolled border on the head and neck region (Figure 14-6)

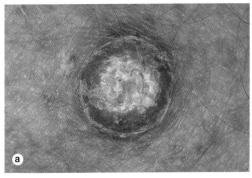

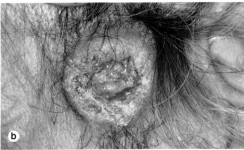

Figure 14-5 a Early keratoacanthoma. **b** Later stage keratoacanthoma

Table 14-4 Keratoacanthoma (KA)				
Surgical candidate		**Medical treatment (not a surgical candidate due to comorbidities, location, large size, or choice)**		
Solitary	**Multiple**	Radiotherapy (difficult to treat locations or large size)	Intralesional or topical 5-fluorouracil (intralesional bleomycin, methotrexate, and interferon-α_{2a} are other options)	Imiquimoid (Aldara) 5% cream Every other day 4–12 weeks
1. Cryosurgery for early, small KAs	1. Cryosurgery for early, small KAs			
2. Shave excision with curettage of the base	2. Surgical excision with pathologic evaluation			
3. For larger lesions, surgical excision	3. Systemic retinoids and close follow-up ± cryosurgery			

- Typically they arise in the elderly; however, they can be seen in younger patients who have extensive sun damage
- Long-standing lesions are often large, locally destructive, and ulcerated, thus the term "rodent ulcer." They may also be pigmented
- Multiple BCCs occur in nevoid BCC syndrome, as well as in Bazex and Rombo syndromes
- Although BCCs were commonly thought to arise in nevus sebaceus, many of these lesions have been reclassified as trichoblastomas

Differential diagnosis

- SCC, AK, sebaceous hyperplasia, seborrheic keratosis, and amelanotic melanoma

Pathogenesis

Key Points

- The pathogenesis is multifactorial, with various environmental (UV and ionizing radiation) and genetic factors playing important roles
- Both in nevoid BCC syndrome and in sporadic BCCs, it has been shown that there are often mutations in the *Patched (PTCH-1)* gene on chromosome 9q22.3 and/or dysregulation of the hedgehog signaling pathway
- Mutations in p53 can also occur

Histological features

As with SCC, there are many histological variants, including nodular, superficial, keratotic, pigmented, fibroepithelioma of Pinkus, micronodular, morpheaform, infiltrative, and metatypical BCCs. The last four variants have a higher risk of recurrence. The most frequent type is the nodular BCC. It is composed of small hyperchromatic cells with scant cytoplasm, which form cords or islands within the dermis and focally connect to the overlying epidermis. Characteristically there is peripheral palisading of the nuclei with retraction of the stroma from the tumor. Mucin can be found within the stromal cleft or within the tumor itself. These findings are less evident in morpheaform, infiltrative, basosquamous, and metatypical variants.

Treatment

Key Points

- Superficial lesions can be treated with topical 5-FU, imiquimod, PDT, excision, or electrodesiccation and curettage (Table 14-5)
- Larger lesions, recurrent lesions, and high-risk lesions should be treated with excision or Mohs micrographic surgery
- Radiation is an alternative treatment for patients unable or unwilling to have surgery, but should be avoided in patients with nevoid BCC syndrome

Prognosis

Approximately 0.1% of BCC metastasize; lesions most often are large, deep, or high-risk (recurrent, micronodular, morpheaform, infiltrative, and metatypical)

Melanoma

Clinical presentation

Key Points

- Typically presents as an enlarging, irregularly pigmented macule, papule, or plaque that is asymmetric with irregular borders (Figure 14-7)
- Nodular melanoma presents as an enlarging pigmented nodule that is more uniform in shape and color, but is often ulcerated
- Amelanotic melanomas are not pigmented and often present as an erythematous nodule or ill-defined plaque
- In adult females, melanomas most commonly arise on the lower extremities, whereas the torso is a more common site for males
- The lifetime risk of melanoma in the United States has risen from 1/1500 in 1930 to 1/63 in 2007
- In 2007, melanoma was the second most common cancer in young Americans aged 15–29

Differential diagnosis

- Melanocytic nevus, recurrent nevus (Figure 14-8) seborrheic keratosis, pigmented basal cell or SCC, amalgam tattoo (Figure 14-9)

Pathogenesis

Key Points

- The etiology of familial melanoma is heterogeneous and complex
- The major genes identified in the pathogenesis include the *CDKN2A* (p16) gene on chromosome 9, the *CDK4* gene on chromosome 12, and a gene on chromosome 1
- Factors that increase a person's risk for developing melanoma include a family history of melanoma (one or more first-degree relatives), having more than 50 typical nevi or having increased numbers of atypical nevi, and having a prior personal history of melanoma
- In addition, patients who are fair (type I/II skin, freckles, light blond or red hair and blue or green eyes), have a history of intermittent high-intensity sun exposure with sunburns, or are immunosuppressed are also at greater risk of developing a melanoma

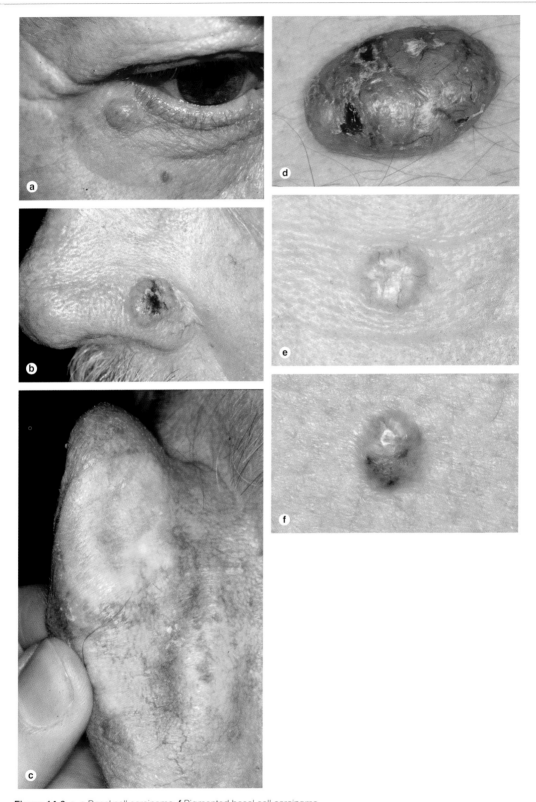

Figure 14-6 a–e Basal cell carcinoma. f Pigmented basal cell carcinoma

Table 14-5 Treatments available for nonmelanoma skin cancers

Type of treatment	Dosage and/or procedure	Indications
Cryotherapy	Freeze times varies	Actinic keratosis; thermocouples required to treat superficial malignancies optimally
Radiation	Varies	Bowen's disease, BCC, SCC, KA
Photodynamic therapy	Blue light for AKs Red light for superficial NMSC	AKs, Bowen's disease, superficial BCC
Skin resurfacing	Carbon dioxide laser	Actinic cheilitis, ± for extensive AKs
Topical 5-fluorouracil	bid for 2–4 weeks	AKs and actinic cheilitis
	bid for 9 weeks	Bowen's
Efudex 5% or	bid for 3–8 weeks	KA
Fluoroplex 1%	bid for 3–6 weeks	Superficial BCC
Carac 0.5%	qd for 1–4 weeks	AK
Topical 3% diclofenac	bid for 60–90 days	AKs
Imiquimod	2 times/week for 16 weeks	AKs
	5 times/week for 6 weeks	Superficial BCC maximum size 2cm
Interferon α (off-label use)	IL: 1.5 MU tiw for 3 weeks	Nonaggressive BCC
	SC: 3 MU/m^2 tiw for 12 months	Advanced head and neck SCC
	IL: 3 MU weeks for 4–6 weeks	KA
Electrodesiccation and curettage	Typically 2–3 successive cycles are employed	Superficial and nodular BCC, Bowen's, superficial SCC
Excisional surgery	Margins are usually 3–5 mm, but up to 2 cm in high-risk tumors, around the clinically apparent tumor. Delayed histological confirmation of margins	BCC, Bowen's, SCC
Mohs micrographic surgery	Removal of the tumor with minimal loss of normal tissue	High-risk BCC or SCC (central face, lip, ear, recurrent lesions and aggressive histologic variants)
	Immediate histological confirmation of margins	

BCC, basal cell carcinoma; SCC, squamous cell carcinoma; KA, keratoacanthoma; AK, actinic keratoses; NMSC, nonmelanoma skin cancer; bid, twice a day; qd, once a day; IL, intralesional; tiw, three times a week; SC, subcutaneous.

Histological features

There are four major histological variants of primary melanoma: superficial spreading, nodular, lentigo maligna melanoma, and acral lentiginous melanoma. Less common variants include desmoplastic or spindle cell melanoma, small cell melanoma, nevoid melanoma, "spitzoid" melanoma, clear cell sarcoma, animal-type melanoma, and malignant blue nevus. The overall silhouette is similar in all histological variants in that the melanocytic proliferation is asymmetric and shows poor lateral circumscription. Cytologically the melanocytes are atypical; the nests are unequal in size, shape, and spacing and are often confluent. Melanocytes arranged as solitary units often predominate over nests and the melanocytes within the nests are not cohesive. The melanocytes within the dermis show no evidence of maturation with progressive descent and melanocytes can be found above the dermal–epidermal junction and extending down adnexa. Immunohistochemical stains expressed by most melanomas include S100 (most sensitive), Mart-1/MelanA (most specific), HMB-45, tyrosinase, and microphthalmia-associated transcription factor (MITF). Desmoplastic melanoma often only stains with vimentin and S-100, but up to 95% of cases have been shown to stain with neuron-specific enolase (NSE).

Melanomas are staged based upon Breslow thickness and Clark's level of invasion, the presence of ulceration, nodal status, and presence of metastases (Table 14-6).

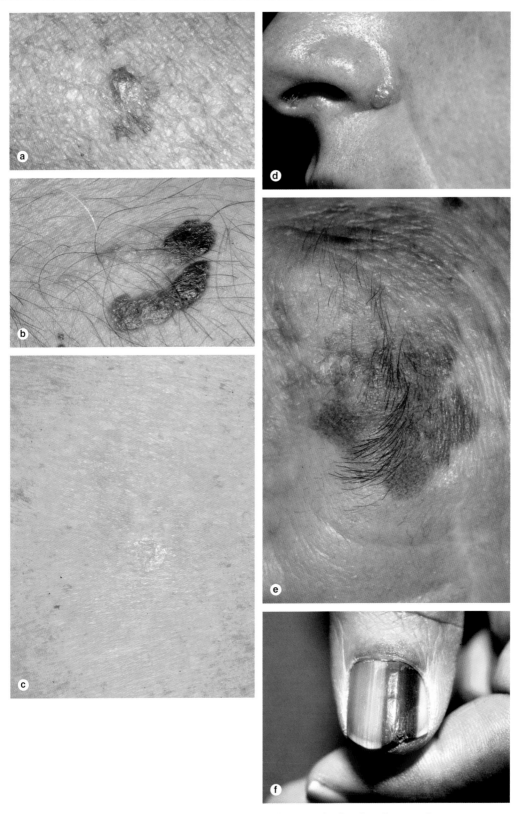

Figure 14-7 a Malignant melanoma with nodule. **b** Malignant melanoma. **c** Amelanotic malignant melanoma.
d Amelanotic malignant melanoma (courtesy of James Keeling MD). **e** Lentigo maligna. **f** Malignant melanoma nail.

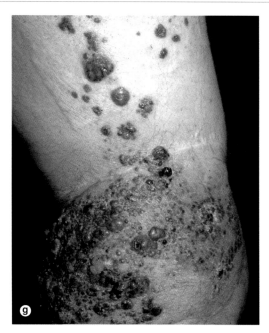

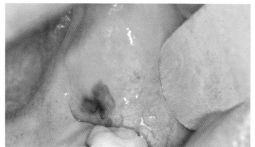

Figure 14-9 Amalgam tattoo (courtesy of Wilford Hall Medical Center teaching file)

Prognosis

The depth of the melanoma, nodal involvement, and the presence of metastases are the most important factors in determining prognosis (Table 14-8).

Controversies

The treatment of metastatic melanoma remains poor. Melanoma fails to respond to most traditional chemotherapies. The use of adjunct therapies, primarily interferon-alpha, remains controversial, as its benefit has been primarily shown to be a small increase in relapse-free survival. Its effect on overall survival remains unclear.

The influence of pregnancy, hormones, and oral contraceptives on melanoma remains controversial. Although early case reports suggested that pregnancy confers a grave prognosis on gravid women diagnosed with melanoma, controlled studies have since shown no adverse effect on survival. Similarly, hormones, including oral contraceptives, have not been proved to affect the outcome of women with melanoma adversely. It is no longer recommended that a woman delay childbearing because of a recent melanoma; however, if the melanoma is high-risk, it may be prudent to delay pregnancy for several years, during which recurrences are most likely to occur. Suspicious pigmented lesions in pregnant women should be biopsied without delay.

The roles of sunscreen in the prevention of melanoma and that of intentional tanning in the etiology of melanoma remain unclear.

Figure 14-7, cont'd g Metastatic malignant melanoma (courtesy of Brooke Army Medical Center teaching file)

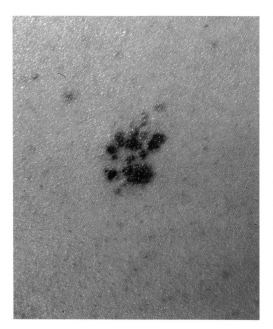

Figure 14-8 Recurrent nevus

Merkel cell carcinoma

Clinical presentation

Key Points

- Most commonly arises in older Caucasian males in sun-damaged skin on the head and neck or upper extremities

Treatment

Excision is the treatment of choice, with surgical margins dependent upon the depth of the tumor (Table 14-7). Sentinel node biopsy is often recommended for intermediate-thickness tumors between 1 and 4 mm in depth.

Table 14-6 Melanoma tumor, metastasis, node (TMN) classification

T classification	Breslow thickness (mm)	Clark's levels and/or presence of ulceration
T1	< 1.0	a: Without ulceration and Clark level II–III
		b: With ulceration or Clark's level IV–V
T2	1.01–2.0	a: Without ulceration
		b: With ulceration
T3	2.01–4.0	a: Without ulceration
		b: With ulceration
T4	> 4.0	a: Without ulceration
		b: With ulceration
N classification	**Number of involved lymph nodes**	**Presence of macroscopic (clinically detectable nodes) or microscopic (histologically identified) positive nodes**
N1	1 node	a: Micrometastasis
		b: Macrometastasis
N2	2–3 nodes	a: Micrometastasis
		b: Macrometastasis
		c: In-transit metastasis or satellite nodes without nodal metastasis
N3	4 or more, or matted nodes, or in-transit metastasis or satellite nodes with nodal metastasis	
M classification	**Site of metastases**	**Serum lactate dehydrogenase**
M1a	Distant skin, subcutaneous or nodal metastases	Normal
M1b	Lung metastases	Normal
M1c	All other visceral metastases	Elevated

Table 14-7 Surgical margins for melanoma based upon Breslow depth

Breslow level	Excision margins
In situ	0.5 cm
< 1 mm	1.0 cm
1–4 mm	2.0 cm
> 4 mm	2.0–3.0 cm

- Presents as a rapidly growing red to violaceous nodule, typically nonulcerated

Differential diagnosis

- Adnexal tumors, SCC, amelanotic melanoma, and cutaneous metastases

Pathogenesis

Since the tumor arises in actinically damaged sites, UV exposure appears to play a role in the tumor's pathogenesis. The ontogeny is not completely understood; however, the tumor is hypothesized to arise from adnexal Merkel cells.

Histological features

Typically a dermal-based tumor composed of small blue cells that exhibit a high nuclear to cytoplasmic ratio. The nuclei are ovoid with dispersed chromatin that characteristically has a "salt-and-pepper" appearance. Throughout the tumor there are often numerous mitoses and focal areas of necrosis. Rare cases show pagetoid extension or are completely intraepidermal. The tumor displays several histological growth patterns, with the most characteristic being the trabecular type with a ribbon-like configuration; however, this pattern is uncommon. The other two patterns, nodular and diffuse, occur more frequently. Immunohistochemical stains show evidence of both neuroendocrine and epithelial differentiation. The tumor stains positively with neural cell adhesion molecule (NCAM), NSE, synaptophysin, and neurofilament, as well as showing a distinctive paranuclear dot or crescentic pattern

Table 14-8 Melanoma staging and estimated 5 year survival

Stage	Survival	Tumor	Node	Metastases
0	100%	Tis	N0	M0
1A	95%	T1a	N0	M0
1B	90%	T1b	N0	M0
		T2a		
IIA	78%	T2b	N0	M0
		T3a		
IIB	65%	T3b	N0	M0
		T4a		
IIC	45%	T4b	N0	M0
IIIA	66%	T1-4a	N1a or 2a	M0
IIIB	52%	T1-4b	N1a or N2a	M0
		T1-4a	N1b or N2b	
		T1-4b	N2c	
IIIC	26%	T1-4b	N1b or N2b	M0
		Any T	N3	
IV	7.5–11%	Any T	Any N	Any M

with epithelial membrane antigen (EMA), CAM 5.2, and most characteristically with CK20 (Table 14-9). Merkel cell carcinoma is negative for thyroid transcription factor-1 (TTF-1) and often for CK7, which characteristically stains small cell carcinoma of the lung, one of the main tumors in the histological differential diagnosis.

Treatment

Either wide excision with 3-cm margins or Mohs micrographic surgery is the preferred treatment. Since there is a high rate of metastases to the regional lymph nodes, sentinel node biopsy has been advocated by some. Adjunctive radiation and chemotherapy have also been suggested, especially for patients with metastatic disease.

Prognosis

This is a highly aggressive malignancy with a high rate of local recurrence and metastasis. Survival at 1, 2, and 3 years respectively is approximately 82%, 72%, and 55%. Indicators of poor prognosis include tumor size greater than 5 mm, invasion into the subcutaneous fat, diffuse growth pattern, small cell size, increased mitotic activity, and a heavy lymphocytic infiltrate.

Controversies

Since the tumor is relatively uncommon, a standard approach to treatment has not been established; sentinel node biopsy and adjuvant therapy are debatable at this time.

SPINDLE CELL TUMORS

Dermatofibrosarcoma Protuberans (DFSP)

Clinical presentation

Key Points

- Nodular or micronodular violaceous to reddish-brown indurated plaque with superimposed nodules that slowly enlarge
- Primarily located on the trunk and proximal extremities of 20–40-year-olds

Differential diagnosis

- Keloid, dermatofibroma, and other soft-tissue neoplasms

Pathogenesis

Molecular studies show that the lesion is associated with a reciprocal translocation and a supernumerary ring involving chromosome 17 and 22. The translocation results in fusion of the two genes COL1A1 and PDGF-beta, which are responsible for the formation of collagen I and platelet-derived growth factor.

Histological features

This is a dermal-based tumor consisting of a monomorphous proliferation of slender spindle cells arranged in long fascicles, often arranged in a "storiform" or "cartwheel" pattern. The cells show

Table 14-9 Immunohistochemical staining pattern of various tumors composed of small round blue cells

	CK20	CK7	CD99	NSE	NFP	EMA	TTF-1	LCA	S100	BER-EP4
MCC	+	−	±	+	+	+	−	−	−	+
Small cell lung	Rare	+	±	+	±	+	+	−	−	−
Small cell amelanotic melanoma	−	−	−	+	−	−	−	−	+	−
Lymphoma/leukemia	−	−	±	−	−	±	−	+	−	−
Ewing's/PNET	−	−	+	+	±	±	−	−	±	−
Carcinoid	+	±	±	+		±	±	−	−	−
BCC	−	±	−	−	−	−	−	−	−	+

NSE, neuron-specific enolase; NFP, neurofilament protein; EMA, epithelial membrane antigen; TTF, thyroid transcription factor-1; LCA, lymphocyte common antigen; BER-EP4, antihuman epithelial antigen; MCC, Merkel cell carcinoma; PNET, primitive neuroectodermal tumor; BCC, basal cell carcinoma.

minimal atypia and there are rare mitotic figures. The tumor extends into and infiltrates the subcutaneous fat in a "honeycomb" pattern. Variants include a pigmented form referred to as Bednar tumor, myxoid, atrophic, sclerosing, and palisaded forms. The cells diffusely stain with CD34.

Treatment

Treatment involves wide excision or Mohs micrographic surgery. Gleevec (imatinib mesylate) is currently in therapeutic trials and is being investigated for use in metastatic disease.

Prognosis

DFSP is an intermediate malignancy that is primarily locally aggressive with a propensity to recur if incompletely excised. Recurrence and incomplete excision are associated with transformation to a fibrosarcoma; this later finding is associated with a greater likelihood for metastases, primarily to the lungs.

Giant cell fibroblastoma

Clinical presentation

Key Points

- A rare tumor that typically presents in early childhood
- Clinically presents as a flesh-colored slow-growing dermal or subcutaneous nodule involving the neck, trunk, or groin

Differential diagnosis

- Cystic hygroma, lipoma, or other soft-tissue neoplasm

Pathogenesis

- Similar to DFSP, associated with a translocation of chromosome 17 and 22

Histological features

Giant cell fibroblastoma is composed of a diffuse sheet of infiltrative spindle cells admixed with multinucleated giant cells within a slightly myxoid stroma. Irregular pseudovascular spaces lined by multinucleated giant cells can be seen throughout the tumor. Immunohistochemical stains show diffuse staining with CD34.

Treatment

- Wide excision or Mohs micrographic surgery

Prognosis

- Local recurrence if incompletely excised

Fibrosarcoma

Clinical presentation

Key Points

- Usually occurs as a slow-growing, occasionally painful subcutaneous mass
- Primarily seen in young to middle-aged adults on the lower extremities, followed by the upper extremities, trunk, and head and neck region
- Represents 1–3% of all adult sarcomas

Differential diagnosis

- Nodular fasciitis and other soft-tissue neoplasms

Pathogenesis

- Currently the pathogenesis is unknown. There is, however, a higher incidence of fibrosarcomas occurring in old burn scars or sites of prior radiation

Histological features

The tumor arises deep to the subcutaneous tissue, but may extend upward and involve the dermis. The tumor is composed of a proliferation of atypical spindle cells arranged as sweeping/intersecting fascicles, creating a "herringbone" pattern; storiform areas may also be seen. The spindle cells have hyperchromatic pleomorphic nuclei with variably prominent nucleoli and scant cytoplasm. Mitotic figures are usually abundant. Immunohistochemical stains are nonspecific and often the tumor primarily stains with vimentin and very focally with smooth-muscle actin. Those arising in a DFSP will have focal areas that are positive for CD34.

Treatment

* Wide excision, which may include amputation. Adjuvant radiation or chemotherapy should be considered in high-grade lesions or in patients with metastatic disease

Prognosis

Behavior is related to tumor grade, size, and depth. The rate of recurrence varies from 12% to 79%, depending upon whether the primary surgical margins were involved. When metastases occur they are usually to the lungs and axial skeleton and rarely to the lymph nodes. Metastasis occurs in 9–63% of patients. The overall 5-year survival is 49–54%.

Atypical fibroxanthoma (AFX)

Clinical presentation

Key Points

* Typically presents in elderly individuals as a solitary rapidly growing ulcerative nodule on actinically damaged skin of the head and neck region
* There is a rare variant that presents in younger patients on the trunk and extremities unrelated to actinic damage

Differential diagnosis

* Chondrodermatitis nodularis helicis, SCC, BCC, amelanotic melanoma, Merkel cell carcinoma, and cutaneous metastases

Pathogenesis

* There is evidence that UV damage plays a role in the tumor's pathogenesis

Histological features

Dome-shaped expansile nodule that centrally has either an attenuated or ulcerated epidermis, and laterally exhibits an epidermal collarette.

Classically within the dermis there is a pleomorphic proliferation of atypical spindle cells in addition to large, markedly atypical, often multinucleated cells associated with extensive solar elastosis. Normal as well as atypical mitotic figures are readily apparent. Histological variants include spindle cell nonpleomorphic AFX, clear cell, osteoclastic, chondroid, granular, and pigmented. If deep invasion, necrosis, vascular, or neural invasion is encountered, the diagnosis of AFX should be called into question. The tumor has nonspecific immunohistochemical staining, and often a diagnosis is made via exclusion of other tumors with a similar histological appearance. Vimentin is diffusely positive in most cases, with a few cases showing focal staining with smooth-muscle actin. The utility of CD99, CD10, and procollagen is still being investigated. The histiocyte-like multinucleated cells can show positive staining with CD68 and/or α1-antichymotrypsin.

Treatment

* Excision

Prognosis

This is a low-grade sarcoma that has a low rate of recurrence if completely excised. Metastases are rare.

Controversies

The histogenesis of this tumor is controversial and there has been debate as to the relationship with a similar-appearing tumor, malignant fibrous histiocytoma (MFH), which occurs in the deeper soft tissues (Table 14-10).

Pleomorphic malignant fibrous histiocytoma

Clinical presentation

Key points

* Typically presents in patients over 40, with a peak incidence in the seventh decade
* Most often arises on the proximal extremities, especially the lower limb
* Typically presents as a large deep-seated tumor which shows progressive and often rapid enlargement; may be painful
* Approximately 5% have metastasis at presentation, most commonly the lung

Differential diagnosis

* Liposarcomas, leiomyosarcomas, and other soft-tissue neoplasms, and nodular fasciitis

Pathogenesis

* Unknown

Table 14-10 Malignant dermal spindle cell tumors

Type of tumor	Age of patient (years)	Location and clinical presentation	Associated findings	Characteristic immunohistochemical stains
Dermatofibrosarcoma protuberans (DFSP)	30–40	Trunk, proximal extremities	t(17;22)	CD34
Giant cell fibroblastoma	Less than 20	Neck, trunk, and groin	t(17;22)	CD34
Fibrosarcoma	30–50	Upper extremity, trunk, head and neck	Prior field of irradiation	Vimentin
Atypical fibroxanthoma (AFX)	40–60	Head and neck	Extensive actinic damage	Vimentin, CD68, CD99, CD10
Malignant fibrous histiocytoma	50–70	Proximal extremities		Vimentin, CD74
Epithelioid sarcoma	10–40	Distal extremities	History of trauma in 20% of cases	CK, EMA, vimentin
Malignant peripheral nerve sheath tumor	30–60	Trunk or extremities	50% found in patient with neurofibromatosis	S100
Kaposi's sarcoma	20–60	Lower extremities, can also be more widely distributed with mucosal involvement	All four clinical variants + HHV8, associated with HLA-DR5	CD31, Podoplanin (D2-40), VEGF-3, VEGFR-3, HHV-8
Angiosarcoma	Over 60	Scalp, chest, abdominal wall, arm	Radiation, lymphedema	CD34, CD31, FLI-1, thrombomodulin

HHV, human herpesvirus; HLA, human leukocyte antigen; EMA, epithelial membrane antigen; VEGF, vascular endothelial growth factor; VEGFR, vascular endothelial growth factor receptor; FLI-1, friend leukemia integration-1.

Histological features

This is typically a diagnosis of exclusion. Histologically the tumors are heterogeneous in appearance, but often resemble an AFX, except for the fact that it arises in the deep soft tissues with occasional extension to the subcutis and dermis. The tumor is often associated with chronic inflammatory cells and focal areas of necrosis, and shows evidence of vascular or neural invasion. Several histological variants have been described: pleomorphic, angiomatoid, myxoid, giant cell, and inflammatory. Immunohistochemical stains are noncontributory. The tumor stains with vimentin and some may show focal staining with CD34, desmin, CD99, and CD74. Although CD68, alpha-antitrypsin, and antichymotrypsin may be positive, it is now accepted that histocytic antigens play no useful role in diagnosis.

Treatment

- Excision

Prognosis

It has been called a high-grade sarcoma with a 5-year survival rate of 50–60%; however, with high-grade myxofibrosarcomas (MFS), the survival rate may be closer to 20%.

Controversies

With the advent of immunohistochemical stains and molecular studies, MFH has currently fallen out of favor as a distinct diagnostic entity, and tumors once diagnosed as MFH have now been shown to be leiomyosarcomas, liposarcomas, MFSs, and malignant peripheral nerve sheath tumors.

Myxofibrosarcoma

Clinical presentation

Key Points

- The most common soft-tissue sarcoma of the elderly
- The tumor shows predilection for the limbs and limb girdle
- Presents as a deep enlarging soft-tissue mass

Differential diagnosis

- Liposarcoma, fibrosarcoma, and metastases

Pathogenesis

- Unknown

Histological features

Characterized by a multinodular, infiltrative proliferation composed of alternating hypercellular and myxoid hypocellular areas. Within the myxoid areas there are spindle and occasionally epithelioid cells, either as single cells or small clusters, intermixed with atypical cells with bubbly cytoplasm reminiscent of lipoblasts. In addition prominent curvilinear vessels are seen. Within the hypercellular areas, there are diffuse sheets of cells with a similar appearance to those in the myxoid, admixed with scattered multinucleated cells. The number of mitoses and degree of necrosis are variable. The tumor has an unremarkable immunohistochemical profile and displays only rare focal staining with pankeratin, desmin, and smooth-muscle actin.

Treatment

- Wide excision with 2-cm surgical margins. Adjuvant radiation therapy can be used in cases with incomplete excision

Prognosis

It has a high risk of developing local recurrence (50–72%) and gives rise to distal metastases to the lung or retroperitoneum in 20–50% of cases. Local recurrence and metastasis appear to be related to the depth and histological grade of the primary tumor.

Controversies

- Previously classified under the rubric of MFH, it is now defined as a distinct tumor

Epithelioid Sarcoma

Clinical presentation

Key Points

- This is a rare tumor that occurs in 10–40-year-old individuals
- Males are more frequently affected 2:1
- The tumor is often initially misdiagnosed as deep granuloma annulare
- Presents as a slow-growing, firm subcutaneous nodule or nodules on the distal extremities, most commonly the flexor surface of the hands and fingers
- Rare variant occurs proximally in the pelvis, perineum,or genital tract. These are typically seen in older adults and are associated with a more aggressive course

Differential diagnosis

- Giant cell tumor of the tendon sheath, rheumatoid nodule, subcutaneous granuloma annulare, and ganglion cyst

Pathogenesis

- A history of trauma is associated with 20% of cases

Histological features

This is a deep subcutaneous tumor, often associated with fascia, tendons, and periosteum. The tumor can be mono- or biphasic, composed of spindle and epithelioid cells. Characteristically the tumor is composed of one or multiple nodules that exhibit central necrosis, surrounded by a palisade of spindle cells and/or round to polygonal cells that have an epithelioid appearance (increased eosinophilic cytoplasm with small uniform nuclei), intermixed with a mixed inflammatory cell infiltrate. Perineural and perivascular infiltration are commonly seen. Immunohistochemical stains are helpful since the tumor uniquely stains with both cytokeratin and vimentin as well as with EMA.

Treatment

Since the tumor is often multifocal and infiltrates deep structures, surgical excision often leads to amputation; however, more recently more conservative surgery with adjuvant radiation has been attempted.

Prognosis

The tumor exhibits frequent recurrences (34–77%) and 40% of cases metastasize, most commonly to the lung, regional lymph nodes, scalp, bone, and brain. Metastases may have a delayed presentation. The 5-year survival rate ranges from 50% to 80%.

Malignant peripheral nerve sheath tumor (Also known as malignant schwannoma, neurosarcoma, or neurofibrosarcoma)

Clinical presentation

Key Points

- Accounts for 2% of all nerve sheath tumors
- Most often seen in the setting of von Recklinghausen's disease (neurofibromatosis); however, sporadic de novo cases also occur
- The lesions usually arise on the trunk or proximal extremities of young to middle aged adults
- Presents as a rapidly expanding mass that can be painful or associated with paresthesia

Differential diagnosis

- Plexiform neurofibroma and other soft-tissue malignancies

Pathogenesis

The tumor typically arises from malignant degeneration of a plexiform neurofibroma with an incidence ranging from 1% to 13%.

Histological features

The histological appearance is variable, but most cases are composed of pleomorphic spindle cells with alternating areas of cellularity. The spindle cells can intersect at acute angles and recapitulate a "herringbone" appearance. The spindle cells are often associated with a myxoid stroma, and nuclear atypia and mitotic figures are variable. The lesion entraps cutaneous appendages rather than destroying them. Tumors that have foci of rhabdomyosarcomatous elements are referred to as malignant Triton tumors. The immunohistochemical staining pattern shows that 50% of cases show reactivity with S-100, 33% with CD57, and 15–20% with myelin basic protein.

Treatment

• Wide excision

Prognosis

Superficial tumors more often recur (80% of cases) then metastasize (20%), but deep tumors have an increased metastatic rate. The mean survival is 2–3 years.

Kaposi's Sarcoma (KS)

Key Points

Clinical presentation

There are four clinical settings in which the tumor is known to occur.
• Classic KS (Figure 14-10) predominantly affects elderly Jewish men of Middle Eastern or Mediterranean descent as multiple red-brown plaques or papules on the distal lower extremities. The lesions may be associated with lymphedema
• African KS is restricted to young adults or children from Africa and presents as nodular lesions that rapidly progress to involve lymph nodes and internal organs
• Transplant-associated KS (iatrogenic immunosuppression) has overlapping features of classic and African KS
• Acquired immunodeficiency syndrome (AIDS)-related KS primarily occurs in homosexual males as ill-defined reddish-brown macules or patches that can affect any cutaneous or mucosal surface. Visceral involvement may also occur

Differential diagnosis

• Lymphangiomas, angiokeratomas

Pathogenesis

Regardless of the clinical setting, all forms of KS are associated with human herpesvirus-8 (HHV-8); however it is felt that a co-infecting virus such as cytomegalovirus, human immunodeficiency virus, or others is required for tumor initiation. Furthermore it has been shown that the human leukocyte antigen (HLA)-DR5 allele is greatly overrepresented in patients with KS.

Histological features

In patch-stage KS the histological findings are subtle. There is a limited proliferation of small, attenuated vascular channels, often with a periadnexal distribution associated with an increased number of spindle cells, extravasated red blood cells, and a lymphoplasmacytic infiltrate. The promontory sign is the term for neovascular channels that form around existing vessels or adnexal structures. As the lesion becomes more developed and plaque-like, there are increased numbers of spindle cells forming small fascicles admixed with slit-like vascular channels. The stroma shows a more exuberant infiltrate consisting of extravasated red blood cells, hemosiderin as well as lymphocytes and plasma cells. Eosinophilic hyaline globules ("erythrophagolysosomes") within the neoplastic endothelial cells may be more recognizable at this stage. In the nodular stage the tumor consists primarily of spindle cells, which have hyperchromatic nuclei and cytoplasmic vacuoles. Immunohistochemical stains show reactivity with CD31 as well as with lymphatic differentiation markers, namely vascular endothelial growth factor (VEGF-3), vascular endothelial growth factor receptor (VEGFR-3), and podoplanin (D2-50).

Treatment

The incidence of AIDS-related KS has significantly diminished with the advent of highly active antiretroviral therapy (HAART). Reduction of immunosuppressant dosage may result in regression of lesions in organ transplant recipients. Because of the multifocal nature of the disease and the risk of recurrence, surgery is generally not advocated except to establish tissue diagnosis. Treatment varies from cryotherapy, radiation, interferon-alpha, intralesional vinblastine to systemic chemotherapy with vincristine, doxorubicin, and bleomycin as the most commonly employed agents. Newer agents include topical alitretinoin gel (Panretin) and gemcitabine. Systemic therapies that inhibit angiogenesis or target HHV-8 are also being investigated.

Prognosis

Classic KS has an indolent course and infrequently causes death. African, transplant-associated, and AIDS-related KS have the potential to evolve rapidly with disseminated lesions, which can be fatal.

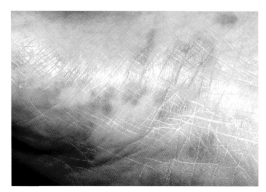

Figure 14-10 Kaposi's sarcoma

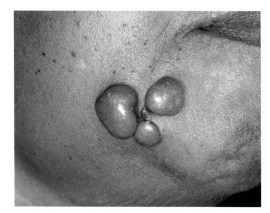

Figure 14-11 Lymphoma

Controversies

It is uncertain whether KS represents a true neoplasm or a reactive vascular hyperplasia to a viral infection.

Angiosarcoma

Clinical presentation

Key Points

- Uncommon neoplasm seen in one of several clinical contexts
- The most common variant clinically presents as an ill-defined bruise-like plaque of the face or scalp of the elderly
- Occurrence in the field of prior therapeutic radiation after a delay of many years. These usually present on the chest or abdominal wall on average 5–7 years following treatment. They appear as erythematous infiltrative plaques or nodules in or near the site of prior radiation
- Stewart–Treves syndrome, which is the development of angiosarcoma within an area of chronic lymphedema that is secondary to mastectomy and lymph node dissection. The duration of lymphedema prior to the appearance of angiosarcoma ranges from 4 to 27 years. The angiosarcoma presents as firm violaceous

nodules that coalesce or as an indurated plaque within a background of nonpitting edema

Differential diagnosis

- Ecchymosis, erysipelas, cavernous hemangioma, and other vascular neoplasms

Pathogenesis

Ionizing radiation and lymphedema are clearly implicated in two of the clinical variants; however, the pathogenesis of the most common type is largely unknown.

Histological features

Within well-differentiated areas there are anastomosing networks of often bloodless, sinusoidal vessels that have jagged lumens; the lumens are lined by moderately atypical endothelial cells that have hyperchromatic nuclei and scant cytoplasm. The vessels are highly infiltrative and dissect between collagen bundles. In less differentiated areas the endothelial cells are more pleomorphic and often pile up and form intraluminal papillary projections. Cutaneous appendages are invariably entrapped or destroyed by the proliferation; hemosiderin and chronic inflammatory cells can be seen in the ensuing stroma. There is also an epithelioid variant in which the vascular channels are often inapparent so that the lesion may be mistaken for a carcinoma. The tumor shows positive staining with CD31 and CD34, with the former being a more sensitive and specific stain for endothelial cells. The tumor also stains with friend leukemia integration-1 (FLI-1) and thrombomodulin.

Treatment

- Excision often followed by radiation

Prognosis

- Usually patients have a poor prognosis, with fewer than 15% of patients surviving 5 years

Cutaneous Lymphomas and Leukemia

There are a variety of T- and B-cell lymphomas (Figure 14-11) that primarily involve the skin with no evidence of extracutaneous disease at the time of diagnosis. In fact, after the gastrointestinal tract, the skin is the second most common site of involvement by extranodal non-Hodgkin's lymphoma. It can be impossible to differentiate many of the lymphomas based solely upon the tumor's clinical appearance; correlation with a person's age, race, the anatomical location of the tumor, and the immunohistological findings help lead to the correct diagnosis (Table 14-11). Primary cutaneous lymphomas have a completely different clinical behavior and prognosis from their systemic counterparts.

T-CELL LYMPHOMAS

Cutaneous T-cell lymphomas represent 75–80% of all primary cutaneous lymphomas. The most common will be discussed in the following section.

Mycosis Fungoides (MF)

Clinical presentation

Key Points

- It is the most common cutaneous lymphoma, accounting for 44% of all cases
- Typically presents in older people, with a median age of 55–60 years, and shows a slight male predominance (1.6-2:1)
- The initial lesion is an erythematous patch with a predilection for the buttocks and other sun-protected areas
- The lesions can slowly progress to plaques and tumors over the course of several years

Differential diagnosis

- Eczema and psoriasis in the initial stages

Pathogenesis

Most cases show a clonal T-cell receptor gene rearrangement. There are several chromosomal abnormalities commonly found in MF, including loss at 10q, 1p, and 17p, gains at chromosome 4q, 18, and 17q, and abnormalities in the p15, p16, and p53 genes.

Histological features

Early lesions show a band-like infiltrate of slightly atypical lymphocytes that line up along the dermal–epidermal junction. As the lesions progress there is progressive epidermotropism of atypical lymphocytes often exhibiting a peripheral halo. Characteristically there are numerous lymphocytes within the epidermis with minimal spongiosis. The most specific finding is focal collections of intraepidermal lymphocytes, referred to as Pautrier microabscesses; however, these are found in only 10% of lesions. In the tumor stage there is less epidermotropism and the atypical lymphocytes diffusely fill the dermis. Variants of MF include folliculotropic (follicular mucinosis), pagetoid reticulosis, and granulomatous slack skin. The neoplastic cells express CD2, CD3, CD4, and CD45RO and are usually negative for CD8 and CD30. There is often loss of expression of pan T-cell antigens (CD2, CD3, CD5, and CD7).

Treatment

Key Points

- Limited cutaneous lesions can be treated with topical steroids, bexarotene gel, PUVA, topical nitrogen mustard, and total electron beam irradiation
- More advanced cases are generally treated systemically with PUVA, topical nitrogen mustard, bexarotene, interferon-alpha, intraleukin-12 and/or denileukin diftitox
- Patients with systemic involvement require multiagent chemotherapy

Prognosis

The prognosis is dependent on stage:

- Patch/plaque stage involving less than 10% total body surface area has a 10-year disease-specific survival of 97–98%
- Patch/plaque stage with more diffuse involvement has a 10-year disease-specific survival of 83%
- Patients with tumor stage disease have a 10-year disease-specific survival of 42%
- Patients with involvement of the lymph nodes have a 10-year disease-specific survival of 20%

Sézary Syndrome

Clinical presentation

Key Points

- The patient typically presents with diffuse erythroderma with marked exfoliation, edema and lichenification, and recalcitrant pruritus
- Generalized lymphadenopathy is common
- Sézary cells are present in the skin, lymph nodes, and in the peripheral circulation, with an absolute peripheral Sézary count of at least 1000 cells/mm^3
- Other findings include alopecia, onychodystrophy, and palmar plantar hyperkeratosis

Differential diagnosis

- Eczema, psoriasis, and a drug eruption

Pathogenesis

This is a leukemic variant of MF and there is clonal rearrangement of the T-cell receptor. Chromosomal abnormalities in 1p, 10q, 14q, and 15q have been identified. Clonal amplification of the *JUNB* gene has been noted.

Histological features

Sometimes similar to MF, but the cellular infiltrates are more monotonous and epidermotropism is often minimal to absent. Approximately 33% of biopsies show a nonspecific histological picture. Involved lymph nodes, however, show a

Table 14-11 Immunohistological findings of different types of cutaneous lymphomas and leukemia

Type of lymphoma	Incidence	Age	Immunophenotype	Clinical presentation	Disease-specific survival
Mycosis fungoides	44–50% of all cutaneous lymphomas	55–60	+CD3, CD4, CD5RO Sometimes +CD8 Aberrant loss of CD2, CD3, CD5, and CD7	Erythematous patch on the buttocks and sun-protected areas	Patch 83–98% Tumor 42% Systemic 20%
Sézary syndrome	<3% of all CTCLs	Adults	+CD3 and CD4 −CD8, CD7, CD26	Erythroderma, generalized lymphadenopathy and presence of peripheral Sézary cells	24%
Adult T-cell leukemia/ lymphoma	Develops in 1–5% of HTLV-1-seropositive patients	Adults	+CD3, CD4, and CD25 −CD8	Hypercalcemia, organomegaly, (lymphadenopathy) osteolytic lesions, skin lesions	Low in the acute form
Primary cutaneous anaplastic large cell lymphoma	12% of all CTCLs	Adults	+CD4 and CD30 + Granzyme B, TIA-1 and perforin −CD CD2, CD3, and CD5	Solitary or multiple localized nodules or tumors	90%
Lymphomatoid papulosis	18% of all CTCLs	35–45	Type A and C: +CD4 and CD30 + Granzyme B, TIA-1 and perforin. Type B: +CD 3 and CD 4, ± CD8, but − CD30	Crops of papules that centrally ulcerate and become necrotic. Spontaneously involute over 3–12 weeks	100%
Subcutaneous panniculitis-like T-cell lymphoma	Fewer than 1% of all CTCLs	Children and young adults	+CD3 and CD8 CD4− + Granzyme B, TIA-1, and perforin	Solitary or multiple erythematous nodules on legs	80%, unless associated with a hemophagocytic syndrome
Extranodal natural killer/ T-cell lymphoma	Uncommon	Adults	+CD56 and CD3ε + granzyme B, TIA-1, and perforin	Ulcerative destructive central facial nodules or, less commonly, similar lesions on trunk or extremities	Median survival of 12 months
Primary cutaneous follicle center lymphoma	41–71% of all B-cell lymphomas	Adults	+CD20 and CD79a +bcl-6 and CD10 with follicle formation, but not when diffuse	Plum-colored nodules on the scalp or trunk	95%
Primary cutaneous marginal zone B-cell lymphoma	10–42%	Adults	+CD19, CD20, CD22, and CD79a. May express bcl-2 and Ig light chains − CD5, CD10, and bcl-6	Violaceous nodules on trunk and extremities (arms), often multifocal	100%
Primary cutaneous diffuse large B-cell lymphoma, leg type	Uncommon	Elderly females	+CD20 and CD79a +sIg and/or cIg +bcl-2 and bcl-6 + MUM-1/IRF4 protein	Erythematous to reddish-brown nodules on legs; occasionally other sites. Often ulcerated	55%

Continued

Table 14-11 Immunohistological findings of different types of cutaneous lymphomas and leukemia—cont'd

Type of lymphoma	Incidence	Age	Immunophenotype	Clinical presentation	Disease-specific survival
Primary cutaneous diffuse large B-cell lymphoma, other	Rare	Adults	+CD20 and CD79a +sIg and/or cIg +bcl-2 and bcl-6 + MUM-1/IRF4 protein	Reddish-brown nodules that can be ulcerated on the head, trunk, and extremities	55–100%
Intravascular large B-cell lymphoma	Rare	Adults	+CD20 and CD79a May coexpress CD10 or CD5 and CD49d	Violaceous plaques or telangiectatic patches on lower legs and trunk	22–56%
Leukemia cutis	30% of cases of AML	Children–adults	CD43, CD45, CD74, myeloperoxidase, TdT	Papules and nodules, often hemorrhagic	Dependent on type of leukemia

CTCL, cutaneous T-cell lymphoma; HTLV-1, human T-lymphotropic virus-1; AML, acute myeloid leukemia; TIA-1, cytotoxic granule-associated RNA-binding protein; Ig, immunoglobulin; TdT, terminal deoxynucleotidyl transferase.

dense monotonous infiltrate of Sézary cells that efface the normal lymph node architecture. The neoplastic cells are positive for CD3 and CD4 and negative for CD8, with a CD4/CD8 ratio greater than 10. In two-thirds of patients there is a loss of CD2, CD3, CD4, CD5, CD7, and/or CD26.

Treatment

Extracorporeal photophoresis either alone or in combination with interferon has been shown to have a 30–80% overall response rate. Systemic chemotherapy (chlorambucil, prednisone, and methotrexate) may be beneficial, but complete response is uncommon.

Prognosis

- Median survival is 2–4 years with a 5-year disease-specific survival of 24%

Adult T-cell leukemia/lymphoma (ATLL)

Clinical presentation

Key Points

- Found where human T-leukemia virus-1 (HTLV-1) is endemic, such as in southwest Japan, the Caribbean islands, South America, and parts of Central Africa
- Develops in 1–5% of seropositive patients after two or more decades of viral persistence
- Hypercalcemia, organomegaly (inclusive of lymphadenopathy), osteolytic skin lesions, and skin lesions are present in approximately 50% of patients
- Skin lesions can be plaques, papules, or nodules with varying numbers of lesions

Differential diagnosis

- MF, other lymphomas or cutaneous metastases

Pathogenesis

- A T-cell receptor gene arrangement and clonal integrated HTLV-1 genes are found in all cases

Histological features

- Superficial to diffuse infiltrate of medium-sized to large T cells with pleomorphic nuclei, which often display epidermotropism. The neoplastic cells express CD3, CD4, and CD25 and are negative for CD8

Treatment

- Systemic chemotherapy

Prognosis

In the acute form, survival ranges from 2 weeks to 1 year. The chronic form has a more protracted course, but there may be transformation to the acute form.

PRIMARY CUTANEOUS CD30 LYMPHOPROLIFERATIVE DISORDERS

This is the second most common group of cutaneous T-cell lymphomas, accounting for 30% of cases. This group consists of several variants, including primary cutaneous anaplastic large cell lymphoma, lymphomatoid papulosis (LyP), and borderline cases, where there is a discrepancy between clinical features and the histological appearance. LyP and anaplastic large cell lymphoma may be two ends of a spectrum of disease; however, in typical cases, the clinical appearance, course, and prognosis differ.

Primary cutaneous anaplastic large cell lymphoma

Clinical presentation

Key Points

- Primarily occurs in adults, with a male female ratio of 2–3:1
- Most present with solitary or localized lesions in the form of nodules or tumors that are often ulcerated
- Multifocal lesions seen in 20% of patients
- Extracutaneous dissemination, mainly to regional lymph nodes, occurs in 10% of cases

Differential diagnosis

- Other lymphomas or cutaneous metastases

Pathogenesis

- Clonal rearrangement of the T-cell receptor genes

Histological features

Diffuse sheets of large atypical cells that have round or irregular-shaped nuclei, prominent eosinophilic nuclei, and abundant cytoplasm. Reactive lymphocytes are often found at the periphery of the lesion. Approximately 20–30% of the neoplastic cells are not anaplastic in appearance. The cells are CD4- and CD30-positive with loss of CD2, CD3, and CD5. There is often expression of granzyme B, cytotoxic granule-associated RNA-binding protein (TIA-1), and perforin. Unlike systemic anaplastic lymphoma there is no expression of EMA or activin receptor-like kinase-1 (ALK-1), to indicate a t(2;5)(p23;q35) translocation.

Treatment

Treatment involves radiotherapy or surgical excision for localized disease. Patients with multifocal lesion can be treated with low-dose methotrexate, but patients with extracutaneous disease require doxorubicin-based multiagent chemotherapy.

Prognosis

The 10-year disease-free survival rate exceeds 90%; however patients may experience skin relapses, even following cyclophosphamide, hydroxyrubicin (Adriamycin), Oncovin (vincristine), prednisone (CHOP) therapy. Spontaneous regression has also been reported.

Lymphomatoid papulosis

Clinical presentation

Key Points

- Characterized by crops of red-brown papules that undergo central necrosis, most commonly on the trunk and limbs
- Lesions spontaneous involute over the course of 3–8 weeks
- There may be lesions at various stages of development present at the same time
- It may occur at any age; average age range is 35–45 years old
- Male to female ratio of 1.5:1

Differential diagnosis

- Folliculitis, arthropod bites, pityriasis lichenoides et varioliformis acuta

Pathogenesis

- Approximately 60–70% of patients exhibit clonal rearrangement of T-cell receptor genes

Histological features

There are three main histological variants:

- LyP type A consists of a wedge-shaped dermal infiltrate composed of a mixed population of inflammatory cells (large CD30+ atypical cells that have a Reed–Sternberg-like appearance, histiocytes, lymphocytes, neutrophils, and eosinophils)
- LyP type B is the least common (less than 10%) and is characterized by epidermotropic band-like infiltrate of small atypical cells with a cerebriform nuclei similar to those seen in MF
- LyP type C is composed of diffuse sheets of large atypical CD30+ cells intermixed with only a few scattered reactive inflammatory cells, similar to the histology of anaplastic large cell lymphoma
- The large atypical cells seen in type A and C are CD4- and CD30-positive as well as positive for granzyme B, TIA-1, and perforin. The atypical cells in type B are CD3 and CD4-positive and CD8 and CD30-negative

Treatment

Since none of the available treatment modalities has been shown to affect the natural course of the disease, the short-term benefit of active treatment must be balanced against the side-effects. The most effective therapy to suppress the development of new lesions is low-dose oral methotrexate (5–20 mg/week). Some benefit is also seen with PUVA, topical mechlorethamine or carmustine and low-dose etoposide; however lesions typically recur once the treatment is discontinued.

Prognosis

- 100% 5-year disease-free survival; however in up to 20% of cases another type of cutaneous lymphoma may precede or follow the diagnosis of LyP

Controversies

There is debate as to whether this is a malignant, premalignant, or reactive condition.

Subcutaneous panniculitis-like T-cell lymphoma

Clinical presentation

Key Points

- Typically presents as solitary or multiple erythematous tender nodules and plaques primarily affecting the legs
- Approximately 40% of cases are associated with fever, fatigue, myalgia, and weight loss
- Occurs in both children and adults and equally occurs in both sexes

Differential diagnosis

- Erythema nodosum or erythema induratum

Pathogenesis

- The neoplastic cells show a clonal T-cell receptor gene rearrangement

Histological features

The epidermis and dermis are typically spared, with the primary process occurring in the subcutaneous adipose. There is a diffuse infiltrate surrounding the adipocytes composed of small, medium, and sometimes large pleomorphic lymphocytes, often with many macrophages simulating panniculitis. Rimming of the individual adipocytes by neoplastic lymphocytes is a helpful diagnostic feature. Necrosis, karyorrhexis, and cytophagocytosis are common findings. The lymphocytes stain positively with CD3 and CD8 with expression of cytotoxic proteins. Under the new combined World Health Organization (WHO)–European Organization for Research and Treatment of Cancer (2005) classification of cutaneous lymphomas, cases are by definition positive for T-cell receptor alpha/beta.

Treatment

- Doxorubicin-based chemotherapy and radiotherapy. Some patients may be controlled with systemic corticosteroids

Prognosis

In some cases a hemophagocytic syndrome occurs, and these patients experience a rapidly fatal course. Other patients have a more protracted course. The overall 5-year survival rate is 80%.

Controversies

Under the new WHO–EORTC (2005) classification of cutaneous lymphomas, cases express the alpha-beta T-cell receptor and generally have a good prognosis. It is thought that the rapidly fatal cases are the ones that express the gamma-delta T-cell receptor, and these cases now fall under the provisional diagnosis of gamma-delta T-cell lymphomas.

Extranodal NK/T cell lymphoma (formerly called lethal midline granuloma)

Clinical presentation

Key Points

- Primarily occurs in adult males, more often seen in Asia, Central America, and South America
- Patients present with multiple plaques or tumors on the trunk and extremities or as central facial nodules that are ulcerative and destructive
- Systemic symptoms such as fever, malaise, and weight loss may be present

Differential diagnosis

- Other lymphomas, Wegener's granulomatosis, fungal infection

Pathogenesis

- Strong association with Epstein–Barr virus

Histological features

This is a dense dermal infiltrate that often extends to the subcutis, consisting of variably sized atypical lymphocytes. The neoplastic cells exhibit angiocentricity and angiodestruction, which accounts for the necrosis that is seen clinically. Epidermotropism may be encountered. The immunophenotype is as follows: CD56+ and + granzyme B, TIA-1, and perforin. Cytoplasmic CD3 (CD3-epsilon) is expressed, but not surface CD3.

Treatment

- Systemic chemotherapy, but the disease is often refractory to treatment

Prognosis

This is a highly aggressive condition with survival less than 12 months. Extracutaneous involvement portends a poor outcome. Patients with lesions restricted to the skin have a median survival of 27 months, compared to 5 months for patients with extracutaneous disease.

Cutaneous B-cell lymphomas

Cutaneous B-cell lymphomas represent 18.8–26.6% of all cutaneous lymphomas in a Dutch registry, and an even smaller percentage, 4.5%, of cases from the United States. Regional variations are also seen between the different types of B-cell lymphomas.

Primary cutaneous follicle center B-cell lymphoma (PCFCL)

Clinical presentation

> **Key Points**
>
> - Solitary or grouped plum-colored papules, plaques, and tumors, often surrounded by a patch of erythema, preferentially on the scalp, forehead, and trunk
> - Multifocal lesions may occur and are not associated with a worse prognosis
> - Tumors located on the back have been referred to in the past as Crosti's lymphoma or reticulohistiocytoma of the dorsum
> - The lesions are asymptomatic and ulceration is uncommon

Differential diagnosis

- Cutaneous metastases

Pathogenesis

Clonally rearranged immunoglobulin genes are present with somatic hypermethylation of the variable region of the heavy- and light-chain genes. It is not associated with the t(14;18) translocation and bcl-2 rearrangement that is found in systemic follicular lymphomas. Inactivation of p15 and p16 is reported in 10% and 30% of PCF-CLs respectively.

Histological features

PCFCLs can show a diffuse or nodular pattern, both of which have a Grenz zone between the neoplastic cells and the epidermis. A follicular pattern is more often seen in lesions from the scalp. Lesions consist of a mixture of centrocytes (small and large cleaved follicular centered cells) with few centroblasts (large noncleaved follicular center cells with prominent nucleoli) admixed with a proliferation of reactive T cells. When follicle formation is present it typically consists of malignant bcl-6+ follicular cells intermixed with CD21 and CD35 follicular dendritic cells. The follicles lack tingible-body macrophages and do not have a defined mantle zone. The neoplastic B cells express CD19, CD20, CD79a, and surface immunoglobulins. When the tumor shows follicular growth pattern CD10 is positive. Unlike

nodal follicular lymphomas, rarely is the typical t(14,18) translocation or bcl-2 protein expressed. Multiple myeloma-1 (MUM-1)/interferon-regulatory factor 4 (IRF4), expressed in diffuse B-cell lymphoma, is not expressed and CD5 and CD43 are negative.

Treatment

In patients with one or several isolated lesions, radiotherapy is preferable. Anthracycline-based chemotherapy is only required for extensive disease. Systemic or intralesional anti-CD20 antibody (rituximab) may be of benefit.

Prognosis

The overall prognosis is excellent, with a 5-year survival of more than 95%; however, recurrences can occur in 20–50% of cases. Expression of bcl-2 in PCFCLs with a diffuse large cell histological pattern is associated with a more unfavorable prognosis.

Primary cutaneous marginal-zone B-cell lymphoma (PCMZL), includes Borrelia associated immunocytoma

Clinical presentation

> **Key Points**
>
> - Usually presents with red to violaceous papules, plaques, or nodules on the trunk and extremities, especially the arms
> - Multifocal lesions are common
> - A small percentage of European cases are associated with *Borrelia burgdorferi*
> - The association with autoimmune disease is primarily seen with systemic marginal-zone lymphoma

Differential diagnosis

- Cutaneous metastases

Pathogenesis

Immunoglobuin H (IgH) is clonally rearranged in 70% of cases. A t(11;18) involving the *API2/MLT* gene is not found in PCMZL, but is common in gastric MZL. However, 33% of PCMZL have a t(14;18)(q32;q21) translocation involving the *IGH* and *MALT1* genes.

Histological features

Within the dermis there is a nodular or diffuse infiltrate of medium-sized lymphocytes that have irregular nuclei, inconspicuous nucleoli, and abundant pale cytoplasm, reminiscent of marginal-zone B cells. Some cells have a monocytoid or plasmacytoid appearance. At scanning magnification there is a classic "inverse pattern," typified by dark centers surrounded by a zone of pale-staining cells. Reactive germinal centers are common; however, they can be obscured by colonization by neoplastic cells. In areas where there are high numbers of plasma cells and lymphoplasmacytoid cells, pseudointranuclear (Dutcher bodies) and intracytoplasmic (Russell bodies) inclusions of immunoglobulin can be seen. The neoplastic cells have the following phenotype: they express CD19, CD20, CD22, CD79a, bcl2 and sometimes clonal restriction of immunoglobulin light chains. Colonized follicles can be identified by expression of CD21 by the follicular dendritic cells and bcl-6 in the germinal centers. Mature plasma cells express CD79a and CD138 but not CD20. They do not express CD5, CD10, or bcl-6.

Treatment

Solitary lesions can be treated with radiotherapy or surgical excision. If there is evidence of a *B. burgdorferi* infection, antibiotics should be initiated. For multifocal lesions, chlorambucil or intralesional or subcutaneous interferon-alpha produces complete response in 50% of patients. Anti-CD20 antibody (rituximab) has enjoyed some success. In patients with frequent relapses, topical or intralesional steroids can be employed.

Prognosis

Spontaneous resolution may occur, leaving a focal area of anetoderma. The 5-year survival rate approaches 100%.

Primary cutaneous diffuse large B-cell lymphoma, leg type (PCLBCL)

Clinical presentation

Key Points

- Primarily affects elderly females on the distal leg or legs; rarely seen at other sites
- Presents as erythematous or reddish-brown nodules that can be solitary or a small cluster
- Ulceration is common
- More often disseminate to extracutaneous sites

Differential diagnosis

- Cutaneous metastases

Pathogenesis

Although bcl-2 is strongly expressed, the t(14;18) translocation is not found. Inactivation of p15 and p16 is seen in 11% and 44% of cases respectively. Chromosomal imbalances have been identified in 85% of cases, with gains in 18q and 7p and loss in 6q the most frequent.

Histological features

There is diffuse infiltration of the dermis extending into the subcutaneous tissue, consisting of a monotonous population of large B-cells resembling centroblasts or immunoblasts. A thin Grenz zone separates the neoplastic cells from the epidermis. Adnexal structures are usually destroyed. Mitotic figures are frequently seen. Usually there are reactive T and B cells, often limited to perivascular areas. The neoplastic cells express surface immunoglobulin or cytoplasmic immunoglobulin, as well as CD20 and CD79a. Both bcl-2 and bcl-6 are also strongly expressed, as is MUM-1/IRF4 protein. CD5 and CD10 are not expressed.

Treatment

These lymphomas should be treated with anthracycline-based chemotherapy, similar to the treatment of systemic diffuse B-cell lymphomas. Systemic use of rituximab may also be an effective alternative, either as a single agent or in combination with chemotherapy. Patients who have an isolated lesion can be treated with radiotherapy.

Prognosis

This cutaneous B-cell lymphoma has the worst prognosis of all cutaneous B-cell lymphomas, and, when located on the leg, PCLBCL has a worse prognosis than when it occurs elsewhere. The overall 5-year survival is 55%; when there is a single lesion on the leg, the 5-year survival approaches 100%, but when multiple lesions are present, survival ranges from 36% to 45% depending upon whether or not one or both legs are involved.

Primary cutaneous diffuse large B-cell lymphoma, other

This term is used for large B-cell lymphomas that do not fit into the previous category. They are composed of large transformed B cells, have a diffuse growth pattern, and are most commonly located on the head, trunk, or extremities. Non-leg PCLBCL may overall have a slightly better prognosis; however, more important prognostic indicators include the number of lesions present and whether or not bcl-2 and MUM1/IRF4 are expressed, with expression of these markers indicative of a better outcome.

Intravascular large B-cell lymphoma, also known as angioendotheliomatosis, intravascular lymphomatosis, and Tappeiner–Pfleger syndrome

Clinical presentation

Key Points

- Rare, highly malignant large cell lymphoma; although most are B-cells, a T-cell variant has been described
- The lymphoma primarily manifests in the skin and nervous system
- Indurated violaceous plaques or telangiectatic patches (reticular erythema and livedo reticularis) on lower legs and trunk are seen in 33% of patients
- Many patients have neurologic defects, including dementia

Differential diagnosis

- Panniculitis or purpura

Pathogenesis

- Rearrangement of IgH genes and structural aberrations in chromosomes 1, 6, 18, and 1p

Pathogenesis

Defects in the homing receptors (CD29/ß1 integrin) and adhesion molecules (CD54/intercellular adhesion molecule-1 (ICAM-1)) on the neoplastic cells and endothelial cells are hypothesized to be responsible for vascular trapping of the neoplastic cells.

Histological features

There is proliferation of large atypical lymphoid cells occluding the lumens of capillaries and post-capillary venules. Extravascular involvement can occur in 20% of cases. Vessels are occluded, but not destroyed, by the process. The neoplastic cells express CD20 and CD79a and coexpress CD10 or CD5 and CD49d. Most overexpress bcl-2.

Treatment

- Systemic chemotherapy

Prognosis

Patients with lesions limited to the skin have a 56% 3-year survival, whereas those with disseminated disease only have a 22% 3-year survival.

Controversies

Formerly classified as a vascular neoplasm, phenotype and genetic analysis allowed for reclassification as a peculiar variant of non-Hodgkin's lymphoma.

Leukemia cutis

Clinical presentation

Key Points

- Can be seen in a variety of different leukemias
- In children it is most often secondary to acute lymphatic leukemia; in adults it is more likely to be due to acute and chronic myeloid leukemia; and in the elderly, chronic lymphatic leukemia and hairy cell leukemia are most prevalent
- The incidence of leukemia cutis is highest among children, with 25–30% of children with congenital leukemia having cutaneous infiltrates. The cutaneous appearance of the nodular infiltrates has been likened to a blueberry muffin. Cutaneous infiltrates in this situation do not alter the prognosis
- In adults cutaneous infiltrates occur late in the disease and portend a poor prognosis
- Cutaneous lesions are most common in acute myeloid leukemia, with an incidence of about 13%. Chronic myeloid leukemia, chronic lymphatic leukemia, and hairy cell leukemia have an incidence of cutaneous lesions in approximately 8% of patients
- The lesions are nonspecific, but tend to be firm red to purple papules and nodules that may become hemorrhagic or ulcerate
- Marked gingival hypertrophy and oral petechiae can also be seen
- Chloroma, also known as granulocytic sarcoma, is a type of leukemia cutis that presents as a dermal nodule. Chloromas are unique in that, when exposed to air, they have a blue-green hue secondary to the presence of myeloperoxidase

Differential diagnosis

- Infection, drug eruption, vasculitis, vascular neoplasm, erythema nodosum, and cutaneus metastases

Pathogenesis

Leukemia results from an abnormal proliferation of lymphocytes in the bone marrow, but the exact mechanism as to how and why the leukemic cells migrate to the epidermis is unknown. Many of the leukemias are associated with chromosomal abnormalities; most notable is the Philadelphia chromosome seen in chronic myeloid leukemia which occurs as a result of a translocation between chromosomes 9 and 22.

Histological features

Histological features vary depending on the type of leukemia, but in general there is a diffuse infiltrate that extends throughout the dermis and spares the epidermis. The neoplastic cells resemble that seen in the bone marrow and often they infiltrate between the collagen bundles as single cells and are distributed around vessels and adnexa. Naphthol AS-D chloroacetate (Leder) stain helps identify cells with myeloid differentiation. Terminal deoxynucleotidyl transferase (TdT) is helpful in identifying lymphoblastic cells.

Treatment

- Systemic chemotherapy

Prognosis

- Dependent upon the type of leukemia
- Adults often have a worse outcome when compared to children

Metastatic lesions to the skin

Cutaneous metastases are relatively rare, occurring in 0.7–10.4% of patients with metastatic cancer.

Clinical presentation

Key Points

- Approximately 88% of patients have a known primary; however, the cutaneous metastasis can be the first sign of an occult malignancy
- Overall, melanoma is the most common malignancy to metastasize to the skin. The second most common is SCC from the head and neck
- In women, the most common metastatic tumor is breast cancer, with lung cancer falling closely behind
- In men, the most common metastatic tumors are lung and colorectal carcinoma
- Ages 50–70 are most commonly affected
- Metastatic cancer of unknown origin accounts for 5–10% of cases
- The clinical presentation is nonspecific. Tumors which access the skin via direct extension often present as indurated plaques with atypical cells either infiltrating in a single-cell pattern between collagen bundles or forming a discrete mass
- Metastases arising from the blood stream often present as focal erythematous patches or with telangiectases. Metastases arising from the lymphatics often present with local edema
- Commonly the patient presents with a firm, painless, erythematous papule or nodule that may ulcerate. Most metastases are solitary, with a minority of cases having multiple lesions
- Most metastases occur close to the site of the primary tumor. Breast and lung cancers frequently metastasize to the chest wall and gastrointestinal and genitourinary cancers metastasize to the abdominal wall. Metastatic nodules that occur around the umbilicus are called Sister Mary Joseph nodules
- The scalp, presumably because of its rich vascular supply, is a common site of metastasis for tumors, particularly from renal, thyroid, and melanoma primaries
- Neonates can present with a "blueberry muffin" appearance from metastases secondary to neuroblastoma, leukemia, or rhabdomyosarcoma.

Differential diagnosis

- Inflammatory dermatoses, melanoma, BCC, KA, adnexal tumor, and soft-tissue neoplasms

Histological features

Most show neoplastic cells throughout the dermis and often extending into the subcutaneous tissues, often with "Indian filing" of neoplastic cells between collagen bundles. Often there is intravascular or intralymphatic invasion by neoplastic cells. In general, there is no epidermal involvement; however, some tumors show pagetoid extension, and other tumors cause ulceration of the epidermis.

To determine the primary site of malignancy, a basic immunohistochemical panel should be performed to separate the lesion into three basic categories: carcinoma, sarcoma, and lymphoma (Table 14-12).

An important histological distinction is between a metastatic lesion and an adnexal tumor; useful stains include p63, cytokeratin 5/6, and B72.3 (Table 14-13).

Treatment

- Treatment is directed against the primary malignancy

Prognosis

- Usually cutaneous metastases portend a poor prognosis

Paget's disease and extramammary Paget's

Clinical presentation

Key Points

- Both types occur more commonly in females as indistinct scaly erythematous plaques that slowly expand; occasionally, they may be pigmented
- Extramammary Paget's disease (Figure 14-12) usually affects areas with numerous apocrine glands, most commonly the anogenital region, but also the axilla, auditory canal, and eyelid. Rare cases have been reported on the buttock, extremities, abdomen, and chest
- Intractable pruritus is common

Differential diagnosis

- Eczema or other inflammatory dermatoses

Pathogenesis

Key Points

- Paget's of the breast occurs as a result of direct extension of an underlying intraductal adenocarcinoma

Table 14-12 Basic immunohistochemical panel for metastatic lesions to the skin

	Cytokeratin	Vimentin	LCA (CD45)
Carcinoma	+	–	–
Sarcoma	–	+	–
Lymphoma	–	–	+

Table 14-13 Distinguishing between an adnexal tumor and a metastatic lesion

	P63	B72.3
Adnexal tumors	96% +	72% –
Metastases	78% –	84% +

- Only 25% of patients with extramammary Paget's have an underlying adnexal carcinoma
- Approximately 80% of patients with perianal Paget's have an underlying adnexal or visceral malignancy
- If extramammary Paget's is found elsewhere, only 10–15% of patients have an underlying internal carcinoma, most commonly of the rectum, prostate, or bladder

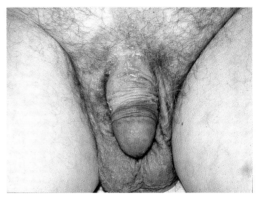

Figure 14-12 Extramammary Paget's disease

Histological features

Paget's cells have abundant pale cytoplasm with large pleomorphic nuclei. Occasionally signet-ring cells or glandular formation with intraluminal mucin can be seen. Mitoses are usually present. The epidermis is typically hyperplastic, and in early lesions, cells crowd the lower epidermis and can spread to neighboring adnexal structures. Uncommonly, Paget cells can be seen scattered throughout the dermis.

The immunohistochemical staining profile can be helpful in differentiating Paget's from extramammary Paget's as well as from other malignancies that have pagetoid extension.

In general:

- Mammary Paget's expresses CK7 but not CK 20, and stains with gross cystic disease protein (GCDFP), cathepsin B, EMA, and variably with carcinoembronic antigen. Estrogen/progesterone receptor status and Her2-neu stains can be performed to help guide treatment
- Primary extramammary Paget's has a similar profile to mammary Paget's disease; however, GCDFP is usually negative and abundant mucin (+ mucicarmine, alcian blue at pH 2.0, Hale's colloidal iron, and periodic acid–Schiff) is seen in most cases of extramammary Paget's

- Secondary extramammary Paget's (i.e., those associated with an internal malignancy) shows variable staining with CK7 and CK20 depending upon the underlying primary. Lung carcinoma is CK7+/CK20–, colon carcinoma is CK7–/CK20+, urinary bladder carcinoma is CK7+/CK20+, and prostate carcinoma is CK7–/CK20– (Table 14-14).

Treatment

- Mammary Paget's is treated by treating the underlying malignancy
- In extramammary Paget's, a thorough search for an underlying carcinoma must be performed, and if found it should be treated appropriately. If there is no underlying malignancy and the lesion is resectable, excision is the preferred treatment. Mohs micrographic surgery has been used successfully. Alternative therapies include PDT and topical imiquimod; however these are not approved by the Food and Drug Administration.

Prognosis

Patients with an underlying malignancy have 50% mortality. Patients with extramammary Paget's without an underlying malignancy fare much better; however local recurrence is common.

Table 14-14 Immunohistochemical staining profile differentiating Paget's from extramammary Paget's and other malignancies with pagetoid extension

	CK7	CK20	CEA	EMA	GCDFP	S100	CD4
Paget's	+	−	±	+	+	−*	−
Extramammary Paget's	±	±	+	+	−	−*	−
Bowen's	+	−	−	+	−	−*	−
Melanoma	−	−	−	−	−	+	−
Sebaceous carcinoma	+	−	−	+	−	−	−
Pagetoid reticulosis	−	−	−	−	−	−	+
Merkel cell carcinoma	−	+	−	+	−	−	−

CEA, carcinoembryonic antigen; EMA, epithelial membrane antigen; GCDFP, gross cystic disease protein.

*S-100-positive cells can be seen in Paget's, extramammary Paget's, and Bowen's if the tumor is colonized by melanocytes.

Further reading

Balch CM, Buzaid AC, Soong SJ, et al. Final version of the American Joint Committee on Cancer staging system for cutaneous melanoma. J Clin Oncol 2001;19:3635–3648.

Cassarino DS, Derienzo DP, Barr RJ. Cutaneous squamous cell carcinoma: a comprehensive clinicopathologic classification. J Cutan Pathol 2006; 33:191–206, 261–279.

Fisher C, van den Berg E, Molenaar WM. Adult fibrosarcoma. In: Fletcher CDM, Unni KK, Mertens F, eds. Pathology and Genetics. Tumors of Soft Tissue and Bone. Lyon: IARCPress, 2002:110–111.

Fletcher CDM, van den Berg E, Molenaar WM. Pleomorphic malignant fibrous histiocytoma/Undifferentiated high grade pleomorphic sarcoma. In: Fletcher CDM, Unni KK, Mertens F, eds. Pathology and Genetics. Tumors of Soft Tissue and Bone. Lyon: IARCPress. 2002:120–122.

Miller SJ, Moresi JM. Actinic keratosis, basal cell carcinoma and squamous cell carcinoma. In: Bolognia JL, Jorrizzo JL, Rapini RP, eds. Dermatology, London: Mosby, 2003:1677–1696.

Mott RT, Smoller BR, Morgan MB. Merkel cell carcinoma: a clinicopathologic study with prognostic implications. J Cutan Pathol 2004;31:217–223.

Nascimento AF, Bertoni F, Fletcher CDM. Epithelioid variant of myxofibrosarcoma: Expanding the clinicomorphologic spectrum of myxofibrosarcoma in a series of 17 cases. Am J Surg Pathol 2007; 31:99–105.

Nestle FO, Kerl H. Melanoma. In: Bolognia JL, Jorrizzo JL, Rapini RP, eds. Dermatology. London: Mosby, 2003:1789–1815.

Sariya D, Ruth K, Adams-McDonnell R, et al. Clinicopathologic correlation of cutaneous metastases. Arch Dermatol 2007;143:613–620.

Satter EK, Schaffer JW, Andea A, et al. Scar carcinoma (Marjolin ulcer) and bullous disease. Pathol Case Rev 2005;10:287–295.

Sober AJ, Burstein JM. Precursors to skin cancer. Cancer 1995;75:645–650.

Weedon D. Skin Pathology, 2nd ed. London: Churchill Livingstone, 2002:883–884, 934–939, 987–991

Willemze R, Jaffe ES, Burg G, et al. WHO-EROTC classification for cutaneous lymphomas. Blood 2005;105:3768–3785.

Wolverton SE. Comprehensive Dermatologic Drug Therapy, 2nd edn, Philadelphia: Saunders, 2007:302–307, 484, 643–645

Benign skin tumors

Donna Marie Vleugels and James E. Sligh

EPIDERMAL

Seborrheic keratosis

Key Points

- Appear as stuck-on keratotic lesions
- May be pigmented
- When the diagnosis is uncertain, a biopsy is necessary

Clinical presentation

Seborrheic keratoses (SKs, Figure 15-1) are common, benign keratinocyte neoplasms. They present as 2-mm to 2-cm skin-color, brown, or black, "stuck-on-appearing," well-demarcated macules, papules, or plaques, depending on the stage of development. They are oval to round, often with a "greasy," "waxy," or verrucous appearance. The presence of surface horn pseudocysts, which represent keratin-filled pits, is virtually pathognomonic. Common sites include the face, trunk, and upper extremities; mucous membranes, palms, and soles are generally spared. Lesions may become irritated or excoriated from rubbing or trauma. SKs usually arise in individuals over 30 years of age, and the number of lesions increases with age. Clinical and histological variants include common SK, reticulated SK, clonal SK, irritated SK, stucco keratosis, dermatosis papulosa nigra, and melanoacanthoma (Table 15-1).

Diagnosis

- Diagnosis is usually made by clinical presentation alone

Differential diagnosis

SKs must be distinguished clinically and histologically from acrochordons, verrucae, solar lentigines, actinic keratoses, melanocytic nevi, lentigo maligna, epidermal nevi, pigmented basal cell carcinomas (BCCs), and melanoma.

Histological Features

Biopsy shows characteristic keratin-filled pseudocysts with uniform intraepidermal proliferation of small, benign squamous and basaloid cells. Biopsy is necessary when the appearance is obscured by inflammation or when clinical appearance alone cannot exclude an atypical melanocytic neoplasm.

Pathogenesis

SKs can have a familial predisposition with an autosomal-dominant inheritance pattern. Sun exposure is thought to be a risk factor, although they do occur in sun-protected areas. Studies revealing monoclonal origin of the majority of SKs suggest

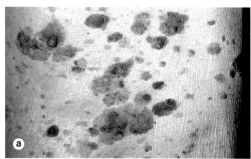

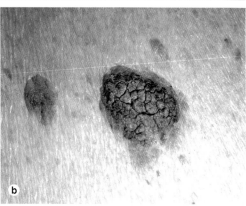

Figure 15-1 a, b Seborrheic keratoses

Table 15-1 Clinicopathologic seborrheic keratosis (SK) variants

Clinicopathologic SK variant	Clinical presentation	Histology
Common SK	Classic lesion	Prominent keratin horn pseudocysts
		Acanthosis – accumulation of benign squamous and basaloid cells
		+ 'String sign' – well demarcation at base
Reticulated SK (adenoid SK)	Similar to classic SK	Fewer horn pseudocysts
		Reticulated cords of basaloid epithelial cells
Clonal SK	Similar to classic SK	Well-defined nests of basaloid cells within epidermis
Irritated SK (inflamed SK)	SK with eczematous changes	Inflammatory infiltrate at dermis
		Eosinophilic squamous eddies, ± cytologic atypia and mitotic figures
		Often lack a clear 'string sign'
Stucco keratosis	Multiple 'stuck-on' small gray to white papules on lower legs	Hyperkeratosis
		Papillomatosis, + 'church spire' pattern
		Horn pseudocysts absent
Dermatosis papulosa nigra	Multiple small, pedunculated, pigmented papules on the face of dark-skinned individuals	Similar to common SKs
Melanoacanthoma (pigmented SK)	Darkly pigmented SK, no malignant potential	Proliferation of dendritic melanocytes with melanin (versus melanin within keratinocytes in other variants)

a neoplastic rather than hyperplastic process. Epidermal growth factors (EGFs) have been implicated, including tumor-derived growth factors with the sign of Leser–Trélat.

Treatment

No treatment is necessary unless lesions are irritated, if biopsy is needed to rule out malignancy, or if removal is desired for cosmetic purposes. Topical treatment with keratolytic agents such as ammonium lactate lotion (AmLactin, LacHydrin) and trichloroacetic acid (Tri-Chlor) flatten SKs and may improve their appearance (Table 15-2). The preferred surgical methods are destruction or shave removal with curettage. Excision is not usually necessary and may cause scarring. Destructive methods include cryotherapy with liquid nitrogen or light electrodesiccation. Although these are efficient and effective methods to remove SKs, they do not permit histopathological verification of the clinical diagnosis. If the clinical diagnosis is in doubt, or if the spectrum of clinical diagnoses includes atypical melanocytic proliferations, the lesion should be submitted for histologic evaluation.

Pharmaceuticals

Keratolytic agents:
- Ammonium lactate lotion (AmLactin, LacHydrin)
- Trichloroacetic acid (Tri-Chlor)

Controversies

The sudden appearance of multiple SKs, referred to as the sign of Leser–Trélat, is purported to be a cutaneous sign of internal malignancy, often of an adenocarcinoma of stomach, ovary, uterus, or breast. The existence of this entity, however, is a matter of debate. Insurance carriers frequently do not cover removal of noninflamed SKs, which they consider to be a cosmetic procedure.

Skin tag (acrochordon, cutaneous papilloma)

Key Points

- Common and generally harmless
- Can be removed if inflamed or necrotic

Clinical presentation

Skin tags (Figure 15-2) are common, soft, 1–10-mm, tan to flesh-colored, pedunculated, fleshy papules with irregular or smooth surfaces. They occur in middle age and in the elderly and are asymptomatic unless trauma or torsion makes them tender. Irritated or injured skin tags can become necrotic, crusted papules. Skin tags are more common in female and obese patients. They occur at sites of body folds and friction (axillae, inframammary folds, groin, neck, and eyelids).

Table 15-2 Treatment of seborrheic keratosis (SK)

Noninflamed SK		Inflamed SK (or suspicious for melanoma)
Medical treatment	**Physical destruction**	Shave excision with curettage: avoid later if melanoma is suspected
1. Ammonium lactate lotion	1. Cryotherapy	
2. Trichloroacetic acid	2. Light electrodesiccation and curettage	Histopathologic evaluation of a deep shave or punch biopsy specimen is preferred if atypical nevus or melanoma is a diagnostic possibility
Results in flattening and lightening of lesions	3. Curettage alone	
	4. Shave excision (allows for histologic evaluation)	
	5. Laser (carbon dioxide)	
	6. Dermabrasion	

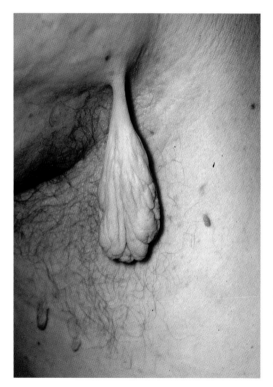

Figure 15-2 Acrochordon

They become larger and more numerous over time, including during the second trimester of pregnancy. Perianal skin tags are associated with Crohn's disease.

Diagnosis

Diagnosis is usually based solely on clinical presentation. A skin biopsy may be necessary to confirm the diagnosis if other entities are in the differential diagnosis, or to remove large or necrotic skin tags. Histopathology reveals slightly hyperplastic epithelium with an underlying dermal stalk composed of loose collagen and capillaries.

Differential diagnosis

Skin tags must be differentiated from pedunculated SKs, dermal or compound nevi that usually develop earlier in life, neurofibromas that invaginate or "buttonhole" with palpation, and molluscum contagiosum with central umbilication. Very rarely, BCC or squamous cell carcinoma (SCC) resembles skin tags.

Pathogenesis

The exact cause of skin tags is unknown. Because they are a frequent finding in obese patients and are considered a cutaneous marker for noninsulin-dependent diabetes mellitus, skin tags may result from increased concentrations of insulin or insulin-like growth factors acting on cutaneous epithelial cells or from their interaction with EGF and its receptors. Skin tags have also been linked to colonic polyps in highly selected referral populations, but not in the general population.

Treatment

Removal by simple scissor excision, electrodesiccation, or cryosurgery is only necessary if lesions become irritated. Local anesthesia is often unnecessary.

Cutaneous horn

Key Points

- Most commonly arise from an actinic keratosis or wart
- Biopsy often necessary

Clinical presentation

The term "cutaneous horn" (Figure 15-3) does not refer to a specific diagnosis, but rather to the clinical presentation of a conical projection composed of compact keratin above the surface of the skin. These lesions, ranging from a few millimeters to several centimeters, are most commonly found on

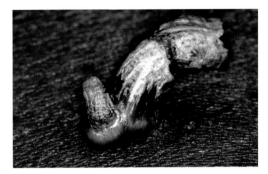

Figure 15-3 Cutaneous horn

Table 15-3 Differential diagnosis of lesions underlying a cutaneous horn

Benign	Premalignant/malignant
Verrucae (20%)	Hypertrophic actinic keratosis (30%)
Seborrheic keratosis	Squamous cell carcinoma (20%)
Benign lichenoid keratosis	Keratoacanthoma
Trichilemmal cyst	Kaposi's sarcoma
Dermatofibroma	Bowen's disease
Discoid lupus	Paget's disease
Epidermoid cyst	Basal cell carcinoma
Epidermal nevus	Sebaceous carcinoma
Pyogenic granuloma	Metastatic renal carcinoma
Sebaceous adenoma	
Angiokeratoma	
Angioma	

sun-exposed areas in elderly patients. Cutaneous horns arise from a wide range of underlying epidermal lesions. Thirty percent are associated with underlying hypertrophic actinic keratoses, 20% with verrucae, and 20% with malignancy, usually SCC. Large size and tenderness at the base favor an underlying malignancy. Less frequent associations include SK, pyogenic granuloma, trichilemmoma, keratoacanthoma, and BCC.

Diagnosis

The cutaneous horn is purely a clinical diagnosis based on gross morphology; the diagnosis of the underlying lesion is made by histopathological evaluation.

Differential diagnosis

See Table 15-3.

Pathogenesis

- Hyperkeratosis at the affected epidermal region results in horn formation.

Treatment

Cutaneous horns can and should be removed by shave biopsy, ensuring sufficient tissue depth to allow for evaluation of possible dermal invasion. When malignancy is diagnosed, additional treatment may be needed to ensure adequate margins.. Although cryotherapy may successfully remove the cutaneous horn, it prevents tissue diagnosis and may not remove the entire base of the lesion.

Corn (Clavus)

Key Points

- Occur at pressure points
- Can be quite symptomatic
- Surgical or chemical debridement often necessary

Clinical presentation

A corn is a localized area of epidermal thickening occurring at locations of chronic friction or pressure, often on the feet as a result of ill-fitting shoes, bony prominences, or repetitive trauma in athletes. These occasionally painful lesions present as well-demarcated, firm papules or nodules with a central translucent hyperkeratotic core. Hard corns occur on dry, external aspects of the foot, whereas soft corns are found between toes and may be macerated from perspiration.

Diagnosis

- Diagnosis is made by clinical appearance, often aided by paring the surface with a scalpel blade

Differential diagnosis

These common lesions are rarely misdiagnosed, but they must be differentiated from plantar warts. Paring of the surface demonstrates intact skin lines with a translucent core, confirming the diagnosis. In contrast, warts have interrupted skin lines, pinpoint hemorrhages, and papilliform surfaces. A callus (tyloma) – diffuse thickening of the stratum corneum due to broad-based friction or pressure – lacks the central core characteristic of corns.

Laboratory testing

- Consider a plain X-ray of the foot to look for bony abnormalities underlying persistent or recurrent corns

Pathogenesis

Chronic pressure and friction due to ill-fitting footwear, bony protuberances, or repetitive athletic activity result in hyperkeratinization and thickening of the stratum corneum. Whereas a callus forms when pressure forces are broadly distributed, a corn forms when the pressure is localized to a small area.

Treatment

Treatment begins with prevention, because lesions will persist until the underlying cause is removed. Paring down the surface with a scalpel blade relieves pain in the short term. Hard corns can be softened with salicylic acid preparations (10–40%). It is important to ensure that salicylic acid plasters correspond exactly to the size of the lesion so as to minimize damage to surrounding skin. These should be used cautiously in patients with peripheral neuropathies as patients may fail to notice pain from improperly placed patches. Other helpful keratolytic agents include lactic acid (AmLactin, Lac-Hydrin, Lactinol) and urea (Aquadrate, Carmol). Reduce friction with properly fitting shoes, soft cushions, and orthotic devices. When these measures fail, consider surgical correction of foot deformities. Treatment avoids potential complications and is especially necessary in diabetic patients in whom lower-extremity amputation is a concern.

Pharmaceuticals

* Salicylic acid plaster 40%
* Salicylic acid 10–20% in petrolatum

Epidermal nevus

Key Points

* The term "nevus" refers to abnormal structure or cellular composition of the skin
* Epidermal nevi are cutaneous hamartomas
* 80% present in the first 12 months of life
* May occur along skin tension lines (lines of Blaschko)
* The epidermal nevus syndrome is characterized by abnormalities of other organ systems (skeletal, neurologic, etc.)

Clinical presentation

The term "epidermal nevus" (Figure 15-4) refers to a group of cutaneous hamartomas composed of structures derived from embryonal ectoderm (keratinocytes, hair follicles, and apocrine, eccrine, and sebaceous glands: Table 15-4). They are not related to melanocytic nevi that are characterized by a proliferation of melanocytes. Most appear in the first year of life as well-circumscribed hyperpigmented papules or plaques, commonly in a linear array, sometimes along lines of Blaschko. Some demonstrate characteristic midline demarcation. Extension beyond the original distribution occurs in approximately one-third of cases. Epidermal nevi variants are classified according to the predominant structure and have a predilection for certain locations (Table 15-4).

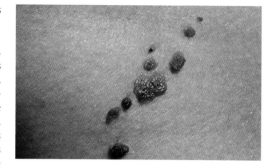

Figure 15-4 Linear epidermal nevus

Association with malignancy is rare, but occurs most commonly with nevus sebaceus. *Inflammatory linear verrucous epidermal nevus* (ILVEN: Figure 15-5) refers to a linear (following Blaschko's lines) epidermal nevus that is more common in females. The *epidermal nevus syndrome* refers to any variant of epidermal nevi associated with abnormalities in other organ systems, most commonly musculoskeletal, neurologic, or ocular. Other benign cutaneous lesions are also associated with the epidermal nevus syndrome (Table 15-5).

Diagnosis

A diagnosis of epidermal nevus is often made clinically. Biopsy confirms the diagnosis, with histologic features demonstrating the variants of epidermal nevi.

Differential diagnosis

An epidermal nevus must be differentiated from SK, verruca vulgaris, psoriasis, acrokeratosis verruciformis, lichen striatus, ichthyosis, and other linear dermatoses depending on clinical presentation.

Histological features

Histologic evaluation of epidermal nevi reveals some degree of epidermal hyperplasia, hyperkeratosis, and acanthosis. Multiple variants exist, with some cases showing a mixed histology. ILVEN is characterized by a psoriasiform histology.

Pathogenesis

These hamartomas arise from multipotent cells in the embryonic epidermis. Growth factors that induce hyperproliferation are suggested to play a role in their development, and studies show that genetic mosaicism in keratin genes leads to clinical mosaicism in the form of epidermal nevi that develop along the lines of Blaschko.

Treatment

Treatment is difficult because lesions often recur after surgical removal unless the excision extends deep into the dermis. Therefore, it is important to inform the patient that scarring is expected and may

Table 15-4 Comparison of epidermal nevus variants

Epidermal nevus	Clinical presentation	Hamartoma, predominant structure	Location
Verrucous epidermal nevus	Flesh-colored to brown verrucous Psoriasiform ± pruritis Female > male	Surface epidermis	Localized or diffuse, often on unilateral limb
Nevus sebaceus (Figure 15-6)	Yellow, verrucous, with linear configuration 20% associated with malignant transformation	Sebaceous glands	Scalp with alopecia, face, neck, or trunk
Nevus comedonicus	Grouped comedones Often linear Can become inflamed and/or infected	Hair follicles	Face, neck, upper arm, chest
Eccrine nevus	Varies, nondescript papule	Eccrine sweat glands	Head, neck, and trunk
Apocrine nevus	Varies, nondescript papule	Apocrine sweat glands	Scalp, axillae, chest

Table 15-5 Epidermal nevus syndrome findings

Cutaneous	Skeletal	Neurologic
Benign		
Hemangioma	Bone cysts	Magnetic resonance
Café-au-lait spots	Kyphosis/scoliosis	Seizures
Hypopigmentation	Spina bifida	Developmental delay
Melanocytic nevi	Skull asymmetry	Cerebrovascular accidents
Malignant		
Keratoacanthoma	Short stature	Cortical atrophy
Basal cell carcinoma	Syndactyly, polydactyly	Cranial nerve palsies
Squamous cell carcinoma	Bone hyperplasia	Hemiparesis

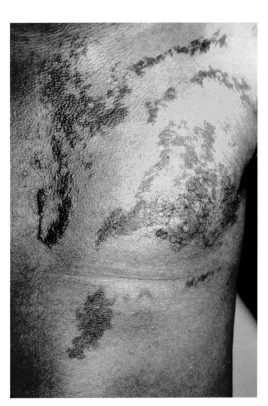

Figure 15-5 Inflammatory linear verrucous epidermal nevus

be complicated by hypertrophic scarring or even keloid formation. Treatment of ILVEN is especially difficult, but both pulsed-dye laser and long-term management with a combination of topical retinoids and 5-fluorouracil have been effective in some cases. All patients with extensive epidermal nevi should have a thorough initial evaluation, as well as regular follow-up, for possible systemic abnormalities associated with the epidermal nevus syndrome.

Clear cell acanthoma

Key Points

- Typically present as a red plaque with peripheral white scale on a leg
- Benign

Clinical presentation

Clear cell acanthomas are slow-growing, pink to brown, well-defined, dome-shaped papules or plaques with a "stuck-on" appearance similar to that of an SK. There is a wafer-like collarette of scale at the periphery. They are most often asymptomatic solitary papules on the legs that develop during middle age. Multiple lesions rarely occur and may be associated with ichthyosis.

Diagnosis

Clear cell acanthomas, demonstrating clear, glycogen-containing epidermal cells with positive periodic acid–Schiff staining and scattered neutrophils, are easily distinguished histologically from other lesions such as pyogenic granuloma, inflamed SK, hemangioma, psoriasis, verruca vulgaris, and xanthogranuloma.

Pathogenesis

Research has failed to discover a link between clear cell acanthomas and environmental trauma, drugs, toxic substances, or viruses. Enzyme deficiency (cytoplasmic phosphorylase within keratinocytes) allows glycogen accumulation within keratinocyte cytoplasm. Cells within these lesions also lack cytochrome oxidase and succinic dehydrogenase.

Treatment

Clear cell acanthomas do not spontaneously regress. Removal is most commonly achieved by shave biopsy with or without electrofulguration. Good results have also been shown with cryotherapy, and lesions do not tend to recur.

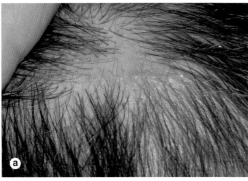

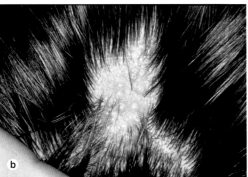

Figure 15-6 **a** Prepubertal nevus sebaceus. **b** Nevus sebaceus

CYSTS

Key Points

- Cysts are common cutaneous lesions
- True cysts have an epithelial lining, whereas pseudocysts do not
- Cysts are classified according to anatomic location, embryologic derivation, and histologic features
- Steatocystomas are the only true sebaceous cysts (Table 15-8)

Epidermoid cyst (Epidermal inclusion cyst, follicular cyst, infundibular cyst)

Clinical presentation

Epidermoid cyst is the most common type of cutaneous cyst. These benign, keratin-containing cysts are often incorrectly termed "sebaceous cysts"; however, they have no sebaceous component. They appear as flesh-colored, mobile, dome-shaped cysts with a characteristic central punctum. Common locations include the face, neck, upper trunk, and scrotum in young to middle-aged adults. The majority of these thin-walled cysts are slow-growing and asymptomatic; however, they may rupture and become inflamed and/or infected. A cream-colored, keratinaceous material with a characteristic rancid odor will be expressed upon spontaneous or intentional rupture. Scrotal lesions may calcify. Multiple epidermoid cysts presenting in atypical locations or epidermoid cysts with pilomatrical differentiation should suggest Gardner's syndrome, a rare autosomal-dominant condition characterized by numerous colonic polyps that undergo malignant transformation. Other associations include fibromas and osteomas. Patients with nevoid BCC syndrome may also have multiple epidermoid cysts.

Diagnosis

The clinical appearance of a discrete, mobile cyst with a central punctum is generally sufficient for diagnosis. Expression of malodoraous keratinaceous debris will confirm the diagnosis. Inflamed cysts are commonly misdiagnosed as infected cysts. Biopsy and histologic evaluation is definitive, but not usually necessary.

Differential diagnosis

An epidermoid cyst may be mistaken for a trichilemmal cyst (pilar cyst). Location on the scalp, a thicker wall, and lack of a central punctum favor the diagnosis of trichilemmal cyst. Lipomas are deeper and more rubbery than epidermoid cysts. Steatocystoma multiplex is characterized by numerous lesions containing an oily yellow fluid. Rapidly enlarging subcutaneous nodules without an obvious punctum may need biopsy to exclude malignancy.

Laboratory testing

Inflamed cysts are rarely infected. When infection is suspected, the contents of an epidermoid cyst may be sent for culture and sensitivity. Colonization with *Staphylococci epidermidis* and *Propionibacterium acnes* is common. A positive culture alone does not indicate infection. Inflamed cysts respond to drainage and intralesional triamcinolone. Infected cysts require antibiotic therapy. The microbiology of infected epidermoid cysts with abscess formation is shown in Table 15-6. It is important to recognize the prevalence of mixed infections. The microbiology of inflamed but uninfected epidermoid cysts is discussed below.

Pathogenesis

The majority of epidermoid cysts result from pilosebaceous follicle occlusion. The cyst wall is made of a keratin-producing epithelial lining derived from the infundibulum of a hair follicle. Cystic enclosure leads to accumulation of keratinaceous material and a cystic mass. The origin and etiology of palmoplantar epidermoid cysts are thought to be distinctive because of the lack of pilosebaceous units in these locations. Human papillomavirus and characteristic verrucous histologic changes have been reported to be present in these cysts. Although controversial, this infection in combination with trauma or mechanical pressure may contribute to the formation of cysts on the palms and soles.

Treatment

Treatment of an epidermoid cyst depends on whether the cyst is quiescent, inflamed, or infected. An inflamed, noninfected cyst can be treated with intralesional corticosteroids. Tetracycline and erythromycin have been considered for anti-inflammatory effects, but their use is not routine. An infected cyst should be incised, drained, and cultured. If surrounding cellulitis is present or with minimal to no improvement of the cyst, systemic antibiotics should be started. Empirical treatment should target the most common pathogen, *S. aureus*, and follow-up with culture and sensitivity data is important. When excision is undertaken, it is imperative to remove the entire cyst wall lining to prevent recurrence. In addition, all excised cysts should be sent for evaluation by a pathologist to confirm the diagnosis.

Treatment algorithm

See Table 15-7.

Pharmaceuticals

- Triamcinolone suspension for injection
- Antibiotics, empiric treatment to cover *S. aureus*

Dosage tables

- Triamcinolone 3–10 mg/mL intralesional; may repeat in 4–6 weeks

Controversies

Inflamed epidermoid cysts are often mistaken for infected cysts and subsequently incised, drained, and treated with systemic antibiotics. A study examining the microbiology of both inflamed and uninflamed cysts revealed no difference in the frequency of positive cultures or in the number of bacteria. *S. aureus*, the most likely potential pathogen, was uncommon and equally distributed between both groups. Because inflammation likely results from cyst wall rupture and extrusion of contents into the dermis rather than from infection, systemic antibiotics are not necessary when treating an inflamed cyst.

Trichilemmal cyst (Pilar cyst, isthmus catagen cyst)

Clinical presentation

Trichilemmal cysts are the second most common type of cutaneous cyst. They appear as smooth, mobile, firm, 0.5–5.0-cm nodules to tumors, with over 90% occurring on the scalp. Middle-aged females are most frequently affected. If the cyst is large, there may be overlying alopecia. These cysts are multiple 70% of the time and characteristically lack a central punctum. Inflammation and rupture are uncommon as the cyst wall is usually thicker than that found in epidermoid cysts. They contain dense, homogeneous keratin that often calcifies. A *proliferating trichilemmal cyst* can develop in the elderly as a rapidly growing, lobulated mass that may ulcerate. These are locally destructive, and cases of malignant transformation have been reported. Multiple cysts, usually developing at an earlier age, are inherited as an autosomal-dominant trait.

Table 15-6 Microbiology of inflamed epidermoid cysts with abscess formation		
Aerobes	44%	*Staphylococcus aureus*
		Group A streptococci
		Escherichia coli
Anaerobes	30%	*Peptostreptococcus*
		Bacteroides
Mixed	26%	26%

Table 15-7 Cyst treatment algorithm

Quiescent cyst		Inflamed, noninfected	Infected cyst
Freely mobile	Slightly mobile or nonmobile	Warm compresses + intralesional triamcinolone (3 mg/mL face, 10 mg/mL trunk)	Incision and drainage:
↓	↓		1% lidocaine (may cause cyst rupture if injected into cyst cavity)
Punch or incise	Dissect or excise	↓ ↓	↓
(Removal of cyst lining imperative)	(Removal of cyst lining imperative)	May resolve Surgical excision	Culture and sensitivity studies
		(wait 4–6 weeks after inflammation has resolved; removal of cyst lining imperative)	↓
			Consider wound packing with iodoform gauze
			Consider replacement if not draining effectively after 24 hours
			Infected wounds should not be sutured
			↓
			Systemic antibiotics
			Consider antibiotics with staphylococcal coverage if mild or no improvement, immunocomprised, or evidence of local/systemic spread
			↓
			± Excision at a later time

Table 15-8 Follicular derivation of cysts

Infundibulum	Epidermal cyst, milium
Sebaceous duct	Steatocystoma multiplex and simplex
Outer-root sheath	Trichilemmal cyst

Diagnosis

Diagnosis can be made by clinical presentation. Histological evaluation is confirmatory.

Differential diagnosis

The differential diagnosis is the same as for epidermoid cysts. Location on the scalp favors the diagnosis of a trichilemmal cyst. Proliferating trichilemmal cysts with severe atypia may represent trichilemmal carcinoma.

Histological features

Trichilemmal cysts are characterized by a stratified squamous epithelial lining that lacks an inner granular layer. The outer layer resembles the outer root sheath of a hair follicle.

Pathogenesis

Because trichilemmal cysts are found predominantly at sites of dense hair follicle concentration and resemble the outer root sheath, it is hypothesized that they originate as a structural abnormality, possibly genetically determined, given the frequent autosomal-dominant inheritance pattern.

Treatment

An uncomplicated cyst can frequently be removed intact without difficulty because of the thick wall. Proliferating trichilemmal cysts must be excised with adequate margins to ensure complete removal.

Milium

Clinical presentation

Milia are small, superficial epidermoid cysts. They are most common on the face and have a predilection for the periorbital region of thin skin. Clinically, they appear as 0.5–2.0-mm superficial, white to yellow papules. They contain keratin, may be solitary or multiple, and can occur at any age. Milia occurring on the palate of infants are referred to as Epstein's pearls. Primary and secondary forms exist (see pathogenesis section, below), but both are morphologically identical.

Diagnosis

Diagnosis is made on the clinical presentation of milia. Acne vulgaris, syringomas, and trichoepitheliomas should also be considered in the differential diagnosis.

Pathogenesis

Primary milia arise de novo from multipotential cells in epidermal or adnexal epithelium at a pilosebaceous follicle. Secondary milia develop after injury (blistering dermatoses, dermabrasion, burns, radiotherapy, etc.) and may arise from a hair follicle, sweat duct, sebaceous duct, or epidermis.

Treatment

Removal of milia involves incision with a scalpel blade or needle and expression of contents via compression with a comedone extractor. When numerous milia are present, treatment with superficial electrodesiccation may be successful. After the charred epidermal surface sloughs off, the keratin core can be removed. Recurrence of milia is common.

Steatocystoma multiplex

Clinical presentation

Steatocystoma multiplex is characterized by the presence of multiple sebum-containing dermal cysts with an epithelial lining containing sebaceous glands. These flesh-colored to yellow, smooth, firm, cystic papules and nodules begin to appear in adolescence or early adulthood. The most common locations are the trunk and proximal extremities, but they can be found anywhere. These are the only true cysts that contain sebaceous glands in their lining, and after lancing, a characteristic oily or creamy fluid is discharged. Cysts are typically asymptomatic, but may become inflamed or infected and heal with scarring. *Steatocystoma simplex* describes the presence of a solitary lesion with no hereditary tendency.

Diagnosis

Diagnosis is made by the combination of clinical presentation, morphological appearance, and family history.

Differential diagnosis

Given the similar anatomic distribution and timing of presentation, steatocystoma multiplex is easily confused with eruptive vellus hair cysts. Scarring acne vulgaris, milia, and syringoma are also in the differential diagnosis.

Histological features

Laboratory testing and biopsy are rarely required. Histopathological examination reveals characteristic sebaceous glands in the cyst wall.

Pathogenesis

Steatocystoma multiplex may have an autosomal-dominant inheritance pattern. Steatocystoma simplex has no hereditary predisposition. Given the association with sebaceous gland development and the appearance at puberty, a hormonal etiology has been suggested.

Treatment

Individual cysts may be surgically excised. Carbon dioxide laser has been reported to be effective in treating multiple lesions. An inflamed lesion should either be excised or treated with incision and drainage with or without intralesional steroids.

Dermoid cyst

Clinical presentation

Dermoid cysts present at birth or early childhood as solitary subcutaneous nodules located along embryonal fusion planes, including the lateral third of the eyebrows, nose, and scalp. These uncommon cysts are smooth, mobile, and firm and they slowly grow with time. They may contain tufts of hair and a cheesy material. Complications include inflammation and infection. Dermoid cysts can be complicated by intracranial extension, which may lead to serious neurologic complications.

Diagnosis

Diagnosis should be suspected on clinical presentation. Histological evaluation is confirmatory.

Differential diagnosis

Other types of cysts, glioma, encephalocele, fibrosarcoma, rhabdomyosarcoma, and hemangiomas are in the differential (Table 15-9). Early appearance of the cyst is often helpful in leading to the correct diagnosis.

Histological features

Biopsy of a dermoid cyst will show a wall with an epidermal lining containing different types of skin appendages, including hair follicles, sweat glands, and sebaceous glands. The presence of hairs within and projecting from the cyst is characteristic. Evaluation for possible intracranial communication with consultation and/or imaging studies may be necessary.

Pathogenesis

Dermoid cysts develop as a result of the sequestration of epithelium along lines of embryonic fusion.

Treatment

Surgical excision is the treatment of choice, but commonly requires advanced imaging and the involvement of a neurosurgeon. To prevent recurrence, it is important to ensure removal of any possible underlying sinus tract.

MELANOCYTIC

Key Points

- Common acquired melanocytic nevi can be junctional, compound, or intradermal
- The significance of numerous atypical nevi is controversial, but has been associated with an increased risk of developing melanoma and these patients should therefore be followed closely
- Other variants of melanocytic nevi (Spitz nevus, blue nevus, halo nevus, and nevus spilus) are benign, but must be differentiated from melanoma

Common acquired melanocytic nevus (Nevus cell nevus, nevocellular nevus, pigmented nevus, pigmented mole, common mole, melanocytic nevus, cellular nevus)

Clinical presentation

The common acquired melanocytic nevus (Figure 15-7) is a collection of melanocytes in the epidermis (junctional nevus), dermis (intradermal nevus), or both (compound nevus). Their appearance varies significantly, but in general they have an orderly, homogeneous surface with symmetry

Table 15-9 Comparison of cysts

	Epidermoid cyst	Trichilemmal cyst	Milium	Steatocystoma multiplex	Dermoid cyst
Clinical appearance	± Central punctum Pressure expresses cheesy material with rancid odor	Often indistinguishable from epidermoid cysts Lack central punctum Overlying alopecia when large	Single or multiple 0.5–2 mm white to yellow papules Primary and secondary: milia clinically indistinguishable	Multiple flesh-colored to yellow smooth cystic papules or nodules	Solitary, smooth, mobile ± tufts of hair Express cheesy material
Location	Face, upper trunk, scrotum Palms and soles	90% on scalp	Primary: Eyelids, cheeks, forehead in pilosebaceous follicles Secondary: Sites of trauma	Chest, axillae, and groin, but can occur anywhere	Around the eyes (lateral one-third of eyebrows, nose, and scalp)
Epidemiology	Most common cutaneous cyst	Less common than epidermoid cysts	Present in approx. half of infants. All ages affected	Appear in adolescence and early adulthood	Appear at birth or early childhood
Pathogenesis	1. Occlusion of pilosebaceous follicles 2. Trapping of epidermal cells in dermis status posttraumatic implantation (palmoplantar) 3. Trapping of epidermal cells along embryonal fusion planes	Structural abnormality at hair follicle Genetic role	Primary: Arise de novo at pilosebacous follicle Secondary: status postinjury: blistering dermatoses, dermabrasion, burns, radiation, etc.	Multiplex shows genetic predisposition versus steatocystoma simplex, which does not Possible hormonal influence	Epithelial sequestration along embryonic lines of fusion
Contents	Laminated keratin, cream-colored with rancid odor	Keratin: very dense, pink, homogeneous, often calcified	Laminated keratin	Oily fluid, only true sebaceous cyst	Cheesy material ± hairs within and projecting from cyst

Continued

Table 15-9 Comparison of cysts—Cont'd

	Epidermoid cyst	Trichilemmal cyst	Milium	Steatocystoma multiplex	Dermoid cyst
Wall lining histology (all lined with stratified squamous epithelium)	+ Granular layer	No granular layer\n\nKeratinization of outer-root sheath of hair follicle	Same as small epidermoid cyst, + granular layer	+ Granular layer\n\nCrenulated pink lining\n\n+ Small sebaceous lobules in or adjacent to cyst wall	Epidermis with various mature epidermal appendages (hair follicles, sweat glands, and sebaceous glands)
Complications	→ Basal cell carcinoma/ squamous cell carcinoma very rarely	Proliferating trichilemmal cyst (elderly women)		Inflammation and/or infection	Inflammation and/or infection\n\nIntracranial communication
Treatment	See Table 15-7	Same as for epidermoid cysts; see Table 15-7\n\nEnsure adequate margins with proliferating trichilemmal cysts	1. Incise with needle or scalpel and express contents with comedone extractor\n\n2. Multiple – laser ablation and electrodesiccation\n\n3. Multiple facial – topical retinoids	When single/few: treatment same as for epidermoid cysts (see Table 15-7)\n\nWhen multiple: surgical excision difficult, carbon dioxide laser	Similar to treatment for epidermoid cysts unless CNS connection is present; see algorithm\n\nImaging studies to exclude connection to CNS
Associations, inheritance	1. Gardner's syndrome (familial adenomatous polyposis)\n\n2. Nevoid basal cell carcinoma syndrome	Multiple lesions may be inherited in autosomal-dominant fashion	Secondary: Milia associated with blistering dermatoses	Autosomal-dominant\n\nPachyonychia congenital type II	Connection to CNS

CNS, central nervous system.

and a regular, well-defined border. Nevi can be elevated, polypoid, or sessile. Skin lines and hair may or may not be present. Acquired nevi develop after birth, with most appearing by age 20. The onset of puberty is often accompanied by rapid development of newly acquired nevi. These will slowly enlarge, stabilize, and gradually involute before disappearing by the seventh or eighth decade. Males and females are affected equally, and the average adult has 20 nevi. The prevalence depends on race and environmental factors, with higher numbers of nevi present in fair-skinned individuals who have had significant ultraviolet exposure. Common locations are listed in Table 15-10, but any nevi can be found on all areas of skin, including the palms and soles, nail beds, and conjunctivae. Both Turner's and Noonan's syndromes are characterized by numerous nevi of large size.

Diagnosis

Diagnosis of common acquired melanocytic nevi is usually made by clinical presentation alone (see Figure 15-7). Histopathologic evaluation is confirmatory.

Differential diagnosis

Malignant melanoma is the most important diagnosis to exclude. Junctional, compound, and intradermal nevi have distinct differential diagnoses given their different appearances (see Table 15-10).

Histological features

Histologic evaluation of nevi must include assessment of both the architecture and cytology of the melanocytes. Whenever possible, the entire pigmented lesion should be removed and examined, as partial biopsies limit the assessment of symmetry and circumscription of the lesion. Benign nevi have regular collections of melanocytes in the epidermis, dermis, or both.

Pathogenesis

The proliferation of melanocytes, derived from the neural crest, within the epidermis leads to the formation of junctional nevi. With subsequent "drop-off" of these cells into the dermis, compound and eventually intradermal nevi are formed. Whether nevi represent hamartomas

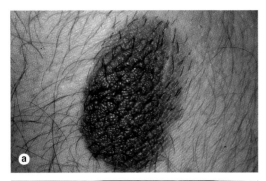

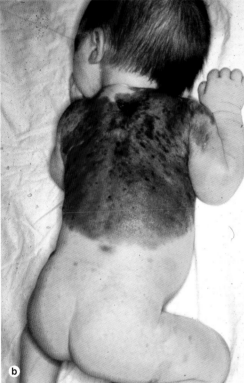

Figure 15-7 a Melanocytic nevus. b Congenital nevus

or benign neoplasms is debated. Solar nevogenesis is thought to be due to ultraviolet-induced alterations in cytokine production and melanocyte adhesion molecules. A genetic role is supported by a strong correlation of nevi with fair skin color, blond and red hair, and light-colored eyes. The eruptive growth of nevi in adolescence and pregnancy results from increased pigmentation induced by increased levels of melanocyte-stimulating hormone.

Treatment

The majority of common acquired melanocytic nevi do not require treatment. Indications for removal include cosmetic concerns, chronic irritation with itching and/or bleeding, changes in appearance (color, size, or shape), and an

appearance suspicious for melanoma. Nevi can be removed by shave technique, punch or elliptical excision, or by deep tangential excision. Recurrent lesions may demonstrate clinical and histological irregularity and can sometimes be difficult to distinguish from melanoma. All biopsied nevi should be examined histopathologically. Destructive methods, including cryotherapy, electrodesiccation, dermabrasion and laser treatment, are not recommended. The use of a photographic record can be useful in the monitoring of nevi for changes over time.

Atypical melanocytic nevus (Dysplastic nevus, Clark's nevus, B-K mole, atypical mole, nevus with architectural disorder)

Clinical presentation

Atypical melanocytic nevi (AMN) are single or multiple and have atypical morphological features, including large size, asymmetry, borders, and/or color variation. It is thought that atypical nevi occupy an intermediate position on the continuum from common acquired nevi to malignant melanoma (Table 15-11). In contrast to common acquired nevi, which typically appear before age 20 and eventually involute, atypical nevi may arise at any age and do not regress. The trunk is the most common site, with the scalp and buttocks as other favored locations. Five percent of the general population develops at least one AMN in a lifetime. Patients with the familial atypical mole syndrome (FAMS) have an increased risk of melanoma that is 150 times that of the general population. Criteria for the FAMS include: (1) a first- or second-degree relative with malignant melanoma; (2) presence of greater than 50 nevi, some of which are atypical; and (3) nevi that demonstrate certain histologic features. Although the precise clinical and histologic criteria for recognition and the exact biological significance of AMN are unclear, the lesions serve as a marker for an increased risk of melanoma in both the solitary and multiple forms.

Diagnosis

AMNs are recognized clinically. The combination of several atypical clinical findings (asymmetry, size, borders, color, "pebbled" surface, accentuation of skin markings) favor the diagnosis. Dermoscopy performed by trained individuals may be helpful. Excision and histopathological evaluation are necessary for definitive diagnosis, because not all atypical-appearing nevi demonstrate an atypical histology.

Table 15-10 Comparison of junctional, compound, and intradermal nevi

	Junctional nevus	Compound nevus	Intradermal nevus
Melanocyte location	Epidermis	Epidermis and dermis	Dermis
Primary lesion	Macule	Papule (smooth or rough)	Papule
Color	Light to dark brown	Pigmented > flesh-colored	Flesh-colored
Anatomic locations	Trunk, extremities, face	Face, scalp, trunk, extremities	Face/neck > extremities
Differential diagnosis	Solar lentigo	Seborrheic keratosis	Basal cell carcinoma
	Lentigo maligna	Dermatofibroma	Neurofibroma
	Café-au-lait macule	Atypical nevus	Trichoepithelioma
	Melanoma	Spitz nevus	Sebaceous hyperplasia
	Atypical nevus	Blue nevus	Dermatofibroma
	Congenital nevus	Melanoma	Acrochordon
		Atypical nevus	Verruca
			Nodular melanoma
			Clear cell acanthoma
			Appendageal tumors

Table 15-11 Comparison of common acquired nevi, atypical nevi, and malignant melanoma

Feature	Common acquired nevi	Atypical nevi	Malignant melanoma
Age of onset	Usually evident by age 20	May develop new lesions throughout life	Any age
Primary lesion type	Junctional nevi – macules Compound and dermal nevi – papules	Macules or papules with elevated portions, especially at center	Macule – lentigo maligna Plaque – superficial spreading or lentigo maligna melanoma Nodules – superficial spreading, lentigo maligna melanoma, or nodular
Anatomic distribution	Anywhere (? with sparing of sun-protected areas)	Trunk, arms, and legs. Rarely on the face. Sun-protected and unprotected areas	Anywhere. Upper back, legs, trunk, and arms most common
Size	Usually < 5–6 mm	Usually > 5 mm, may be smaller	Usually > 10 mm
Color	Flesh-color, tan, light or dark brown	Tan, light or dark brown, black, or pink	Brown, black, red, gray, blue, or white
Color pattern – naked eye versus dermoscopy	Uniform, regular	Variegated, haphazard. Usually more than two shades	Variegated
Shape	Symmetrical, round or oval	Asymmetrical, round or oval, ellipsoid	Asymmetrical, round, oval, ellipsoid
Border	Well-defined, regular	Ill-defined, irregular	Ill-defined, irregular
Surface (oblique lighting) and skin markings	Usually papular, accentuated skin markings	Macular component, "pebbling"	Macular, raised nodular Accentuation, obliteration, ulceration

Differential diagnosis

The differential diagnosis of AMN includes common melanocytic nevus, congenital nevus, malignant melanoma, lentigo maligna, Spitz nevus, blue nevus, solar lentigo, SK, pigmented actinic keratosis, pigmented BCC, angioma, pyogenic granuloma, dermatofibroma (DF), sclerosing hemangioma, and nevus spilus.

Histological features

Histopathological evaluation is necessary to confirm the diagnosis of AMN and to rule out malignant melanoma. AMNs have abnormal melanocytic architecture with variable cytologic atypia.

Pathogenesis

Atypical nevi occurring in the familial syndromes have been mapped to genetic alterations at chromosome loci 1p36 and 9p21. An effect of ultraviolet radiation has been suggested; however, the direct effect has not been proven.

Treatment

Any lesion suspicious for melanoma should be completely excised and sent for histological evaluation. Saucerization (scoop or deep tangential removal) is often the preferred method. Lesions with significantly atypical features or those in difficult-to-monitor locations such as the scalp may also warrant removal. Prophylactic removal of all AMNs results in unnecessary surgery and can be cosmetically disfiguring. Where available, use of serial photography and dermoscopy may enhance the monitoring of patients with atypical nevi. Sun protection, monthly self-examination, and screening of relatives for atypical nevi and melanoma are other important aspects of treatment. The use of lasers and other physically destructive methods that prohibit histological evaluation is not recommended.

Treatment algorithm

See Figure 15-8.

Controversies

Exactly what atypical nevi are, and the best way to manage patients with them, have yet to be defined. Five percent of the Caucasian population have at least one AMN and never develop melanoma. Pathologists disagree on the precise description of atypical nevi and several terms, including "nevus with architectural disorder," are commonly used (Table 15-11).

Spitz nevus (Benign juvenile melanoma, epithelioid cell – spindle cell nevus)

Clinical presentation

A Spitz nevus is a clinically benign 2-mm to 2-cm well-defined pink to pigmented papule or nodule that histologically mimics melanoma. Approximately one-half appear in children; persons over 40 years of age are rarely affected. A history of recent onset or rapid growth can often be elicited. They may occur anywhere, but the face, trunk, and extremities are common locations. Lesions are typically solitary, but they may be numerous.

Diagnosis

Definitive diagnosis must be confirmed with histologic evaluation by an expert pathologist.

Differential diagnosis

Spitz nevi clinically can mimic dermal melanocytic nevi, AMN, pyogenic granulomas, hemangiomas, juvenile xanthogranulomas, DFs, and verrucae.

Histological features

The histology of a Spitz nevus is often misleading because of atypical features (mitotic figures, melanocytes at all epidermal levels) similar to those found in melanoma. A skilled dermatopathologist will be able to distinguish between a Spitz nevus and melanoma in most cases, although approximately 8% of cases are equivocal. Spitz nevi have large and/or spindle-shaped melanocytes with maturation of the cellular

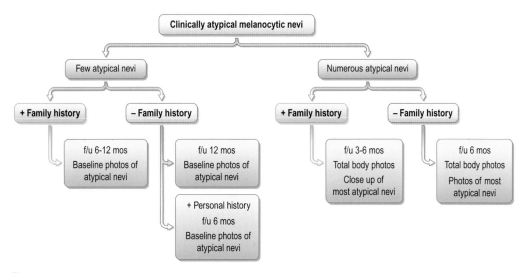

Figure 15-8 Atypical melanocytic nevus treatment algorithm

elements toward the base. Genetic evaluation for mutations and chromosomal rearrangements may prove useful in the future to differentiate Spitz nevi from melanomas.

Pathogenesis

The cause of Spitz nevi is unknown; however, human immunodeficiency virus (HIV), Addison's disease, and treatment with chemotherapy have been associated with eruptive, widespread lesions. A hormonal etiology has also been suggested because of the association with pregnancy and puberty.

Treatment

Treatment involves surgical excision and histologic evaluation of the entire lesion if possible. Complete removal of the Spitz nevus is important because they may be difficult to distinguish from melanoma and 10–15% recur following incomplete excision. Follow-up in 6–12 months is recommended.

Blue nevus

Clinical presentation

Blue nevi (Figure 15-9) are blue to blue-gray, firm, well-demarcated papules or nodules acquired in childhood and adolescence. These asymptomatic, solitary, benign lesions are composed of melanin-producing melanocytes in the dermis. The dorsa of hands and feet, scalp, and sacral region are typical locations. Prevalence is 3–5% in Asians, compared to only 1–2% in Caucasians. Two recognized subtypes are the common blue nevus and the less common cellular blue nevus, which is larger (1–3 cm) and associated with malignant melanoma in rare cases. Multiple blue nevi are associated with LAMB syndrome (lentigines, atrial myxomas, mucocutaneous myxomas, and blue nevi).

Diagnosis

Diagnosis is made on clinical presentation.

Differential diagnosis

The differential diagnosis of blue nevus includes primary or metastatic melanoma, pigmented spindle cell nevus, atypical nevus, sclerosing hemangioma, DF, pigmented BCC, and nevi of Ota and Ito.

Laboratory testing

When diagnosis is uncertain, biopsy with histologic evaluation is necessary to rule out malignant processes. Blue nevi should be biopsied when a lesion appears de novo, undergoes a sudden change, or has a multinodular or plaque-like appearance.

Pathogenesis

Blue nevi represent the ectopic accumulation of melanocytes in the dermis after failure to migrate from the neural crest to epidermal sites.

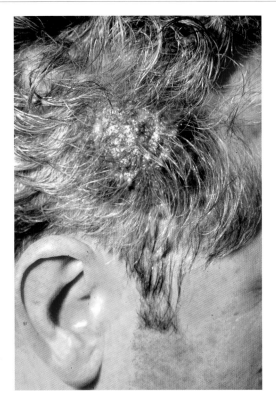

Figure 15-9 Giant blue nevus

Collections of melanocytes are normally found in the fetal dermis; however, these typically involute later in gestation. The blue color is a result of the Tyndall phenomenon, in which short blue wavelengths do not penetrate deep enough into the dermis to be absorbed by melanin, and are therefore reflected back to the observer's eye.

Treatment

Treatment of unchanging, stable blue nevi is unnecessary. With new onset or sudden change in a lesion, histologic evaluation is recommended. Because of a small risk of malignant transformation of cellular blue nevi, complete resection, including subcutaneous fat to ensure removal of dermal melanocytes, is recommended.

Halo nevus

Clinical presentation

Halo nevus (Figure 15-10) is a nevomelanocytic nevus surrounded by a symmetric halo of macular depigmentation with sharply defined borders. Its development often indicates the beginning of regression of the central nevus. Halo nevi are most commonly found on the posterior trunk in teenagers, and multiple lesions may occur simultaneously. Halo nevi typically develop in several stages. First, a halo arises around a pre-existing nevus over the course of several months. The nevus then regresses over months to years and is followed by repigmentation of the halo. Halo nevi are associated with vitiligo, and depigmentation may rarely develop around a primary malignant melanoma.

Diagnosis

Diagnosis of halo nevus is made clinically by the presence of macular depigmentation surrounding a nevus.

Differential diagnosis

The halo is actually a reaction pattern that can occur around both melanocytic and nonmelanocytic lesions, including blue nevus, Spitz nevus, primary melanoma, verruca plana, DF, neurofibroma, hypopigmented sarcoidosis, and papular urticaria.

Laboratory testing

The central lesion should be evaluated like any other pigmented lesion, and biopsy is only required in the presence of worrisome features. Examination with Wood's lamp is often useful.

Pathogenesis

The pathogenesis of halo nevi is poorly understood. The halo of depigmentation represents a decrease of melanin at the dermoepidermal junction, likely due to a combination of both humoral and cellular immunologic phenomena that result in the destruction of nevus cells.

Treatment

Patients with a halo nevus should have a thorough skin exam to rule out atypical nevi, malignant melanoma, and vitiligo. If the central lesion has no worrisome features, no treatment is required and spontaneous regression often occurs.

Nevus spilus (Speckled lentiginous nevus, zosteriform lentiginous nevus)

Clinical presentation

Nevus spilus (Figure 15-11) (Greek *spilos*, meaning "spot") is a well-circumscribed tan macule or patch with many smaller dark brown macules or papules scattered throughout the hyperpigmented background. Most are acquired during infancy or childhood, with approximately 2–3% of the adult Caucasian population affected. The trunk and extremities are common locations. A nevus spilus does not disappear with time, and increased speckling may occur with ultraviolet exposure. Malignant melanoma and/or atypical nevi rarely arise within these lesions. Larger varieties occur

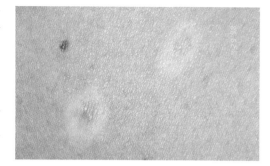

Figure 15-10 Halo nevus

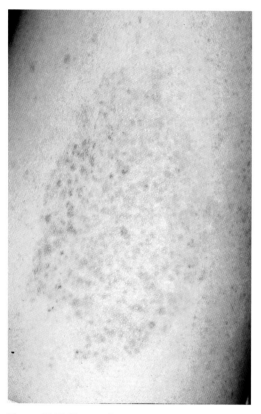

Figure 15-11 Nevus spilus

and are occasionally found in a segmental or zosteriform distribution.

Diagnosis

Clinical features are usually sufficient for diagnosis. Biopsy may be necessary to confirm the diagnosis or to evaluate atypical areas for melanoma.

Differential diagnosis

The nevus spilus may be mistaken for a café-au-lait spot, congenital nevus, or lentigo. Biopsy may reveal the small internal hyperpigmented macules and papules to be lentigines, junctional or compound nevi, spindle cell nevi, blue nevi, dyplastic nevi, or melanoma.

Histological features

The pathology of nevus spilus shows increased melanocytes similar to a lentigo simplex. Smaller internal areas are often junctional or compound nevi. Rarely, atypical nevi are present.

Pathogenesis

How nevus spilus differs from other melanocytic nevi in its pathogenesis is unknown. It may represent a localized defect in neural crest melanoblasts. Familial cases have not been reported, but genetic factors may play a role. Mosaicism has been suggested to explain the zosteriform variant.

Treatment

Patients with nevus spilus should be followed regularly with photography. A biopsy or excision of areas with change or atypical appearance should be done, following the same guidelines for evaluation of other nevi. To prevent recurrence of hyperpigmenation, the entire area must be excised. Cosmetically, laser treatment of nevus spilus has not been promising.

Controversies

The association between nevus spilus and melanoma is not well understood. At least 20 cases of melanoma arising within nevus spilus have been reported. In terms of serving as a risk marker for melanoma, one study reveled 4.8% of melanoma patients compared to 2.3% of dermatological outpatients to be affected by nevus spilus.

Becker's nevus (Becker's melanosis, pigmented hairy epidermal nevus)

Clinical presentation

Becker's nevus is an acquired unilateral, well-demarcated, but irregularly shaped, hyperpigmented macule or patch, most commonly found on the shoulder region of males around the time of puberty. It often has hypertrichosis. On rare occasions, there are associated developmental abnormalities, including smooth-muscle hamartomas, hypoplasia of underlying structures, and other soft-tissue and bony abnormalities.

Diagnosis

Diagnosis is made by clinical appearance and history.

Differential diagnosis

Becker's nevi are often mistaken for congenital melanocytic nevi, which are more elevated and are present since birth. Epidermal nevi, also hamartomas, more commonly appear along lines of Blaschko. If hypertrichosis is not present, lesions may be confused with café-au-lait patches or postinflammatory hyperpigmentation.

Pathogenesis

The pathogenesis is unknown; however, androgen hypersensitivity may be a factor given the onset with puberty, male predominance, hypertrichosis, and reports of an increased number of androgen receptors in the affected skin.

Treatment

Biopsy should be done, if needed, to rule out a hairy congenital nevus. Because Becker's nevus is a purely benign lesion, removal is for cosmetic purposes only. Q-switched ruby lasers are successful for treating hyperpigmentation and hypertrichosis. Surgical excision is unnecessary and may result in extensive scarring.

Deep pentrating nevus

Clinical presentation

Deep penetrating nevus (DPN) is a benign melanocytic lesion that may be mistaken for malignant melanoma. Typically, DPN is a solitary, darkly pigmented, dome-shaped, papule (< 1 cm) on the face, neck, or shoulders of young adults.

Diagnosis

Diagnosis is made by clinical appearance and histopathological evaluation.

Differential diagnosis

Clinical and histopathological features of DPN may be confused with primary and metastatic malignant melanoma, pigmented nevus, common blue nevus, and Spitz nevus. In one series, 29% of DPN were misdiagnosed as melanoma. When compared to melanoma, DPN is well demarcated and symmetrical with an outline resembling a bulbous finger pushing into the dermis. Nuclei are uniform and hyperchromatic with a smudged chromatin pattern and inconspicuous nucleoli. Other distinguishing features include the absence of pagetoid epidermal involvement, absence of mitotic figures, and absence of the characteristic host responses of fibroplasia and lymphoplasmacytic infiltrate found in melanomas.

Histological features

Histologically, DPN is a wedge-shaped lesion that extends into the deep reticular dermis and sometimes into the subcutaneous fat. The upper portion is well circumscribed, containing nests and fascicles of pigmented spindle-shaped melanocytes that can be associated with blood vessels, nerves, and adnexal structures. Low-grade cellular atypia is present; however, mitotic figures are extremely rare.

Treatment

Although a benign lesion, treatment of DPN by surgical excision is often necessary to rule out malignant melanoma.

SOFT TISSUE

Dermatofibroma (Fibrous histiocytoma)

Key Point

* Firm dermal papules that dimple when the adjacent skin is compressed

Clinical presentation

DFs are common dermal nodules that typically occur on the lower extremities of young adult women. They appear as 5–10-mm firm, light tan to dark brown papules. Palpation reveals the fibrotic and indurated nature of these slightly elevated asymptomatic or tender lesions. Lateral compression with the thumb and index finger demonstrates the characteristic and specific "dimple sign," evidenced by central depression of the lesion. *Dermatofibrosarcoma protuberans* (DFSP) should be considered with large, slowly growing DFs with irregular borders. This low-grade, malignant, fibrous tumor rarely metastasizes, but demonstrates continued local growth. DFs are typically solitary; however, a variant with multiple (> 15) DFs has been described with associated immune dysfunction such as HIV, leukemia, or systemic lupus erythematosus.

Diagnosis

The diagnosis of DF is generally made by clinical features. Biopsy to rule out malignancy should be done if the diagnosis is uncertain.

Differential diagnosis

Because DFs are frequently hyperpigmented, nevus and melanoma are in the differential diagnoses. Others include Spitz nevus, scar, metastatic carcinoma of the skin, and neurilemmoma. DFSP should also be considered with large, slowly growing lesions with irregular borders.

Histological features

A number of well-described histologic variants of DF exist. In general, histologic evaluation reveals a focal proliferation of densely packed bands of collagen, often with an overlying hyperplastic epidermis. Immunohistochemical staining reveals CD34–/factor XIIIa+ cells, in contrast to CD34+/factor XIIIa– cells in cases of DFSP. In the presence of multiple DFs (> 15), screening for autoimmune diseases and causes of altered immunity should be completed.

Pathogenesis

The exact mechanism of development is unknown. DFs have been classified as both reactive and neoplastic processes. Trauma, such as an insect bite, may initiate the reactive growth of a DF. The persistent nature of DFs and demonstration of clonal proliferative growth both support a neoplastic process.

Treatment

Treatment of a DF is not indicated unless biopsy or excision to rule out melanoma is necessary. Up to 20% recur after simple biopsy. The remaining scar may be more evident than the original lesion, making routine removal for cosmetic purposes on any part of the body unfavorable.

NEURAL LESIONS

Key Points

* Benign neural growths are of neuroectodermal origin, as are melanocytic growths
* Hamartomatous processes include neuromas and neurofibromas, while schwannomas, nerve sheath myxomas, and granular cell tumors represent true neoplastic growths (Table 15-12)
* Associated syndromes include neurofibromatosis 1 (NF-1) and NF-2

Neuromas (Traumatic/ amputation neuroma, palisaded encapsulated neuroma)

Neuromas are nonneoplastic, hamartomatous proliferations of Schwann cells and axons. There are two major subtypes. *Traumatic (amputation) neuromas* result from injury when regenerating nerve fibers proliferate in a chaotic tangle. They appear as flesh-colored, firm papules or nodules with variable symptoms ranging from severe pain, itching, to tingling. Histologically, neuromas demonstrate an encapsulated, but disorganized, proliferation of axons and Schwann cells with fibrosis.

Palisaded encapsulated neuroma (PEN) is an asymptomatic flesh-colored to pink, rubbery papule or nodule on the face of adults. It represents primary hyperplasia of peripheral nerve fibers and is not associated with injury. Treatment of both types of neuromas is simple excision.

Table 15-12 Benign neural hamartomas and tumors

	Traumatic neuroma	Palisaded encapsulated neuroma (PEN)	Neurofibroma	Schwannoma	Nerve sheath myxoma
Location	Site of previous trauma	Face (90%)	Trunk, head	Head, flexor aspect of extremities	Head and upper extremities
Clinical appearance	Flesh-colored, firm papules or nodules	Flesh-colored to pink, rubbery, firm papules or nodules	Flesh-colored papules or nodules, often pedunculated, "buttonhole sign"	Smooth, soft nodules or tumors	Soft, flesh-colored papules and nodules
Symptoms	Tingling, itching, and/or pain	Asymptomatic	Asymptomatic	Rarely painful or with paresthesias	Asymptomatic
Differential diagnosis	Hypertrophic scar Keloid DF Granuloma	Intradermal nevus Basal cell carcinoma Neurofibroma Adnexal tumors	Neuromas DF Intradermal nevi Skin tags	Lipoma Angiolipoma Adnexal tumors Dermoid cysts Leiomyoma Ganglion cysts Melanocytic nevi	Myxoid cyst Ganglion cyst Intradermal nevi Adnexal tumors DF Keloid Hemangioma
Association	None	Multiple seen in MEN2B	NF if multiple	NF2 rarely	None
Histology	Poorly organized tangles of nerve fasicles, axons, areas of fibrosis	Incomplete encapsulation, palisading of nuclei usually not well developed	Unencapsulated; rare axons	Encapsulated spindle cell proliferation; palisading of nuclei and Verocay bodies; axons absent	Axons absent; lobular/fascicular pattern
Hamartoma/tumor	Hamartoma	Hamartoma	Hamartoma	Tumor	Tumor
Treatment	Simple excision	Excision/enucleation	Simple excision; consider evaluation for NF1	Excision/enucleation	Simple excision; recur if removal incomplete

DF, dermatofibroma; MEN2B, multiple endocrine neoplasia-2B; NF, neurofibromatosis.

Schwannoma (Neuriliemmoma)

Schwannomas are deep encapsulated benign nerve sheath neoplasms that consist of proliferating Schwann cells with no axons. They appear as nondescript papules or nodules on the flexural aspects of extremities along the distribution of a peripheral nerve. Although typically asymptomatic, they may become painful and have associated motor disturbances or parasthesias. Approximately 90% are solitary. The remaining 10% are multiple and may be associated with NF-2 and meningiomas. Psammomatous melanotic schwannoma is associated with the Carney complex.

Neurofibroma

Neurofibromas are flesh-colored to tan papules or nodules that are often pedunculated. They characteristically demonstrate the "buttonhole sign," described as invagination of the lesion with lateral pressure. Solitary neurofibromas are common in young adults and have no anatomic predilection. Multiple neurofibromas are typically located on the trunk and extremities and may be associated with NF-1, or von Recklinghausen disease. In contrast to schwannomas, both solitary and multiple neurofibromas demonstrate the proliferation of several cell types. Variants include diffuse, pigmented, and plexiform neurofibromas. The plexiform variant, a pedunculated mass covered by hyperpigmented skin, is pathognomonic for NF-1 and carries a higher risk of malignant transformation. Treatment is with simple excision with consideration of evaluation for NF-1.

Nerve sheath myxoma

Nerve sheath myxoma is a proliferation of nerve sheath cells within a myxomatous stroma. They appear as flesh-colored papules and nodules on the head and neck of young to middle-aged women. These benign lesions are susceptible to local recurrence after incomplete excision. Three variants based on the amount of myxomatous stroma exist and include the classic, myxoid, and cellular types.

Pyogenic granuloma

Key Points

- Exophytic friable lesions
- Often crusted
- Bleed easily

Clinical presentation

The term "pyogenic granuloma" is misleading, since these lesions are neither pyogenic nor granulomatous. They present as a rapidly developing red to violaceous or brown to black papule or nodule that frequently arise at sites of minor trauma. Pyogenic granulomas (Figure 15-12) are composed of benign blood vessels, frequently bleed or ulcerate, and are usually pedunculated. Common sites include face, fingers, toes, and the trunk. They appear in children and young adults, but can occur at any age. Gingival lesions are found during pregnancy.

Diagnosis

Diagnosis is made by clinical presentation. Histopathologic evaluation confirms the diagnosis.

Differential diagnosis

Because of their rapid growth and appearance, it is important to rule out nodular or amelanotic melanoma by histology. Other entities in the differential include SCC, glomus tumor, nodular BCC, bacillary angiomatosis, Kaposi's sarcoma, and hemangiomas.

Laboratory testing

Histopathologic evaluation is important to rule out an amelanotic malignant melanoma.

Pathogenesis

Although the precise cause is unknown, trauma, arteriovenous malformations, hormonal influences, and the production of angiogenic growth factors may play a role in this reactive process.

Treatment

As they do not regress spontaneously, removal is required to stop bleeding or to rule out malignancy. Shave excision with electrodesiccation at base with local anesthesia is an acceptable removal method. Pulsed-dye laser is successful for small lesions, especially in children. Lesions tend to recur, and on occasion, smaller satellite lesions form after surgical removal.

Angiofibroma (Fibrous papule, pearly penile papule)

Key Points

- Solitary lesions common
- Multiple facial lesions should raise suspicion of tuberous sclerosis

Clinical presentation

Angiofibromas (Figure 15-13) are small, flesh-colored to red-brown, shiny, smooth papules commonly found on the nose and medial cheeks. Solitary lesions are common and resemble BCC. They may also occur as pearly penile papules on the glans penis, which can be mistaken for condyloma acuminata. Finally, multiple facial angiofibromas (referred to as adenoma sebaceum) are associated

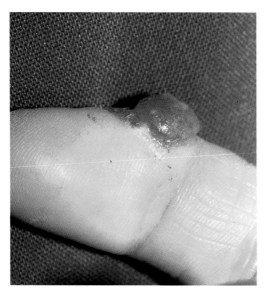

Figure 15-12 Pyogenic granuloma

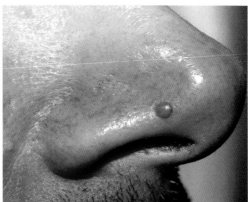

Figure 15-13 Fibrous papule

with tuberous sclerosis. Their presence occurs in 75% of patients with the disease, with onset during childhood. Multiple angiofibromas may also be associated with multiple endocrine neoplasia type I, Birt–Hogg–Dube syndrome, or be inherited/sporadic as an isolated finding with no other stigmata. Acquired digital fibrokeratoma (Figure 15-14) is a closely related lesion that occurs on the fingers, toes, palms, and soles.

Diagnosis

Definitive diagnosis is made by biopsy.

Differential diagnosis

Solitary angiofibromas can be mistaken for BCC because of the shiny, smooth nature of these papules. They also mimic small intradermal nevi, as well as appendageal tumors.

Histological features

Biopsy is unnecessary unless other processes need to be ruled out. Histopathology shows dermal proliferation of fibroblasts with increased number of dilated blood vessels.

Pathogenesis

Fibrous papules may represent the end-stage of involuted nevi or possibly a hamartoma.

Treatment

Shave excision or electrodesiccation is used to remove angiofibromas completely for cosmetic purposes. Histologic evaluation is necessary to exclude BCC in certain clinical presentations.

Lipomas and associated syndromes

Key Points

- Common benign soft-tissue tumors
- Angiolipomas are often spontaneously painful

Clinical presentation

Lipomas are benign tumors of mature fat found at any subcutaneous site, commonly the neck and trunk. These rubbery, mobile, round to lobulated nodules are typically slow-growing and asymptomatic with a normal overlying epidermis. They appear most often in middle-aged adults. Lipomas may be single or multiple. Multiple lipomas may be a clue to one of the following underlying syndromes.

Familial multiple lipomas is an autosomal-dominant syndrome with hundreds of well-circumscribed nontender lipomas appearing in the third decade of life. There is a widespread distribution, with significant involvement of the extremities, including the forearms. *Diffuse*

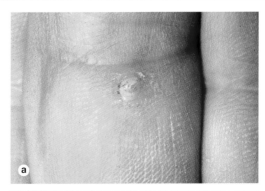

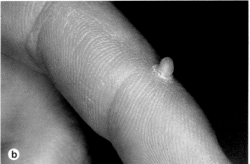

Figure 15-14 a, b Acquired digital fibrokeratoma

lipomatosis syndrome is characterized by a widespread involvement of poorly circumscribed lipomas. In this form, recurrence of the lipomas is common, because complete resection of the nonencapsulated lipomas is difficult. *Dercum's disease*, also known as *adiposis dolorosa*, presents as multiple tender lipomas appearing in middle-aged, often obese women. *Madelung's disease*, or *symmetric lipomatosis*, typically affects middle-aged men. In this nonhereditary syndrome, multiple large and nontender lipomas appear on the head, neck, or upper trunk as symmetrical fat deposits. The lipomas may coalesce, forming what is known as a "horse collar" on the neck that is not only disfiguring but may also lead to limitations in range of motion and respiration. Multiple lipomas appear in several other syndromes, including Proteus, Gardner's, and Bannayan–Zonana syndromes.

Diagnosis

Diagnosis is generally made by clinical presentation alone.

Differential diagnosis

Angiolipomas resemble lipomas, but develop as numerous mobile tender nodules at the forearms and trunks of young adults and have a vascular component. Liposarcomas are extremely rare and tend to be asymmetric and infiltrative when compared to the well-circumscribed lipomas. An epidermoid cyst often demonstrates a characteristic punctum, which is lacking in lipomas.

Histological features

Further evaluation with fine-needle aspiration may be necessary to rule out a liposarcoma. In addition, computed tomography scanning is indicated if lipsarcoma is suspected. When sent for histological evaluation, lipomas resemble normal fat and demonstrate sheets of mature adipocytes within a thin fibrous capsule. Several variants exist, including spindle cell, pleomorphic, chondroid, and myolipomas.

Pathogenesis

Little is known about the pathogenesis of lipomas, but their prevalence is increased in individuals with obesity, diabetes, and/or elevated cholesterol levels. Studies show clonal chromosomal aberrations in up to two-thirds of patients with lipomas and a possible role of the *HMGI-C* gene located at 12q13-15.

Treatment

Lipomas can be excised or "shelled out" surgically, especially when well circumscribed. Diffuse lipomatosis syndrome is an exception, as lesions frequently recur. When lipomas grow in size (up to 15 cm) they become increasingly difficult to excise. However, because lipomas are not precursors to liposarcomas, removal is not mandatory. Liposuction has also been shown to be effective for removing lipomas. Management of the pain of Dercum's disease may require medical treatment with lidocaine, steroids, and analgesics.

Connective tissue nevus (Collagenoma, elastoma, shagreen patch in tuberous sclerosis)

Clinical presentation

Connective tissue nevi are hamartomas that typically present at birth or during early childhood as firm, flesh-colored papules, nodules, or plaques. They may be solitary or multiple and occur in a grouped, linear, or irregular distribution. The shagreen patch of tuberous sclerosis is a variant with a "pigskin"-like plaque on the lower back. Buschke–Ollendorff syndrome, an autosomal-dominant disorder, is characterized by the appearance of multiple flesh-colored to yellow papules at an early age. Osteopoikilosis, or scattered areas of increased bone density, is characteristically found on X-ray in affected patients. Multiple other medical syndromes have been associated with connective tissue nevi.

Diagnosis

Clinicopathologic evaluation leads to the diagnosis of connective tissue nevi.

Histological features

Biopsies should be taken at the edge of connective tissue nevi to allow for comparison of the surrounding normal skin. Affected areas demonstrate an ill-defined increase of dermal collagen or elastin. No laboratory studies are indicated unless there is suspicion of an underlying syndrome. For example, patients suspected of having Buschke–Ollendorff syndrome should have appropriate radiographs. Brain imaging, electroencephalogram, renal ultrasound, and echocardiogram are indicated for patients with tuberous sclerosis.

Pathogenesis

The pathogenesis of connective tissue nevi is unknown.

Treatment

Because connective tissue nevi are benign lesions, surgical excision is not recommended. Patients with associated syndromes may require other forms of therapy.

Hypertrophic scar, keloid

Key Points

* Normal scars are flat, whereas hypertrophic scars and keloids are raised
* Hypertrophic scars are confined to original wound margins, may regress spontaneously, and have a good response to treatment
* Keloids extend beyond original wound margins, do not regress, and have a poor response to treatment
* See Chapter 22

Benign adnexal tumors

Key Points

* Epidermally derived skin appendages include eccrine, apocrine, and sebaceous glands and hair follicles (Table 15-13)
* Histopathology is required for definitive diagnosis because most lesions derived from skin appendages are clinically indistinct
* Anatomic distribution reflects high-density areas of involved structures
* Because most are benign lesions with little or no risk for malignant transformation, treatment is mainly for cosmetic purposes
* Eccrine and apocrine-derived lesions have been considered as separate categories historically; however, clear distinction is often not possible
* When multiple, adnexal tumors are often markers for an associated syndrome

Table 15-13 Comparison of lesions derived from epidermal skin appendages

	Differentiation	Clinical	Location	Associations/complications	Treatment – typically for cosmetic purposes
Trichoepithelioma	Hair follicle	Papules with solitary, multiple, and desmoplastic variants	Nose, upper lip, and cheeks	Brooke–Spiegler syndrome	Surgical excision, carbon dioxide laser and electrodesiccation for multiple lesions
Trichofolliculoma	Hair follicle	Dome-shaped papule or nodule with central ostium and vellus hair	Face, scalp, upper trunk	Folliculosebaceous cystic hamartoma: a large, cystic variant	None required; consider surgical excision
Syringoma	Eccrine or apocrine	Multiple flesh-colored to yellow, firm papules; familial and eruptive variants	Eyelids, face	Increased in patients with Down's syndrome; scalp syringomas may cause scarring alopecia	Surgical excision if solitary; laser ablation for eruptive form; electrodesiccation and curettage for multiple
Poroma	Eccrine or apocrine	Flesh-colored to pigmented papules, plaques, nodules; widespread variant	Palms and soles, head, neck, and trunk		Surgical excision
Cylindroma	Poorly differentiated	Papules, nodules or tumors; solitary and multiple variants	Scalp, head, or neck	Brooke–Spiegler syndrome	Surgical excision
Sebaceous hyperplasia	Sebaceous (hyperplasia, not neoplasia)	Yellowish papules ± central pore and telangiectasias	Forehead, face	Rosacea – rhinophyma	None required. Cryosurgery, surgical excision if solitary; long-term topical and oral retinoids if multiple

Trichoepithelioma (Dermal trichoblastomas)

Clinical presentation

Trichoepitheliomas are benign neoplasms with follicular differentiation. There are three distinct clinical presentations: solitary, multiple, and desmoplastic. Solitary lesions appear as 5–8-mm flesh-colored papules with a predilection for the nose, upper lip, and cheeks of adults. Multiple trichoepitheliomas occur in adolescents as small papules on the face that may coalesce to form plaques, nodules, or tumors. These may be associated with multiple cylindromas and the autosomal-dominant Brooke–Spiegler syndrome. The desmoplastic variant is a small firm papule or plaque on the face of young to middle-aged adults.

Diagnosis

Biopsy is required for definitive diagnosis given the indistinct clinical presentation.

Differential diagnosis

Trichoepitheliomas clinically mimic BCC, milia, cylindromas, trichilemmal cysts, syringomas, steatocystoma multiplex, and trichofolliculomas.

Histological features

Biopsy reveals a well-circumscribed dermal tumor with aggregates of basaloid cells surrounded by fibrous stroma.

Pathogenesis

Trichoepitheliomas demonstrate hair follicle differentiation. The cause of solitary lesions is unknown. The familial, multiple form is liked to a gene on chromosome 9p21. Cases associated with Brooke–Spiegler syndrome demonstrate mutations of the cylindromatosis oncogene (*CYLD*), which maps to16q12-q13.

Treatment

Solitary lesions may be treated with surgical excision, but removal is not required. Multiple, lesions may respond better to destruction with carbon dioxide laser or electrodesiccation.

Trichofolliculoma

Clinical presentation

A trichofolliculoma typically appears as a small, solitary, dome-shaped papule or nodule on the face, scalp, or upper trunk of an adult. The lesion may have a central follicular ostium and/or wooly white hairs protruding from the surface. Rarely, trichofolliculomas are large nodules or cysts. *Folliculosebaceous cystic hamartoma* may represent a large, cystic sebaceous trichofolliculoma variant.

Diagnosis

Biopsy is required for definitive diagnosis, given the indistinct clinical presentation.

Differential diagnosis

Trichofolliculomas may be confused with BCC, epidermoid cysts, and intradermal nevi.

Histological features

Biopsy demonstrates several small secondary follicles radiating from a central dilated primary follicle.

Pathogenesis

Trichofolliculomas likely represent follicular hamartomas, rather than a true neoplastic process.

Treatment

Although treatment is not required for these benign lesions, surgical excision for definitive diagnosis or cosmetic purposes is often done.

Syringoma

Clinical presentation

Syringomas (Figure 15-15) are benign adenomas of eccrine or apocrine ducts. They often present as multiple 1–2-mm flesh-colored to yellow, firm papules. Although they can present anywhere, favored locations include the eyelids and face. Scalp involvement may produce a scarring alopecia. Syringomas develop during puberty and are more common in women than men. Familial and eruptive forms exist. Eruptive syringomas are

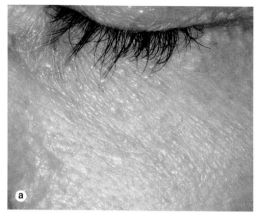
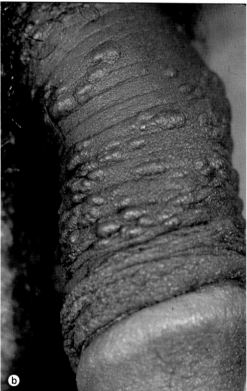

Figure 15-15 a Syringomas. **b** Eruptive syringomas

more common in black males and often involve the chest or penis.

Diagnosis

The diagnosis of syringoma may be favored by the clinical presentation, but histological evaluation is necessary for definitive diagnosis.

Differential diagnosis

Syringomas on the face clinically mimic trichoepitheliomas and BCC, whereas eyelid lesions can be mistaken for xanthelasma. Eruptive syringomas may resemble disseminated granuloma annulare, especially on the trunk.

Histological features

The typical histologic pattern demonstrates numerous small solid, tubular, and cystic structures in the upper dermis. "Tadpole" or comma-like tails are used to describe the characteristic morphology of tumor islands.

Pathogenesis

The exact cause of syringomas is unknown. On occasion, they are associated with Down's syndrome.

Treatment

Syringomas are benign lesions with no true proliferative capacity. Treatment for these potentially disfiguring lesions is often done for cosmetic purposes. Single lesions may be surgically excised. Patients presenting with the eruptive form may be treated with laser ablation. Electrodesiccation with curettage is also useful for the treatment of multiple lesions.

Controversies

Syringomas have historically been categorized as neoplasms of eccrine lineage; however, with current immunohistochemical and histological techniques it is impossible to differentiate between apocrine and eccrine lineage.

Poroma (Acrospiroma, hidradenoma)

Clinical presentation

The term "poroma" refers to a group of cutaneous appendageal tumors with terminal ductal differentiation. Historically classified as derivatives of eccrine glands, evidenced by the frequent use of the term "eccrine poroma," they may also derive from apocrine glands. Poromas present as clinically indistinct solitary, slow-growing, flesh-colored or pigmented papules, plaques, or nodules. They may become red, itchy, or painful. Typical locations include the head, neck, palms, and soles, but they may occur at any site. Subtypes are discussed below. Rarely, multiple poromas will develop in an acral or widespread distribution, a condition known as poromatosis.

Diagnosis

Definitive diagnosis is made with biopsy and histological evaluation.

Differential diagnosis

Clinical appearance may be similar to a pyogenic granuloma, especially when acral skin is involved.

Histological features

Poromas are well-circumscribed nodular aggregations of uniform basaloid cells. The subtype is determined by the location in relation to the epidermis. Intraepidermal poromas are known as *hidroacanthoma simplex*, while intradermal poromas are known as *dermal duct tumors* or *hidradenomas*. A third form, with epidermal and papillary dermal involvement, is termed *juxtaepidermal poroma*.

Pathogenesis

When occurring at cutaneous sites with many eccrine structures such as the palms and soles, poromas likely represent a true eccrine neoplasm. Other lesions are more likely to represent apocrine poromas, such as those developing within a nevus sebaceus (Figure 15-6).

Treatment

Treatment with surgical excision is curative. Poromas may transform into porocarcinomas.

Cylindroma

Clinical presentation

Cylindromas are poorly differentiated adnexal neoplasms. Two clinical forms exist. The more common solitary form presents as a papule or nodule on the scalp, head, or neck of adults and is more common in women. Lesions grow slowly over time and may become painful. The multiple form involves numerous papules, nodules, or tumors, also typically located on the scalp, head, and neck. These lesions may coalesce, and the term "turban tumor" is used to describe involvement of a large portion of the scalp. Multiple cylindromas have a familial tendency and are inherited in an autosomal-dominant fashion. Brooke–Spiegler syndrome describes the association of multiple cylindromas, trichoepitheliomas, milia, and spiradenomas. Malignant cylindromas are extremely rare, but may develop within the solitary or multiple variants.

Diagnosis

Biopsy is required for definitive diagnosis as clinical presentation is often indistinct for solitary lesions.

Histological features

Histopathological evaluation reveals a well-circumscribed lesion with a distinctive "jigsaw puzzle" pattern of nests of basaloid cells.

Pathogenesis

The familial form is inherited in an autosomal-dominant fashion and has been linked to the gene *CYLD* on 16q12-13. The cause of sporadic, solitary cylindromas is unknown but may also be linked to the *CYLD* locus.

Treatment

Solitary cylindromas lack the capacity to proliferate, making treatment unnecessary. Aggressive local spread and malignant transformation, which warrant excisional surgery, have been reported rarely with multiple cylindromas, especially in the case of turban tumors of the scalp. Brooke–Spiegler syndrome should be considered with multiple cylindromas and a positive family history.

Sebaceous hyperplasia

Clinical presentation

Sebaceous hyperplasia, a relatively common benign condition, describes sebaceous lobule enlargement around the follicular infundibulum. Sebaceous hyperplasia presents as solitary or multiple 1–3-mm, yellowish papules on the face, especially the forehead of adults. Often the papule contains a central pore, representing the follicular infundibular ostium, and overlying telangiectasia. Lesions may be clinically mistaken for BCC. Other presentations include a linear or "beaded lines" form, and rhinophyma, nasal sebaceous hyperplasia that may occur as a prominent feature in patients with rosacea. Sebaceous hyperplasia is more common in men than in women.

Diagnosis

Diagnosis can be made clinically, but biopsy may be indicated to rule out BCC.

Differential diagnosis

It is important either clinically or histopathologically to differentiate sebaceous hyperplasia from BCC. Yellow color, the presence of a central pore, and expression of a sebum globule with compression all favor sebaceous hyperplasia. In addition, BCCs tend to be firmer on palpation. Xanthomas, fibrous papule of the face, milia, sebaceous adenoma, syringoma, trichopethilioma, and trichofolliculomas should also be included in the differential diagnosis. Sebaceous adenomas have a greater proportion of undifferentiated cells and may be associated with Muir–Torre syndrome.

Histological features

Histopathologic evaluation reveals large and mature sebaceous lobules surrounding a central infundibulum.

Pathogenesis

Sebaceous glands are found on all locations of the skin except for the palms and soles. The majority of these androgen-sensitive holocrine glands are located on the face, chest, back, and upper arms.

With aging and decreasing androgen levels, sebocyte turnover slows, resulting in their crowding within the sebaceous gland and hyperplasia. Ultraviolet radiation and immunosuppression have also been considered to be cofactors in causing sebaceous hyperplasia.

Treatment

Treatment of sebaceous hyperplasia is either for cosmetic purposes or to rule out BCC. Solitary lesions may be surgically excised or treated with liquid nitrogen cryosurgery, while multiple lesions may respond more favorably to light electrodesiccation. The addition of long-term topical retinoids may also improve the appearance of multiple lesions. Oral isotretinoin is effective in clearing sebaceous hyperplasia because of its ability to shrink sebaceous glands; however, recurrence is common upon discontinuation. Isotretinoin should only be considered for disfiguring cases.

Further reading

Alfadley A, Hainau B, Al Robace A. Becker's melanosis: a report of 12 cases with a typical presentation. Int J Dermatol 2005;44:20.

Atiyeh BS, Costagliola M, Hayek SN. Keloid or hypertrophic scar, the controversy: Review of the literature. Ann Plast Surg 2005;54:676–680.

Berman B, Bienstock L, Kuritzky L. Actinic keratoses: sequelae and treatments. Suppl J Fam Pract 2006;May:1–8.

Brook I. Microbiology of infected epidermal cysts. Arch Dermatol 1989;125:1658–1661.

Cordain L, Eades MR, Eades MD. Hyperinsulinemic diseases of civilization: more than just syndrome X. Comp Biochem Physiol A Mol Integr Physiol 2003;136:95–112.

Diven DG, Dozier SE, Meyer DJ. Bacteriology of inflamed and uninflamed epidermal inclusion cysts. Arch Dermatol 1998;134:49–51.

Feigin I. Skin tumors of neural origin. Am J Dermatopathol 1983;5:397–399.

Gould BE, Ellison RC, Greene HL, et al. Lack of association between skin tags and colon polyps in the primary care setting. Arch Intern Med 1988;148:1799–1800.

Happle R. Lethal genes surviving by mosaicism: a possible explanation for sporadic birth defects involving the skin. J Am Acad Dermatol 1987;16:899–906.

Harris AO, Levy ML, Goldberg LH. Nonepidermal and appendageal skin tumors. Clin Plast Surg 1993;20:115–130.

Kopf AW. Congenital nevus-like nevi, nevi spili, and café-au-lait spots in patients with malignant melanoma. J Dermatol Surg Oncol 1985;11:275.

Krengel S. Nevogenesis – new thoughts regarding a classical problem. Am J Dermatopathol 2005;27:456–465.

Manuskiatti W, Fitzpatrick RE. Treatment response of keloidal and hypertrophic sternotomy scars. Arch Dermatol 2002;138:1149–1155.

Mehregan DA, Mehregan AH. Deep penetrating nevus. Arch Dermatol 1993;129:328.

Mooney MA, Janniger CK. Pyogenic granuloma. Pediatr Dermatol 1995;55:133.

Mooney MA, Barr RJ, Buxton MG. Halo nevus or halo phenomenon: a study of 142 cases. J Cutan Pathol 1995;22:342.

Mutalik S. Treatment of keloids and hypertrophic scars. Ind J Dermatol Venereol Leprol 2005;71: 3–8.

Rogers M, McCrossin I, Commens C. Epidermal nevi and the epidermal nevus syndrome, a review of 131 cases. J Am Acad Dermatol 1989;20: 476–488.

Sage RA, Webster JK, Fisher SG. Outpatient care and morbidity reduction in diabetic foot ulcers associated with chronic pressure callus. J Am Podiatr Med Assoc 2001;91:275.

Schwartz RA. Keratoacanthoma: A clinico-pathologic enigma. Dermatol Surg 2004;30:326–333.

Seab JA, Graham JH, Helwig EP. Deep penetrating nevus. Am J Surg Pathol 1989;13:39–44.

Sharad M. Treatment of keloids and hypertrophic scars. Ind J Dermatol Venereol Leporl 2005;71: 3–8.

Tucker MA, Halpern A, Holly EA. Clinically recognized dysplastic nevi: a central risk factor for cutaneous melanoma. JAMA 1997;277:1439.

Wetherington RW, Cockerell CJ. The "dysplastic" nevus: an update at 25 years. Adv Dermatol 2003;19:237–248.

Genodermatoses 16

Robin P. Gehris and Laura Korb Ferris

Ichthyosis

> **Key Points**
>
> - Ichthyosis can be a primary disorder or a feature of a syndrome
> - Presence of a collodion membrane at birth is suggestive of lamellar ichthyosis or nonbullous congenital ichthyosiform erythroderma (NBCIE)
> - Treatment options include emollients and, in some cases, oral retinoids

Clinical presentation

Ichthyosis is characterized by the presence of fish-like scales on the skin (Table 16-1). The quality and distribution of the scales can be suggestive of the type of ichthyosis, as described below. Ichthyosis usually presents at birth or in the neonatal period. The presence of a collodion membrane, or paper-like skin, at birth is suggestive of lamellar ichthyosis or NBCIE (Table 16-2), although this presentation has also been described in infants who were subsequently found to have ichthyosis vulgaris or who had no apparent skin disease later in life (so-called self-healing collodion babies).

Diagnosis

Diagnosis is usually made by a combination of clinical presentation and skin biopsy. Examination of family members may help point to an etiology as well, such as an X-linked recessive inheritance pattern (X-linked ichthyosis) or the presence of atopic dermatitis or scaling of the legs (ichthyosis vulgaris). In patients with suspected BCIE/epidermolytic hyperkeratosis (EHK), the finding of an epidermal nevus in a parent may clarify the diagnosis, since a parent with an epidermal nevus may have a child with BCIE/EHK due to genetic mosaicism for mutations in keratin 1 or 10. Certain clinical findings can be helpful as well. An adherent brown-colored scale, especially on the lateral neck, suggests X-linked ichthyosis (Figure 16-1). The presence of palmar hyperlinearity and plate-like scales on the lower leg suggests ichthyosis vulgaris (Figure 16-2). Ectropion is most commonly

seen in patients with lamellar ichthyosis. A corrugated appearance of the flexural skin suggests the diagnosis of EHK (Figure 16-3).

Histopathologically, all these disorders are characterized by hyperkeratosis. Certain histologic features may suggest a specific diagnosis. For example, the epidermis of patients with ichthyosis vulgaris has an absent granular layer, whereas the granular layer is increased in X-linked ichthyosis and BCIE. Massive orthokeratosis is seen in lamellar ichthyosis. In BCIE/EHK, hyperkeratosis is prominent, as is keratinocyte vacuolization. The differential diagnosis of patients with ichthyosiform dermatitis includes severe xerosis, syndromes with ichthyosis as a feature (Table 16-3), or acquired ichthyosis (Box 16-1).

Pathogenesis

Proteins that are important for normal keratinocyte differentiation are mutated in patients with ichthyosis. The outcome of this is a disruption in the barrier function of the skin. Transglutaminase-1, mutated in lamellar ichthyosis and some cases of NBCIE, catalyzes the cross-linking of structural proteins to form an insoluble protein envelope in the cornified layer of skin. In self-healing collodion babies, a mutation in transglutaminase-1 makes this protein sensitive to increased hydrostatic pressures found in utero, decreasing its activity. However, after birth, the change in hydrostatic pressure allows this protein to regain normal function. The condition resolves without long-term sequelae. Filaggrin, which is defective in patients with ichthyosis vulgaris, is found in keratohyalin granules and is important for the aggregation of keratin filaments prior to their cross-linking to form the cornified envelope of the skin. The lipoxygenases encoded by *ALOXE3* and *ALOX12B* are critical for the formation of the cutaneous lipid barrier; these enzymes are defective in NBCIE and in some cases of lamellar ichthyosis. The ABCA12-encoded lipid transporter, the gene for harlequin ichthyosis, is important for formation of a proper

Table 16-1 Primary ichthyoses

Disease	Inheritance	Gene/protein	Features
Ichthyosis vulgaris	Autosomal recessive	Filaggrin	Fine scales on legs, arms
			Hyperlinear palms
			Keratosis pilaris
			High prevalence of atopic dermatitis
			Histopathology shows absent granular layer
Lamellar ichthyosis	Autosomal recessive	*TGM1*: transglutaminase-1	Thick plate-like scales diffusely
		ALOXE3: lipoxygenase 3	Collodion baby
		ALOX12B: 12R-lipoxygenase	Decreased sweating
			Ectropion
			Nail dystrophy
			Histopathology shows massive orthokeratosis
X-linked ichthyosis	X-linked recessive	*STS*: steroid sulfatase	Dark adhesive large scales on extensor surfaces, lateral trunk and neck, cheeks
			Cryptorchidism
			Comma-shaped corneal opacities
			Failure of progression of maternal labor
			May be associated with Kallman syndrome (anosmia, mental retardation) or chondrodysplasia punctata due to contiguous gene deletions
			Accumulation of serum cholesterol sulfate
Nonbullous congenital ichthyosiform erythroderma (NBCIE)	Autosomal recessive	*TGM1*: transglutaminase 1	Collodion baby at birth
		ALOXE3: lipoxygenase 3	Erythroderma and fine white scaling
		ALOX12B: 12R- lipoxygenase	Hyperkeratosis of palms and soles
		Loricrin gene	
Bullous congenital ichthyosiform erythroderma (BCIE), epidermolytic hyperkeratosis (EHK)	Autosomal dominant	*KRT1* and *KRT10*: keratins 1 and 10	Congenital erythrodema with blisters
			Palmoplantar hyperkeratosis
			Corrugated scale, especially at flexures
			Histopathology shows epidermolytic hyperkeratosis
Ichthyosis bullosa of Siemens	Autosomal recessive	*KRT2E*: keratin 2e	May have erythema and scaling at birth
			Superficial peeling (Mauserung or molting phenomenon)
			Brown discoloration of extremities due to hyperkeratosis
Harlequin ichthyosis	Autosomal recessive	*ABCA12* (lipid transporter)	Plates of armor-like scaling (red plates with deep fissures) at birth
			Frequently lethal in the neonatal period
			Severe ectropion and eclabium

Table 16-2 Diagnostic clues in the classification of patients with ichthyosis

Finding	Suggests diagnosis of:
History	
Only males in family affected	X-linked recessive ichthyosis
Failure of maternal labor to progress	X-linked recessive ichthyosis
Collodion baby	Lamellar ichthyosis
	NBCIE
Strong family history of atopic dermatitis	Ichthyosis vulgaris
Heat intolerance	Lamellar ichthyosis
	CIE
Photosensitivity	(Photosensitivity); icthyosis; brittle hair; impaired intelligence; decreased fertility; and short stature
Associated malignancies	
Testicular cancer	X-linked ichthyosis
Acute lymphoblastic leukemia	X-linked ichthyosis
Physical exam	
Thick plate-like scales, ectropion, eclabium	Lamellar ichthyosis
Fine white scale	NBCIE
Hyperlinear palms	Ichthyosis vulgaris
	X-linked ichthyosis
	Refsum disease
Persistently "dirty" appearance to neck	X-linked ichthyosis
Comma-shaped corneal opacities	X-linked ichthyosis
Flexural skin with corrugated scale	EHK
Double-edged scale	Netherton's syndrome
Limb abnormalities	Conradi–Hunermann–Happle syndrome
	CHILD syndrome
Bullae/blisters	BCIE/EHK
	Ichthyosis bullosa of Siemens
Retinitis pigmentosa	Refsum disease
Perifoveal glistening white dots	Sjögren–Larson disease
Laboratory abnormalities	
Elevated serum cholesterol sulfate	X-linked ichthyosis
Increased mobility of low-density B lipoproteins	X-linked ichthyosis
Low serum cholesterol	CHILD syndrome
	Conradi–Hunermann–Happle syndrome
Elevated serum immunoglobulin E	Netherton's syndrome
Elevated phytanic acid in body fluids	Refsum's disease

NBCIE, nonbullous congenital ichthyosiform erythroderma; CIE, congenital ichthyosiform erythroderma; EHK, epidermolytic hyperkeratosis; CHILD, congenital hemihypertrophy, unilateral ichthyosiform nevus, limb defects.

lipid barrier. The *STS* gene, mutated in X-linked ichthyosis, encodes steroid sulfatase. Absence of this gene results in the accumulation of cholesterol-3 sulfate in the skin, which may inhibit transglutaminase-1 activity. Mutated keratins are responsible for BCIE/EHK (keratins 1 or 10) and ichthyosis bullosa of Siemens (keratin 2e).

Treatment

Emollients are useful in the treatment of ichthyosis to decrease transepidermal fluid loss. To decrease scale, glycolic acid, lactic acid, or salicylic acid can be used. However, caution should be used when applying salicylic acid over a large body

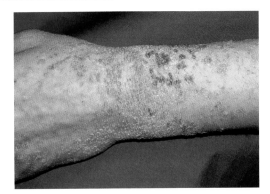

Figure 16-1 X-linked ichthyosis

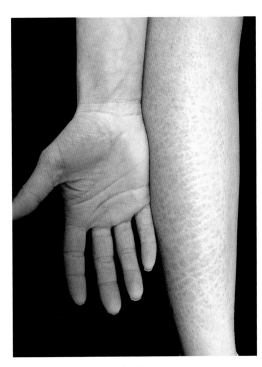

Figure 16-2 Ichthyosis vulgaris

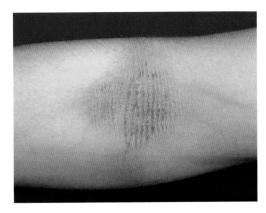

Figure 16-3 Epidermolytic hyperkeratosis

surface area, as salicylism (salicylate toxicity) can result. Urea, ammonium lactate, and propylene glycol are also helpful. Calcipotriol ointment has been reported to be beneficial in Sjögren–Larson syndrome and in lamellar ichthyosis. Topical retinoids, particularly tazarotene, may be effective in the treatment of ichthyoses, although they can cause some irritation. Oral retinoids are useful in the treatment of some ichthyoses, particularly lamellar ichthyosis and EHK, and are life-saving in patients with harlequin ichthyosis. Studies have shown that acetretin may be more effective than isotretinoin for treatment of lamellar ichthyosis. In EHK, high doses of systemic retinoids can cause epidermal blistering. Dosing of isotretinoin should begin at 0.5 mg/kg per day and be slowly increased as tolerated to minimize this risk.

Palmoplantar keratodermas (PPK)

Key Points

* Characterized by focal or diffuse hyperkeratosis of the palms and/or soles
* May be primary (genetic) or secondary to inflammatory skin diseases
* Subtypes can be distinguished from one another by the presence or absence of transgrediens, and by associated extracutaneous features such as deafness, cardiomyopathy, gum disease, or cancer (Table 16-4)
* May be painful with weight-bearing
* Patients may experience hyperhidrosis or foul odor secondary to overgrowth of bacteria within the hyperkeratotic skin

Clinical presentation

The subcategorization *diffuse keratodermas* demonstrates either confluent or discontinuous keratoderma of the palms and soles without any specific geometric pattern.

Epidermolytic PPK, or Vorner syndrome, is secondary to an autosomal-dominant mutation in the keratin-9 gene. It presents with a waxy yellow keratoderma and characteristic erythematous border that is often present at birth or in early infancy. Patients may experience significant hyperhidrosis.

Nonepidermolytic PPK, or Unna–Thost syndrome (Figure 16-4), results from mutations in genes that encode keratins 1 and 16 and similarly presents with a waxy yellow keratoderma and hyperhidrosis.

Vohwinkel syndrome (Figure 16-5) is transmitted in an autosomal-dominant fashion and can present in two different forms, which are now known to be both clinically and genetically distinct. Mutations in *GJB2* lead to abnormal connexin 26 and result in deafness and keratoderma,

Table 16-3 Disorders with ichthyosis as a feature

Disease	Inheritance	Gene/protein	Features
Refsum disease	Autosomal recessive	Phytanic acid oxidase	Milder ichthyosis
			Retinitis pigmentosa
			Sensorimotor polyneuropathy
			Cranial nerve dysfunction
			Electrocardiogram changes
			Cardiomyopathy
			Renal tubular dysfunction
			Epiphyseal dysplasia
Neutral lipid storage disease with ichthyosis (Chanarin–Dorfman syndrome)	Autosomal recessive	*ABHD5* gene (lipid hydrolase)	Oil red O-positive lipid droplets in tissues and leukocytes
			Pruritic ichthyosiform erythroderma
			Hepatosplenomegaly
			Cataracts
			Horizontal nystagmus
			Growth retardation
			Myopathy
			Ataxia
			Hearing loss
Ichthyosis hystrix	Autosomal dominant	Keratin 1 (some cases)	Verrucous porcupine quill-like growths
Netherton syndrome (ichthyosis linearis circumflexa)	Autosomal recessive	*SPINK5*/LEKTI serine protease inhibitor	Serpiginous red plaques with double-edged scale
			High serum immunoglobulin E and anaphylaxis to foods
			Trichorrhexis invaginata
Sjögren–Larsson syndrome	Autosomal recessive	*FALDH*/fatty aldehyde dehydrogenase	Spastic paralysis
			Mental retardation
			Glistening white dots in retina
Keratitis, ichthyosis, deafness (KID) syndrome	Autosomal recessive	GJB2 (connexin 26)	Keratitis
			Ichthyosis
			Deafness
Trichothiodystrophy (photosensitivity); icthyosis; brittle hair; impaired intelligence; decreased fertility; and short stature Tay syndrome	Autosomal recessive	*ERCC2*/XPD *ERCC3*/XPB	Often collodion baby at birth, fine white to large yellow-brown scale later in life
			Photosensitivity
			Decreased fertility
			Intellectual impairment
			Brittle hair
			Short stature
Congenital hemihypertrophy, unilateral ichthyosiform nevus, limb defects (CHILD) syndrome	X-linked dominant	*NSDHL* (3β-hydroxysteroid dehydrogenase)	Male lethal
			Congenital hemihypertrophy, unilateral ichthyosiform nevus, limb defects
Conradi–Hunermann–Happle syndrome	X-linked dominant	*EBP* (emopamil-binding protein)	Linear ichthyosis
			Chondrodysplasia punctata (focal epiphyseal calcifications)
			Cataracts
			Short stature

BOX 16-1

Causes of acquired ichthyosis

Malignancy

Most commonly Hodgkin's lymphoma

Autoimmune disorders

Systemic lupus erythematosus

Sarcoidosis

Graft-versus-host disease

Dermatomyositis

Nutritional deficiency

Metabolic disease

Diabetes

Hypothyroidism

Renal failure

Infection

Human immunodeficiency virus

Human T-lymphotrophic virus -I and -II

Medications

Cimetidine

Clofazimine

Hydroxyurea

but no ichthyosis. Conversely, mutations in *LOR* result in abnormal loricirin and a keratoderma with mild ichthyosis, but normal hearing. Both variants of Vohwinkel syndrome exhibit a clinically unique keratoderma characterized by a stippled or honeycombed pattern with starfish-like keratoses on the knuckles and dorsal hands and the potential for the development of digital constriction bands or pseudoainhum, which, if left untreated, can lead to autoamputation. Other mutilating keratodermas (Figure 16-6) are still awaiting molecular characterization.

Clouston syndrome or hidrotic ectodermal dysplasia will be fully discussed in the ectodermal dysplasia section of this chapter, but is briefly included here as it can present with a diffuse palmoplantar keratoderma, hyperhidrosis, and paronychia.

Mal de Meleda is an autosomal-recessive syndrome typified by a classic painful and malodorous "stocking-and-glove" keratoderma with transgrediens that is accompanied by fissuring, hyperhidrosis, and the potential to form digital constriction bands, or pseudoainhum.

Olmsted syndrome is a similarly mutilating keratoderma whose hallmark is its association with thickening and fissuring of the periorifical region that can begin in infancy. The genetic mutation is presently unknown.

Naxos disease is an autosomal-recessive syndrome secondary to a mutation in the gene that encodes plakoglobin and presents with a diffuse palmoplantar keratoderma, as well as wooly hair and cardiac arrhythmias.

The focal keratodermas (Figure 16-7) present with patterned, geometric, or discrete, as opposed to confluent, hyperkeratosis.

Striate PPK results from an autosomal-dominant mutation in either desmoplakin or desmoglein-1 and appears as a focally streaked or linear keratoderma on the palms and soles.

A striated keratoderma can also occur in association with dilated cardiomyopathy and wooly hair secondary to a mutation in desmoplakin and is transmitted in an autosomal-recessive fashion.

Papillon–Lefèvre syndrome is an autosomal-recessive keratoderma that results from a mutation in cathepsin C and presents with a classically malodorous keratoderma accompanied by gingivitis, alveolar bone resorption, and eventual loss of teeth. These patients are prone to frequent cutaneous and systemic bacterial and fungal infections and can also have dural calcification. A variant of Papillon–Lefèvre syndrome known as Haim Munk presents in a similar fashion, but has the additional feature of nail dystrophy.

Richner–Hanhart syndrome is secondary to an autosomal-recessive mutation in tyrosine transaminase and presents with a focal and painful keratoderma with overlying bullae, as well as hyperkeratotic plaques of the knees and elbows. Patients with this syndrome may exhibit tearing secondary to a pseudoherpetic keratitis.

Howel–Evans syndrome is a malignancy-associated, late-onset keratoderma that affects skin only in weight-bearing areas. The keratoderma arises in the second decade, and there is a significantly increased risk of mucosal squamous cell carcinoma, especially esophageal carcinoma, starting after the third decade.

Punctate keratoderma is characterized by focal crenulations of keratoderma within the creases of the soles and palms, leading to pain with walking and pressure. The classic keratoderma in this category is keratosis punctata palmaris et plantaris (see Figure 16-7), which is due to an unknown genetic mutation and is transmitted in an autosomal-dominant fashion.

Diagnosis

Diagnosis of the keratodermas is based on a constellation of characteristic physical findings, associated extracutaneous manifestations, and confirmation of the appropriate genetic mutation

Table 16-4 Classification of palmoplantar keratodermas

A Diffuse keratodermas

Disease subtype	Disease synonyms	Gene mutation	Protein	Key clinical features	Inheritance	Trans-gradiens
Epidermolytic PPK	Vorner	K9	Keratins 9	Waxy yellow congenital keratoderma with an erythematous border, hyperhidrosis	Autosomal dominant	No
Nonepidermolytic PPK	Unna–Thost	K1, 16	Keratin 1, 16	Waxy yellow congenital keratoderma with an erythematous border, hyperhidrosis	Autosomal dominant	No
Vohwinkel syndrome	Keratoderma hereditaria mutilans or PPK mutilans	1. GJB2 2. LOR	1. Connexin 26 2. Loricrin	1. Deafness, no ichthyosis 2. Normal hearing, mild icthyosis. Both variants show a honeycombed PPK, pseudoainhum, and starfish-shaped keratoses	1. Autosomal dominant 2. Autosomal dominant	
Clouston syndrome	Hidrotic ectodermal dysplasia	GJB6	Connexin 30	Sparse hair, thickened nails with paronychia, palmoplantar keratoderma	Autosomal dominant	Yes
Mal del Meleda	Keratosis palmoplantaris transgradiens	SLURP	Secreted Ly-6/uPar-related protein 1	Erythema followed by malodorous stocking-glove keratoderma, painful fissures, hyperhidrosis, possible contractures and pseudoainhum	Autosomal recessive	Yes
Olmsted syndrome	Mutilating PPK with periorifical plaques	Unknown		Mutilating PPK beginning in infancy, thickening and fissuring of periorifical area	Autosomal dominant	
Naxos disease	Keratosis palmoplantaris with arrhythmogenic cardiomyopathy	PKGB	Plakoglobin	Diffuse keratoderma, cardiac arrhythmias and woolly hair	Autosomal recessive	

B. Focal keratodermas

Disease subtype	Disease synonyms	Gene mutation	Protein	Key clinical features	Inheritance	Trans-gradiens
Striate PPK		DSP DSG1	Desmoplakin Desmoglein-1	Focal streaks of keratoderma on soles and palms	Autosomal dominant	No
Dilated cardiomyopathy with keratoderma		DSP	Desmoplakin	Striate PPK, dilated cardiomyopathy, woolly hair	Autosomal recessive	
Papillon–Lefevre syndrome	PPK with periodontitis	CTSC	Cathepsin C	Malodorous keratoderma, periodontitis, gingivitis, alveolar bone resorption, loss of teeth, dural calcification, frequent bacterial and fungal infections. Variant Haim–Munk has nail dystrophy	Autosomal recessive	Yes
Richner–Hanhart syndrome	Tyrosinemia type II	TAT	Tyrosine transaminase	Painful focal keratoderma with bullae, hyperkeratotic plaques on elbows and knees, tearing from pseudoherpetic keratitis	Autosomal recessive	No

Continued

Table 16-4 Classification of palmoplantar keratodermas—Cont'd

Disease subtype	Disease synonyms	Gene mutation	Protein	Key clinical features	Inheritance	Trans-gradiens
Howel–Evans syndrome	Tylosis	*TOC*	Tylosis and esophageal cancer gene product	Late-onset focal (not diffuse) weight-bearing keratoderma in second decade, mucosal squamous cell carcinoma after third decade	Autosomal dominant	No
C. Punctate keratodermas						
Keratosis punctata palmaris et plantaris		Unknown		PPK in the creases of hands and feet, leading to pain with pressure and walking	Autosomal dominant	No

PPK, palmoplantar keratodermas.

when possible. Given the patterns of inheritance, in many cases it is helpful when evaluating an infant or toddler with early keratoderma to examine family members for the typical fully evolved clinical manifestations. Biopsy can occasionally help distinguish between some of the keratodermas; for example, when differentiating nonepidermolytic from epidermolytic keratoderma.

Pathogenesis

Much of the current classification of the PPKs is now driven by their pathogenesis. Important structural proteins of the stratum corneum which can lead to keratoderma include loricrin, the various keratins, and the desmosomal proteins. Other components whose mutations may lead to abnormalities in the cornified envelope are the connexins, which form intercellular gap junctions and regulate ionic calcium signals that are necessary for the expression of the proteins that form the cell envelope, and cathepsins, which mediate enzymatic processes necessary for the formation and dissolution of the cell envelope. See Table 16-4 for a specific grouping of the genetic mutations that lead to the various keratodermas.

Treatment

Treatment of the various types of keratodermas currently consists primarily of symptomatic therapies that chemically and physically debulk the hyperkeratosis. These include soaks followed by application of keratolytic agents such as salicylic acid and urea, either alone or under occlusion, and manual debridement. Intermittent bedrest may be necessary for conditions such as Howel–Evans syndrome, in which the hyperkeratosis can be painful. Accompanying hyperhidrosis can be treated with aluminum chloride, botulinum toxin injections, or iontophoresis, and the foul odor can be remedied with repeated

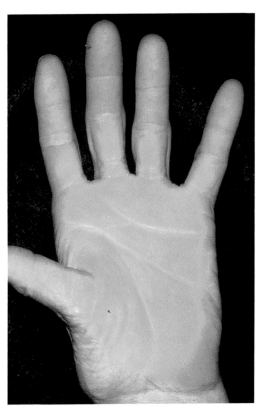

Figure 16-4 Unna–Thost syndrome

treatments of topical antibacterial agents such as clindamycin or diluted Clorox bleach soaks (2 tablespoons per tub). Both of these reduce bacterial counts, but need to be repeated on a regular basis. Patients who suffer from recurrent fungal superinfection or colonization may benefit from regular courses of topical antifungal creams. Use of systemic retinoids should be considered for the more debilitating subtypes of keratoderma, specifically Vohwinkel, mal

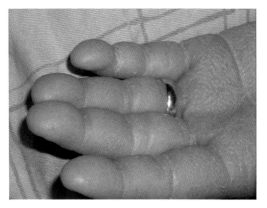

Figure 16-5 Vohwinkel syndrome

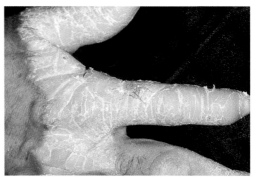

Figure 16-6 Mutilating keratoderma

de Meleda, and Olmsted syndromes, in which pseudoainhum formation can threaten the viability of affected digits. Retinoids may halt progression of the pseudoainhum and minimize development of further hyperkeratosis.

If medical therapy alone is unsuccessful, surgery may be needed to release constriction bands and prevent autoamputation. Subspecialty care should also be sought at an early stage in the subtypes of keratoderma that can occur in association with extracutaneous systemic disease. For example, patients with suspected Naxos disease or striate PPK that appears to be transmitted in an autosomal-recessive fashion should be referred to cardiology, those with Papillon–Lefèvre syndrome should be followed regularly by a dentist, patients with Richner–Hanhart syndrome should be cared for by ophthalmology and those with Howel–Evans by an internist who is aware of the potential for development of mucosal malignancy.

Ectodermal dysplasias

Key Points

* Can be classified as hidrotic (characterized by normal sweating) or hypo- or anhidrotic (with decreased or absent sweating: Table 16-5)
* Evaluation for associated hair, dental, and craniofacial abnormalities can help make the diagnosis

Clinical presentation

Hypohidrotic ectodermal dysplasia in many cases presents with dry, scaling skin in the neonatal period, but it has also been reported to present with features of a true collodian membrane. Affected infants have sparse hair and frontal bossing, as well as periorbital wrinkling and hyperpigmentation, a finding that is very characteristic of this disorder. Dentition is abnormal, with hypo- or anodontia, and peg-shaped or conical incisors are often seen (Figure 16-8).

Patients with hypohidrotic ectodermal dysplasia may develop frequent respiratory infections. In general, nails changes are absent or minimal and there is no keratoderma.

Hidrotic ectodermal dysplasia is characterized by normal sweating and dentition but sparse, fine hair, palmoplantar keratoderma with transgrediens, dystrophic nails with frequent paronychial infections and swollen, tufted distal phalanges. Due to the normal eccrine content in skin, overheating is not a feature of this disorder, but the palmar and nail changes cause the most morbidity.

Ectrodactyly–ectodermal dysplasia–cleft lip/palate (EEC) syndrome has features similar to those of hidrotic ectodermal dysplasia, with normal sweating and dystrophic nails, but patients also demonstrate lacrimal duct abnormalities, clefting of the lip and/or palate and musculoskeletal deformities, the most common of which is a "lobster-claw deformity" or ectrodactyly. Unlike patients with pure hidrotic ectodermal dysplasia, those with EEC syndrome may also have conductive hearing loss and abnormal dentition.

Ankyloblepharon filiforme adenatum–ectodermal dysplasia–cleft palate (AEC) syndrome has as its hallmark ankyloblepharon filiforme adenatum, a fusion of the eyelids with stranding of skin between the lids. This occurs in association with dry skin, sparse hair, and an often recurrent and erosive scalp dermatitis, a feature not found in the other subtypes of ectodermal dysplasia. Like patients with EEC syndrome, those with AEC syndrome can also have clefting and abnormal lacrimal ducts, as well as ear malformations and conductive hearing loss.

Diagnosis

Hypohidrotic ectodermal dysplasia may be detected in the newborn period by the presence of periorbital wrinkling. The presence of dry skin, abnormal hair, or dentition in the mother helps support the clinical suspicion. Infants and toddlers with this disorder may have recurrent unexplained fevers, and they may exhibit bizarre behaviors aimed at self-cooling as their lack of

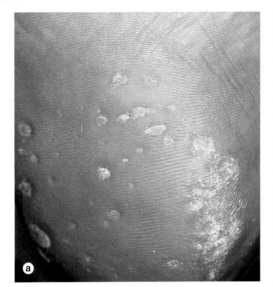

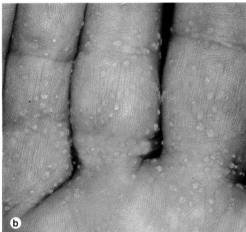

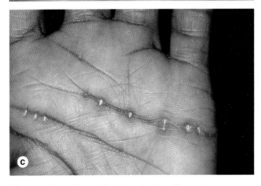

Figure 16-7 a Keratosis plantaris. b, c Punctate keratoderma

hair, keratoderma, nail dystrophy, and tufted, swollen terminal phalanges. The diagnosis is confirmed through genetic testing that reveals the connexin-30 gene mutation.

Both EEC and AEC syndromes can be detected upon recognition of their unique clinical aspects, but confirmatory genetic testing for the p63 mutation can be done.

Pathogenesis

Various defects in the stream of NFkappaB signaling, whose proper function is crucial to the development of cutaneous structures, teeth, and palate formation appear to contribute to the pathogenesis of many of the ectodermal dysplasias. Ectodysplasin is a similar tumor necrosis factor (TNF) superfamily member whose signaling is necessary to activate the transcription factor NFkappaB.

Treatment

Treatment for all subtypes of ectodermal dysplasia is aimed at symptomatic relief. The most essential of these measures is in patients with the hypohidrotic subtype, in whom avoidance of overheating is of paramount importance to prevent febrile seizures. Early and regular dental care with avoidance of tooth extraction is needed to preserve the alveolar ridge for future implants. Patients with the hidrotic subtype should be seen regularly by a dermatologist to receive topical keratolytic therapy for keratoderma and possible nail matrix ablation to treat the pain associated with the tufted phalanges and nail dystrophy. In contrast to patients with the other subtypes, those with EEC and AEC syndromes specifically need ophthalmologic care as well as possible intervention by specialized surgeons for any clefting that may be present. Both dental and skin care are essential in these subtypes as well.

Epidermolysis bullosa

Key Points

* Epidermolysis bullosa (EB) is the prototypic mechanobullous disorder characterized by genetic transmission, mechanical fragility, and recurrent blister formation
* The epidermis and dermis of normal skin are bound by several crucial cytoskeletal components, which pathologically are lacking in the skin of patients with EB
* The ultrastructural level of blister formation determines the severity of blistering in EB and is the major factor driving the classification of various EB subtypes
* Although there is a wide range of intricate EB classification systems, it is the authors' view that Uitto and Richard's classification is the most practical and clinically and scientifically relevant

sweating leaves them at risk of overheating. The diagnosis is confirmed by a punch biopsy of palmar skin that should demonstrate the absence of eccrine ducts.

Hidrotic ectodermal dysplasia should be suspected in patients with the constellation of sparse

Table 16-5 Classification of ectodermal dysplasias

Disease subtype	Disease synonyms	Gene mutation	Protein	Key clinical features	Inheritance
Hypohidrotic ectodermal dysplasia	Anhidrotic ectodermal dysplasia; Christ–Siemens–Touraine syndrome	EDA (encodes ectodysplasin A) EDAR (encodes ectodysplasin A Receptor) EDADD (ectodysplasin A receptor associated death domain)	Ectodysplasin Eda-A1 receptor Ectodysplasin A2 Eda-A2 receptor NF-κB essential modulator	Sparse hair, hypo- or anhidrosis, abnormal dentition with conical incisors, frontal bossing and periorbital wrinkling, saddle nose, normal nails, no keratoderma. Immunodeficiency may be present in association with *NEMO* mutations	X-linked recessive Autosomal recessive or autosomal dominant
Hidrotic ectodermal dysplasia	Clouston syndrome	*GJB6*	Connexin 30	Sparse hair, normal sweating and dentition, palmoplantar keratoderma, nail dystrophy with chronic paronychia	Autosomal dominant
Ectrodactyly–ectodermal dysplasia–cleft lip/palate (EEC) syndrome		p63, *EEC1, EEC2, EEC3*	Tumor suppressor proteins important in morphogenesis	"Lobster-claw deformity," cleft palate and/or lip, sparse hair, normal sweat, hypodontia, some with lacrimal duct abnormalities	Autosomal dominant
Ankyloblepharon filiforme adenatum–ectodermal dysplasia–cleft palate (AEC) syndrome	Hay–Wells syndrome	*p63 SAM* (sterile alpha-motif) domain	Tumor suppressor protein important in morphogenesis	Collodion membrane at birth, sparse hair, chronic erosive scalp dermatitis with secondary bacterial infection, dystrophic nails, fusion of eyelids, lacrimal duct atresia, abnormal dentition, cleft palate and/or lip	Autosomal dominant

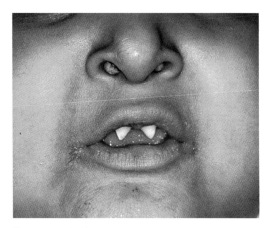

Figure 16-8 Anhidrotic ectodermal dysplasia

Clinical presentation

EB simplex (EBS) (Figure 16-9) is the most superficial EB variant. It results from an autosomal-dominant mutation in keratins 5 and 14, the keratin intermediate filaments that normally provide internal structural support to the epidermal basal keratinocyte. Bullae in EBS occur intraepidermally in the lower half of the basilar keratinocyte. Patients with EBS are typically free of other systemic manifestations and heal without scarring. This disease can, nonetheless, be debilitating because of chronicity. Three clinical subtypes of EBS are recognized: (1) EBS Weber–Cockayne, which presents with palmoplantar bullae and hyperhidrosis that worsen in warm temperatures; (2) generalized EBS or Koebner type, which is characterized by generalized bullae and also worsens in warm climates; and (3) EBS Dowling–Meara, in which widespread bullae group in a herpetiform pattern and may be accompanied by palmoplantar keratoderma and nail dystrophy. EBS Dowling–Meara has the highest morbidity and mortality within the first few months of life, but may improve somewhat with a warmer environment.

A more recently recognized subtype is the *EB hemidesmosomal subtype*. This was first proposed by Pulkkinen and Uitto in 1998 and was subsequently included in the formal classification of EB by Uitto and Richard in 2004. Hemidesmosmoal EB includes three disorders in which blistering occurs within the hemidesmosome, which is located at the interface between the basal cell keratinocyte and the lamina lucida:

1. EB with pyloric atresia, a type of EB previously classified under dominant dystrophic EB (DEB), which results from a mutation in alpha-6 beta-4 integrin. Patients with this subtype suffer severe blistering, as well as morbidity or mortality from gastrointestinal abnormalities. If they survive the neonatal period, they often improve with age. There is a risk of hydronephrosis and possible renal failure secondary to stricture formation in these patients
2. Generalized atrophic benign EB (GABEB), previously classified as "non-Herlitz" junctional EB (JEB), is caused by mutations in the collagen XVII gene and results in a typically normal lifespan with recurrent blistering that is often associated with hair, nail, and dental abnormalities; it may abate with age
3. EBS with muscular dystrophy results from an autosomal-recessive mutation in plectin. These patients do not have severe blistering, but do present with a later onset of muscular weakness

The newer hemidesmosomal classification is helpful because of its genetic precision and its clinical prognostic value, specifically its ability to predict phenotypic severity and disease progression among individual patients and their families.

JEB comprises a group of patients with autosomal-recessive mutations in the ultrastructural components of the lamina lucida, namely laminin 5 and BPAg2 (collagen XVII). The split in JEB occurs through the lamina lucida, a region of the basement membrane so named for its clear appearance on electron microscopy. Patients with JEB present with generalized blistering at birth and are at high risk of developing blistering of other epithelial surfaces, such as the respiratory, gastrointestinal, and genitourinary systems. JEB

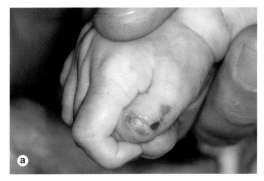
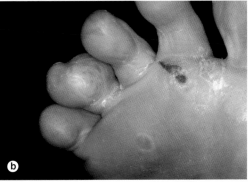

Figure 16-9 a, b Epidermolysis bullosa simplex

patients often have coexistent malnutrition and stricture formation, leading to failure to thrive and anemia; they may also have abnormal dentition and multiple caries. Many patients with the "Herlitz" or more severe variant of JEB exhibit exuberant periorificial granulation tissue, have abnormal teeth and enamel defects, and shed nails. Death within the first year of life from sepsis and multisystem organ failure is common. As previously mentioned, the "non-Herlitz" variant or GABEB has been reclassified under the hemidesmosomal type of EB.

DEB (Figure 16-10), the most disabling of the EB subtypes, results from either an autosomal-dominant (dominant DEB or DDEB) or autosomal-recessive (recessive DEB or RDEB) mutation in collagen VII, the major collagen that forms the anchoring fibrils in the dermis. Patients with RDEB are more severely affected than are patients with DDEB. The cleft in both forms of DEB occurs in the sublamina densa region. DEB patients heal with scarring, atrophy, and milia. It is important to note that, whereas milia are classically seen in the DEB subtypes, milia have been described, albeit less commonly, in all subtypes of EB. As with any chronic cicatricial skin condition, patients with DEB have a dramatically increased risk of developing cutaneous squamous cell carcinomas, even at a young age, within scar tissue. This can be fatal if undetected, so it is important to biopsy any nonhealing site on these highly vulnerable patients.

Patients with DDEB may have extensive mucous membrane involvement, including bullae and resultant scarring of the buccal mucosa, tongue, palate, esophagus, pharynx, and larynx. They may also develop contractures of the gingivolabial sulcus, as well as symptoms of dysphagia from scarring of the esophagus.

RDEB is the most severe of the DEB subtypes and in its gravest form has been called the "Hallopeau–Siemens" variant. The hallmark of these patients is pseudosyndactyly or the "mitten deformity," which occurs as the end result of repeated bullae with re-epithelialization of the adjacent digits.

Diagnosis

Several methods may be useful in confirming the diagnosis of EB. Routine skin biopsy after blister induction with a light, rotating motion of a pencil eraser will show the basic level of bulla formation and is helpful in distinguishing EB simplex from the other subtypes. Electron microscopy and immunomapping with monoclonal antibodies remain the gold standard for precise diagnosis, especially when JEB or DEB is suspected. Genetic testing for the specific mutations can be performed by genotypic analysis. It is important when evaluating any bullous process to exclude viral and bacterial etiologies, as well as autoimmune bullous dermatoses.

Pathogenesis

See Table 16-6.

Treatment

Current treatment of EB is largely supportive and is aimed at minimizing excessive heat and friction and maximizing wound healing in order to prevent contractures and infection. A neonate with suspected EB must be treated with extreme care, as even gentle manipulation can lead to bullae formation. In patients with RDEB, it is important to monitor the skin for possible development of squamous cell carcinomas. Also, these patients are at high risk for development of esophageal and laryngeal strictures, which frequently require dilation. Close attention to nutritional requirements is crucial in the more

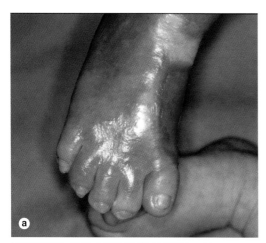

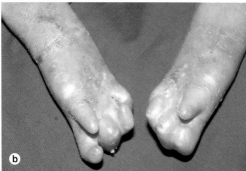

Figure 16-10 a Dominant dystrophic epidermolysis bullosa. **b** Recessive dystrophic epidermolysis bullosa

Table 16-6 Epidermolysis bullosa (EB) subtypes			
EB subtype	Genetic mutation	Level of defect	Inheritance
EB simplex	Keratins 5 and 14	Intraepidermal	Autosomal dominant (rarely autosomal recessive)
EB hemidesmosomal			
EB with pyloric atresia	Alpha-6 beta-4 integrin	Hemidesmosome	Autosomal recessive
Generalized atrophic benign EB	Laminin 5, bullous pemphigoid antigen 2 (collagen XVII)	Hemidesmosome	Autosomal recessive
EB simplex with muscular dystrophy	Plectin	Hemidesmosome	Autosomal recessive
Junctional EB	Laminin 5, BPAg2 (collagen XVII)	Lamina lucida	Autosomal recessive
Dystrophic EB (DEB)			
Dominant DEB	Collagen VII	Sublamina densa	Autosomal dominant
Recessive DEB	Collagen VII	Sublamina densa	Autosomal recessive

severe forms of EB, as these patients may have increased metabolic needs. Extra caloric and protein intake via tube feeding, as well as iron supplementation, may be required. Early surgical consultation is of paramount importance for subtypes of EB, such as EBS with pyloric atresia, in which extracutaneous manifestations may be life-threatening.

Waardenburg syndrome

Key Points

- Clinical features include hair and/or skin hypopigmentation, deafness, dystopia canthorum, synophrys, Hirschsprung's disease, and/or limb abnormalities
- Four clinical subtypes result from different gene mutations in transcription factors (Table 16-7)

Clinical presentation

There are four types of Waardenburg syndrome (WS) that are classified as WS1–4.

WS1

Up to 50% of patients with WS1 will have a white forelock (Figure 16-11) (although on occasion the forelock may be red or black). They may also have poliosis (premature graying of scalp or body hair). Skin may show patchy leukoderma. Because there are neural crest cells in the cochlea, many patients have hereditary sensorineural deafness that can be unilateral or bilateral. Heterochromia irides can be unilateral (irises of two different colors; Figure 16-12) or bilateral (isohypochromia, or bilateral pale blue eyes; Figure 16-13). Dystopia canthorum (an increased distance between inner canthi) is also a very common finding, present in up to 99% of patients with WS1. Patients may exhibit synophrys (medial eyebrow confluence or hyperplasia). Facial dysmorphism is frequent with hypoplasia of the nasal bone, hypoplastic alae nasi, shortened philtrum, and shortening and displacement of the maxilla being characteristic.

WS2

Patients with WS2 lack dystopia canthorum and are more likely than those with WS1 to be deaf and have heterochromia irides.

WS3

WS3 is also called Klein–Waardenburg syndrome. Patients with WS3 have many of the clinical features of WS1 but also have upper-extremity limb deformities, particularly contractures.

WS4

WS4, also called Shah–Waardenburg syndrome, is characterized by the presence of Hirschsprung's disease (aganglionic megacolon). Patients are frequently deaf and have a white forelock and heterochromia irides. Dystopia canthorum is rare.

Diagnosis

The diagnosis of WS should be considered in families with more than one deaf member. The presence of other findings, such as unusual eye color, poliosis, or white forelock, helps the clinician make the correct diagnosis. A white forelock with leukoderma can also be seen in individuals with piebaldism and the two conditions can be differentiated by the absence of other associated

Table 16-7 Classification of Waardenburg syndrome (WS)

Disease subtype	Gene mutation	Protein	Key clinical features
WS1	PAX3	PAX3 transcription factor	White forelock Patchy leukoderma Dystopia canthorum Heterochromia irides Deafness Synophrys
WS2	1. MITF 2. SLUG (SNA12)	1. MITF transcription factor 2. SLUG Zn-finger transcription factor	Like WS1 but no dystopia canthorum, heterochromia irides and deafness more common
WS3 (Klein–Waardenburg)	PAX3	PAX3 transcription factor	Like WS1, but with limb deformities
WS4 (Shah–Waardenburg)	1. SOX10 2. EDN3 3. EDNRB	1. SRY-box containing gene 10 2. Endothelin 3 3. Endothelin B receptor	Like WS1, but with Hirschsprung's disease, rare dystopia canthorum

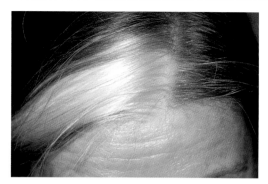

Figure 16-11 Waardenburg syndrome, white forelock

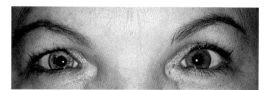

Figure 16-12 Waardenburg syndrome

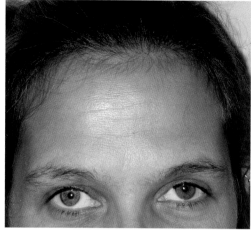

Figure 16-13 Waardenburg syndrome

findings in piebaldism. Genetic testing can be done to help to make the diagnosis and classify the subtype of WS. Examination of family members for features of WS can be helpful as well.

Pathogenesis

WS results from abnormal migration and differentiation of neural crest cells. The absence of melanocytes in hair causes the white forelock and the absence in skin results in leukoderma. The deafness seen in WS patients is due to the absence of cochlear melanocytes. Impairments in ganglion cell migration to the hindgut results in Hirshprung's disease in WS4 patients. The specific genes involved in the subtypes of WS have been identified and characterized.

WS1 and WS3 are due to mutations in the *PAX3* gene. *PAX3* encodes a transcription factor that is responsible for the migration and differentiation of mesenchymal cells and melanocytes from the neural crest. If one copy of *PAX3* is mutated, the affected individual will have WS1. In individuals with WS3, both autosomal-dominant and autosomal-recessive inheritance have been described. WS3 appears to result from more severe *PAX3* deficiency, which can be the result of a dominant negative mutation or of a mutation in both copies of the gene. WS2 is most commonly caused by a mutation in *MITF*, which encodes a melanocyte transcription factor important for, among other functions, tyrosinase transcription, and is inherited in an autosomal-dominant fashion. The *SLUG* gene encodes a Zn-finger transcription factor expressed in migratory melanocytes and has been found to be mutated in some patients with WS2 who have a normal *MITF* gene.

Autosomal-dominant, or less commonly autosomal-recessive, inheritance of mutations in *SOX10*, *EDN3*, and *EDNRB* all result in WS4. These genes regulate the differentiation and migration of melanoblasts and ganglion precursor cells from the neural crest, explaining the pigment abnormalities and aganglionic megacolon seen in these patients. *EDNRB* encodes the receptor for the *EDN3* gene product endothelin B. The expression of *EDNRB* is regulated by the *SOX10* gene. *MITF* expression is also regulated by *SOX10* and *PAX3*, possibly explaining how mutations in multiple genes causes a similar phenotype.

Treatment

The role of the dermatologist in the management of patients with WS largely involves referral to the appropriate specialists to help in the management of deafness or Hirschsprung's disease.

Oculocutaneous albinism (OCA)

Key Points

- A group of related disorders caused by low or absent melanin production (Table 16-8)
- Patients are at high risk of ultraviolet light-induced cutaneous malignancy
- Defective melanin production also results in misrouting of the optic nerve during eye development, causing poor vision, nystagmus, and strabismus

Clinical presentation

The clinical presentation of patients with OCA is variable and can be suggestive of their specific subtype of OCA. Due to their impaired melanin synthesis, all patients are at increased risk of cutaneous malignancy induced by ultraviolet light.

Table 16-8 Classification of oculocutaneous albinism (OCA)

Type	Gene	Defect	Phenotype
OCA1A (tyrosinase-negative OCA)	TYR	Absent tyrosinase activity	White hair Pink skin Red pupils
OCA1B (yellow-mutant OCA)	TYR	Decreased tyrosinase activity	Neonates look like those with OCA1A, but develop some pigment over time. Yellow hair, some pigment in eyes and skin
OCA1TS (temperature-sensitive OCA)	TYR	Decreased tyrosinase activity centrally due to temperature sensitive mutation	Develops darker hair on cooler extremities beginning at puberty
OCA2	P	P protein, may play a role in transporting tyrosinase into the melanosome	Variable loss of melanin
OCA3 (Rufous OCA)	TYRP1	Tyrosinase-related protein 1, may stabilize tyrosinase	Light brown skin, primarily in patients of African descent
OCA4	MATP	Function of membrane-associated transporter protein is unknown	Variable loss of melanin

OCA1A

Patients with OCA1A, or tyrosinase-negative albinism, have an absence of pigment in their hair, skin, and eyes throughout life due to a lack of tyrosinase, an enzyme critical in the initial steps of the melanin biosynthesis pathway. Also, because of a complete lack of melanin production they do not develop lentigines or nevi. Eyes are typically blue in color with red pupils, and visual acuity is poor. Other ocular manifestations include nystagmus, strabismus that is exacerbated by light, iris transillumination, hypopigmentation of the uveal tract and retinal pigment epithelium, foveal hypoplasia, and abnormal decussation of the optic nerve fibers at the optic chiasm, resulting in a lack of binocular vision.

OCA1B

Patients with OCA1B have limited tyrosinase activity and thus, although they appear identical to OCA1A patients at birth, they do develop some skin pigmentation and hair becomes yellow to light brown with time. Similarly, these patients can develop lentigines and nevi. The ocular manifestations of nystagmus and strabismus tend to persist however. This subtype is most commonly seen in Amish individuals in the United States.

OCA1TS

A very rare form of OCA1, referred to as temperature-sensitive OCA or OCA1TS, is due to a mutation in tyrosinase that makes it unstable at temperatures greater than 35°C. Patients have white hair in warm areas of the body such as the scalp and axillae but have darker hair in cooler areas of the body such as the scalp. They typically have ocular manifestations similar to those seen in patients with OCA1A.

OCA2

Patients with OCA2 carry a mutation in the P gene. They may have some hair and skin pigmentation at birth. Hair may be yellow to light brown and skin may be light but not white. They may also have congenital nevi. There is an association of OCA2 with the genetic disorders Prader–Willi syndrome and Angelman syndrome. Approximately 1% of patients with these syndromes, which result from deletion of portions of chromosome 15q near the P-gene locus, will have OCA2 and up to half will have decreased pigmentation, suggesting hemizygosity of the P-gene allele.

OCA3

This form of albinism, also called rufous albinism, was initially thought to be restricted to African blacks. However, one case of albinism in a Caucasian and a second in a Pakistani patient due to a mutation in the tyrosine-related protein 1 (TYRP1) gene has been reported. Black patients have light brown to bronze skin, ginger-red hair, and blue-green irides. Nystagmus in these patients is mild or absent.

OCA4

The clinical presentation of patients with OCA4, the most recently described form of OCA, varies from a complete absence of pigment as seen in OCA1 to a decrease in pigment with some ability to tan and the presence of nevi. Nystagmus and poor visual acuity are present in some but not all patients. The phenotypic presentation can be correlated with specific mutations in the *MATP* gene.

Diagnosis

The diagnosis of albinism is usually made at or soon after birth based on the characteristic clinical presentation. However, other syndromes of abnormal pigmentation can present similarly to tyrosinase-positive OCA. Skin biopsy will show the presence of melanocytes, but the absence of melanin granules. The activity of dihydroxyphenylalanine (DOPA) oxidase can be measured in the hair bulb in vitro using a quantitative hair bulb tyrosinase assay. By electron microscopy, melanosomes in patients with a complete absence of tyrosinase will be predominantly in stage I or II. One report found that, by treating skin samples with DOPA prior to performing electron microcroscopy, the sensitivity for detecting stage III and IV melanomsomes is increased, allowing patients to be classified as having tyrosinase-negative versus positive OCA. Genetic studies must be performed for definitive diagnosis. Diagnosis may also be done prenatally using fetal skin biopsies to look for failure of melanogenesis in hair bulb or skin melanocytes by light microscopy or electron microscopy and by chorionic villus sampling to detect specific mutations.

Tyrosinase-negative albinism has a unique phenotype that is unlikely to be confused with other disorders of pigmentation. However, some forms of albinism in which there is some melanogenesis can be confused clinically with pigmentary dilution disorders such as Hermansky–Pudlak syndrome, Elejalde syndrome, Chédiak–Higashi syndrome, and Griscelli syndrome. Patients with phenylketonuria who are not following a low-phenylalanine diet may have impaired melanogenesis. The end stages of widespread vitiligo may resemble OCA clinically; however, onset is not at birth.

Pathogenesis

OCA1 results from absent or reduced melanin synthesis due to a defect in tyrosinase, an enzyme involved in melanogenesis. In OCA1A, tyrosinase is completely absent. In OCA1B, tyrosinase levels are significantly reduced. Inheritance is in an autosomal-recessive fashion. OCA2 results from a mutation in the P gene which most likely regulates the processing of tyrosinase and its localization to the melanosome. OCA3 is due to a mutation in the *TYRP1* gene. The function of *TYRP1* in humans is most likely to stabilize tyrosinase. The *MATP* gene has been found to be mutated in patients with OCA4 and it is predicted, based on its structure, to function as a membrane transport, but its role in melanogenesis is not yet understood.

Treatment

In the management of patients with OCA, the importance of photoprotection should be emphasized as these patients are at high risk for cutaneous malignancy, especially squamous cell carcinomas. Also, because most will also have decreased visual acuity, nystagmus, and/or strabismus, involvement of ophthalmology is necessary as well.

Controversies

While the high prevalence of nonmelanoma skin cancers is well described, it is interesting to note that to date there are only 27 reported cases of cutaneous melanoma in patients with OCA. Although the absence or decrease in skin pigment in this patient population would be predicted to result in an increase in melanoma, this would not appear to be the case based on the available literature. This may be due to a lower incidence of melanoma, underreporting of the disease, or to more missed diagnoses due to the fact that melanomas in these patients are amelanotic or hypopigmented.

Darier's disease

Key Points

* Synonyms: keratosis follicularis, dyskeratosis follicularis, Darier–White disease
* Autosomal-dominant disorder due to mutation in the *ATP2A2* gene
* Characterized by greasy papules in a seborrheic distribution
* Viral and bacterial superinfection of skin lesions is a common problem
* Most effectively treated with oral retinoids

Clinical presentation

Darier's disease most commonly presents in childhood or adolescence and is chracterized by greasy hyperkeratotic brown-yellow papules in a seborrheic distribution. Lesions are often pruritic and exacerbated by heat and/or ultraviolet light. Oral manifestations include cobblestoning of mucosa, fine white papules on the hard palate, and the presence of salivary duct stones. Acral keratoses are commonly seen. Other palmar findings include palmar pitting and hemorrhagic macules. Nail findings include longitudinal red and white lines, nail fragility, and V-shaped nicking of the free nail edge (Figure 16-14). The disease may fluctuate in severity but remissions typically do not occur.

Several unusual morphologies of Darier's disease have been described, including cornifying, hypertrophic, comedonal, and linear subtypes.

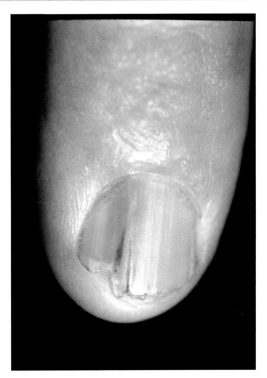

Figure 16-14 Darier's disease

Cornifying Darier's disease typically presents as hypertrophic plaques on the lower legs and is characterized by the presence of cutaneous horns. Hypertrophic Darier's disease most commonly presents in intertriginous areas. Comedonal Darier's disease presents as an acneiform eruption on the head and neck and resembles small warty dyskeratomas clinically and histopathologically. Linear, or localized, Darier's disease is often unilateral and most likely the result of genetic mosaicism due to a postzygotic mutation.

Complications of Darier's disease are generally infectious in nature. Skin may become malodorous in the setting of bacterial overgrowth, a condition that causes many patients significant social discomfort. More concerning, patients may experience cutaneous infection with bacteria or viruses. Of particular concern is the risk of Kaposi's varicelliform eruption, superinfection of skin with herpes simplex virus. This condition should be considered in any patient experiencing fever or changes in lesion morphology.

Diagnosis

Diagnosis of Darier's disease is usually based on histopathologic confirmation of biopsy of typical skin lesions. Some unusual variants of Darier's disease may be difficult to diagnose in the absence of other typical clinical findings and biopsy is particularly helpful in these cases. Histopathologically, Darier's disease is characterized by acanthosis, dyskeratosis, and the presence of dyskeratotic cells, referred to as "corps ronds and grains."

The initial manifestation of Darier's disease is often the presence of acral keratoses. These are clinically identical to the lesions of acrokeratosis verruciformis of Hopf. This has led some to debate whether acrokeratosis verruciformis is simply a forme fruste of Darier's disease. Some studies have found mutations in the *ATP2A2* gene in lesions of acrokeratosis verruciformis, seemingly supporting this hypothesis, while others have not found this mutation to be present. Differential diagnoses of comedonal Darier's disease include multiple warty dyskeratomas and familial dyskeratotic comedones. Histologically, Grover's disease can appear similar to Darier's disease, but the focal and transient nature of Grover's disease makes it relatively simple to distinguish clinically from Darier's disease.

Pathogenesis

Darier's disease is an autosomal-dominant disease that results from a mutation in the *ATP2A2* gene which encodes the sarcoplasmic/endoplasmic calcium adenosine triphosphatase (SERCA2). The SERCA2 pump helps to modulate cytosolic Ca^{2+} levels in keratinocytes by mediating the transfer of Ca^{2+} between the cytosol and the endoplasmic reticulum. Intracellular Ca^{2+} concentration helps to regulate the assembly of desmosomes and cultured keratinocytes from patients with Darier's disease show impaired trafficking and localization of desmoplakin to the desmosome. This finding may explain the acantholysis seen histologically in Darier's disease.

In addition, studies from a canine skin disease due to mutant SERCA2 that is similar to Darier's disease clinically reveal that cells that harbor a mutant SERCA2 fail to upregulate the p21^{WAF1} gene and exit the cell cycle under stress. This can result in the increased apoptosis, correlating histologically with corps ronds and grains seen in lesional Darier's skin. Further, this failure to exit the cell cycle can result in the accumulation of secondary mutations, which the authors speculate may be responsible for the formation of persistent lesions.

Treatment

Darier's disease can be difficult to treat and remission of the disease is not seen. Because disease activity is typically exacerbated by sunlight and heat, avoidance of these measures is helpful. Topical steroids may offer some symptomatic relief in patients with Darier's disease. A frequent concern of Darier's patients is the malodor of their skin that can develop due to bacterial overgrowth. This can be reduced by the use of topical antibiotics and/or antiseptic washes. Topical retinoids may reduce hyperkeratosis, but are often irritating.

This irritation can be reduced by the concomitant use of topical steroids and emollients. Other topical treatments that have been reported to be effective in small series include topical 5-fluorouracil, topical tacrolimus, and photodynamic therapy. For patients with significant disease, systemic retinoids offer the best reported efficacy, with approximately 75–90% of patients reporting improvement in disease activity with their use. The two used most commonly today are acitretin and isotretinoin.

Treatment is often limited by mucocutaneous side-effects. Retinoids must be used with extreme caution in females of reproductive age because of the well-known teratogenicity of these drugs. Other systemic drugs useful in patients with Darier's disease include oral antibiotics and antivirals that are used in cases of secondary infection of involved skin. Case reports or small case series of surgical treatments of Darier's disease include electrosurgery and laser ablation with carbon dioxide and erbium: yttrium aluminum garnet (YAG) lasers.

Controversies

The coexistence of neuropsychiatric morbidity, including seizures and mental illness, has been reported by some. However, other studies refute this finding or find that genetic loci associated with psychiatric disease are in close proximity to, but distinct from the SERCA2, gene. Given the significant psychosocial morbidity caused by Darier's disease, the etiology of this association, if it does indeed exist, is difficult to determine.

Hailey–Hailey disease

Key Points

- Synonyms: familial benign chronic pemphigus
- Characterized by blisters and erosions at sites of friction
- Autosomal-dominant disorder, cause by a mutation in the *ATP2C1* gene

Clinical presentation

The typical age of onset of Hailey–Hailey disease is in the second to fourth decade. Skin disease can vary in severity and is characterized by erythematous and erosive plaques primarily in the intertriginous areas, including the axilla, groin, and neck folds. However, involvement of the trunk and extremities has been reported as well. Some patients will have thick, vegetative plaques or vesicles. Up to 70% of patients will also have longitudinal white lines on the fingernails. Lesions are often quite uncomfortable. This disease fluctuates in its course and patients may experience sustained relapses or remissions. Heat, sweating, friction, and microbial infection exacerbate the disease.

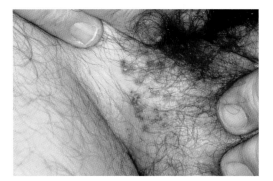

Figure 16-15 Hailey–Hailey disease

Diagnosis

Diagnosis of Hailey–Hailey disease (Figure 16-15) is usually made by biopsy of typical lesions. Histopathologically, Hailey–Hailey disease is characterized by suprabasilar acantholysis that has been described as having an appearance like a "dilapidated brick wall." Differential diagnosis includes pemphigus vegetans, inverse psoriasis, *Corynebacterium* infection, and axillary granular parakeratosis. Histopathologically, Grover's disease can show a Hailey–Hailey-like form but the two entities are quite different clinically. Also, the acantholysis seen in biopsies of lesional skin from patients with Darier's disease can look similar to that seen in Hailey–Hailey disease, although the acantholysis tends to be more suprabasilar and dyskeratosis is not a prominent feature in Hailey–Hailey disease.

Pathogenesis

The gene for Hailey–Hailey disease has been identified as *ATP2C1* and encodes SPCA1, a endoplasmic reticulum-Golgi Ca^{2+}/Mn^{2+} ATPase that sequesters Ca^{2+} into the Golgi. Keratinocytes from patients with Hailey–Hailey disease have a higher resting cytoplasmic Ca^{2+} concentration but a decreased ability to mobilize Ca^{2+} to the cytoplasm from the Golgi upon stimulation when compared to keratinocytes from healthy individuals. The epidermal calcium gradient is important in epidermal differentiation, desmosome assembly, and profilaggrin processing. Interestingly, this gradient is higher in suprabasilar than basilar keratinocytes, perhaps explaining the confinement of acantholysis to this part of the epidermis.

Treatment

Treatment of Hailey–Hailey disease is primarily with topical or oral steroids to reduce secondary inflammation. Topical tacrolimus ointment has been reported to induce remission of disease. Other treatments reported to be effective in some cases include calcitriol and photodynamic therapy. Because Hailey–Hailey disease is exacerbated by sweating, some have tried and reported success with treatment of affected areas with botulinum toxin type A. Reports of the efficacy of oral retinoids are conflicting. Surgical treatments include wide local excision of the affected area with the placement of split-thickness skin grafts, carbon dioxide laser ablation, or treatment with the pulsed-dye laser. Antibiotics, both systemic and topical, are important treatment adjuvants, as disease is often exacerbated by infection.

Controversies

There have been a few case reports of squamous cell carcinoma arising within lesions of Hailey–Hailey disease, all in the genital area. In one report, the tumor was found to be positive for oncogenic strains of human papillomavirus. These malignancies may be secondary to chronic inflammation or to the increased susceptibility of these patients to infection with human papillomavirus infection due to their impaired skin barrier.

Acknowledgments

The authors would like to thank Drs. Joseph English, Matthew Zirwas, Timothy Patton, and Dirk Elston for providing some of the photographs used in this chapter.

Further reading

Burge SM. Hailey–Hailey disease: the clinical features, response to treatment and prognosis. Br J Dermatol 1992;126:275–282.

Burge SM, Wilkinson JD. Darier–White disease: a review of the clinical features in 163 patients. J Am Acad Dermatol 1992;27:40–50.

Dhitavat J, Macfarlane S, Dode L, et al. Acrokeratosis verruciformis of Hopf is caused by mutation in ATP2A2: evidence that it is allelic to Darier's disease. J Invest Dermatol 2003;120:229–232.

DiGiovanna JJ, Robinson-Bostom L. Ichthyosis: etiology, diagnosis, and management. Am J Clin Dermatol 2003;4:81–95.

Gabriele R. Molecular genetics of the ichthyoses. Am J Med Genet Part C: Semin Med Genet 2004;131C:32–44.

Horn HM, Tidman MJ. The clinical spectrum of dystrophic epidermolysis bullosa. Br J Dermatol 2002;146:267–274.

Hu Z, Bonifas JM, Beech J, et al. Mutations in ATP2C1, encoding a calcium pump, cause Hailey–Hailey disease. Nat Genet 2000;24:61.

Kimyai-Asadi AKL, Jih MH. The molecular basis of hereditary palmoplantar keratodermas. J Am Acad Dermatol 2002;47:3.

König A, Happle R, Bornholdt D, et al. Mutations in the NSDHL gene, encoding a 3-hydroxysteroid dehydrogenase, cause CHILD syndrome. Am J Med Genet 2000;90:339–346.

O'Driscoll J, Muston GC, McGrath JA, et al. A recurrent mutation in the loricrin gene underlies the ichthyotic variant of Vohwinkel syndrome. Clin Exp Dermatol 2002;27:243–246.

Paller AS. The genetic basis of hereditary blistering disorders. Curr Opin Pediatr 1996;8:367–371.

Patel N, Spencer LA, English JC 3rd, et al. Acquired ichthyosis. J Am Acad Dermatol 2006;55:647–656.

Raghunath M, Hennies HC, Ahvazi B, et al. Self-healing collodion baby: a dynamic phenotype explained by a particular transglutaminase-1 mutation. J Invest Dermatol 2003;120:224–228.

Read AP, Newton VE. Waardenburg syndrome. J Med Genet 1997;34:656–665.

Rubeiz N, Kibbi AG. Management of ichthyosis in infants and children. Clin Dermatol 2003;21:325–328.

Shwayder T. Disorders of keratinization: diagnosis and management. Am J Clin Dermatol 2004;5:17–29.

Smith FJ, Irvine AD, Terron-Kwiatkowski A, et al. Loss-of-function mutations in the gene encoding filaggrin cause ichthyosis vulgaris. Nat Genet 2006;38:337–342.

Spritz RA, Strunk KM, Giebel LB, et al. Detection of mutations in the tyrosinase gene in a patient with type IA oculocutaneous albinism. N Engl J Med 1990;322:1724–1728.

Thomas AC, Cullup T, Norgett EE, et al. ABCA12 is the major harlequin ichthyosis gene. J Invest Dermatol 2006;126:2408–2413.

Uitto J, Richard G. Progress in epidermolysis bullosa: genetic classification and clinical implications. Am J Med Genet C Semin Med Genet 2004;131C:61–74.

Chapter 17

Perforating dermatoses

Jonathan Cotliar

The perforating disorders share the similar histologic feature of transepidermal elimination of dermal substances (Table 17-1). While a variety of disorders can display transepidermal elimination, there are four main diseases that consistently have transepidermal elimination as a histologic finding. These diseases are: (1) acquired perforating dermatosis (APD); (2) elastosis perforans serpiginosa; (3) reactive perforating collagenosis of childhood; and (4) perforating pseudoxanthoma elasticum.

Acquired perforating dermatosis

Clinical presentation

> **Key Point**
>
> • APD is characterized by pruritic, hyperkeratotic papules and nodules, often in association with diabetes mellitus and/or renal failure

Kyrle disease, perforating folliculitis, perforating disorder of renal failure (Figure 17-1) and reactive perforating collagenosis were previously classified as distinct dermatoses, based on the clinical variability of the skin lesions in these conditions. However, APD is the term that now unifies these entities, based on the specific histologic finding of transepidermal elimination of dermal substances (collagen, elastic fibers) seen in all these diagnoses. Although there is also an inherited, familial form of reactive perforating collagenosis, APD includes the noninherited, adult-onset variant of this disorder. Patients typically present with intensely pruritic, hyperkeratotic papules and/or nodules that may be either follicular or nonfollicular, with or without umbilication. Lesions most commonly occur on the arms and legs, but may present on any portion of the body, sometimes near or within areas of excoriation. Koebnerization has been described. Although the majority of cases are associated with diabetes mellitus and/or renal

failure, APD has been associated with a variety of systemic illnesses (Box 17-1).

Diagnosis

> **Key Points**
>
> • Suspect APD in diabetic or renal failure patients with pruritus and multiple hyperkeratotic lesions
> • Confirm diagnosis with skin biopsy that reveals transepidermal elimination of amorphous, degenerated material

Patients with diffuse pruritus and hyperkeratotic papules or nodules should raise a high index of suspicion for APD, particularly those with underlying diabetes mellitus and/or renal failure.

The hallmark of APD is the histologic finding of transepidermal elimination of one or any combination of keratin, collagen, or elastic fibers. Skin biopsy results may vary with the location of APD (follicular or nonfollicular), chronicity of the lesions, and the amount of excoriation that has resulted from scratching. Typically, lesions are hyperkeratotic with epidermal acanthosis. They may also have a verrucous appearance on low power. A horny plug with a central parakeratotic column may extend and perforate into the dermis, although this may not be present in all cases. In early lesions, suppurative inflammation may be seen at the site of perforation, while older lesions may have chronic inflammation or foreign-body granulomas. Necrotic and/or amorphous material may be visualized extruding through follicles (if follicular lesions are present) or areas of epidermal perforation. Characterization of this amorphous material as collagen, elastic fibers, or both is best done with the use of Verhoeff-Van Gieson staining.

Differential diagnosis

> **Key Point**
>
> • Skin biopsy is necessary to exclude clinical imitators of APD

Table 17-1 The perforating disorders

Disease	Perforating substance	Associations	Clinical lesions	Age of onset
Acquired perforating dermatosis (APD)	Elastic tissue and/or collagen	Diabetes mellitus Renal failure	Keratotic papules, nodules on legs, arms	Adulthood
Elastosis perforans serpiginosa (EPS)	Elastic tissue	Penicillamine Genetic diseases	Serpiginous or annular papules/plaques on neck, face, arms, flexural regions	First or second decade
Reactive perforating collagenosis of childhood	Collagen	Trauma	Keratotic papules on extremities, face, buttocks	Childhood (inherited)
Perforating pseudoxanthoma elasticum	Altered elastic fibers	Multiparity in women, obesity	Keratotic papules on the abdomen near the umbilicus	Middle-aged women

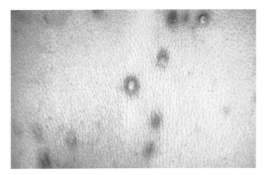

Figure 17-1 Perforating disorder of renal failure

Skin biopsy should be performed on clinical lesions suggestive of APD to exclude other dermatoses and/or neoplasms which may clinically mimic APD (Box 17-2). Missing these diagnoses in patients with renal failure and diabetes mellitus may have deleterious consequences.

Pathogenesis

Key Point

• Pruritus is likely an important factor

Many of the associated diseases cause pruritus of the skin, and lesions may be induced by scratching. Several theories have been proposed for the etiology of APD, including dermal microvasculopathy, serum vitamin A alterations, increased serum and extracellular fibronectin levels, and alterations in dermal collagen and elastic fibers, although no single cause has been proven.

Laboratory testing

Key Point

• Evaluate renal function and serum glucose and/or hemoglobin A1C levels in patients with suspected APD

While APD has been described with a variety of underlying systemic illnesses, diabetes mellitus and renal failure are by far the most common. APD lesions may herald the onset of worsening renal function in those patients with a history of chronic kidney disease. In the absence of diabetes or renal disease, a search for other causes of pruritus or careful medication history should be undertaken.

Treatment

Key Point

• Treatment goals are to minimize pruritus and hyperkeratosis of lesions

No controlled randomized trials have been done to evaluate the efficacy of various treatment modalities for any of the perforating dermatoses. Thus, anecdotal reports must be used to extrapolate what might be best suited for an individual patient. Box 17-3 summarizes reported treatment options for APD. Most therapies are directed either toward relieving the pruritus associated with these skin diseases or minimizing the hyperkeratosis, which tends to be a common clinical feature.

Controversies

Key Point

• Dermatology texts and journals have not universally adopted APD as the preferred nomenclature

Though the term APD has been widely accepted to include Kyrle disease, perforating folliculitis, and the acquired variant of reactive perforating collagenosis, there is not uniform acceptance across the body of dermatology literature. In fact, various case reports and texts still maintain that the clinical variability and etiology of the skin lesions should preclude such grouping. Thus, confusion

BOX 17-1

Systemic illnesses associated with acquired perforating dermatosis

Most common

Diabetes mellitus

Renal failure

Endocrine diseases

Hypothyroidism

Acanthosis nigricans

Hyperparathyroidism

Malignancy

Hodgkin's lymphoma

Myelodysplastic syndrome

Prostate cancer

Pancreatic cancer

Infectious diseases

Human immunodeficiency virus (HIV)/acquired immunodeficiency syndrome (AIDS)

Tuberculosis

Aspergillosis

Medications

Tumor-necrosis factor-alpha inhibitors

Salt-water application

Other

Primary sclerosing cholangitis

Hypertension

Rheumatoid arthritis

Pulmonary fibrosis

Poland syndrome

Trauma

BOX 17-2

Differential diagnosis: other diagnoses that mimic acquired perforating dermatosis

Sarcoidosis

Secondary syphilis

Prurigo nodularis

Pityriasis lichenoides

Arthropod bites

Flegel's disease (hyperkeratosis lenticularis perstans)

Scabies

Keratoacanthomas

Dermatofibromas

Folliculitis

Neurotic excoriations

Hypertrophic lichen planus

BOX 17-3

Reported treatment options for acquired perforating dermatosis

Corticosteroids (topical, intralesional, systemic)

Antihistamines

Retinoids (topical, systemic)

Phototherapy (psoralen ultraviolet A, ultraviolet B, narrowband ultraviolet B)

Cryotherapy

Doxycycline

Rifampin

Allopurinol

Thalidomide

Salicylic acid

Sulfur

Benzoyl peroxide

Emollients

Methotrexate

Charcoal

Excision

Renal transplantation

Carbon dioxide laser

Capsaicin

regarding APD remains pervasive. Recognition of the disease associations, clinical presentation, and microscopic findings of APD should eventually resolve this controversy.

Elastosis perforans serpiginosa

Clinical presentation

Key Points

* Elastosis perforans serpiginosa generally presents as hyperkeratotic papules in a serpiginous pattern

* Lesions are commonly located on the nape of the neck
* Patients are typically young, adult males

Characteristic hyperkeratotic papules in a serpiginous pattern (Figure 17-2) are found most

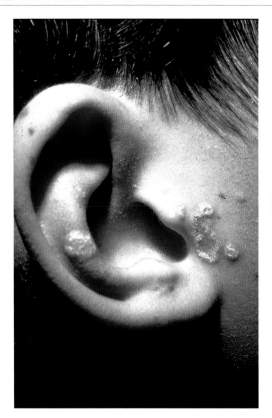

Figure 17-2 Elastosis perforans serpiginosa

commonly in young adult males on the nape of the neck. Lesions may also occur on the trunk or extremities and generally are asymptomatic or only mildly pruritic. Lesions may spontaneously resolve in months to years, sometimes with no sequelae or atrophic scarring.

Diagnosis

Key Points

- A potassium hydroxide scraping of the skin may reveal elastic fibers
- Biopsy will show typical findings of elastic fibers perforating the epidermis

The appearance of hyperkeratotic papules in a serpiginous pattern in those patients with a history of Down's syndrome, Rothmund–Thompson syndrome, Marfan's syndrome, or oral penicillamine use should prompt the consideration of elastosis perforans serpiginosa. Skin biopsy reveals tortuous channels of elastic tissue perforating through an acanthotic epidermis.

In the absence of known penicillamine use or underlying genetic disease, several skin diseases may clinically mimic elastosis perforans serpiginosa (Box 17-4). Skin biopsy will ultimately differentiate elastosis perforans serpiginosa from these other dermatoses.

Pathogenesis

Key Point

- Elastosis perforans serpiginosa is associated with underlying genetic disease or penicillamine use

Elastosis perforans serpiginosa is a skin disease that results from alterations in elastic fibers, usually in association with any number of underlying genetic diseases or treatment with oral penicillamine (Box 17-5). How exactly such diseases or medications alter elastic fibers to produce these skin lesions is not well understood. There is some evidence that penicillamine may interfere with copper-dependent lysyl oxidase, an enzyme involved with cross-linking of elastin.

Laboratory testing

Key Point

- Biospy demonstrates a narrow serpiginous path through the epidermis with transepidermal elimination of elastic fibers (Figure 17-3).

Treatment

Key Point

- Treatment options are largely based on anecdotal case reports (Box 17-6)

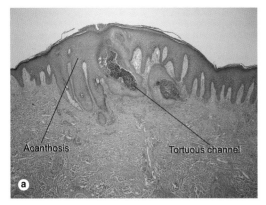

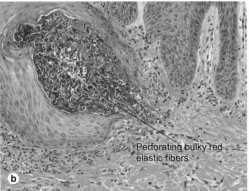

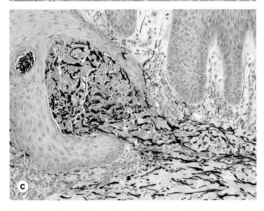

Figure 17-3 a–c Elastosis perforans serpiginosa

Reactive perforating collagenosis of childhood

Clinical presentation

Key Points

* Hyperkeratotic to umbilicated papules on extremities, face, buttocks
* Children in their first and second decades are affected
* Lesions may be in linear arrays

These hyperkeratotic, umbilicated papules occur in children in their first and second decades, often

following superficial trauma from scratching or a bug bite. The lesions are most commonly on the extremities and tend to resolve within 4–8 weeks. Lesions may come in crops.

Diagnosis

Key Point

* Biopsy typically shows a shallow depression with collagen fibers perforating the base (Figure 17-4)

Pathogenesis

Key Point

* An abnormal response to superficial trauma is thought to cause the lesions

Laboratory testing

Key Point

* No single laboratory test is useful

Treatment

Key Point

* Lesions generally resolve spontaneously and do not need treatment

Perforating pseudoxanthoma elasticum

Clinical presentation

Key Points

* Yellowish plaques with keratotic papules
* Lesions are commonly on the abdomen
* Patients are typically obese middle-aged women with a history of multiple gestations

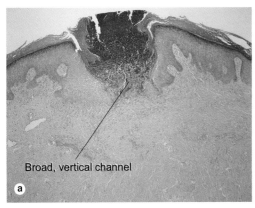

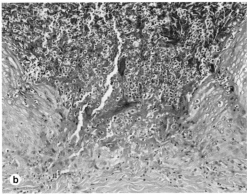

Figure 17-4 a, b Reactive perforating collagenosis

This disease has also been termed perforating calcific elastosis. Yellowish plaques that resemble the "chicken skin" of pseudoxanthoma elasticum can be seen on the abdomen. In this perforating variant, the plaques have superimposed keratotic papules. Obese or multiparous women are most often affected.

Diagnosis

Key Point

- Biopsy shows altered elastic fibers in the dermis and perforating the epidermis

Pathogenesis

Key Point

- Multiple episodes of trauma to the abdominal skin may be a cause

Laboratory testing

Key Point

- No single laboratory test is useful

Treatment

Key Point

- No specific treatment exists

BOX 17-7

Perforating variants of other dermatoses

Cutaneous infections

Secondary to *Mycobacterium abscessus*

Secondary to varicella-zoster virus

Botryomycosis

Leprosy

Chromomycosis

Cryptococcosis

Leishmaniasis

Schistosomiasis

Aspergillosis

Granulomatous diseases

Granuloma annulare

Necrobiosis lipoidica

Sarcoidosis

Papulosquamous diseases

Psoriasis

Atopic dermatitis

Connective tissue diseases

Discoid lupus erythematosus

Morphea

Rheumatoid nodule

Tumor/malignancy

Cutaneous T-cell lymphoma

Melanoma

Keratoacanthoma

Pilomatricoma

Other

Acne keloidalis

Porokeratosis

Paget's disease

Melanocytic nevi

Amyloidosis

Chondrodermatitis nodularis helicis

Gout

Scabies

Follicular hybrid cyst

Lichen nitidus

Calcinosis cutis

Pseudoxanthoma elasticum

Wood splinters

Miscellaneous

- Perforating variants of other primary dermatoses or cutaneous infections/infestations may occur

Many other primary skin disorders can feature histologic evidence of perforation on routine biopsy. These include neoplasms such as keratoacanthomas, infestations such as scabies, infections such as herpes zoster, and inflammatory conditions such as granuloma annulare (Box 17-7). These dermatoses have no characteristic clinical appearance.

Further reading

Basak PY, Turkmen C. Acquired reactive perforating collagenosis. Eur J Dermatol 2001;11:466–468.

Herzinger T, Schirren CG, Sander CA, et al. Reactive perforating collagenosis–transepidermal elimination of type IV collagen. Clin Exp Dermatol 1996;21:279–282.

Kovich O. Acquired perforating disorder. Dermatol Online J 2004;10:16.

Saray Y, Seckin D, Bilezikci B. Acquired perforating dermatosis: clinicopathological features in twenty-two cases. J Eur Acad Dermatol Venereol 2006;20:679–688.

Satchell AC, Crotty K, Lee S. Reactive perforating collagenosis: a condition that may be underdiagnosed. Australas J Dermatol 2001;42:284–287.

Acne, rosacea, and hidradenitis suppurativa

18

Jonette E. Keri and Linda S. Nield

Acne

Clinical presentation

Key Points

- Disease of the pilosebaceous unit
- Characterized by open and closed comedones, papules, pustules, and nodules, with severe cases progressing to cystic lesions, possible fistula tracts, and scarring
- Primarily a disease of adolescence, but can last into adulthood
- Social and psychological implications

Acne is a common condition affecting more than 50 million people in the United States. Women are more affected than men, and 79–95% of teenagers will have acne. Acne may also begin during the adult years (20–30 years old) and approximately 12% of women and 3% of men will have acne until their mid-40s. Clinically, acne is characterized by open comedones ("blackheads"), closed comedones ("whiteheads"), papules, and pustules. More severe acne may have deep inflammatory nodules, cysts, and even fistula tracts, and significant, permanent scarring may result. It most commonly involves the face, but can also affect the neck, chest, back, and upper arms.

Diagnosis

Key Points

- Acne is usually easily diagnosed by its clinical appearance
- The comedone (Figure 18-1) is the clinical hallmark of acne; its absence should prompt consideration of other conditions that resemble acne (including rosacea and perioral dermatitis)

Acne is a common disease that is easily recognized by most physicians. The primary lesion is the comedone. Inflammatory papules, nodules, and cysts (Figure 18-2) may be present. However, other conditions can imitate acne and those are included in Box 18-1. If the classic comedones are not seen, a history should be taken; this should include the length of duration of the condition, exacerbating factors, and response to previous treatments. If a patient has been using corticosteroids on the face, a diagnosis of rosacea or periorificial dermatitis should be considered. These conditions lack comedones. Any history of photosensitivity should prompt consideration of laboratory testing for lupus. Resistant pustules that are unresponsive to systemic antibiotics should be cultured for Gram-negative organisms. If the patient has small, pink/brown perinasal and perioral papules that are unresponsive to treatment, a biopsy should be considered. Multiple facial adnexal tumors are often associated with an inherited syndrome. Angiofibromas (adenoma sebaceum; Figure 18-3) are associated with tuberous sclerosis complex, multiple endocrine neoplasia syndrome type I and Birt–Hogg–Dube syndrome. Birt–Hogg–Dube syndrome is also associated with fibrofolliculomas. Trichoepitheliomas are associated with Brooke–Spiegler syndrome.

Pathogenesis

Key Points

- Multifactorial disease of the pilosebaceous unit
- Characterized by:
  - Increase in sebum production
  - Follicular hyperkeratinization
  - *Propionibacterium acnes*
  - Inflammation (Box 18-2)

Acne is a multifactorial disease, and many of the contributing factors first arise or are exacerbated during puberty (Box 18-3). Under the influence of androgens that rise during puberty, sebum production increases. Keratinocytes within the pilosebaceous unit become more cohesive and create the follicular plug or comedo. *Propionibacterium acnes* propagates in this environment and secretes many proinflammatory factors, including

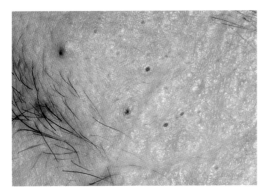

Figure 18-1 Comedonal acne

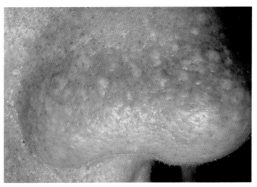

Figure 18-3 Angiofibromas

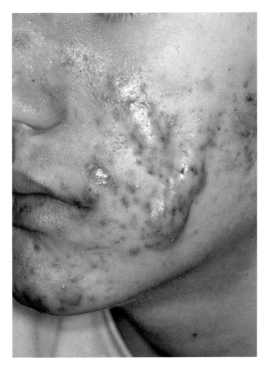

Figure 18-2 Nodulocystic acne

BOX 18-2

Four key components of acne development

1. Follicular plugging and excessive sebum production
2. Enlargement of sebaceous glands and development of microcomedones
3. *Propionobacterium acnes* in microcomedones triggers inflammatory process
4. Release of cytotoxic and chemotactic agents leads to further inflammation

BOX 18-3

Emotional impact of acne

Anxiety

Depression

Social withdrawal

Poor body image

Poor self-esteem

BOX 18-1

Differential diagnosis of acne

Adenoma sebaceum

Pityrosporum folliculitis

Rosacea

Gram-negative folliculitis

Steroid use–abuse dermatitis

Tinea barbae

proteases, lipases, and other chemotactic factors which result in inflammation. Rupture of the follicle may also release sebum and other irritating chemicals into the dermis, also contributing to the inflammation characteristic of "pimples."

Recently, Toll-like-receptors have been implicated in the pathogenesis of acne. These receptors are found on keratinocytes and sebocytes in the pilosebaceous unit. *P. acnes* has been found to trigger inflammatory cytokine responses by activating such Toll-like-receptors.

Treatment

Key Points

- Treatment should be directed to the type and severity of acne
- The age, gender, and lifestyle of the patient may influence treatment choices
- Compliance issues must be considered
- Retinoids are the mainstay of treatment for comedonal acne
- Topical benzoyl peroxide helps prevent resistance to topical and oral antibiotics

Remembering that acne is a multifactorial disease, most patients will benefit from simultaneous use of at least two forms of treatment (Table 18-1). For comedonal acne, topical retinoids should be the mainstay of treatment (Tables 18-2 and 18-3). All patients should be educated about the proper use of retinoids. Those who identify themselves as having "sensitive skin" should be offered alternative ways of applying retinoids. Every-other-day or twice-weekly applications with a gradual increase in frequency may be an appropriate way to begin therapy in such patients. Prior application of a dimethicone-containing moisturizer may improve tolerance in adult patients who "sting" with any topical. Short-contact therapy with tazarotene used for as little as 30 seconds daily has been reported to have beneficial results.

Benzoyl peroxide alone or topical antibiotics in combination with benzoyl peroxide are good treatment choices for mild to moderate inflammatory acne. The addition of benzoyl peroxide reduces the risk of antibiotic resistance. Efficacy is improved when a retinoid is added. Ordinary tretinoin breaks down in the presence of benzoyl peroxide. Adapalene is stable in the presence of

benzoyl peroxide; microencapsulated tretinoin is relatively stable. There are fewer data about tazarotene, but it is probably stable.

Moderate inflammatory acne may require the use of systemic agents (Table 18-4). Oral antibiotics generally provide good results and can be initiated at higher doses that can be decreased after several months of use. The tetracyclines have long been considered effective oral acne treatments. Tetracyclines should not be used in children under the age of 8 years, in patients with deciduous teeth, or in women who are pregnant or breastfeeding. Patients should be cautioned about photosensitivity with all tetracycline drugs, particularly doxycycline. Severe side-effects of tetracyclines are rare. These include esophageal ulceration with doxycycline, and rare fulminant hepatitis, pneumonitis, lupus-like syndrome, vasculitis, and serum sickness with minocycline. Doxycycline monohydrate has a lower incidence of esophageal problems, and sustained-release minocycline is establishing a good safety record, with little potential for otovestibular side-effects and data suggesting no statistical increase in antinuclear antibody positivity. Subantimicrobial-dose doxycycline has been

Table 18-1 Antibiotic treatments for acne

Medication	Formulation	Dose
Topical		
Clindamycin	1% solution, gel, lotion, foam, pledget	Daily or bid
Erythromycin	2% solution, gel, ointment	bid
Topical combination		
Clindamycin plus BP	5% BP/1% clindamycin gel	Daily or bid
Erythromycin plus BP	5% BP/3% erythromycin gel	bid
Clindamycin plus tretinoin	Clindamcyin phosphaste 1.2% /tretinoin 0.025% gel	Daily
Oral (alphabetical order)		
Azithromycin	250, 500, 600 mg capsule and/or tablet	Daily
	100 mg or 200 mg per 5 mL suspension	Note: Efficacy no better than tetracycline and resistance issues more significant
Doxycycline	20, 40, 50, 75, 100 mg capsule or tablet	100 mg daily or bid
		Notes: Monohydrate forms are better tolerated. Always dose with meals, but not dairy. Never take at bedtime
Erythromycin	250, 500 mg capsule or tablet	500 mg bid Note: Many drug interactions. Efficacy may be lower than other agents
Minocycline	50, 75, 100 mg capsule and/or tablet	Typically 100 mg daily or bid
	Sustained-release formulation	1 mg/kg or 90 mg for an average adult
		Note: Minocycline shows greater reduction in *Propionibacterium acnes* than other tetracyclines
Tetracycline	100, 250, 500 mg capsule	500 mg bid
Trimethoprim-sulfamethoxazole DS	160 mg trimethoprim/ 800 mg sulfamethoxazole	bid

bid, twice-daily dosing; BP, benzoyl peroxide; DS, double strength.

Table 18-2 Most commonly prescribed topical acne treatments

Medication	Formulation	Dose
Antibiotics	See Table 18-1	See Table 18-1
Benzoyl peroxide	4%, 8% cream	Daily to bid
	6%, 9% gel	May bleach fabric
	4.5%, 6.5%, 8.5% with 10% urea wash	
	8% creamy wash	
	5 and 10% bar	
	7% pledget	
	5%, 10% shaving cream	
Retinoids		
Adapalene	0.1% cream, gel	Daily (or less often to improve tolerance)
Tazarotene	0.1% cream, gel	Daily (short contact may be used to improve tolerance)
Tretinoin	0.025%, 0.04%, 0.05% cream, gel and/or solution, microencapsulated formulations	Daily (or less often to improve tolerance)

bid, twice daily.

Table 18-3 Other topical acne treatments

Medication	Formulation	Dose
Azelaic acid	20% cream (15% gel marketed for rosacea)	Daily to bid (the gel is both more potent and more irritating)
Sodium sulfacetamide	Various ± sulfur	bid
		Note: Marketed for rosacea. Little data in acne

bid, twice daily.

Table 18-4 Other oral acne treatments

Medication	Formulation	Dose
Antibiotics	See Table 18-1	See Table 18-1
Hormonal therapy	0.035 mg/0.18, 0.215, 0.25 mg tablet (norgestimate/ethinyl estradiol)	Daily
		Three forms currently have labeling for acne
	1 mg/0.2, 0.3, 0.35 mg tablet (norethinodrone acetate/ethinyl estradiol)	Note: Any estrogen-containing contraceptive will increase sex hormone-binding globulin and decrease free testosterone.
	3 mg/0.2 mg tablet (drospirenone/ethinyl estradiol)	
Istotretinoin	10, 20, 30, 40 mg capsules	0.1–1mg/kg/day × 20 weeks, cumulative dose 120–150 mg/kg

BOX 18-4

Potential adverse effects of isotretinoin

Birth defects: abnormalities of face, skull, ears, eyes, brain, heart, thymus, parathyroid glands

Cheilitis

Corneal opacities

Hearing impairment

Hematologic dyscrasias

Hepatitis

Hypersensitivity reactions

Hypertriglyceridemia

Inflammatory bowel disorders

Pancreatitis

Premature birth

Pseudotumor cerebri

Psychiatric disorders (possibly depression and suicidal ideation)

Skeletal hyperostosis

Spontaneous abortion

approved for the treatment of periodontal disease (20 mg) and rosacea (40 mg).

Isotretinoin remains the most effective drug for severe, scarring, cystic acne. Isotretinoin, a derivative of vitamin A, has many potentially severe side-effects, including teratogenicity and possibly depression (Box 18-4). Users of isotretinoin in the United States must participate in a mandatory regulatory registry, called the iPledge program, in which patients, prescribers, pharmacists, and distributors of the drug must be registered. The standard dosing regimen for isotretinoin is 1 mg/kg per day for a total of 20 weeks, although many physicians begin the drug at a lower dose to prevent flaring, and use cumulative dosing 120–150 mg/kg as a goal.

Female patients with persistent, recurrent, or severe acne should be evaluated for clinical evidence of hyperandrogenism. Irregular menses, hirsuitism, female-pattern alopecia, deepening of the voice, and clitoromegaly may be indicative of elevated androgens. Most of these patients have polycystic ovarian syndrome (PCOS). The diagnosis of PCOS is established by the presence of anovulation (fewer than 9 periods per year or periods greater than 40 days apart), signs of hyperandrogenism, and exclusion of other causes. Laboratory examination is essential in those with new-onset virilization, but may also be considered in women whose acne is resistant to conventional therapy, those who relapse quickly after a course of isotretinoin, or when there is sudden onset of severe acne. Screening tests serve to exclude a virilizing tumor. These include serum dehydroepiandrosterone sulfate (DHEAS) and testosterone, obtained 2 weeks before the onset of menses. DHEAS levels are typically very high in adrenal tumors (> 8000 ng/mL) and less dramatic in congenital adrenal hyperplasia (4000–8000 mg/mL). Ovarian tumor is suggested by testosterone levels above 200 ng/dL. Many patients with late-onset congenital adrenal hyperplasia will have normal screening DHEAS and 17-hydroxyprogesterone levels.

Although adrenocorticotropic hormone stimulation tests have been used in this setting, they may result in overdiagnosis of the syndrome. As these patients generally respond well to empiric therapy for acne and hirsutism, it is not clear that screening for adult-onset 21-hydroxylase deficiency improves patient outcome. A 24-hour urine cortisol is appropriate for any patient with signs of Cushing's disease.

The use of oral contraceptives and antiandrogens such as spironolactone can be beneficial in the management of acne in patients with acne and hirsutism. Evening doses of dexamethasone have been used, but may increase the risk of steroid withdrawal complications and do not appear to perform any better than spironolactone.

Recently a variety of laser and light techniques have been employed in the treatment of acne. They may be useful for patients resistant to systemic agents, or in whom other agents are contraindicated. These modalities include photodynamic therapy with aminolevulinic acid, nonablative lasers, and blue light therapy.

Controversies

Key Points

- The contribution of diet to acne has yet to be fully defined
- In most patients, diet plays little role

Early studies of the role of chocolate, milk, peanuts, and cola showed no correlation, but the studies were noted to have design flaws. More recently, high-carbohydrate western diets composed largely of foods with a high glycemic index or ingestion of large quantities of milk have been implicated. Diet may be an etiologic factor in those patients with insulin resistance, such as is seen in PCOS. Treatment of the insulin resistance in some of these patients has resulted in an improvement in their acne.

Rosacea

Clinical presentation

Key Points

- Common condition characterized by facial flushing, telangiectasia, papules, and pustules
- Ocular rosacea is common
- Severe rosacea can result in rhinophyma
- Most commonly affects Caucasians of Northern or Eastern European heritage
- A disease of adults

Rosacea is a common condition that affects about 13 million adults in the United States. All races and both sexes can be affected, but it is more commonly seen in fair-skinned individuals. Women are more frequently affected then men, although men are more likely to develop rhinophyma. Rosacea is usually diagnosed between the ages of 30 and 50. Risk factors in addition to heritage include actinic damage, relatives with rosacea, and a propensity to flush. Recently, rosacea has been characterized into four subtypes: (1) erythematotelangiectatic; (2) papulopustular; (3) phymatous; and (4) ocular (Box 18-5). Transition between forms is unusual.

Diagnosis

Key Points

- Common skin conditions such as acne, telangiectasia, simple flushing, and seborrheic dermatitis are often incorrectly labeled as rosacea
- A thorough history, including review of symptoms, should be done to exclude other conditions

The diagnosis of rosacea is based upon the identification of the four subtypes. Chin acne in adult women (Figure 18-4) is a variant of rosacea. In general, these four subtypes are thought to be distinct. In the past it was thought that rosacea went through a progression of stages from milder to more severe disease, with rhyinophyma (Figure 18-5) being the most severe form. Although patients with severe rosacea can progress to develop rhinophyma, most patients will maintain their clinical subtype. They may experience disease exacerbations within their subtypes, however. Patients with inflammatory rosacea may progress from papular (Figure 18-6) to papulopustular (Figures 18-7 and 18-8) forms. Although flushing is a major characteristic of rosacea, sudden new-onset flushing or flushing in association with systemic symptoms warrants evaluation for other causes. Other causes of flushing include emotion, menopause, carcinoid syndrome, mastocytosis, lupus erythematosus, dermatomyositis, mixed

Standard classification of rosacea subtypes

Erythematotelangiectatic

Flushing, central facial edema with or without telangiectasia

Papulopustular

Persistent central facial erythema

Papules/pustules usually on the central face

Phymatous

Thick skin

Irregular surface nodularities

Enlargement of the central face, forehead, and ears

Ocular

Foreign-body sensation

Burning/stinging

Dryness/itching of the eyes

Blurred vision

Inflamed eyelids

Styes

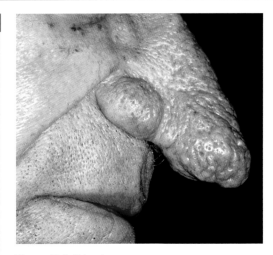

Figure 18-5 Rhinophyma

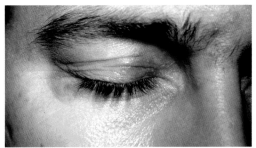

Figure 18-6 Papular rosacea

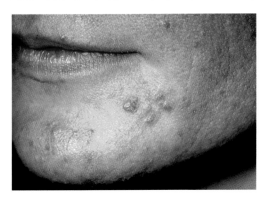

Figure 18-4 Chin acne

connective tissue disease, photosensitivity from medications, and allergic contact dermatitis.

Pathogenesis

- Etiology remains unknown
- Multifactorial condition
- Associated with vascular lability, photoaging, dermal connective tissue damage, pilosebaceous abnormalities, and responses to chemical and ingested agents
- Association with *Demodex* mites remains controversial

Rosacea begins in most patients with flushing. This prolonged vascular response can lead to dilation of vessels with telangiectasia. The flushing

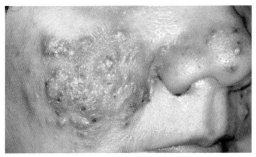

Figure 18-7 Papulopustular rosacea

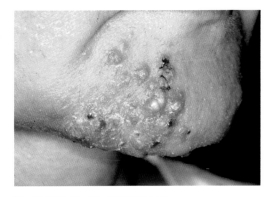

Figure 18-8 Papulopustular rosacea

Rosacea: potential aggravating factors

Chemicals

Alcohol

Caffeine withdrawal

Medications

Environmental exposures

Cold

Heat

Humidity

Sun

Wind

Foods

Chocolate

Dairy products

Hot temperature or spicy foods or drinks

Marinated meat, liver

Soy sauce

Vanilla

Vinegar

Physical exertions

Chronic cough

Lift and load maneuvers

Valsalva maneuver

Stress

Basics of treatment of rosacea

Use topical treatments for mild to moderate disease

Add oral antibiotics and/or other oral agents for moderate to severe disease

Avoid or modify aggravating factors

Topical treatments for rosacea

Antibiotics

    Clindamycin ($\pm$ benzoyl peroxide)

    Erythromycin ($\pm$ benzoyl peroxide)

    Metronidazole

Azelaic acid

Immunomodulators (pimecrolimus, tacrolimus)

Retinoids

Sulfur

Sodium sulfacetamide

can also cause edematous skin, a common finding in rosacea. Because flushing is not unique to rosacea, other factors are thought to contribute to the development of rosacea (Box 18-6).

Treatment

Key Points

- Identify the type of rosacea
- Provide patient education about exacerbating factors
- Give patients reasonable expectation of response to treatment
- Tetracyclines remain the mainstay for papulopustular disease

Identification of the type of rosacea is important in the treatment of the disease (Box 18-7). Sun avoidance is important for all types of rosacea, as many patients identify the sun as an aggravating factor. Erythematotelangiectatic disease is best treated with laser and light modalities, but improvement in the erythema is often modest at best. Papulopustular rosacea can be treated with topical agents, systemic antibiotics and, in severe cases, with isotretinoin. Effective topical therapies include metronidazole, azelaic acid, sulfur and sodium sulfacetamide preparations, and topical antibiotics. Retinoids and benzoyl peroxide should be used cautiously in rosacea patients, as they may be irritating and may increase erythema (Box 18-8). They may be valuable, but frequency of application should seldom be daily initially. Patients are more likely to tolerate them every other day or twice per week with gradual increases in the frequency of application. Prior application of a dimethicone-containing moisturizer may improve tolerance. Ocular rosacea may respond to oral antibiotics (Boxes 18-9 and 18-10). Rhinophyma can be surgically treated.

Controversies

Key Points

- Data supporting a role of *Helicobacter pylori* is controversial
- Treatment for *H. pylori* will help some rosacea patients, but this does not prove causation

There is controversy concerning the role of *H. pylori* in rosacea patients as *H. pylori* infection is the most common infection seen in humans.

BOX 18-9

Oral treatments that may be effective in the treatment of rosacea

Antibiotics

Ampicillin

Azithromycin

Doxycycline

Erythromycin

Metronidazole

Minocycline

Tetracycline

Trimethoprim

Other

Aspirin

Beta-blockers

Clonidine

Dapsone

Estrogen

Flax seed oil

Isotretinoin

Prednisone

Selective serotonin reuptake inhibitors

BOX 18-10

Other treatments for rosacea

Carbon dioxide resurfacing

Dermabrasion

Hot-loop electrocoagulation

Intense pulsed light

Vascular laser/pulsed dye laser

There are studies supporting both sides of the argument. Some patients will see an improvement in their rosacea during treatment for *H. pylori*.

Hidradenitis suppurativa

Clinical presentation

Key Points

- A disease of the follicle secondarily affecting apocrine sweat glands
- Chronic disease predominantly affecting the intertriginous areas of the body
- Characterized by inflamed abscesses, nodules, fistulas, and scarring

Hidradenitis suppurativa (HS) is a chronic, relapsing inflammatory disease associated with follicular occlusion in apocrine gland areas. The disease is characterized by painful nodules and abscesses, usually in the intertriginous areas, that drain, form sinus tracts, and lead to scarring. HS occurs in about 1/300 adults and is more prevalent in females than males, and in African Americans. It usually occurs after puberty and before age 40. The average duration of disease is approximately 19 years.

Diagnosis

Key Points

- Disease affects areas of the body with apocrine glands, including the axillae, groin, and buttocks. It can also involve breasts, shoulders, and neck and can occur in association with nodulocystic acne and dissecting cellulitis of the scalp.
- Ulcerated lesions can be confused with pyoderma gangrenosum and bacterial pyodermas

HS can be diagnosed by its location and clinical presentation. Initially cultures should be obtained to rule out simple pyodermas. Cultures in HS are often sterile, but over time wounds may be colonized with staphylococcal species and Gram-negative organisms. Rarely, pyoderma gangrenosum has been associated with long-standing HS.

Pathogenesis

Key Points

- Hidradenitis suppurativa is part of the follicular occlusion tetrad that includes acne conglobata, dissecting cellulitis of the scalp, and pilonidal cysts
- Because of the timing of the onset of the disease, it is thought that androgens may play a role in the pathogenesis

HS is a disease of the hair follicle and apocrine gland in which follicular plugging causes obstruction with resultant inflammation, bacterial overgrowth, and abscess formation. It occurs more commonly in obese individuals, and friction and occlusion are thought to contribute to its development.

Treatment

Key Points

- Multiple therapies have been tried, with no consistent response
- Many patients respond to oral tetracyclines together with intralesional corticosteroid injections
- Individual chronic sinus tracts can be unroofed, curetted, and allowed to heal by secondary intention

Treatment of hidradenititis suppurativa

Adalimumab

Antibiotics – doxycycline, tetracycline, minocycline, amoxicillin, ampicillin

Corticosteroids – intralesional and systemic

Cyclosporine

Dapsone

Entanercept

Infliximab

Isotretinoin

Local wound care (incision and drainage)

Oral contraceptives

Surgical excision with skin grafting

Photodynamic therapy

Radiation therapy

Spironolactone

Finasteride

- Some patients respond to oral retinoids or tumor necrosis factor-alpha biologics
- Surgical excision is a definitive treatment option, but the extent and location of the disease must be considered

Mild HS can be managed by wearing loose clothing, topical antibiotics including antibacterial washes, and minimal intervention (Box 18-11). More severe cases can be treated with systemic antibiotics. Intralesional corticosteroids can be very helpful and local incision and drainage can be beneficial as well, although repeated incision and drainage has also been associated with sinus tract formation. Systemic corticosteroids may provide a good initial response, but the condition relapses when they are discontinued. Isotretinoin has also been shown to help some patients. Recently, antiandrogens, including finasteride and spironolactone, have been used with some success. Photodynamic therapy, as well as newer biologic agents that block tumor necrosis factor-alpha, including infliximab, etanercept, and adalimumab, are novel treatment options being tried in some patients with severe disease. Surgical excision with or without skin grafting and radiation therapy has also been used. Depending on the severity of the disease, surgery may consist of ablation of individual sinus tracts or excision of the entire axilla.

Controversies

Key Point

- Controversies in this condition include which treatment is the best and the timing of surgical treatment

Further reading

Baldwin HE. The interaction between acne vulgaris and the psyche. Cutis 2002;70:133–139.

Crawford GH, Pelle MT, James WD. Rosacea: I. Etiology, pathogenesis and subtype classification. J Am Acad Dermatol 2004;51:327–341.

Crosson J, Stillman MT. Minocycline-related lupus erythematosus with associated liver disease. J Am Acad Dermatol 1997;36:867–868.

Cusack C, Buckley C. Etanercept: Effective in the management of hidradenitis suppurativa. Br J Dermatol 2006;154:726.

Gollnick H, Cunliffe W, Berson D, et al. Global Alliance to Improve Outcomes in Acne. Management of acne: a report from a Global Alliance to Improve Outcomes in Acne. J Am Acad Dermatol 2003;49(Suppl):S1–S37.

Harper JC, Thiboutot DM. Pathogenesis of acne: recent research advances. Adv Dermatol 2003;19: 1–10.

Heyman WR. Toll-like receptors in acne vulgaris. J Am Acad Dermatol 2006;55:691–692.

James WD. Clinical practice. Acne. N Engl J Med 2005;352:1463–1472.

Kagan RJ, Yakuboff KP, Warner P, et al. Surgical treatment of hidradenitis suppurativa: A 10-year experience. Surgery 2005;138:734–741.

Keri JE. Acne: improving skin and self-esteem. Pediatr Ann 2006;35:174–179.

Leyden JJ. Therapy for acne vulgaris. N Engl J Med 1997;336:1156–1162.

Nield LS. Managing adolescents. Pediatr Ann 2006;35:149–151.

Pelle MT, Crawford G, James WD. Rosacea: II. Therapy. J Am Acad Dermatol 2004;54:499–512.

Schachner LA, Hansen RC. Pediatric Dermatology. 3rd edn. Philadelphia: Mosby, 2003: 976–978.

Slade DE, Powell BW, Mortimer PS. Hidradenitis suppurativa: pathogenesis and management. Br J Plast Surg 2003;56:451–461.

Strauss RM, Pollock B, Stables GI, et al. Photodynamic therapy using aminolaevulinic acid does not lead to clinical improvement in hidradenitis suppurativa [letter]. Br J Dermatol 2005;152: 803–804.

Thiboutot DM. Acne and rosacea. New and emerging therapies. Dermatol Clin 2000;18:63–71.

Thiboutot D. Acne: hormonal concepts and therapy. Clin Dermatol 2004;22:419–428.

Wilkin J, Dahl M, Detmar M, et al. Standard classification of rosacea: report of the National Rosacea Society Expert Committee on the Classification and Staging of Rosacea. J Am Acad Dermatol 2003;46:584–587.

Zane LT, Leyden WA, Marqueling AL, et al. A population-based analysis of laboratory abnormalities during isotretinoin therapy for acne vulgaris. Arch Dermatol 2006;142:1016–1022.

Granuloma faciale **19**

Steven Chow and Kimberly Bohjanen

Clinical presentation

Key Points

- Granuloma faciale (GF) typically presents as a solitary reddish-brown asymptomatic facial lesion with prominent follicular openings
- It is an uncommon and benign condition
- It predominantly affects elderly Caucasian males
- Eosinophilic angiocentric fibrosis occurs in the oral and nasal mucosa and may be an extracutaneous form of GF

GF typically presents as a solitary, well-defined, indurated, brown-red plaque on the face (Figure 19-1). Lesions range in size from 0.5 to 8 cm, with a mean diameter of 1.9 cm. Although generally asymptomatic, some patients complain of tenderness, pruritus, and hyperpigmentation with sun exposure. The lesion may persist for a period of months to as long as 8 years. Lesion duration does not correlate to plaque size.

The most commonly affected site is the face. Commonly involved regions include the forehead (38%), cheek (30%), nose (27.5%) or eyelid (10.5%). A minority of patients may have multiple sites of involvement and/or extrafacial lesions. Extrafacial lesions may occur anywhere on a patient's body, even on non sun-exposed regions. Sunlight has been reported to increase the pigmentation of these extrafacial lesions. Disseminated GF has also been reported, but is relatively rare.

Caucasians have the highest incidence of GF, although cases have also been reported in African-Americans and Asians. The male to female ratio of GF is 1.7:1, and the mean age of GF presentation is 53 years, with an age range of from childhood to 85 years.

An extracutaneous form of GF may also exist. Eosinophilic angiocentric fibrosis, a rare lesion that generally occurs in the nasal septum and sinus mucosae, has been postulated to be a mucosal variant of GF. Patients are generally middle-aged women and may present with both entities concurrently. Similar to GF, eosinophils are prominent, but unlike GF, perivascular, whorled fibrosis is always seen and vasculitis is not present. Patients with upper-airway symptoms (i.e., obstruction) and GF should be evaluated for potential eosinophilic angiocentric fibrosis and referred to the ear, nose, and throat department for evaluation.

Diagnosis

Key Points

- GF can be difficult to diagnose clinically
- A biopsy of the lesion may be necessary for proper diagnosis
- GF may be associated with a mild peripheral eosinophilia

GF has a nonspecific clinical appearance. One retrospective analysis indicated that it was initially diagnosed correctly only 15% of the time. Common misdiagnoses include sarcoidosis, discoid lupus erythematosus, and cutaneous lymphoma. Biopsy of suggestive lesions will lead to the correct diagnosis.

Histologically, GF displays a dense polymorphous infiltration of inflammatory cells in the papillary and upper dermis beneath a grenz zone (Figure 19-2). The infiltrate is generally composed of neutrophils, eosinophils, lymphocytes, histiocytes, and plasma cells. Fibrinoid necrosis of vessel walls, nuclear dust, and extravasation of erythrocytes around vessels may also be present (Figure 19-3). "Onion-skin" fibrosis may present in long-standing lesions.

Differential diagnosis

- Sarcoidosis
- Cutaneous lymphoma
- Lupus erythematosus
- Benign lymphocytic infiltrate of Jessner
- Pseudolymphoma
- Polymorphous light eruption
- Basal cell carcinoma
- Fixed drug eruption
- Rosacea

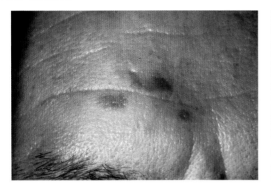

Figure 19-1 Granuloma faciale

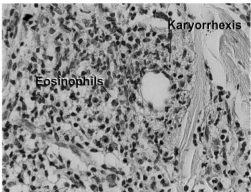

Figure 19-3 Granuloma faciale

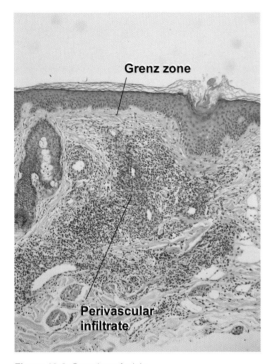

Figure 19-2 Granuloma faciale

Laboratory testing

Mild peripheral eosinophilia may be found in some patients with GF, but there does not appear to be a strong or consistent correlation.

Pathogenesis

Key Point

* GF has an unknown etiology

Treatment

Key Points

* GF is resistant to therapy, and combined treatment modalities may be necessary (Table 19-1)

* Treatment is focused on maximizing the cosmetic outcome
* Pulsed-dye laser (PDL) has been effective, even in long-standing lesions

Recent investigations have focused on the utilization of lasers that minimize scarring, such as the PDL or potassium titanyl phosphate (KTP) laser. The benefit of these newer lasers is their selective photothermolysis and decreased risk of scarring during treatment. With the PDL, purpura must be achieved. In the past, carbon dioxide and argon lasers were utilized for treatment of GF lesions, but these types of laser are less often utilized due to the hypopigmentation and scarring that may result.

Topical and/or intralesional corticosteroids may also be useful in some patients with GF. Dowlati et al. reported that combination intralesional triamcinolone with cryotherapy resulted in clearance in 9 of 9 patients. Recently, scattered case reports have indicated that tacrolimus 0.1% ointment used alone, or in conjunction with laser therapy, has resulted in clinical clearance of GF. Like topical corticosteroids, tacrolimus suppresses proinflammatory cytokines necessary for lesion development. In contrast to topical steroids, however, tacrolimus has no risk of skin atrophy. Open-spray and contact cryoprobe cryosurgery at 3-month intervals for the treatment of GF have also been attempted. Utilizing this technique, Panagiotopoulos et al. reported clearance in 9 of 9 patients, with transient hypopigmentation occurring in 2 patients. Utilization of topical psoralen and ultraviolet A for the treatment of GF has been described. Another case report described improvement in a patient's GF lesions during prostate cancer treatment with cyproterone acetate 300 mg intramuscularly every 2 weeks and leuproline acetate 3.75 mg intramuscularly every month. Systemic therapies like chloroquine, clofazimine, isoniazid, and dapsone have also been utilized for the management of GF. The potential

Table 19-1 Treatment modalities	
Treatment	**Schedule**
Topical steroids	
Tacrolimus 0.1%	bid
Intralesional (IL) corticosteroid injections	2.5–5 mg/mL
Cryotherapy	
Combination cryotherapy and IL corticosteroid injections	Every 3 weeks: 1 cryotherapy cycle for 20–30 seconds duration Triamcinolone acetonide (5 mg/mL)
Topical psoralen with ultraviolet A (PUVA)	
PUVA	Weeks 1–6: 0.5 joules 3×/week Weeks 7–8: 1 joule 3×/week Weeks 9–10: 1.5 joules 3×/week
Pulsed-dye laser (PDL)	8–8.5 joules/cm² with pulse duration of 0.45 ms
V-beam PDL	8–12 joules/cm² with pulse duration of 0.45–3 ms
Potassium titanyl phosphate (KTP) laser	20 joules/cm² with pulse duration of 15 ms
Dapsone	100–200 mg PO qd
Clofazimine	300 mg PO qd
Carbon dioxide laser	
Surgical excision	

bid, twice daily; PO, orally; qd, once a day.

side-effect profiles of some of these medications may outweigh the benefits, however, and should be discussed with the patient prior to treatment.

Controversies

Key Point

- Among investigators, there is debate on whether erythema elevatum diutinum and GF are part of the same disease

Erythema elevatum diutinum is a disease that presents on the bilateral-extremity extensor surfaces, and is associated with other systemic diseases. Some individuals believe that the similar histological features between erythema elevatum diutinum and GF indicate that these two conditions are part of the same disease that present on different body regions. Other investigators feel that erythema elevatum diutinum and GF could be members of the same disease family but not the same disease.

Further reading

Ammirati CT, Hruza GJ. Treatment of granuloma faciale with the 585-nm pulsed dye laser. Arch Dermatol 1999;135:903–905.

Cecchi R, Paoli S, Giomi A. Granuloma faciale with extrafacial lesions. Eur J Dermatol 2002;12:438.

Cheung ST, Lanigan SW. Granuloma faciale treated with the pulsed-dye laser: a case series. Clin Exp Dermatol 2005;30:373–375.

Dinehart SM, Gross DJ, Davis CM, et al. Granuloma faciale: comparison of different treatment modalities. Arch Otolaryngol Head Neck Surg 1990;116:849–851.

Dowlati B, Firooz A, Dowlati Y. Granuloma faciale: successful treatment of nine cases with a combination of cryotherapy and intralesional corticosteroid injection. Int J Dermatol 1997;36:548–551.

Elston DM. Treatment of granuloma faciale with the pulsed dye laser. Cutis 2000;65:97–98.

Gomez-de la Fuente E, del Rio R, Rodriguez M, et al. Granuloma faciale mimicking rhinophyma: response to clofazimine. Acta Dermatol Venereol 2000;80:144.

Guill MA, Aton JK. Facial granuloma responding to dapsone therapy. Arch Dermatol 1982;118:332–335.

Holme SA, Laidler P, Holt PJ. Concurrent granuloma faciale and eosinophilic angiocentric fibrosis. Br J Dermatol 2005;153:851–853.

Marcoval J, Moreno A, Peyr J. Granuloma faciale: a clinicopathological study of 11 cases. J Am Acad Dermatol 2004;51:269–273.

Mitchell D. Successful treatment of granuloma faciale with tacrolimus. Dermatol Online J 2004;10:23.

Panagiotopoulos A, Anyfantakis V, Rallis E, et al. Assessment of the efficacy of cryosurgery in the treatment of granuloma faciale. Br J Dermatol 2006;154:357–360.

Disorders of pigmentation

Chapter 20

Clarissa Yang

Basic science

Key Points

- Melanocyte: neural crest-derived cell at the dermoepidermal junction involved in producing melanin
- Melanin: pigmented product from conversion of tyrosine. Three types: eumelanin (brown-black, ellipsoid), pheomelanin (yellow-red, spherical), neuromelanin (black)
- Epidermal-melanin unit: functional unit of one melanocyte to 36 keratinocytes. Melanosomes synthesized by the melanocytes can be transferred to the keratinocytes
- Melanosomes: packaged melanin in lysosomes
- Hypomelanosis: decrease of melanin in the skin
- Amelanotic/depigmented: absence of melanin in the skin
- Hypermelanosis: increase of melanin in the skin
- Tyrosine → dopa → melanin. First step is mediated by tyrosinase enzyme.

Disorders of hypopigmentation

Clinical presentation/diagnosis

Key Points

See Tables 20-1–20-9.

- The diagnostic algorithm can be based on the clinical presentation (Figure 20-1)
- The disorders can also be divided into melanocytopenic (decreased or absent melanocytes) and melanopenic (decreased or absent melanin) (Figure 20-2)
- Wood's lamp examination: helpful, particularly in lighter-skinned individuals to identify involved areas. Depigmented lesions enhance more brightly blue-white than hypopigmented lesions. It is also helpful to distinguish nonmelanotic causes of hypopigmentation since these lesions will not enhance
- Chemical leukodermas are due to exposures to specific chemical compounds that are cytotoxic to melanocytes

Table 20-1 Drug-induced hypopigmentation

Melanocytopenic	Melanopenic
Catechols	Arsenicals
Monobenzylether of hydroquinone	Chloroquine
Para-substituted phenols	Glucocorticoids
Sulfhydryls	Hydroxychloroquine/chloroquine
	Hydroquinone
	Mercaptoethylamines
	Mephenesin (lightening of the hair)
	Triparanol (lightening of the hair)
	Valproic acid (lightening of the hair)
	Retinoids

Table 20-2 Hypopigmentation associated with systemic disease

Systemic condition	Key points
Nutritional deficiency	
Melanocytopenic	
Vitamin B$_{12}$ deficiency	Pernicious anemia associated with vitiligo
Melanopenic	
Kwashiorkor	"Flag sign" – alternating horizontal light and dark hair
(nutritional protein deficiency)	"Flaky-paint skin" – red skin with exfoliation then hypopigmentation
	Predominantly on the face and pressure points
Other forms of low protein	Malabsorption, nephrotic syndrome, inflammatory bowel disease
Selenium deficiency	Pigmentary dilution of hair and skin, nail changes
	Peripheral myopathy, cardiomyopathy, increased liver enzymes and creatine phosphokinase
Endocrine	
Melanopenic	
Addison's disease	Associated with vitiligo, but typically there is hyperpigmentation of skin
Hypopituitarism	Reversible hypomelanosis from low melanocyte-stimulating hormone and adrenocorticotrophic hormone production
Hypothyroidism	Associated with vitiligo
Renal	
Melanopenic	
Hemodialysis	Generalized hypopigmentation of the hair and skin in uremic patients

Table 20-3 Hypopigmentation associated with inflammatory disorders

	Key points
Melanocytopenic	
Alopecia areata	Associated with vitiligo
	Poliosis can occur in regrowth of hair
Halo nevus	Depigmented ring around nevus that can be benign or associated with melanoma
Pityriasis lichenoides chronica	Successive crops of asymptomatic, red-brown, oval to round lichenoid papules with centrally adherent scale that subside, leaving hypopigmented macules
Chemical leukoderma	Toxic free radical formation and interference with melanogenesis
Physical leukoderma	Burns, physical injury, freezing, X-rays, ionizing, ultraviolet irradiation
	External injury resulting in loss of functional melanocytes
Melanopenic	
Discoid lupus erythematosus	Red-violaceous plaques with scale, particularly perifollicular, that heal with white scars
	Mostly photodistributed
Lichen sclerosus et atrophicans	Hypopigmented atrophic skin; occasional fissuring
	Predilection for the anogenital skin; pruritus is common
	Scarring can ensue with loss of normal architecture of the vulva in women, phimosis in men
Pityriasis alba	Thought to be a postinflammatory reaction to an eczematous dermatitis with very subtle to no erythema that fades, leaving macules with powdery scale
	Face most common, but also neck, trunk, back, limbs, scrotum
Postinflammatory	Off-white macules following resolution of pre-existing inflammatory disorder

Table 20-3 Hypopigmentation associated with inflammatory disorders—cont'd

	Key points
Progressive macular hypomelanosis	Mainly young adult women
	Hypopigmented macules on the central trunk
	Follicular red fluorescence with Wood's lamp
	Propionibacterium acnes may be causative agent
Sarcoidosis	Rare form of sarcoidosis
	More common in dark-skinned people
Scleroderma	"Salt-and-pepper" skin – diffuse hyperpigmentation with localized areas of complete pigment loss that spares the perifollicular skin
	Most common on upper trunk, face, and areas of pressure

Table 20-4 Infectious causes of hypopigmentation

Disease	Organism	Clinical key points
Melanocytopenic		
Onchocerciasis	*Onchocerca volvulus* Vector: black fly	Late feature of disease
		Pretibial skin depigmentation most common
		Leopard-like skin
Pinta	*Treponema carateum* (treponematosis)	Skin-only disease
		Phases:
		Erythema or copper color
		Slate-blue
		Mottling with hyper- and hypopigmentation over bony prominences
Yaws	*Treponema pallidum pertenue* (treponematosis)	Healed primary lesions result in atrophic loss of pigmentation
		Can occur in secondary stage, but most common in tertiary stage
Leprosy	*Mycobacterium leprae*	Anesthetic hypomelanotic macules
		Can be associated with enlarged nerve trunk
		Decreased sweating
		Decreased or absent melanocytes and melanosomes
		Immune system destroys nevus cells
Melanopenic		
Post kala-azar	*Leishmania infantum, L. donovani, L. chagasi* Vector: sand fly	Pinpoint hypopigmented macules that enlarge to 1 cm
		Mostly spares the skin from the waist to the feet
		Later-stage lesions become raised and are asymptomatic
Nonvenereal syphilis (bejel)	*Treponema pallidum* (treponematosis)	Bejel is the nonvenereal form of syphilis
		Late stage resembles pinta
Tinea versicolor	*Malassezia furfur/ Pityrosporum ovale* (yeast)	Lesions have very fine scale typically on back, chest
		Can also be associated with erythema or hyperpigmentation
		Hypopigmentation is due to yeast inhibition of tyrosinase

Table 20-5 Neoplastic conditions with hypopigmentation

Melanocytopenic	Key features
Halo nevus	Halo around a pigmented lesion
Leukoderma acquisitum centrifugum	Neuroectodermal-derived tumors associated with leukodermic halos
	Multiple halo nevi
	Has been associated with malignant melanoma
	Decreased melanocyte and melanosome
Mycosis fungoides/ Cutaneous T-cell lymphoma	Hypopigmented lesions in darker skin types
	Resembling tinea versicolor or pityriasis alba

Table 20-6 Genodermatoses with melanocytopenic hypopigmentation

Disease	Gene defect	Key features
Melanocytopenic		
Ataxia telangiectasia (Louis–Bar syndrome)	ATM	Autosomal recessive
		Associated with premature graying hair and hypomelanotic macules
		Ataxia, bulbar and cutaneous telangiectasias, café-au-lait macule, nystagmus, sinopulmonary infections, lymphoma, breast carcinoma (heterozygotes)
Piebaldism (Figure 20-3)	c-kit	Autosomal dominant
		White forelock, vitiligo-like depigmentation centrally and anteriorly sparing the dorsal spine
		Involves midarms and legs, but spares distal extremities and periorificial areas which are more characteristic of vitiligo
Vitiligo (Figure 20-4)	Associated with VIT1, catalase	Patches of depigmentation in characteristic and trauma-prone distribution (see Table 20–11)
Alezzandrini syndrome		Syndrome of facial vitiligo, poliosis, deafness, unilateral tapetoretinal degeneration
Vogt–Koyanagi–Harada syndrome		Rare disease with vitiligo, poliosis, uveitis, dysacousia, alopecia; typically darker-skinned individuals (Asians, Native Americans, Latin Americans, or African)
Waardenburg's syndrome		White forelock, premature graying of hair, hypopigmented macules resembling piebaldism that are localized or generalized; most common on the forehead, neck, anterior chest, abdomen, anterior knees, arms, dorsal hands; iris heterochromia; sensorineural deafness; facial dysmorphism – wide-spaced inner canthi, broadened nasal root
Type I	PAX3	Autosomal dominant
		Associated with dystopia canthorum (classic form)
Type II	MITF	Autosomal dominant
		High rate of deafness and heterochromia, but no dystopia canthorum
Type III	PAX 3	Autosomal dominant
		Associated with limb defects and dystopia canthorum
Type IV	SOX10, EDN3, EDNRB	Autosomal recessive
		Similar to type III, but with Hirschprung's disease
Xeroderma pigmentosa	XPA – XPG, and XPV	Autosomal recessive
		Defective DNA repair upon exposure to ultraviolet radiation
		Acute sun sensitivity with sunburns, pigmented and achromic macules, and telangiectasias in photodistribution; narrowing of mouth, nares
		Increased risk of skin cancers; photophobia, other eye disturbances
Ziprkowski–Margolis syndrome		X-linked recessive
		Deaf–mute, heterochromic irides, piebaldism-like hypomelanosis of skin and hair;
		At birth skin is completely amelanotic, but hyperpigmented macules develop on the trunk and extremities, but retains white hair

Table 20-7 Genodermatoses with melanopenic hypopigmentation

Disease	Gene defect	Key features
Melanopenic		
Chédiak–Higashi syndrome	LYST	Autosomal recessive
		Abnormal giant peroxidase-positive lysosomal granules affecting neutrophils, melanocytes, neurons
		Hypopigmentation of the skin, eyes, and silvery hair
		Prolonged bleeding times, easy bruisability, recurrent infections, abnormal natural killer cell function, and peripheral neuropathy. Mortality results from frequent bacterial infections or from a lymphoproliferative "accelerated phase"
Cross–McKusick–Breen syndrome		Ocular and generalized cutaneous hypopigmentation
		Severe mental retardation with spastic tetraplegia, and athetosis; growth retardation, dolichocephaly, cataracts, high arched palate, small, widely spaced teeth, psychomotor retardation, progressive neurological manifestations, and hypochromic anemia
Griscelli's syndrome	RAB27A, MYO5A MLPH (melanophilin)	Autosomal recessive
		Silvery hair and pale skin (mild form of albinism)
		Large clumps of pigment in hair shafts
		Accumulation of melanosomes in melanocytes
Hermansky–Pudlak syndrome	HPS1, HPS 2, HPS 3, HPS 4 (total seven genes)	Autosomal recessive; Puerto Rico, Netherlands, India
		Variable depigmentation of the skin, eyes, hair
		Pigmented nevi, squamous cell carcinoma, basal cell carcinoma
		Petechiae, ecchymoses, bleeding associated with platelet dysfunction; lysosomal ceroid storage defects affecting the lung (interstitial fibrosis), gut (granulomatous colitis) and cardiac muscle (cardiomyopathy)
		Eye defects similar to oculocutaneous albinism
Histidinemia	Histidase	Autosomal recessive
		Fair skin, blue eyes, red hair
		Central nervous system: mental retardation, speech difficulties, ataxia, convulsions
Homocystinuria	Cystathionine synthetase	Autosomal recessive
		Fine blond hair, blue eyes, fair skin, Marfan-like features, ectopia lentis (downward), skeletal abnormalities, thromboembolic events
Hypomelanosis of Ito		Mostly sporadic; chromosomal or gene mosaicism
		Present at birth or early childhood
		Blaschkonian whorled and streaked marble-cake hypopigmentation that is unilateral or bilateral
		Alopecia, seizures, strabismus, hypertelorism, scoliosis, anodontia
Incontinentia pigmenti	NEMO	X-linked dominant, lethal in males
		Swirls/streaks of hypopigmentation in lines of Blaschko
		Four stages: vesiculobullous, verrucous, hyperpigmented, hypopigmented
		Scarring alopecia, dystrophic nails, peg teeth/anodontia, cataracts and other eye findings, seizures, mental retardation
Menkes kinky hair	MNK	X-linked recessive
		Wiry depigmented hair with pili torti, trichorrhexis nodosa
		Hypopigmentation, doughy skin, Cupid's bow of the upper lip
		Progressive central nervous system degeneration, growth retardation, tortuous arteries, hypothermia, skeletal abnormalities, urogenital abnormalities
		Death by age 2–3 years

Continued

Table 20-7 Genodermatoses with melanopenic hypopigmentation—cont'd

Disease	Gene defect	Key features
Multiple endocrine neoplasia type 1 (Wermer syndrome)	MEN1 (Menin)	Autosomal dominant
		Facial angiofibromas, collagenomas, lipomas, confetti-like hypopigmented macules, café-au-lait macules
		Pituitary, parathyroid, pancreatic tumors
Nevus depigmentosus (Figure 20-5)	Cutaneous mosaicism; decreased dopa activity	Three clinical forms: isolated, circular/rectangular, quasidermatomal, systematized whorled or streaked forms
		Most common on the trunk and typically does not cross the midline
Oculocutaneous albinism		Autosomal recessive
		Eye findings: nystagmus, photophobia, decreased visual acuity, abnormal iris pigment, foveal hypoplasia, abnormal optic tract development, iris translucency
Type IA	Tyrosinase-negative	Cannot make melanin
		Complete lack of pigment in the skin and hair, blue eyes, red nevi
		High risk for squamous cell carcinoma > basal cell carcinoma > melanomas
Type IB (yellow albinism)	Decreased tyrosinase activity	Very little or no pigment at birth, then varying amounts of melanin in first to second decade of life
		Hair becomes yellow, light blond, and can eventually turn blond or brown. Eyes can also become light tan or brown. Pigmented lesions develop
Type TS (temperature-sensitive)		Scalp and axillary hair color is white at birth and remains white, but arm and leg hair pigments
Type 2 (tyrosinase-positive)	P gene (pink-eye dilution gene)	Melanosome transfer defect; slight residual pigment
		Creamy white skin, blue-gray eyes, yellow hair
		"Goosefoot" lentigines and nevi
Type 3 (Rufous albinism)	Tyrosinase-related protein-1 (Trp1) gene	Minimal reduction in pigment found in people of African descent
		Hair and skin are light brown, gray to tan eyes at birth
Type 4	Membrane-associated transporter protein (MATP) gene	Similar presentation to oculocutaneous albinism type 2
Phenylketonuria	Phenylalanine hydroxylase deficiency	Autosomal recessive
		Generalized hypopigmentation, blond hair, blue eyes, sclerodermoid skin changes, eczema
		Central nervous system: seizures, hyperreflexia, psychomotor delay, mousy odor to urine
Phylloid hypomelanosis	Mosaic trisomy 13	Round or oval hypomelanotic macules
		All have central nervous system defects (mental retardation, absence of corpus callosum), conductive hearing loss, choroidal and retinal coloboma, craniofacial defects, brachydactyly, camptodactyly, skeletal abnormalities
Tietz's syndrome	MITF	Autosomal dominant
		Generalized cutaneous hypomelanosis and histologic absence of melanin; light blond hair, blue eyes without ocular dysfunction, deaf-mutism, eyebrow hyperplasia
Tuberous sclerosis (Figure 20-6)	Hamartin (TSC1) Tuberin (TSC2)	Autosomal dominant; up to 66% spontaneous mutations
		Off-white macules in 82–100% by age 2 that can occur as: lance-ovate/ash-leaf macules, polygonal macules, confetti spots, and dermatomal hypomelanosis
		Poliosis and macular hypopigmentation of the retina and iris may occur. Other features: adenoma sebaceum/angiofibromas – small red-brown or skin-colored 1–3 mm papules on the sides of nose and medial cheeks
		Koenen tumors – periungual fibromas
		Central nervous system tubers with seizures, gray or yellow retinal plaques, heart rhabdomyomas, hamartomas of the kidneys, liver, thyroid, testes, gastrointestinal tract

MITF, microphthalmia-associated transcription factor.

Table 20-8 Miscellaneous causes of hypopigmentation

Melanopenic	Key features
Idiopathic guttate hypomelanosis	Well-demarcated porcelain white macules
	Typically in the sun-exposed areas of the extremities sparing the face
	Two types: actinic and familial
	More prominent in darker-skinned individuals, but occurs in all skin types
	Decreased melanocytes and melanin
Vagabond's leukoderma	Older, ill-kempt individuals with poor hygiene, inadequate diet, and alcohol abuse
	White macules in light-brown patches on the waist, groin, buttocks, axilla, back, neck
	Attributed to multiple ectoparasitic infections with phagocytosed melanosomes Reversible with good hygiene and diet
Disseminated hypopigmented keratoses Leukoderma punctatum:	Slightly raised lichenoid hypomelanotic, hyperkeratotic papules on trunk and extremities of young patients
	< 1 cm macules in patients on psoralen and ultraviolet A for vitiligo (phototoxic effect)

Table 20-9 Nonmelanotic hypopigmentation

Nonmelanotic	Key features
Nevus anemicus (Figure 20-7)	Focal increased blood vessel sensitivity to catecholamines
	Most common on trunk
	Cold, heat, or friction fails to induce erythema in the leukoderma areas
Bier spots	Benign physiologic vascular anomaly, vascular mottling
	Light macules on legs > arms > trunk with erythematous blanchable intervening skin
	Young adults
Woronoff's ring	Hypomelanotic ring around psoriatic lesion under treatment
	Secondary to vascular changes

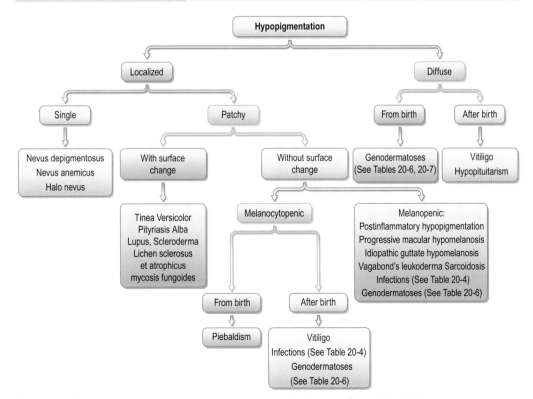

Figure 20-1 Diagnostic algorithm based on clinical presentation for disorders of hypopigmentation

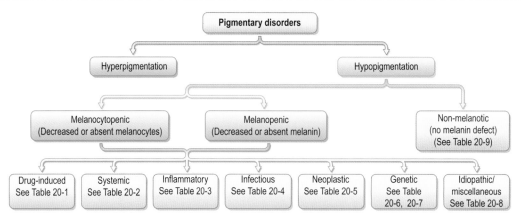

Figure 20-2 Diagnostic algorithm divided into melanocytopenic and melanopenic for disorders of hypopigmentation

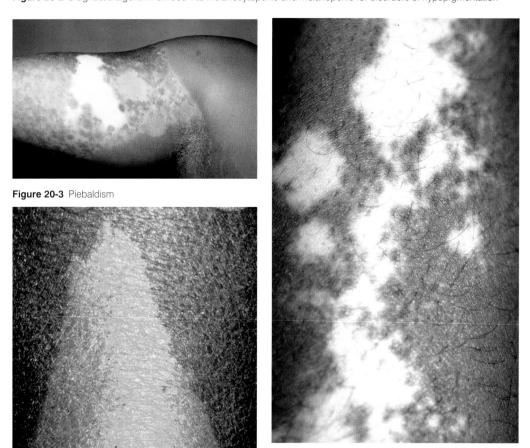

Figure 20-3 Piebaldism

Figure 20-4 Vitiligo

Figure 20-5 Nevus depigmentosus

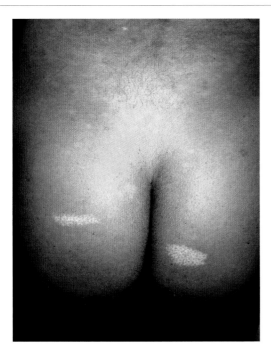

Figure 20-6 Ash-leaf macules of tuberous sclerosis

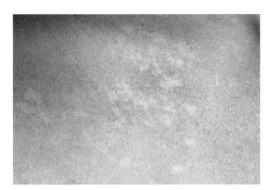

Figure 20-7 Nevus anemicus

- These chemicals can be found in disinfectants, germicides, rubber dish trays, adhesives, bands, rubber products, neoprene
- Other medications may cause pigment dilution or inhibit melanosome transfer
- Nonmelanotic hypopigmentation is usually due to vascular constriction. In this case there would be no enhancement of hypopigmentation with Wood's lamp examination

Vitiligo

Clinical presentation

Key Points

See Tables 20-10 and 20-11.
- Thyroid disease, diabetes, pernicious anemia, Addison's disease, and alopecia areata have been associated

Diagnosis

Key Points

- Progressive, symmetric acquired chalk-white macules in typical distribution
- Wood's lamp examination will enhance involved skin, especially in sun-protected areas

Differential diagnosis

Key Points

- Chemical leukoderma
- Leprosy
- Lupus erythematosus
- Melanoma-associated leukoderma
- Piebaldism
- Pityriasis alba
- Postinflammatory hypomelanosis
- Tinea versicolor
- Tuberous sclerosis
- Waardenburg's syndrome
- Nevus depigmentosus

Laboratory testing

Key Points

- If a biopsy reveals a decreased number of melanocytes compared to normal margin; the changes are consistent with, but not diagnostic for vitiligo
- Screen with complete blood count (pernicious anemia), thyroid-stimulating hormone (thyroid disease), fasting glucose (diabetes), and adrenocorticotropic hormone (Addison's disease) if signs or symptoms are present.

Pathogenesis

Key Point

- Both genetic and environmental factors influence disease

See Table 20-12.

Treatment

Key Point

See Table 20-13.

DISORDERS OF HYPERPIGMENTATION

Clinical presentation/diagnosis

Key Points

- Wood's lamp examination: Epidermal pigment is darker under Wood's lamp, but dermal pigment gets only minimally darker

- Hyperpigmented disorders can be classified into melanocytic (increased melanocytes), melanotic (increased melanin) or non-melanotic (see Figure 20-9)

Table 20-10 Colors of vitiligo

Typical	Milk-white, scalloped bordered macules and patches
Trichrome	Presence of intermediate tan color between normal skin and typical vitiligo macule
Quadrichrome	Presence of a fourth color of perfollicular or marginal hyperpigmentation
Pentachrome	Presence of a fifth color of blue occurring in postinflammatory hypermelanosis
Inflammatory	Erythematous, raised border similar to tinea versicolor
Confetti	Typical in color, but 1–2 mm color randomly or perifollicular

Table 20-11 Distribution of vitiligo

Focal	Macules are limited in size and number
Segmental	Unilateral, in a dermatomal or quasidermatomal distribution; trigeminal > neck > trunk
Generalized	Symmetric, widespread involving extensor surfaces, interphalangeal joints, elbows, knees
Acrofacial	Involves digits and periorificial facial areas
Universal	Widespread with few remaining normal macules
Artifactual	Corresponds exactly to an area of injury, which is koebnerization
Hair	Associated with leukotrichia/poliosis (Figure 20-8), prematurely gray hair, alopecia areata
Mucosa	Genitalia, nipples, lips, gingival
Ocular	Iris and retinal pigmentary abnormalities, choroidal abnormalities, iritis, visual acuity normal

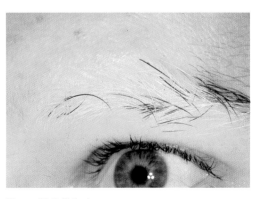

Figure 20-8 Poliosis

Key Points (Table 20-15)

- Tyndall effect: dermal pigmentation that is perceived as blue-gray because there is decreased reflectance in the longer-wavelength (red) region compared with surrounding areas
- Dermal hypermelanosis is common in East Indians and Asians, but rare in Caucasians
- Infrared photography can accentuate cerulodermas, but Wood's lamp is not useful

Table 20-12 Pathogenesis of vitiligo

Autoimmune hypothesis	Aberrant regulation of inflammatory cells that destroy melanocytes
Neurogenic hypothesis	Destruction of melanocytes or inhibition of melanin products by neurochemical mediators
Self-destruct hypothesis	Destruction of melanocytes from a metabolite of melanin synthesis
Genetic hypothesis	Inherent inability of melanocytes to survive conditions for normal melanocytes

Table 20-13 Treatment of vitiligo

Sunscreens	Protection from sunburns and possible koebnerization; sun protection factor > 30 with zinc oxide and/or titanium dioxide
Cosmetics	Blending with makeup or sunless tanners
Topicals	Glucocorticoids qd × 3 weeks then 1 week rest, then resume × 2 months
	Macrolides (tacrolimus, pimecrolimus)
Systemic	Short-term low-dose or pulse steroids; however, risks and benefits of long-term use must be evaluated
Phototherapy	Narrowband ultraviolet B, psoralen plus ultraviolet A ± calcipotriol, excimer laser
Surgical	Punch grafts, minigrafts, suction blisters, autologous melanocyte cultures
Depigmentation	If widespread vitiligo, consider monobenzylether of hydroquinone to bleach remaining pigmented skin

qd, every day.

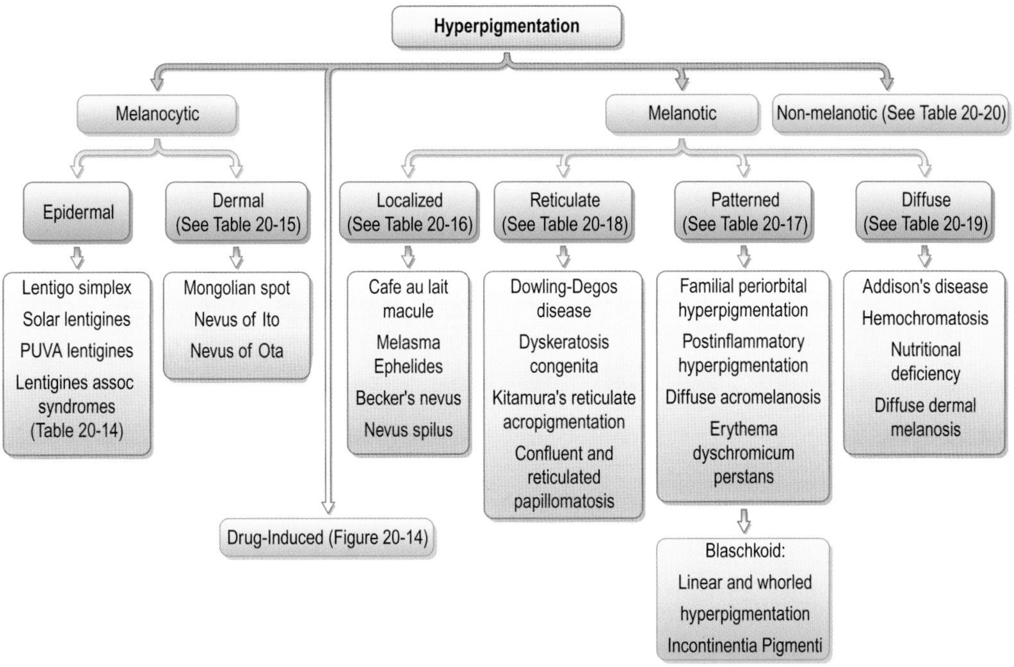

Hyperpigmentation

```
Hyperpigmentation
├── Melanocytic
│   ├── Epidermal
│   │   └── Lentigo simplex
│   │       Solar lentigines
│   │       PUVA lentigines
│   │       Lentigines assoc
│   │       syndromes
│   │       (Table 20-14)
│   └── Dermal (See Table 20-15)
│       └── Mongolian spot
│           Nevus of Ito
│           Nevus of Ota
├── Melanotic
│   ├── Localized (See Table 20-16)
│   │   └── Cafe au lait macule
│   │       Melasma
│   │       Ephelides
│   │       Becker's nevus
│   │       Nevus spilus
│   ├── Reticulate (See Table 20-18)
│   │   └── Dowling-Degos disease
│   │       Dyskeratosis congenita
│   │       Kitamura's reticulate acropigmentation
│   │       Confluent and reticulated papillomatosis
│   ├── Patterned (See Table 20-17)
│   │   └── Familial periorbital hyperpigmentation
│   │       Postinflammatory hyperpigmentation
│   │       Diffuse acromelanosis
│   │       Erythema dyschromicum perstans
│   │       └── Blaschkoid: Linear and whorled hyperpigmentation
│   │           Incontinentia Pigmenti
│   └── Diffuse (See Table 20-19)
│       └── Addison's disease
│           Hemochromatosis
│           Nutritional deficiency
│           Diffuse dermal melanosis
└── Non-melanotic (See Table 20-20)
Drug-Induced (Figure 20-14)
```

Figure 20-9 Diagnostic algorithm for disorders of hyperpigmentation. PUVA, psoralen with ultraviolet A

Table 20-14 Lentigines and associated syndromes	
Disorders	**Key points**
Localized	
Lentigo simplex	Hyperpigmented macule irrespective of sun exposure
Bannayan–Riley–Ruvalcaba	PTEN mutation
	Lentigines or café-au-lait macules of the glans penis, macrocephaly, multiple lipomas, vascular malformations
Centrofacial neurodysraphic lentiginosis	Lentigines limited to the medial face, neuropsychiatric problems, dysraphic malformations
Inherited pattern	Autosomal dominant
	Familial periorbital – dark circles around the eyes starting at puberty
Laugier–Hunziker syndrome	Macular hyperpigmentation of the lips, buccal mucosa, palms, and soles with hyperpigmented nail streaks
	Patients have no associated disease
Peutz–Jeghers syndrome	Autosomal dominant; *LKB1/STK11* gene mutation
	Lentigines on buccal mucosa, lips, fingers, toes
	Hamartomatous gastrointestinal polyps; increased risk of ovarian, breast, pancreatic cancers
Photodistributed	
Solar lentigines	Often less than 5 mm pigmented macules in sun-exposed areas
Psoralen with ultraviolet A lentigines	Large solar lentigines in patients receiving psoralen with ultraviolet A > 2–3 years
Xeroderma pigmentosum (XP)	Autosomal recessive; XPA through XPG, and XPV
	Defective DNA repair upon exposure to ultraviolet radiation
	Acute sun sensitivity with sunburns, pigmented and achromic macules, and telangiectasias in photodistribution; narrowing of mouth, nares
	Increased risk of skin cancers; photophobia, other eye disturbances
Segmental	
Partial unilateral lentiginosis	Numerous lentigines involving one-half of the body starting early in life

Continued

Table 20-14 Lentigines and associated syndromes—cont'd

Generalized	
Arterial dissection with lentiginosis	Familial syndrome of multiple lentigines, arterial dissection
Carney complex (NAME/ LAMB) syndrome (Figure 20-10)	Autosomal dominant; *PRKAR1A* gene mutation
	LAMB syndrome: lentigines, atrial myxomas, mucocutaneous myxomas (skin, breast), blue nevi
	NAME syndrome: nevi, atrial myxomas; myxoid neurofibromas, ephelides
	Rare pigmented adrenocortical disease, acromegaly, testicular tumors, schwanommas, endocrine hyperactivity
Cronkite Canada syndrome	Lentigines on upper and lower extremities, face, palms, soles
	Adenomatous polyps of the stomach to rectum
	Diarrhea, abdominal pain, and weight loss are presenting symptoms
	Patchy alopecia, dystrophic nails
Eruptive lentiginosis	Development of several hundred lentigines over months to years
	Young adults without internal disease
Faces syndrome	Hereditary syndrome of multiple lentigines, café-au-lait macules
	Anorexia, cachexia, eye and skin anomalies
LEOPARD syndrome (Moynahan's)	Autosomal dominant; *PTPN11* gene mutation
	Acronym for: Lentigines generalized except mucous membranes, Electrocardiogram conduction defects, Ocular hypertelorism, Pulmonic stenosis, Abnormal genitalia, Retardation of growth, Deafness
Tay's syndrome	Autosomal recessive
	Multiple lentigines, vitiligo, café-au-lait macules, premature canities
	Growth and mental retardation, cirrhosis, hypersplenism, skeletal defects

Table 20-15

Dermal melanocytosis	Key points
Mongolian spot (Figure 20-11)	Asians most common
	Blue-gray macules on the lumbosacral, buttock, back area in babies
	Disappears in childhood
Hori's nevus	Acquired circumscribed dermal melanocytosis of the face
	Bilateral blue-brown macules on forehead, temples, eyelids, malar areas, nose
	Middle-aged Asian women
Nevus of Ota (Figure 20-12)	Oculodermal melanocytosis
	Unilateral blue-gray-black macules intermixed with small brown macules in the first or second branches of the trigeminal nerve
	Intensity of pigmentation can vary daily and with menstruation
	Eye fundus may be involved
Nevus of Ito	Analogous to Ota, but less mottled and more diffuse, distributed along lateral supraclavicular and lateral branchial nerves

Table 20-16

Localized melanosis	Key points
Becker's nevus	Large pigmented plaque from smooth-muscle hyperplasia, often with hypertrichosis appearing around puberty
	Shoulders, submammary or back
	May be associated with tissue hypoplasia (breast or limb)
Café-au-lait macule	Discrete, pale brown, well-circumscribed lesions > 5 mm in infants, > 1.5 cm in adults
Ephelides, "freckles"	Less than 0.5 cm brown macules on sun-exposed skin
	First 3 years of age and darken with sun
Fixed drug eruption	Red-violaceous, desquamative plaques, followed by reddish-brown or slate-gray macule that erupts in the exact same distribution upon re-exposure to the same drug
	Often in the mouth, anogenital, axilla
	Can be bullous
	Most common drugs: tetracyclines, sulfonamides, nonsteroidal anti-inflammatory drugs, barbiturates, phenolphthalein
Macular amyloid	Brown-gray pigmentation most common on upper back, buttocks, chest, breast, shins, forearms (areas of rubbing)
	From amyloid deposition and melanophages in papillary dermis
Melasma	Symmetric facial hyperpigmentation: centrofacial, malar, or mandibular
	In sun-exposed areas, darker-skinned women
	Exacerbated by sun, pregnancy, oral contraceptive pill, epilepsy drugs
Nevus spilus	Junctional or compound nevi within a congenital café-au-lait macule
Tar melanosis (melanodermatitis toxica)	Industrial workers, patients with photosensitivity reaction from tar
	Erythema, edema, vesiculation, pruritus, reticulate hyperpigmentation, and hyperkeratosis

Table 20-17

Patterned melanosis	Key points
Diffuse acromelanosis	Autosomal dominant
	Diffuse hyperpigmentation of the fingers
	Starting in early childhood that later includes flexor creases of large joints
Erythema dyschromicum perstans (ashy dermatosis)	Most common in Spanish or Indian descent
	Slate gray or blue-brown macules that start out erythematous
	Primarily over trunk, face, neck, proximal upper extremites
Hypomelanosis of Ito	Blaschkoid hyperpigmented macules appearing weeks after birth
	May be associated with peripheral eosinophilia
Incontinentia pigmenti	X-linked dominant seen almost exclusively in females; lethal in males
	Blaschkonian distribution in four stages:
	1. Vesiculobullous (birth to 1–2 weeks linear)
	2. Verrucous stage (weeks 2–6)
	3. Whorls of hyperpigmentation over trunk and extremities that darken until age 2 years, then fade in adolescence
	4. 14% develop fourth stage of hypopigmentation
	Note: pigmentation does not correspond exactly to areas of other stages, and therefore, are not postinflammatory
Pellagra	Niacin deficiency
	Photosensitivity in areas that are susceptible to mechanical trauma (thickening, pigmentation of dorsal hands, bony areas), neck (Casal's necklace), nasal bridge, scalp
Postinflammatory hyperpigmentation	Following various dermatitides that can persist for months

Table 20-18

Reticulate melanosis	Key points
Cantu syndrome	Reticulate pigmentation of the face, forearms, feet
	Palmoplantar keratoderma
Confluent and reticulated papillomatosis of Gougerot and Carteaud	Hyperkeratotic and papillomatous pigmented papules on the central chest and reticulate at the periphery
Dowling–Degos disease	KRT 5 defect
	Acquired reticulate hyperpigmented macules in the axilla, groin, progressing to intergluteal, inframammary folds, neck, trunk, arms
	Comedones, facial pitted scars
Dyskeratosis congenita	X-linked recessive
	Dyskerin or telomerase mutation
	Reticular hyperpigmentation on the trunk around 1 cm islands of white atrophic patches, nail atrophy, palmoplantar keratodermas, increased sweating, thin hair, premalignant leukoplakia, Fanconi-type pancytopenia, mental retardation
Erythema ab igne	Reticulate hyperpigmentation in livedo reticularis pattern from heat
Naegeli–Franceschetti–Jadassohn syndrome	Autosomal dominant
	Reticulate hyperpigmentation around age 2, fading by adolescence
	Hypohidrosis, dental anomalies, palmoplantar hyperkeratosis, loss of dermatoglyphics
Prurigo pigmentosus	Asians; reticulate macules and papules on the trunk
Reticulate acropigmentation of Kitamura	Autosomal dominant; two-thirds Japanese
	Reticular, freckle-like pigmentation starting on the dorsal hand, spreading over the body; palmar pits
X-linked reticulate pigmentary disorder (Partington syndrome type II)	Reticulate Blaschkonian pigmentation in women and more generalized pattern in men
	Men have severe systemic complications with early mortality

Table 20-19

Diffuse melanosis	Key points
Addison's disease	Generalized brown hyperpigmentation, "summer tan not fading"
	May involve eyes, nipples, palmar creases, axilla, anogenital, gingiva/buccal
	Primarily adrenocorticoid deficiency with weakness, fatigue, anorexia, nausea. Old scars, mucosal surfaces, and nevi may darken (Figure 20-13)
Hemochromatosis	Autosomal dominant
	Bronze diffuse hyperpigmentation from deposition of hemosiderin or melanin
	Can precede diabetes or cirrhosis by years
Nutritional deficiency	Ashy discoloration accompanied by eczematous or psoriasiform scaling
POEMS	Acronym for: Polyneuropathy, Organomegaly, Endocrinopathy, M protein, Skin changes (diffuse hyperpigmentation, especially over extensor surfaces, back, neck, axilla, sclerodermatous changes, hirsutism, hyperhidrosis, acquired angiomas)
Progressive systemic sclerosis	Hyperpigmentation and sclerodermoid skin changes

Table 20-20

Nonmelanotic pigmentation	Key points
Carotenemia	Heavy ingestion of carrots, oranges, mangoes, apricots, green vegetables, and exogenous beta-carotene
	Most prominent on palms, soles, under tongue, behind ears
Jaundice	Increased bilirubin that has high affinity for elastic tissue
	Deposited in the dermis and sclera

Table 20-20—cont'd

Nonmelanotic pigmentation	Key points
Ochronosis (alkaptonuria)	Autosomal recessive
	Deficiency of homogentisic acid oxidase
	Accumulation of dark pigment (homogentisic acid) resulting in blue-gray pigment of pinna, nose tip, sclera, extensor tendons of the hands
	Dark urine causing black underwear after washing with alkaline soap
	Dark ear wax
Xanthomas	Yellow-orange intracellular and dermal lipid deposition in the skin
Argyria	Silver deposition in the skin, especially in sun-exposed areas
	Nails, sclerae can be involved
Arsenic	Bronze-colored hyperpigmentation on trunk with possible superimposed raindrops
	Keratoses of palms and soles
Bismuth	Blue-gray pigmentation of face, neck, dorsal hands, oral mucosa, gingiva
Chrysiasis	Gold deposition from parenteral administration
	Prominent color around eyes and sun-exposed areas
Iron	Brown pigment at injection site or application site
Lead	"Lead line" in the gingiva, nail pigmentation
Mercury	Pigmentation from topical exposures
	Gingival pigmentation from systemic administration

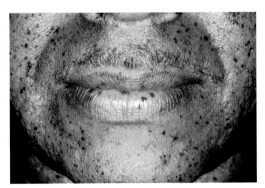

Figure 20-10 Lentigines (LAMB Syndrome)

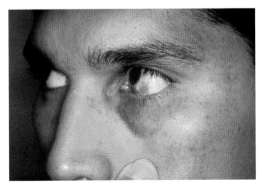

Figure 20-12 Nevus of Ota

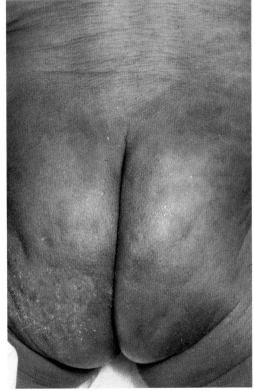

Figure 20-11 Mongolian spot

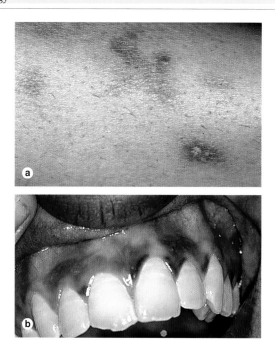

Figure 20-13 a Addison's pigment. **b** Addison's

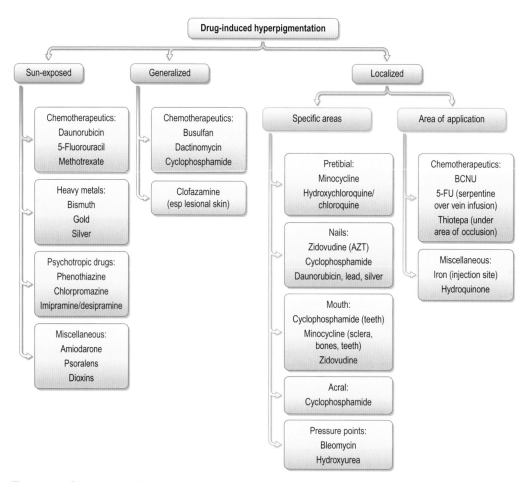

Figure 20-14 Diagnostic algorithm for drug-induced hyperpigmentation

Table 20-21 Treatments for hyperpigmentation

Treatments	Key points
Topicals	
Sunscreens	Cornerstone to management
	Inhibits stimulation of melanin synthesis
	Decreases transfer of melanosomes from melanocytes to keratinocytes
Alpha hydroxy acids	Water soluble; Glycolic acid, Citric acid, Malic acid, Lactic acid
	Decreases corneocyte cohesion
	Faster desquamation of pigmented keratinocytes
Beta hydroxy acids	Lipid-soluble; salicylic acid is most common
	An exfoliant, anti-inflammatory agent, comedolytic
	Not particularly known to decrease pigment, but helps due to exfoliation
Arbutin	β-D-glucopyranoside derivative of hydroquinone, but less toxic
	Dose-dependent reduction in tyrosinase activity and decreased melanin in melanocytes
	May cause paradoxical hyperpigmentation at higher concentrations
	Used for postinflammatory hyperpigmentation and hyperactive melanocytes
Azelaic acid	Derived from *Pityrosporum* species
	Competitively inhibits tyrosinase. Inhibits DNA synthesis and mitochondrial enzymes, inducing direct cytotoxic and antiproliferative effects on melanocytes
	Selective effect on abnormal melanocytes
	No effect on normally pigmented skin, freckles, senile lentigines, and nevi
	Effective for hypermelanosis caused by physical or photochemical agents, lentigo maligna melanoma as well as other disorders characterized by abnormal proliferation of melanocytes such as hyperpigmentation in acne
Chemical peels	Glycolic acid, trichloroacetic acid, Jessner's solution
Hydroquinone	Reversibly inhibits tyrosinase, reducing the conversion of dopa to melanin
	Other possible mechanisms: destruction of melanocytes, degradation of melanosomes, and the inhibition of the synthesis of DNA and RNA
	May cause paradoxical hyperpigmentation at higher concentrations
	Used for postinflammatory hyperpigmentation and hyperactive melanocytes
Kojic acid	Derived from certain species of *Acetobacter*, *Aspergillus*, and *Penicillium*
	Inhibits production of free tyrosinase
	Efficacy similar to hydroquinone
	Can cause contact dermatitis and erythema
	Used more commonly in Japan
Licorice extract	Not yet available in North America, but used particularly in Egypt
	Glabridin is main ingredient that affects the skin
	Mechanism of action similar to kojic acid; no effect on DNA synthesis
	Inhibits melanogenesis and inflammation
Monobenzone	Monobenzyl ether of hydroquinone, a topical phenolic agent
	Permanently depigment normal skin after 6–12 months
	Used only for final depigmentation of disfiguring vitiligo covering >50% of body
Resorcinol	Isomeric with hydroquinone
	Bactericidal
	Used in postinflammatory hyperpigmentation, melasma, acne
	Not to be used in darker skin types

Continued

Table 20-21 Treatments for hyperpigmentation—cont'd

Treatments	Key points
Retinoids	Reduces epidermal melanin, possibly from inhibition of tyrosinase
	Moderate side-effects of desquamation and erythema
	Darker-skinned patients who develop a dermatitis may develop secondary postinflammatory hyperpigmentation
	Used for melasma, postinflammatory hyperpigmentation
Soy	Inhibits PAR-2, a G-protein-coupled receptor that regulates the ingestion of melanosomes by keratinocytes in culture
	Prevents ultraviolet-induced pigmentation in vitro and in vivo; antioxidant
	Can reduce skin color clinically and decrease melanin histologically
Vitamin C	Most are unstable, except for magnesium-l-ascorbyl-2-phosphate
	Can also use iontophoresis to increase penetration
	Depigmenting agent, antioxidant, stimulates collagen synthesis
	Used for melasma or senile lentigines
Combination topical therapy	To improve efficacy. Tretinoin + hydroquinone ± corticosteroid
	Tretinoin reduces atrophy of corticosteroid, may decrease melanosome transfer to keratinocytes and facilitates epidermal penetration of hydroquinone
	The tretinoin-induced irritation is reduced by the corticosteroid
	Corticosteroid may suppress biosynthesis and secretory functions of the melanocyte. The first triple combination topical therapy approved by the US Food and Drug Administration for melasma: fluocinolone acetonide 0.01%, hydroquinone 4%, and tretinoin 0.05%
	Used for melasma, postinflammatory hyperpigmentation
Lasers and lights	
Intense pulsed light	Broadband visible light that is filtered from a flash lamp
Carbon dioxide ablation	Older ablative mechanism with permanent scarring and hypopigmentation
Q-switched alexandrite, neodymium: yttrium aluminum garnet (Nd:YAG), ruby	Targets small particles of melanin in melanocytes, keratinocytes, macrophages
	Risk of pigmentary alteration and scarring in darker skin types
	Used for lentigines, café-au-lait macules, nevus of Ota/Ito
Fractional resurfacing (Fraxel)	Nonablative resurfacing by depositing microscopic thermal columns of destruction that heals from the intervening normal skin
	Used for treatment of melasma, nonablative rejuvenation
Oral therapy	
Oral hydroquinone	Banned in Europe, highly regulated in Asia because it is a metabolite of benzene and has mutagenic properties
	Most serious complication is pigmentation of the eye and corneal damage
Vitamin E ± C	In vitro inhibits tyrosine hydrolase indirectly; antioxidant
	Reported improvement in facial hyperpigmentation in the Japanese literature
Miscellaneous	
Cryotherapy	Melanocytes are destroyed at −5°C
	Used for lentigines; risk of scar and depigmentation/hyperpigmentation
Tranexamic acid	Pilot study in Korea of localized injection to ultraviolet-induced hyperpigmentation and melasma
Microdermabrasion	Superficial exfoliation with aluminum oxide crystals under vacuum suction
Dermabrasion	Mechanical abrasion that removes epidermis and superficial dermis

Further reading

Bahadoran P, Ortonne JP, King RA, et al. Albinism. In: Freedberg IM, Eisen AZ, Wolff K, et al., eds. Fitzpatrick's Dermatology in General Medicine, 6th edn. New York: McGraw-Hill, 2003:826–836.

Baumann L. Disorders of pigmentation. In: Baumann L, ed. Cosmetic Dermatology Principles and Practice. New York:McGraw-Hill, 2002:63–71.

Baumann L. Depigmenting agents. In: Baumann L, ed. Cosmetic Dermatology Principles and Practice. New York: McGraw-Hill, 2002:99–104.

Halder RM, Richards GM. Topical agents used in the management of hyperpigmentation. Skin Ther Lett 2004; 9:1–3.

Lee JH, Park JG, Lim SH, et al. Localized intradermal microinjection of tranexamic acid for treatment of melasma in Asian patients: a preliminary clinical trial. Dermatol Surg 2006; 32:626–631.

Ortonne JP. Vitiligo and other disorders of hypopigmentation. In: Bolognia JL, Jorrizzo JL, Rapini RP, eds. Dermatology. London: Mosby, 2003:947–973.

Ortonne JP, Bahadora P, Fitzpatrick TB, et al. Hypomelanoses and hypermelanoses. In: Freedberg IM, Eisen AZ, Wolff K, et al., eds. Fitzpatrick's Dermatology in General Medicine, 6th edn. New York: McGraw-Hill, 2003:836–881.

Ortonne JP, Pandya AG, Lui H, et al. Treatment of solar lentigines. J Am Acad Dermatol 2006; 54:S262–S271.

Rendon M, Berneburg M, Arellano I, et al. Treatment of melasma. J Am Acad Dermatol 2006; 54:S272–S281.

Schmults CD, Wheeland RG. Pigmented lesions and tattoos. In: Goldberg DJ, ed. Laser and Lights, vol. 2. London: Elsevier Saunders, 2005:41–66.

Spitz JL. Genodermatoses: A Clinical Guide to Genetic Skin Disorders, 2nd edn. Philadelphia: Lippincott Williams & Wilkins, 2005.

Trout CR, Levine N, Chang MW. Disorders of hyperpigmentation. In: Bolognia JL, Jorrizzo JL, Rapini RP, eds. Dermatology. London: Mosby, 2003:975–1004.

Westerhof W, Relyveld GN, Kingswijk MM, et al. Progressive macular hypomelanosis. Arch Dermatol 2004;140:210–214.

Leg ulcers **21**

Jared Lund and Donald Miech

Clinical presentation

Of the adult population in the United States, 1–3% suffers from chronic leg ulcers. Chronic leg ulcers drastically reduce the patient's quality of life and place a large financial burden on society. An ulcer is defined as loss of both the epidermis and dermis and is classified as chronic when persisting beyond 6 weeks. Venous insufficiency, arterial disease, and neuropathy delay wound healing and predispose patients to develop chronic ulcers. A summary of the clinical features of ulcers associated with these three disease states is presented in Table 21-1.

Venous ulcers (Stasis ulcers) (Figure 21-1)

Venous stasis ulcers are the most common cause of leg ulcerations and account for 70–80% of all leg ulcers. Patients often have signs and symptoms of venous insufficiency, including dependent lower-extremity edema and aching legs, which are both often relieved by elevation. The most common location of ulcer formation is in the gaiter area or area between the ankle and calf. The surrounding skin typically demonstrates hemosiderin staining. Discomfort from the actual ulcer is variable and not related to the surface area. However, deep ulcers, especially those present over the medial malleoli, and those associated with atrophie blanche, are typically more painful. Risk factors for the development of venous ulcers include elderly age, obesity, previous leg injury, venous insufficiency, varicose veins, and history of deep venous thrombosis.

Arterial ulcers (Ischemic ulcers and digital necrosis) (Figure 21-2)

Patients with ischemic ulcers secondary to arterial disease commonly present with symptoms of intermittent claudication. The ulcers are typically located more distally than venous ulcers and commonly affect the digits. They may also overlie bony prominences or areas prone to trauma or pressure. The surrounding skin is typically taut and atrophic with loss of skin markings and hair. Pulses are difficult to palpate and capillary refill is poor. Unlike neuropathic ulcers, they usually do not affect the volar surfaces and lack surrounding hyperkeratosis. The ulcer may appear punched out and round or stellate with an eschar or dry base. Ulceration pain is typically more severe and exacerbated by exertion or leg elevation. Placing the leg in the dependent position increases blood flow to the affected area and decreases pain. Risk factors for development of arterial ulcers include diabetes mellitus, smoking, hypertension, and hypercholesterolemia.

Neuropathic ulcers (Figure 21-3)

Neuropathic ulcers occur in insensate limbs and are typically asymptomatic; however paresthesias of the lower extremities are often present. They occur primarily over the plantar aspects

Table 21-1 Summary of the clinical features of ulcers

Type of ulcer	Location	Ulcer characteristics	Other clinical findings
Venous	Commonly located over the medial malleolus	Typically larger Shallow in depth Irregular "shaggy" margins Granulation tissue at base	Varicosities Venous stasis dermatitis Dependent edema Atrophie blanche Lipodermatosclerosis
Arterial	More distal Common over bony prominences	Typically round and punched out or stellate Well-demarcated borders Little or no granulation tissue Dry base	Absent lower-extremity hair Shiny atrophic skin Cool feet Weak or absent dorsalis pedis pulses Pallor with leg elevation Dependent rubor Delayed capillary refill
Neuropathic	Pressure sites – plantar metatarsal heads, heels, or great toe	Well demarcated May be painless Deep Surrounded by moist malodorous callus Purulent drainage may indicate infection	Parasthesias or numbness of lower extremities Pain improved by exertion Charcot foot

of the foot and toes and commonly overlie the metatarsal heads. Thick surrounding callus is typically present. Debridement of the dead and hyperkeratotic skin reveals the full extent of the ulcer. Ulcers often extend deep into the tissue, reaching bone. Persistent drainage from a deep ulcer may indicate osteomyelitis. The most common underlying disease predisposing patients to neuropathic ulcers is diabetes mellitus. In all, 12–25% of diabetic patients will develop foot ulcers during their lifetime. Such ulcers are both life- and limb-threatening and require immediate attention. Although diabetic ulcers are most often neuropathic in nature, peripheral vascular disease may also be present, creating a neuroischemic process in 15–20% of diabetic patients. Neuroischemic ulcers are commonly seen on the medial first metatarsophalangeal joint or lateral aspect of the fifth metatarsophalangeal joint secondary to friction forces from ill-fitting shoes.

Diagnosis

Key Points

- A thorough history and physical exam including ulcer characteristics and adjacent physical findings will help delineate the underlying etiology
- An ankle–brachial index (ABI) should be measured in the evaluation of leg ulcers
- Diminished peripheral pulses and a reduced ABI require further evaluation for arterial insufficiency
- Appropriate laboratory evaluation will assist in identifying systemic causes of ulceration
- Recalcitrant chronic ulcers or those with abnormal morphology and location should be biopsied and cultured to rule out vasculitis, neoplasia, or infection

The underlying cause must be correctly determined to guide the appropriate treatment regimen. Error in determining the correct etiology may lead to worsening ulceration. While venous ulcers are the predominant type of leg ulcer and often diagnosed on clinical presentation alone, a systematic approach should be taken in each patient presenting with a leg ulcer.

The first step in leg ulcer evaluation is a thorough history and physical examination. Information that should be elicited and pertinent areas to be examined are included in Table 21-2.

An important aspect in leg ulcer evaluation is assessing the arterial competency to the affected limbs. Pulses should always be palpated. However patients with palpable pulses may still have arterial insufficiency or patients with significant edema may not have palpable pulses. It is therefore important to measure an ABI. This is defined as the ratio of the ankle systolic pressure to the brachial

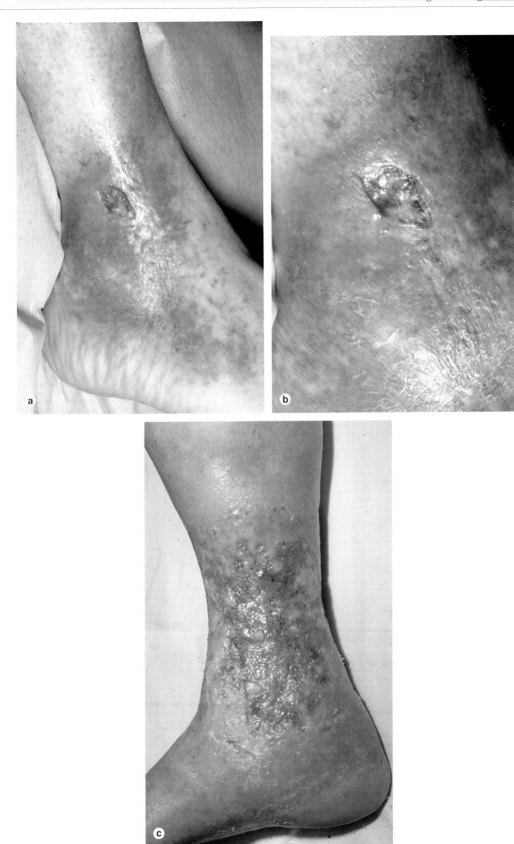

Figure 21-1 a–c Stasis ulcer (courtesy of Geisinger Medical Center teaching file)

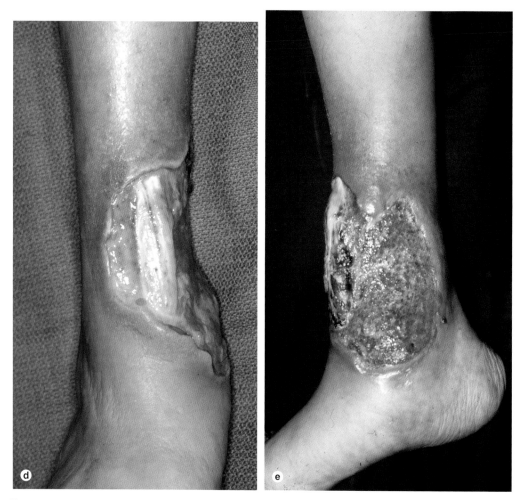

Figure 21-1, cont'd d Venous ulcer extending to tendon. e Venous ulcer with granulation tissue

systolic pressure. Both arms should be measured and the higher systolic pressure used. These measurements are done with the patient in the supine position using a Doppler flow meter. Patients with diabetic microvascular disease may have inelastic vessels and the ABI may be falsely elevated. Therefore, other physical exam findings may suggest arterial insufficiency in diabetic patients in the setting of a normal ABI (Figure 21-4).

Differential diagnosis

Uncommon causes for leg ulceration should be considered if the morphology and location appear unusual on examination. Recalcitrant ulcers should alert the physician to other etiologies, including vasculitis, neoplasia, and invasive infection. Other systemic symptoms and signs elicited on the history and physical examination will assist the physician in narrowing down the numerous etiologies of leg ulcers. A list of causes of leg ulcerations is given in Box 21-1.

Laboratory testing and imaging

Initial laboratory tests include a complete blood count, blood glucose level, and an erythrocyte sedimentation rate to screen for hematologic disease, diabetes mellitus, or inflammatory diseases such as osteomyelitis or connective tissue disease. Factors important in wound healing include albumin, transferrin, iron, and zinc and should be measured and corrected to maximize wound-healing potential.

If unusual causes of leg ulceration are suspected either from the initial assessment or from biopsy results, a more extensive laboratory investigation is indicated (Box 21-2).

Noninvasive vascular studies are useful in assessing the anatomy and function of the venous and arterial systems in the presence of leg ulceration. Color duplex ultrasonography is the "gold standard" in the evaluation of venous insufficiency. It is accurate and reproducible and

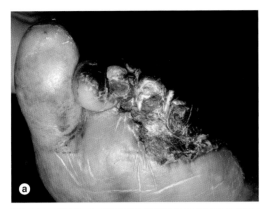

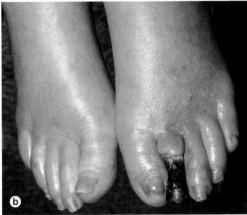

Figure 21-2 a, b Ischemic toes (courtesy of Geisinger Medical Center teaching file)

more reliable tissue cultures compared to simply swabbing the ulcer bed. First excess necrotic tissue should be debrided. Then tissue should be obtained by punch biopsy or curettage at the ulcer base. Histologic evaluation with special stains can also assist in the identification of pathologic organisms.

If ulcers do not show response to appropriate treatment within 6–12 weeks, biopsy is indicated to confirm the diagnosis and rule out other etiologies such as malignancy, vasculitis, or pyoderma gangrenosum. Malignancy may either develop within a chronic ulcer (such as squamous or basal cell carcinoma) or may manifest primarily as an ulcer. Punch biopsies at multiple sites or deep wedge biopsy of the edge and ulcer bed are suggested.

Pathogenesis

Key Points

- Chronic ulcers are characterized by a persistent inflammatory state which impairs wound healing
- Valvular incompetence, venous obstruction, or calf muscle pump dysfunction cause microcirculatory changes which lead to venous ulcerations
- Reduction of arterial flow leads to tissue hypoxia and predisposes patients to developing arterial ulcers
- Repetitive trauma to insensate tissue causes neuropathic ulcers

allows assessment of patency and reflux and identifies incompetent perforator and saphenous veins. Duplex ultrasonography will also provide information on arterial occlusion, stenosis, and atheromatous disease. Plethysmography studies are helpful in quantifying the degree of reflux and calf muscle pump dysfunction in venous insufficiency. In diabetic patients, transcutaneous oxygen measurements can be performed when arterial insufficiency is suspected as the ABI may be falsely elevated due to incompressible vessels.

If osteomyelitis is suspected in patients with diabetic foot ulcers, plain radiographs may be helpful, but magnetic resonance imaging is now considered the best imaging study for confirming the diagnosis. The gold standard however is bone biopsy and culture.

When infection is suspected, either as the primary cause or as a secondary infection of the ulcer, tissue should be submitted for culture and histology. Signs of secondary infection include tenderness, purulent drainage, foul smell, redness, warmth, and induration at the ulcer site. However, Charcot foot in diabetic patients may also present with nonpainful ankle and foot swelling and erythema. Deep tissue specimens produce

Venous hypertension may be associated with superficial, deep, and perforator vein valve incompetence which may be congenital or acquired. Venous obstruction and calf muscle pump dysfunction may also contribute to venous hypertension. Valvular incompetence allows regurgitation into the superficial venous plexus, increasing the pressure and increasing the permeability of the microcirculation. The exact mechanism of the sequence of events leading from venous hypertension to ulceration is unclear. Three plausible hypotheses have been described to account for the underlying etiology behind venous ulceration:

1. Development of pericapillary fibrin cuffs: venous hypertension may lead to capillary distension and leakage of fibrinogen and other macromolecules. It has been suggested that polymerization of these molecules around vessels walls may act as a barrier for diffusion of oxygen and nutrients, leading to tissue hypoxia and ulceration. Conflicting data exist as healing may occur with cuff persistence and the cuffs are discontinuous around the dermal capillaries. Fibrin and fibrinogen have been shown to inhibit production of type 1

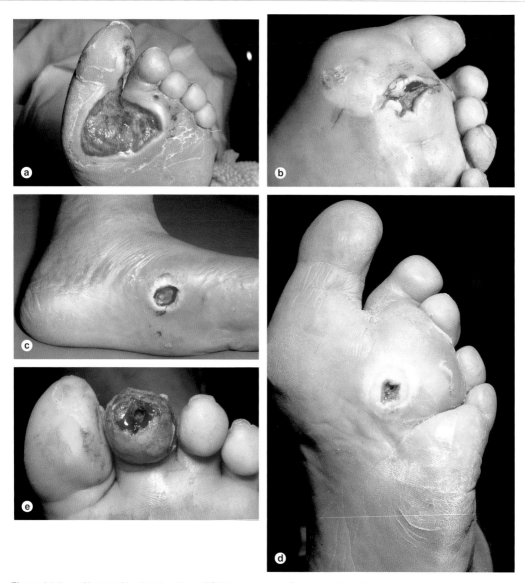

Figure 21-3 a–e Neuropathic ulcer (courtesy of Geisinger Medical Center teaching file)

procollagen in cultures and may impede healing of damaged tissue

2. Leukocyte trapping: reduced flow through capillaries occurs secondary to venous hypertension. Leukocytes are thought to plug the capillaries, leading to tissue ischemia. This occurs more frequently when legs are in the dependent position. Trapping of leukocytes may also lead to activation and release of mediators that increase vascular permeability and cause tissue damage

3. Growth factor trapping: macromolecules such as β_2-macroglobulin enter the dermis from the effects of venous hypertension and may trap important growth factors that are important in maintaining the integrity of the skin

Arterial ulcers are caused by reduction in the arterial flow leading to tissue hypoxia and death. This most commonly results from arteriosclerosis causing narrowing of vessel lumens, but may also be secondary to vasculitis, pyoderma gangrenosum, thrombotic, and embolic phenomena, or other causes of arterial occlusion. Ulceration may manifest after minor traumatic insults to an already compromised limb.

Profound peripheral neuropathy results in the loss of the protective sensation of pain and increases the risk of foot ulceration by sevenfold. Motor neuropathy may alter the patient's gait, leading to repetitive trauma over unusual areas. Autonomic dysfunction also causes anhidrosis which predisposes the skin to fissuring and callus formation. All these factors contribute to

Table 21-2 Information to be elicited and pertinent areas to be examined in leg ulcer

History	Physical
Ulcer-directed history	**Ulcer-directed physical**
Onset (rapid versus slow)	Location and size
Duration and initiating factors	Borders
Current therapies (topical and systemic)	Evaluation of ulcer bed for granulation tissue, fibrin, or malodorous exudate
Certain therapies may delay wound healing or cause allergic contact dermatitis on surrounding skin	Tenderness
Ulcer pain, including alleviating and exacerbating factors	**Perilesional skin**
	Erythema, induration, scale, warmth
Associated features	Scarring from previous ulcerations
Intermittent claudication, ankle swelling, parasthesias	**General lower-extremity exam**
Past medical history/family history	Evaluation for associated clinical findings in Table 21-1
Diabetes mellitus	Extent of lower-extremity edema/varicosities
Coronary or peripheral vascular disease	Capillary refill time
Deep venous thrombosis or leg swelling following surgery or pregnancy	Peripheral pulse evaluation
Connective tissue diseases	Hand-held Doppler to evaluate if necessary
Social history	10 g monofilament, deep tendon reflexes, and vibratory testing
Tobacco use	
Alcohol intake	
Living arrangements (patient may need assistance later on with treatment and dressing changes)	
Review of systems	

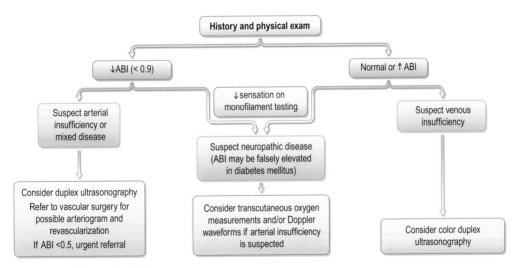

Figure 21-4 Diagnostic algorithm

neuropathic ulcer formation. Inappropriate footwear is the most common cause of repetitive trauma in the diabetic foot. Repetitive trauma to insensate tissue often results in callus formation which precedes development of ulcers. Chronic calluses exert force on the underlying tissue,

causing tissue necrosis with eventual debridement revealing the ulcer.

Diabetic patients also have multiple abnormalities in the wound-healing process. There is impaired neovascularization, collagen synthesis, and fibroblast proliferation.

BOX 21-1

Causes of leg ulcerations

Vascular disease

Venous

Arterial (atherosclerosis, arteriovenous malformations, cholesterol emboli)

Vasculitic (idiopathic, infectious, drug-induced, rheumatoid arthritis, systemic lupus erythematosus, Behçet's disease, polyarteritis nodosa, Wegener's granulomatosis, giant cell arteritis)

Lymphatics (lymphedema)

Other (livedoid vasculopathy, Buerger's disease, calciphylaxis, cryoglobulinemia, cryofibrogenemia)

Neuropathic disease

Diabetes mellitus, alcohol neuropathy, leprosy, tabes dorsalis, syringomyelia, spina bifida, multiple sclerosis, paraplegia, paresis

Infectious disease

Bacterial (ecthyma, ecthyma gangrenosum, mycobacterial, septic emboli, Gram-negative, anaerobic, spirochetal)

Fungal (blastomycosis (Figure 21-5), coccidioidomycosis, sporotrichosis, cryptococcosis, and maduromycosis)

Protozoal (leishmaniasis, amoebiasis)

Metabolic disease

Diabetes mellitus, Gaucher's disease, gout, prolidase deficiency, calcinosis cutis

Hematologic disease

Hereditary spherocytosis, polycythemia vera, sickle-cell anemia, thalassemia, thrombocytosis

Hypercoagulable states (factor V Leiden, antiphospholipid antibody syndrome, antithrombin III deficiency, protein C and S deficiency, prothrombin G20210A mutation)

Neoplastic

Squamous cell carcinoma (Figure 21-6), basal cell carcinoma, cutaneous T- and B-cell lymphoma, angiosarcoma, malignant melanoma, Kaposi's sarcoma, rhabdomyosarcoma, lymphangiosarcoma

Physical

Pressure, trauma, cold injury, burns, factitial, radiation, chemical corrosive agents, sclerotherapy

Medications

Hydroxyurea, vaccinations, methotrexate, leflunomide, halogens including bromides and iodides

Others

Pyoderma gangrenosum (Figure 21-7), vasculitis (Figure 21-8), systemic sclerosis, necrobiosis lipoidica, sarcoidosis, panniculitis, Langerhans cell histiocytosis, ulcerative lichen planus (Figure 21-9)

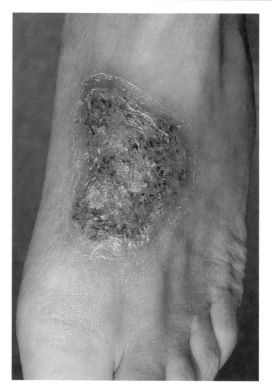

Figure 21-5 Blastomycosis

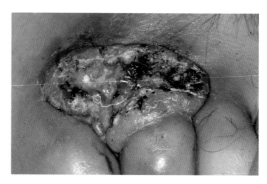

Figure 21-6 Squamous cell carcinoma

Treatment

Key Points

Venous stasis ulcers

- In treating venous ulcers, the primary goal should be to reverse venous hypertension and provide a suitable environment for wound healing
- High compression is more effective than low compression in venous ulcers
- Compression with an Unna boot is often first-line therapy
- Arterial disease must be excluded before compression

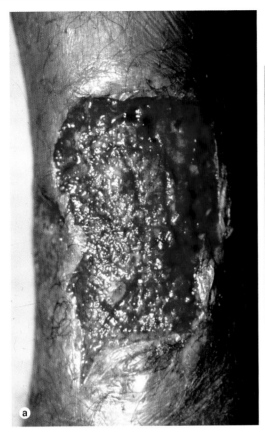
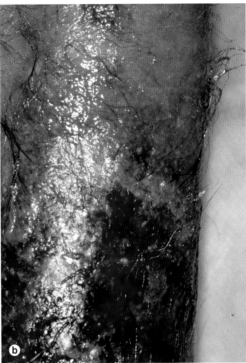

Figure 21-7 a, b Pyoderma gangrenosum

Arterial ischemic ulcers

- Re-establishment of the arterial supply will hasten healing in arterial ulcers
- *Refer to a peripheral vascular surgeon*

Neuropathic ulcers

- Debridement and off-loading of the ulcer site promote healing neuropathic ulcers. Contact casting is commonly used to off-load the ulcer
- Prompt treatment of infection of diabetic foot ulcers may be limb-saving

Venous ulcer therapy: compression therapy

Reduction of edema and reversal of venous hypertension are necessary elements in the treatment of venous ulcers. Leg elevation and bed rest allow swelling to subside and improve venous microcirculation; however many patients find this impractical and such a regimen may not be sufficient in patients with advanced disease. Therefore, compression therapy in combination with leg elevation remains the mainstay in decreasing venous hypertension, controlling edema, promoting venous ulcer healing, and preventing recurrence. Compression providing external ankle pressures of 35–40 mmHg is recommended to prevent capillary exudation in the legs. The first phase of compression therapy is meant to reduce edema. This is effectively done with bandages that exert low resting pressures and higher pressures with muscle contraction. Nonelastic bandages, such as the Unna boot, demonstrate these characteristics and are useful in treating this phase. Short-stretch bandages are considered to be a very rigid elastic bandage and have many of the same characteristics as the Unna boot, such as exerting low resting pressures and higher ambulatory pressures. They can be rewrapped daily as edema decreases.

Elastic bandages are also used to reduce edema and promote healing. They are classified by the amount of pressure they exert and are single or multilayered, long- or short-stretch, and adherent or nonadherent. These bandages are more flexible and comfortable than the Unna boot and maintain compression over extended periods of time. Long-stretch and multilayered bandages are more useful in the initial stages of controlling edema.

Elastic support stockings or elastic compression bandages are useful during the maintenance phase once edema has been controlled and healing of the ulcer has occurred. Lifelong therapy is important in preventing ulcer recurrence.

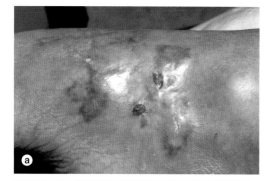

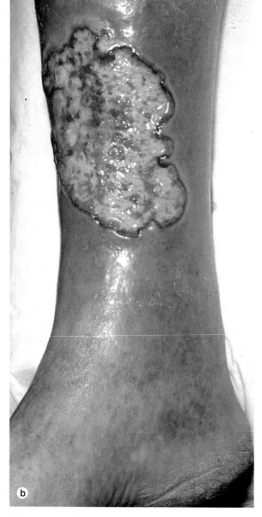

Figure 21-8 **a** Early vasculitic ulcer (courtesy of Gesinger Medical Center teaching file). **b** Rheumatoid vasculitis (courtesy of Geisinger Medical Center teaching file)

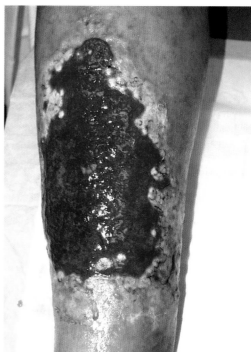

Figure 21-9 Ulcerative lichen planus

BOX 21-2

More extensive laboratory investigation of leg ulcer

Screening laboratory tests

Complete blood count, blood glucose, erythrocyte sedimentation rate

Albumin, transferrin, iron, zinc

Additional laboratory tests

Antinuclear antibodies

Lupus anticoagulant

Antithrombin III

Protein C and S

Cryoglobulins

Cryofibrinogen

Rheumatoid factor

Screening for hepatitis B and C infection

Rapid plasma reagin

Blood cultures in patients with severe infections who are systemically ill

---

Recurrence has been reported in up to 79% of patients who are not compliant with compression hosiery versus 4% who were compliant. Custom fitting and proper education on how to apply the stocking may improve compliance. Patients with higher-grade compression stockings have lower compliance rates. Therefore patients should be offered the strongest appropriate compression stocking which they will wear.

Whenever compression therapy is considered, it is important to ensure arterial insufficiency does not exist. Regardless, care should be taken in applying all of the different forms of compression as excess pressure may lead to necrosis, worsening ulceration, or gangrene. Despite compression therapy, risk factors exist that delay ulcer healing (Box 21-3).

Details of the different compression options are listed in Table 21-3. Other compression methods include intermittent pneumatic compression and specialized Velcro-enforced orthotics.

Topical therapy

Wound dressings and debridement

A moist wound environment accelerates autolysis of necrotic tissue and maintains a fluid medium where many endogenous factors important in wound healing exist. Removal of necrotic tissue promotes granulation tissue formation and re-epithelialization. A dry desiccated wound open to air heals up to 50% slower because keratinocytes only migrate over viable tissue during the re-epithelialization process. Therefore they must burrow under the desiccated debris to encounter the nutrient-enriched moist environment that sustains their survival. Such a process takes considerably more time.

Maintenance of a moist environment may be achieved by performing moist to moist dressing changes with physiologic saline or by using occlusive dressings. Such dressings reduce pain, promote autolytic debridement, and protect the

Table 21-3 Compression choices for venous ulceration

Type	Characteristics	Examples
Nonelastic bandages	Provide low resting pressure and high pressure with muscle contraction	Unna boot
	Effective in ambulatory patients	Moist zinc oxide-impregnated paste bandage that hardens to become inelastic
	Changed weekly or earlier if secondary infection is present	
	Not for high-exudate ulcers as an unpleasant odor may develop	
	Do not accommodate changes in volume of the leg with reduction of edema	
Multilayered elastic bandages	Adaptation possible for wide array of ankle circumference and leg size	Includes a wool absorbing layer, a crêpe layer, and 1–2 elastic layers
	Deliver graded pressures of 40 mmHg at the ankle and 17 mmHg at the knee	Dynaflex: three-layered
	Nonreusable, but cost-effective when compared to other elastic bandages because of faster healing times	Profore: four-layered
		System 4: four-layered
	Useful in wounds with large amounts of exudate	
	Skilled providers need to apply	
Elastic bandages	Conforms to leg easily	Class I: Light-weight, conforming stretch products
	Provide both high working and resting pressures	Class II: Light with minimal elasticity (short-stretch); useful in prevention of edema
	Reusable; allows for frequent dressing changes	
	Patients may not correctly apply decreasing desired compression	Class III: graded by amount of pressure exerted (IIIa–IIId)
Elastic support stockings	Useful in preventing ulcer recurrence	Class I: 20–30 mmHg
	Elasticity decreases over time	Class II: 30–40 mmHg
	Replace every 6 months	Class III: 40–50 mmHg
		Class IV: > 60 mmHg

wound. Infection rates have also been shown to be lower when occlusive dressing are used. It has been proposed that occlusive dressing creates a barrier to exogenous bacteria, increases the amount of neutrophils in the wound, and promotes the accumulation of host factors that inhibit bacterial growth.

Occlusive dressings include hydrogels, alginates, hydrocolloids, foams, and films. There is no evidence to support one type of moist retentive dressing over the other when comparing healing rates. However, numerous factors are considered when choosing an occlusive dressing type, including amount of exudate, area of ulcer, and the cost of the materials (Table 21-4).

Besides enhancing autolytic debridement, mechanical and chemical debridement may also be used to remove necrotic tissue. Mechanical debridement is a fast but nonselective method for removal of necrotic tissue. Because damage may occur to viable tissue, caution should be exercised when performing this method.

Chemical enzyme debridement is easy to perform, painless, and selective for necrotic tissue. However, large randomized controlled studies are needed to prove their effectiveness. Specific examples of each type of debridement are listed in Table 21-5.

Topical antibiotics and steroids

There exists a continuum from contamination to colonization to critical colonization and infection in chronic ulcers. While it is well understood that overt infection delays wound healing, there is controversy over the relationship of bacterial colonization and ulcer healing. Critical colonization represents a state where bacteria have not yet invaded deeper or viable tissue, but there exist increased amounts of secreted toxins and host cytokines and proteases that may impair wound healing. The only signs of critical colonization may be increased exudate, sudden odor, new areas of tissue breakdown, friable or foamy granulation tissue, or just a plateau in the wound-healing process. Although there is currently little evidence to support the use of topical antibiotics to promote healing in clinically uninfected wounds, there is much debate regarding use of topical agents in ulcers that demonstrate the subtle characteristics of critical colonization. Two recently studied preparations that decrease wound bacterial counts include Candexomer iodine preparations and controlled-release silver dressings. Candexomer iodine preparations improved healing time when compared to hydrocolloid and paraffin gauze dressings in a 12-week study. Randomized controlled trials have demonstrated that ulcers that show signs of critical colonization treated with silver foam dressings demonstrate a significant reduction in ulcer area and odor.

Physicians should be aware that many of the topical preparations are cytotoxic and impair re-epithelialization or may cause a contact dermatitis. Such preparations include chlorhexidine, povidone-iodine, neomycin preparations, and acetic acid. Dermatitis secondary to either venous stasis or allergic contact should be treated with a mid-potency topical steroid. Oral corticosteroids may be warranted in severe cases of dermatitis.

Systemic therapy

Pentoxifylline and Daflon (diosmin and flavonoids)

Pentoxifylline is a methyl xanthine derivative that increases flexibility of erythrocytes and inhibits neutrophil adhesion and activation. Aggregation and activation of platelets are also inhibited. A systematic review showed pentoxifylline to be more effective than placebo in substantially improving or completely healing venous ulcers and it offers additional benefit together with compression. Patients with characteristics that delay ulcer healing, those with atrophie blanche (Figure 21-10), or those who do not tolerate compression may benefit from a trial of pentoxifylline.

Daflon, a micronized and purified flavonoidic fraction, may decrease white blood cell plugging in endothelial cells and may reduce vascular permeability. A recent meta-analysis showed it to be effective in adjunct to conventional therapy in ulcers between 5 and 10 cm^2 of area and those of greater duration than 6 months.

Antibiotics

Systemic antibiotics are indicated in patients who have clinically infected ulcers, cellulitis, and fever. Baseline cultures may be helpful in choosing empiric treatment.

Table 21-4 Occlusive dressings	
Ulcer characteristics	Type
Heavy exudates	Foams, alginates
Moderate exudates	Hydrocolloids, foams
Mild exudates	Hydrogels, hydrocolloids

Table 21-5 Methods of debridement	
Autolytic	Enhanced by compression and moist or occlusive dressings
Chemical	Collagenases, papain, and trypsin
Mechanical	Hydrotherapy, irrigation, dextranomers, sharp surgical methods, wet–dry dressings

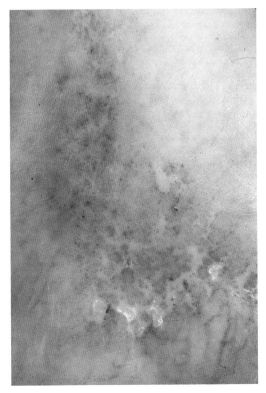

Figure 21-10 Atrophie blanche (courtesy of Geisinger Medical Center teaching file)

Other systemic agents

Faster ulcer-healing rates have been reported with aspirin therapy. Anti-inflammatory or antiplatelet aggregation may be the mechanisms behind the benefits. Stanozolol, an attenuated androgen, has potent fibrinolytic properties. Although this medication is helpful in decreasing pain and skin induration in patients with lipodermatosclerosis, no studies have demonstrated quicker healing ulcer times within affected skin.

Surgical therapy

Surgical treatment of venous ulcers targets either underlying venous hypertension or the ulcer itself via graft placement. The ESCHAR study showed no differences in healing time and rate of ulcers treated with compression alone versus ulcers treated with compression and superficial vein surgery. However, 12-month recurrence rates were significantly lower in the surgery group both in patients with isolated superficial venous reflux and with superficial and deep segmental venous reflux. Recurrence was not statistically different in patients with superficial and total deep reflux who underwent surgery. Other studies have shown decreased recurrence rates in patients followed for 3 years after surgical correction when compared to compression alone. Superficial vein surgery can be performed by a variety of minimally invasive

techniques and should be considered in patients with incompetent isolated superficial reflux and perhaps in patients with segmental deep reflux. This may be very helpful in preventing recurrence, especially in patients who do not tolerate or are noncompliant with compression therapy.

Skin grafts

Skin grafting is also an alternative in the treatment of venous leg ulcers and may be helpful in large, deep, or slow-healing ulcers. A recipient bed free of excess necrotic debris and infection improves graft survival. There are a variety of techniques and graft materials used (Table 21-6). A recent

Table 21-6 Grafts

Type	Features
Pinch grafts	Simple to perform
	Useful for small ulcerations
	Use a 3–4 mm trephine to obtain multiple pieces
	Allow space between each graft for wound exudate drainage
	May be done as outpatient procedure under local anesthesia
	Healing rates reported at 43% at 3 months and 67% at 12 months
Split-thickness skin grafts	Used for large ulcers
	Requires more extensive anesthesia
	Patient will have two wound sites to care for
	Meshed grafts allow drainage of exudate
	Healing rates have been reported at up to 75%
Composite grafts (Apligraf)	Approved by the Food and Drug Administration for the treatment of venous and neuropathic foot ulcers
	Tissue-engineered bilayer composed of dermal fibroblasts and neonatal keratinocytes
	Apligraf and compression therapy versus compression therapy alone
	More patients healed at 6 months
	Significant shortened time to wound closure
Cultured keratinocyte grafts	Autografts: keratinocytes from patient's skin are isolated, grown in culture, and subsequently placed back on the ulcer; cells from patient's own skin
	Allografts: cultured neonatal foreskin keratinocytes
	Thought to stimulate epithelialization and release of growth factors

meta-analysis on skin grafting for venous ulcers showed evidence of increased healing of ulcers using the tissue-engineered bilayer grafts.

Alternative therapies for venous ulcer are given in Box 21-4; see Figure 21-11 for diagnostic algorithm.

Arterial ulcer therapy

The aim of treatment for arterial ulcers is to increase blood flow and oxygen tension by re-establishing an arterial supply to the affected limb. Therefore, consultation with a vascular surgeon is necessary in the treatment of arterial ulcers. The patient should be encouraged to quit smoking and comorbid conditions such as hypertension, diabetes, and hypercholesterolemia should be optimally treated by the patient's primary care physician. Exercise should be encouraged as it promotes the development of collateral circulation; however some patients will not tolerate this because of symptoms of claudication.

Wound infections should be treated with oral antibiotics. The patient should be on antiplatelet

medication (aspirin or Plavix). Medications such as cilostazol and pentoxyfylline are useful in treating claudication symptoms (Table 21-9).

Debridement of eschar is risky as it may extend the ulceration and promote further tissue necrosis. Local wound care with moist dressings should be performed; however, compression is contraindicated in these patients.

Neuropathic ulcer therapy

Prevention of neuropathic ulcers in patients with diabetes is of paramount importance. However, when ulceration develops, prompt aggressive care is necessary to decrease the risk of lower-limb amputation. Aggressive debridement and avoidance of weight-bearing (off-loading) are essential elements in the treatment of diabetic neuropathic ulcers. Wounds that are shallow, present less than 2 months, are less than 2 cm in size, and are not infected have the highest probability of healing. Principles in the management of diabetic foot ulcers are listed in Table 21-7.

Infection and diabetic foot ulcers

Roughly half of all diabetic foot ulcers are infected at the time the patient presents for evaluation. Patients with severe foot infections may not have fever or leukocytosis. They may complain of flu-like symptoms, poor glucose control, local signs of inflammation around the ulcer, foul odor, and increased purulence. If left untreated, infection will progress to involve surrounding structures, including bone, and may evolve to gangrene which usually requires amputation. The most commonly isolated organisms in superficial

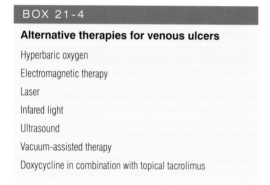

BOX 21-4

Alternative therapies for venous ulcers

Hyperbaric oxygen

Electromagnetic therapy

Laser

Infared light

Ultrasound

Vacuum-assisted therapy

Doxycycline in combination with topical tacrolimus

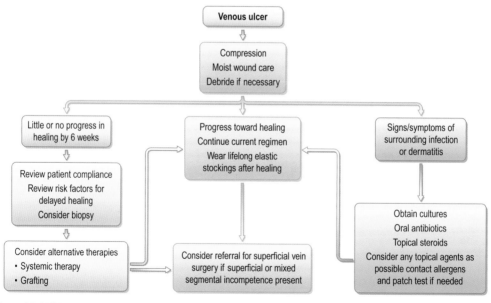

Figure 21-11 Diagnostic algorithm

Table 21-7 Management of diabetic foot ulcers

Debridement	Aggressive removal of all callus and nonviable tissue extending up to 2–3 mm into viable tissue
	Probe ulcer for extension to surrounding tissue and bone
	If bone is visible or easily palpated with probe, suspect osteomyelitis
	Obtain tissue for wound culture
	Surgical resection of all necrotic infected bone if osteomyelitis present
Mechanical off loading	Total contact casts applied properly and changed regularly
	Orthotics evaluation
Moist wound dressings	Physiologic saline moist dressings
	May use occlusive dressings as appropriate based on characteristics of ulcer
Vascular control	If compromise present, consultation with vascular surgery is recommended as revascularization may be necessary for wound healing
Infection control	Clinically infected ulcers require treatment with oral or parenteral antibiotics guided by appropriate cultures
	Patients with osteomyelitis
Adjunctive therapy	**Growth factors**
	Becaplermin (Regranex) is a recombinant platelet-derived growth factor approved by the Food and Drug Administration for treatment of diabetic ulcers
	Improved complete and faster wound healing when compared to placebo
	Tissue-engineered skin
	Apligraf
	Topical tretinoin
	Stimulates angiogenesis and possibly re-epithelialization
	Short contact application (10 minutes daily) generated improved healing of ulcers in one small study

Table 21-8 Classification of diabetic foot infections

Infection severity	Clinical features
No infection	No purulent drainage or manifestations of inflammation
Mild	≥ 2 manifestations of inflammation
	Cellulitis/erythema extends ≤ 2cm around the ulcer
	Limited to skin or superficial subcutaneous layer; patient is not systemically ill
Moderate	Patient with the above *plus* one of the following: cellulitis extending beyond 2 cm, lymphangitic streaking, deep tissue infection, gangrene, or infection of muscle, tendon, joint, or bone
Severe	Systemic toxicity or metabolic instability
	Fever, chills, tachycardia, hypotension, confusion, vomiting, leukocytosis, azotemia, acidosis, and severe hyperglycemia

Adapted from Lipsky BA, Berendt AR, Deery HG, et al. Diagnosis and treatment of diabetic foot infections. Plast Reconstr Surg 2006;117(Suppl):212S–238S.

Gram-negative organisms. Such infections are treated for longer durations with antibiotic therapy (2–4 weeks if involving only soft tissue, 4–6 weeks if involving bone). An executive summary was recently published with guidelines regarding classification (Table 21-8) and management of diabetic foot infections. See Figure 21-12 for diagnostic algorithm.

Prevention of diabetic foot ulcers

Limb amputations occur 10–30 times more often in diabetic patients compared to the general population. Mortality at 5 years after amputation ranges from 39% to 80%. Therefore frequent clinical evaluation and patient education on prevention are mandatory. Important factors to consider in the prevention of diabetic foot ulcers are listed in Box 21-5.

Controversies

• Treatment of ulcers that show signs of critical colonization with topical antimicrobials is a controversial area subject to debate.

Acknowledgment

The authors would like to thank Drs. Erik Stratman and Dirk Elston for their help in assembling images for this chapter.

infections are *Staphylococcus aureus* and hemolytic streptococci. Such infections are usually treated with a 2-week course of oral antibiotics. However, limb-threatening infections may be polymicrobial with the addition of anaerobes and

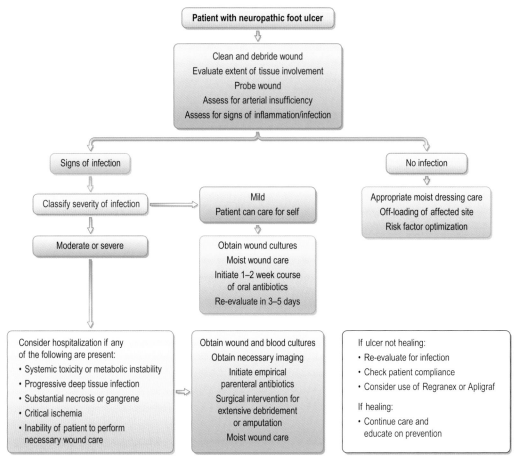

Figure 21-12 Diagnostic algorithm

Prevention of diabetic foot ulcers

Frequent foot examinations

- Yearly if no neuropathy, deformities, or history of previous ulcer
- Every 6 months if neuropathy is present
- Every 3 months if neuropathy and foot deformity present
- Every 1–3 months if there is neuropathy, foot deformity, and Charcot arthropathy, or history of ulcer or amputation

If structural abnormalities exist, refer to foot specialist for custom shoes, orthotics, or prophylactic surgery

Debridement of all calluses

Treatment of fungal infections of the feet

Counsel patient on:

- Smoking cessation, tight blood sugar control
- Daily evaluation of feet, looking for fissures or ulcers
- Proper hygiene
- Proper nail care
- Appropriately fitted shoes
- Measures to avoid trauma (i.e., avoid walking barefoot)
- Prompt reporting of breaks in skin

Table 21-9 Medication table

Generic name	Trade name	Dose	Pregnancy category	Possible side-effects
Pentoxyfylline	Trental Pentoxil Pentopak	400 mg 3–4× daily	C	Nausea, gastrointestinal disturbances, dizziness, headache Caution in patients with severe cardiac disease
Diosmin	Daflon	500 mg 2 tablets daily	B	Gastrointestinal disturbance, insomnia, vertigo, drowsiness, headache
Aspirin	Bayer Ecotrin Entercote	300 mg daily was studied	D	Gastrointestinal disturbances, bleeding, bronchospasm, tinnitus, angioedema, Reye's syndrome
Cilostazol	Pletal	100 mg twice daily	C	Gastrointestinal disturbance, edema, palpitations, tachyarrhythmia, dizziness, headache, vertigo, myalgias, cough

Further reading

Armstrong DG, Lipsky BA. Diabetic foot infections: stepwise medical and surgical management. Int Wound J 2004;1:123–132.

Aronow WS. Drug treatment of peripheral arterial disease in the elderly. Drugs Aging 2006; 23:1–12.

Barwell JR, Taylor M, Deacon J, et al. Surgical correction of isolated superficial venous reflux reduces long-term recurrence rate in chronic venous leg ulcers. Eur J Vasc Endovasc Surg 2000;20:363–368.

Barwell JR, Davies CE, Deacon J, et al. Comparison of surgery and compression with compression alone in chronic venous ulceration (ESCHAR study): randomized controlled trial. Lancet 2004;363:1854–1859.

Bello YM, Phillips TJ. Recent advances in wound healing. JAMA 2000;283:716–718.

Boulton AJ, Kirsner RS, Vileikyte L. Clinical practice. Neuropathic diabetic foot ulcers. N Engl J Med 2004;351:48–55.

Brem H, Sheehan P, Rosenberg HJ, et al. Evidence-based protocol for diabetic foot ulcers. Plast Reconstr Surg 2006;117(Suppl):193S–209S.

Cavanagh PR, Lipsky BA, Bradbury AW, et al. Treatment of diabetic foot ulcers. Lancet 2005;366:1725–1735.

Christiansen J, Ek L, Tegner E. Pinch grafting of leg ulcers. A restrospective study of 412 treated ulcers in 146 patients. Acta Dermatol Venereol 1997;77:471–473.

Dinh TL, Veves A. The efficacy of Apligraf in the treatment of diabetic foot ulcers. Plast Reconstr Surg 2006;117(Suppl):152S–157S.

Ebright JR. Microbiology of chronic leg and pressure ulcers: clinical significance and implications for treatment. Nurs Clin North Am 2005;40:207–216.

Edmonds ME, Foster AV. Diabetic foot ulcers. Br Med J 2006;332:407–410.

Elias SM, Frasier KL. Minimally invasive vein surgery: its role in the treatment of venous stasis ulceration. Am J Surg 2004;188(Suppl):26–30.

Falabella AF. Debridement and wound bed preparation. Dermatol Ther 2006;19:317–325.

Falanga V, Margolis D, Alvarez O, et al. Rapid healing of venous ulcers and lack of clinical rejection with an allogeneic cultured human skin equivalent. Arch Dermatol 1998;134:293–300.

Fivenson D, Scherschun L. Clinical and economic impact of Apligraf for the treatment of nonhealing venous leg ulcers. Int J Dermatol 2003;42:960–965.

Frank C, Bayoumi I, Westendorp C. Approach to infected skin ulcers. Can Fam Physician 2005;51:1352–1359.

Gohel MS, Barwell JR, Earnshaw JJ, et al. Randomized clinical trial of compression plus surgery versus compression alone in chronic venous ulceration (ESCHAR study) – haemodynamic and anatomical changes. Br J Surg 2005;92:291–297.

Grey JE, Harding KG, Enoch S. Venous and arterial leg ulcers. Br Med J 2006;7537:347–350.

Hansson C. The effects of cadexomer iodine paste in the treatment of venous leg ulcers compared with hydrocolloid dressing and paraffin gauze dressing. Int J Dermatol 1998;37:390–396.

Hiatt WR. Pharmocologic therapy for peripheral arterial disease and claudication. J Vasc Surg 2002;36:1283–1291.

Jones JE, Nelson EA. Skin grafting for venous leg ulcers. Cochrane Database Syst Rev 2005;1: CD001737.

Jorgesen B, Price P, Andersen KE, et al. The silver-releasing foam dressing, Contreet Foam, promotes faster healing of critically colonized venous leg ulcers: a randomized, controlled trial. Int Wound J 2005;2:64–73.

Jull AB, Waters J, Arroll B. Oral pentoxifylline for treatment of venous leg ulcers. Cochrane Database Syst Rev 2002;1: CD001733.

Jull A, Waters J, Arroll B. Pentoxifylline for treatment of venous leg ulcers: a systematic review. Lancet 2002;359:1550–1554.

Lipsky BA, Berendt AR, Deery HG, et al. Diagnosis and treatment of diabetic foot infections. Plast Reconstr Surg 2006;117(Suppl):212S–238S.

Mackelfresh J, Soon S, Arbiser JL. Combination therapy of doxycycline and topical tacrolimus for venous ulcers. Arch Dermatol 2005;141:1476–1477.

Mani R, White JE. Pinch skin grafting or porcine dermis in venous ulcers: a randomized clinical trial. Br Med J 1987;294:674–676.

Margolis DJ, Berlin JA, Strom BL. Risk factors associated with the failure of a venous leg ulcer to heal. Arch Dermatol 1999;135:920–926.

Mekkes JR, Loots MA, Van Der Wal AC, et al. Causes, investigation and treatment of leg ulceration. Br J Dermatol 2003;148:388–401.

Miller OF, Phillips TJ. Leg ulcers. J Am Acad Dermatol 2000;43:91–95.

Munter KC, Beele H, Russell L, et al. Effect of a sustained silver-releasing dressing on ulcers with delayed healing: the CONTOP study. J Wound Care 2006;15:199–206.

Nelson EA, Bell-Syer SE, Cullum NA. Compression for preventing recurrence of venous ulcers. Cochrane Database Syst Rev 2000;4: CD002303.

Nelson EA, Iglesias CP, Cullum NA, et al. Randomized clinical trial of four-layer and short-stretch compression bandages for venous leg ulcers (VenUS I). Br J Surg 2004;91:1292–1299.

Nelson EA, Harper DR, Prescott RJ, et al. Prevention of recurrence of venous ulceration: randomized controlled trial of class 2 and class 3 elastic compression. J Vasc Surg 2006;44:803–808.

Obermayer A, Göstl K, Walli G, et al. Chronic venous leg ulcers benefit from surgery: long term results from 173 legs. J Vasc Surg 2006;44:572–579.

Oien RF, Håkansson A, Hansen BU, et al. Pinch grafting of chronic leg ulcers in primary care: fourteen years' experience. Acta Dermatol Venereol 2002;82:275–278.

Ovington L. Bacterial toxins and wound healing. Ostomy Wound Manage 2003;49(Suppl):8–12.

Palfreman SJ, Nelson EA, Lochiel R, et al. Dressing for healing venous leg ulcers. Cochrane Database Syst Rev 2006;3: CD001103.

Phillips TJ. Successful methods of treating leg ulcers: The tried and true, plus the novel and new. Postgrad Med 1999;105:159–180.

Phillips TJ. Current approaches to venous ulcers and compression. Dermatol Surg 2001;27:611–621.

Phillips TJ, Dover JS. Leg ulcers. J Am Acad Dermatol 1991;25:965–987.

Phillips TJ, Machado F, Trout R, et al. Prognostic indicators in venous ulcers. J Am Acad Dermatol 2000;43:627–630.

Ravaghi H, Flemming K, Cullum N, et al. Electromagnetic therapy for treating venous leg ulcers. Cochrane Database Syst Rev 2001;1: CD002933.

Sackheim K, De Araujo TS, Kirsner RS, et al. Compression modalities and dressings: their use in venous ulcers. Dermatol Ther 2006;19:338–347.

Sarker PK, Ballantyne S. Management of leg ulcers. Postgrad Med J 2000;76:74–682.

Schultz GS, Barillo DJ, Mozingo DW, et al. Wound bed preparation and a brief history of TIME. Int Wound J 2004;1:19–32.

Sibbald RG. An approach to leg and foot ulcers: a brief overview. Ost/Wound Manage 1998;44: 28–35.

Simon DA, Dix FP, McColloum CN. Management of venous leg ulcers. Br Med J 2004;328:1358–1362.

Singh N, Armstrong DG, Lipsky BA. Preventing foot ulcers in patients with diabetes. JAMA 2005;293:217–228.

Smith PC. Daflon 500 mg and venous leg ulcer: new results from a meta-analysis. Angiology 2005;56(Suppl 1):S33–S39.

Steed DL. Clinical evaluation of recombinant human platelet-derived growth factor for the treatment of lower extremity ulcers. Plast Reconstr Surg 2006;117(Suppl):143S–149S.

Tom WL, Peng DH, Allaei A, et al. The effect of short-contact tretinoin therapy for foot ulcers in patients with diabetes. Arch Dermatol 2005;141:1373–1377.

Valencia IC, Falabella A, Kirsner RS, et al. Chronic venous insufficiency and venous leg ulceration. J Am Acad Dermatol 2001;44:401–421.

Wang C, Schwaitzberg S, Berliner E, et al. Hyperbaric oxygen for treating wounds. Arch Surg 2003;138:272–279.

Wieman TJ. Principles of management: the diabetic foot. Am J Surg 2005;190:295–299.

Wu SC, Armstrong DG. The role of activity, adherence, and off-loading on the healing of diabetic foot wounds. Plast Reconstr Surg 2006;117(Suppl):248S–253S.

Zalli A. Foot ulceration due to arterial insufficiency: role of cilostazol. J Wound Care 2004;13:45–47.

Keloids

Oliver J. Wisco and Robert T. Gilson

Clinical presentation

Key Points

- Keloids result from excessive proliferation of fibrous tissue at the site of injury to the skin
- Keloids differ from hypertrophic scars in that, while hypertrophic scars remain confined to the site of original injury, keloids extend and grow beyond the original wound margin (Figure 22-1)

Hypertrophic scars tend to resolve spontaneously, whereas keloids progress. Keloids demonstrate thick "bubble gum" collagen bands histologically.

- Common locations include the neck, ears, extremities, and trunk
- Uncommon locations include the central face, palms, and soles
- Occur in all skin types, but have a higher risk in pigmented skin
- Affect males and females equally
- Occur less commonly in children and the elderly
- Highly resistant to treatment with a high recurrence rate

The most common location for a keloid to occur is the sternal region (Figure 22-2). Keloids typically arise from lacerations, surgical wounds, burns, and inflammatory lesions such as acne. They rarely arise spontaneously and are usually delayed (months) in their onset. Early lesions are erythematous, tender, and rubbery plaques whereas established lesions are smooth, glossy, and firm plaques. Lesions may be painful and/or pruritic. Rarely, they may ulcerate or develop sinus tracks. Lesions on the anterior chest and posterior scalp have a higher risk for developing draining sinus tracks.

Earlobe keloids (Figure 22-3) are unique in that they can present in four different ways (Table 22-1).

Acne keloidalis nuchae (AKN) is a scarring condition that occurs predominantly in African American males over the posterior scalp. Histologically, it demonstrates hypertrophic scars, but not true keloidal collagen (Box 22-1).

Diagnosis

Key Points

- Clinical appearance is usually distinctive enough for diagnosis
- Keloids that develop secondary characteristics such as ulceration or sinus tracks may be difficult to distinguish from neoplastic or infectious processes
- Biopsy lesions when suspicious of an alternate or secondary process; perform a 3 or 4-mm punch biopsy of a representative portion of the lesion or remove the entire lesion.
- Biopsy demonstrates thick "bubble gum" collagen within a fibrous nodule (Figure 22-4).
- Cryotherapy or intralesional steroid injection at the time of biopsy can help prevent recurrence
- If surrounding lesions have a different morphology, biopsy one of those representative lesions as well
- Consider fungal stains, fungal culture, and/or wound culture if an infectious process is suspected

PEARL

A Marjolin's ulcer is a malignant neoplasm (typically squamous cell carcinoma) that occurs in a scar

See the diagnostic algorithm set out in Figure 22-5

Laboratory testing

- No specific laboratory work-up is typically needed, except for a biopsy if the diagnosis is unclear

In comparison to normal scars, which have vertically oriented blood vessels with fibrillary collagen arranged parallel to the skin, keloids have thickened, eosinophilic, homogeneous large collagen bundles dispersed in a haphazard pattern in the mid-dermis. Keloids also have increased numbers of fibroblasts like scars, but the fibroblasts in keloids are plumper with prominent nuclei. Whorled, hypertrophic scar tissue may be found at the periphery of a keloid (Box 22-2).

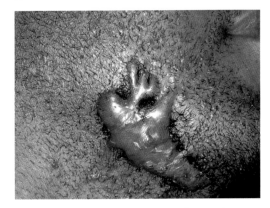

Figure 22-1 Keloid demonstrating claw-like margin

Table 22-1 Earlobe keloids

Type	Description
Button	Broad-based or pedunculated and occur on the anterior or posterior aspect of the earlobe
Dumbbell	A "stalk" through the lobule connects button keloids on the anterior and posterior aspects of the earlobe
Wraparound	A "wreath" or "U-shaped" keloid around the earlobe
Lobular	Occur in the setting where recurrent keloids have completely replaced the earlobe

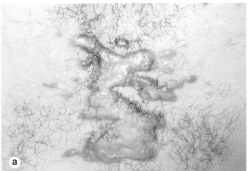

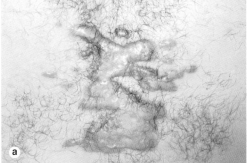

Figure 22-2 a, b Keloid

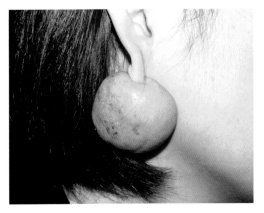

Figure 22-3 Keloid

BOX 22-1

Acne keloidalis nuchae

Partially relates to trauma to the follicles, commonly from short hair cuts causing the hair to curl back into the skin

Some develop only papules, whereas others develop pustules and progressive scarring alopecia similar to folliculitis decalvans

Initially presents as a chronic folliculitis/perifolliculitis

May have an overlap with pseudofolliculitis barbae

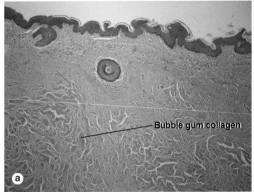

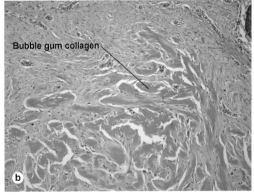

Figure 22-4 a, b Keloid

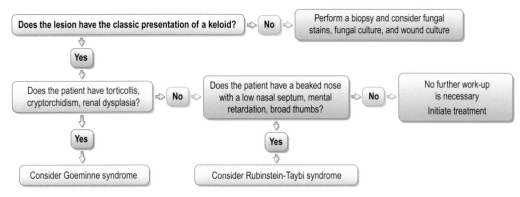

Figure 22-5 Diagnostic algorithm

Keloid: differential diagnoses

Hypertrophic scar

Pink-purple firm plaques that fade back to normal skin color in long-standing lesions

Plaques can be tender and are confined to site of original trauma

Immediate onset after initiating trauma

Treated similarly to keloids

Dermatofibrosarcoma protuberans (DFSP)

Multiple slowly growing painful red-purple nodules

50–60% occur on the trunk, rarely on the proximal extremities and head and neck

Bednar tumors are pigmented DFSPs

Low likelihood of metastasis

Treat with excision with wide margins; Mohs micrographic surgery is recommended

Hypertrophic lichen planus

Reddish-brown to violaceous, hypertrophic, verrucous plaques

Initially evolve from characteristic lichen planus lesions (purple, planar, pruritic, polygonal papules or plaques)

May result from frequent scratching or recurrent trauma to the original lichen planus lesions

Treat with high-potency topical steroids

Prurigo nodules and lichen simplex chronicus

Habitual rubbing or scratching of the skin causes the lesions

Highly pruritic, slightly erythematous, scaly, well-demarcated, firm plaques or nodules with exaggerated skin lines (lichenification)

Classically presents with underlying atopic dermatitis or a history of arthropod bites initiating the chronic lesions

Treat with high-potency topical steroids

Epidermal maturation arrest

Glossy pink exudative plaque of excessive granulation tissue at the site of a wound healing by secondary intention

Occurs 3–4 weeks postoperatively

Theorized to be due to abnormal epidermal migration and/or proliferation

Treat with silver nitrate sticks or topical high-potency steroids

Pathogenesis

Key Points

- The pathogenesis of keloid formation is unknown, but seems to be linked to an increased inflammatory response causing excessive fibrogenesis
- Upregulation of numerous cytokines has been implicated; the most commonly found to be associated is transforming growth factor-beta (TGF-beta) (Figure 22-6)

In the formation of keloids, the sequence of normal scar formation is altered through an unknown mechanism causing excessive fibrogenesis with increased collagen and glycosaminoglycan content. Factors that increase inflammation, such as infection, excessive wound tension, and presence of foreign material, may contribute. TGF-beta is the cytokine most commonly associated with keloids, as it is upregulated in keloid fibroblasts. Many extracellular matrix components are also stimulated by TGF-beta. There are also numerous other inflammatory factors/components implicated; some that have been more closely studied include the upregulation of matrix metalloproteinase (MMP)-1 (interstitial collagenase), MMP-2 (gelatinase-A), tissue inhibitor of metalloproteinase (TIMP)-1, vascular endothelial growth factor (VEGF), connective tissue growth factor (CTGF), urokinase-mediated plasminogen activation (uPA) system, angiotensin-converting enzyme (ACE), and Gli-1.

The role of melanocytes is unclear in keloid formation, but they are felt to be associated, as keloid risk is increased in darker-skinned individuals while there is virtually no risk in albinos. In addition, there may be an autosomal dominant inheritance pattern with incomplete penetrance and variable expression in familial cases.

Treatment

Key Points

- Focus should be on prevention and patient education
- Intralesional corticosteroids at 10–40 mg/ml are the mainstay of treatment
- The use of multiple modalities is typically necessary when treating keloids
- Excisional surgery often has high recurrence rates that can be prevented if using combination therapy

Treating keloids can be very frustrating as there are numerous approaches with no definitive treatment protocol and all options have a relatively high therapeutic failure rate. The most common first approach is the use of intralesional corticosteroids. Other common treatment options include occlusive dressings, compression therapy, cryosurgery, intralesional interferon, excision, radiation, laser therapy, and topical imiquimod. The use of multiple modalities may be necessary when keloids fail to respond to initial treatment with intralesional triamcinolone.

The benefit of excisional surgery is highly variable, with recurrence rates ranging from 50 to 100%. It is primarily used when nonsurgical methods have failed. However, earlobe keloids seem to have a lower recurrence rate following surgical excision than do other forms of keloids: only 41% recur following surgery alone. This recurrence rate can be further reduced by the adjunctive use of intralesional steroids, cryotherapy, or radiation.

Basics of surgical excision of the keloid

- Used when nonsurgical measures have failed
- Better results with pedunculated lesions
- Sessile/broad-based keloids are more difficult to excise

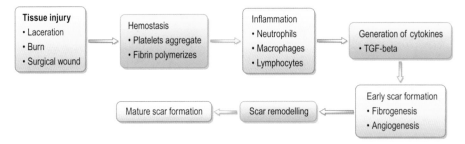

Figure 22-6 Sequence of normal scar formation. TGF-beta, transforming growth factor-beta

- Excise with narrow margins and close with the least amount of tension as possible
- Avoid buried sutures when possible
- Grafting has lower recurrence rates than does primary closure, but there is a risk for donor-site keloids
- Tissue expanders are a preferred method over grafting, as the pressure from the expanders may help prevent excess collagen deposition
- Superficial lesions allowed to heal by second intention may have an improved cosmetic appearance and lower recurrence rates, as there is less tension on the wound than with primary closure

- Multiple modalities, particularly intralesional triamcinolone, should be used following surgery to help prevent recurrence (Table 22-2)

PEARL

Following excision, apply pressure earrings daily for 6–18 months and use other treatment modalities to assist in prevention of recurrence

Treatment modalities

See Table 22-3.

Controversies

Key Points

- Studies on the treatment of keloids show variable results
- Beyond the use of intralesional triamcinolone, data are mixed

The studies published on the treatment of keloid are not definitive in their outcomes. There are numerous articles showing highly variable results as the ability to perform randomized double-blinded controlled studies for the treatment of this entity is difficult. It is not uncommon to see studies demonstrating recurrence rates, with wide ranges such as 50–100% for postsurgical recurrences. While the use of intralesional corticosteroids is considered the first step in treating keloids, beyond that, there is no proven significant advantage of the other modalities. The other modalities are viable options when considering alternate therapies for resistant lesions, but more importantly, their use is most beneficial in the multimodality approach.

Table 22-2 Surgical excision of earlobe keloids

Type	Procedure
Anterior and posterior button	Shave excision followed by second intention healing
Dumbbell	Shave the anterior and posterior aspects, then remove the core using a punch biopsy 1 mm larger than the core
	Close the anterior surface horizontally and the posterior surface vertically
Wraparound and lobular	Use a wedge excision if a remaining functional/cosmetically appropriate lobule can be achieved
	If unable to remove the entire keloids, sculpt the keloids, removing as much as possible, and then use the other treatment modalities to minimize recurrence

Table 22-3 First-line therapies

Modality	Dosage/Application/Notes	Mechanism of action	Adverse drug reactions and cautions
Intralesional (IL) corticosteroids	Use for sessile, flat, or broad keloids; not useful for pedunculated lesions	May increase collagenase and reduce collagenase inhibiting alpha-globulins	Atrophy Hypopigmentation
	Useful as a primary treatment or as a preventive measure after excision		
	Inject triamcinolone 10–40 mg/ml IL with a 30-gauge needle every 2–6 weeks		
	Postoperatively, inject 40 mg/ml into the wound margin the day of surgery and then at 2, 4, 6 weeks; then inject 10-40 mg/ml monthly into lesion or margins as needed		
Topical corticosteroids	Used alone or as an adjunct to other therapies to help soften the lesion between treatments	See above (Intralesional (IL) corticosteroids)	See above
	Apply a class 1 topical steroid bid		

Continued

Table 22-3 First-line therapies—cont'd

Modality	Dosage/Application/Notes	Mechanism of action	Adverse drug reactions and cautions
Occlusive dressing	May be more useful when applied after excision Apply occlusive (with or without silicone) dressing 24 hours/day for 2 months	May decrease epidermal water loss Silicone may cause alterations in static electricity Silicone may reduce keloidal ground substance	Contact irritation
Compression	Used primarily as a preventive measure after excision Apply a compression dressing with > 24 mmHg 24 hours/day for 4–6 months Compression earrings are specifically made for post-earlobe keloid excisions	Pressure may cause hypoxia which results in collagen degradation through fibroblast degeneration	Pressure necrosis Pain
Intralesional interferon-alpha-2b	Useful as a primary treatment or as a preventive measure after excision Sutured wounds: inject 1 million units per linear centimeter into the wound base and margins Injections are to be performed the day of surgery and then 1 week later Second intention wounds: inject 1 million units per square centimeter Limit total dose to 5 million units	Thought to normalize collagen, gylcosaminoglycans, and collagenase production May upregulate native p53 to promote natural cell death of dysfunctional fibroblasts	Flu-like symptoms
Other therapies			
Imiquimod	Useful primarily as a preventive measure after excision Apply bid starting the day of surgery for 8 weeks	See above (under Intralesional interferon-alfa-2b)	Contact irritation
Intralesional 5-fluorouracil	Inject 0.2 to 0.4 ml/cm^2 of 50 mg/ml once a week Limit dose to less than 100 mg May have added benefit when used with IL triamcinolone and/or PDL	Inhibition of fibroblast proliferation	Atrophy
Intralesional bleomycin	Apply 0.1 ml of 1.5 IU/ml to the surface of the keloid with a 25 gauge needle repeatedly spaced 0.5 mm apart on the surface of the keloid to allow penetration of the medication; repeat monthly as needed	May induce apoptosis May decrease collagen synthesis through decreasing lysyl-oxidase, which is required in collagen maturation	Pain Hyperpigmentation
Intralesional verapamil	Inject 2.5 mg/ml with doses ranging from 0.5 to 2.0 ml (depending on the size) on postoperative days 7, 14, 28, and during the second month	Increases procollagenase synthesis resulting in net fibroblast extracellular matrix degradation	Pain Atrophy
Cryosurgery	Useful primarily as an adjunct to other therapies, particularly intralesional techniques, as it can soften the tissue to facilitate the injections Apply for 10–30 seconds and use two freeze–thaw cycles Typically requires more than three treatments Not recommended in patients with darker skin	Direct cell damage and vascular damage causing anoxia and further cell death	Pain and edema Milia formation Infection Hypoesthesia Delayed healing Hypopigmenation

Table 22-3 First-line therapies—cont'd

Modality	Dosage/Application/Notes	Mechanism of action	Adverse drug reactions and cautions
Radiation	Used as a preventive measure after excision only in adults, not used as a primary/solo therapy Do not use in children due to risk of stunting bone growth Use limited due to increased risk for cutaneous or soft-tissue malignancies Similar cure rates for X-radiation, electron beam, and interstitial radiation Consult radiation oncologist for postoperative application	May decrease fibroblast collagen synthesis May decrease vascular hyperplasia	Dyschromias Alopecia Telangiectasias Atrophy
Laser	CO_2 laser: useful in the focused mode ND:YAG: more useful in early lesions PDL: useful in early lesions, but no benefit in mature lesions	CO_2 laser: tissue ablation ND:YAG: inhibition of collagen production PDL: decreases microvasculature and downregulates transforming growth factor-beta 1 expression	Pain Atrophy Dyspigmentation
Surgery	See discussion above		

bid, twice a day; PDL, pulsed-dye laser; CO_2, carbon dioxide; Nd:YAG, neodymium: yttrium aluminum garnet.

Further reading

Baldwin H. Keloid management. In: Robinson JK, Hanke CW, Sengelmann RD, et al., eds. Surgery of the Skin, Procedural Dermatology. Philadelphia (PA): Mosby, 2005:705–716.

Berman B, Zell D, Romagosa R. Keloid scarring. In: Lebwohl MG, Heymann WR, Berth-Jones J, et al., eds. Treatment of Skin Disease. China: Mosby, 2006:314–317.

Burd A, Huang L. Hypertrophic response and keloids diathesis: two very different forms of scar. Plast Reconstr Surg 2005;116:150e–157e.

Burton CS. Dermal hypertrophies. In: Bolognia JL, Jorizzo JL, Rapini RP, eds. Dermatology. Edinburgh: Mosby, 2003:1531–1537.

Fujiwara M, Muragaki Y, Ooshima A. Keloid-derived fibroblasts show increased secretion of factors involved in collagen turnover and depend on matrix metalloproteinase for migration. Br J Dermatol 2006;153:295–300.

Gira AK, Brown LF, Washington CV, et al. Keloids demonstrate high level epidermal expression of vascular endothelial growth factor. J Am Acad Dermatol 2004;50:850–853.

Khoo YT, Ong CT, Mukhopadhyay A, et al. Up-regulation of secretory connective tissue growth factor (CTGF) in keratinocyte–fibroblast coculture contributes to keloids pathogenesis. J Cell Phys 2006;208:336–343.

Kim A, DiCarlo J, Cohen C, et al. Are keloids really "gli-oids"? High-level expressiojn of gli-1 oncogene in keloids. J Am Acad Dermatol 2001;45:707–711.

Kuo YR, Jeng SF, Wang FS, et al. Flashlamp pulsed dye laser (PDL) suppression of keloids proliferation through down-regulation of TGF-beta1 expression and extracellular matrix expression. Lasers Surg Med 2004;34:104–108.

Leake D, Doerr TD, Scott G. Expression of urokinase-type plasminogen activator and its receptor in keloids. Arch Otolaryngol 2003;129:1334–1338.

Palamaras I, Kyriakis K. Calcium antagonists in dermatology: A review of the evidence and research-based studies. Dermatol Online J 2005;11:8.

Saray Y, Gulec AT. Treatment of keloids and hypertrophic scars with dermojet injections of bleomycin: a preliminary study. Int J Dermatol 2005;44:777–784.

Shaffer JJ, Taylor SC, Cook-Bolder F. Keloidal scars: A review with a critical look at therapeutic options. J Am Acad Dermatol 2002;46:S63–S97.

Adverse drug reactions in the skin

David R. Adams

Overview

Key Points

- Differential diagnosis of many cutaneous eruptions includes drug reactions
- Most cutaneous drug eruptions are diagnosed by their clinical features, including morphology and timing
- Most drug reactions are inflammatory, generalized, and symmetrical
- Histology can be helpful, but is not usually diagnostic
- Rechallenge with the offending medication may confirm the diagnosis but is not usually practical and may be unsafe
- Reactions may be allergic or nonallergic in etiology
- There are four types of allergic reactions:
  - Type I: immediate hypersensitivity (immunoglobulin (Ig) E-mediated) – urticaria, angioedema, and anaphylaxis
  - Type II: cytotoxic reactions – drug-induced thrombocytopenia
  - Type III: circulating immune complexes – leukocytoclastic vasculitis (LCV), serum sickness
  - Type IV: delayed hypersensitivity – drug exanthems, allergic contact dermatitis (ACD)
- Patient populations at high risk for drug reactions include those with/on:
  - Human immunodeficiency virus (HIV) infection
  - Other viral infections (mononucleosis)
  - Chemotherapy patients
  - Multiple drug regimens
  - Allergic history
  - Genetic variations in drug metabolism
- Complete drug history should inquire about prescription, nonprescription, herbal, and holistic treatments
- Reporting, publishing, and documenting of drug reactions is an inexact science as many single case reports are "best-guess" scenarios and should be reviewed critically
- Drug lists in this chapter represent the more commonly reported agents. A more complete list is available in the annually updated Drug Eruption Reference Manual by Litt, Jerome Z.

Adverse drug reactions are common and account for many outpatient visits and inpatient consultations in dermatology. In addition to morbilliform

(Figure 23-1) and urticarial rashes (Figure 23-2), drugs may induce immunobullous disease and a host of other dermatologic conditions. The prudent physician always considers the possibility that a drug may be causing or exacerbating a skin eruption. Many ingestants, including herbal preparations may cause adverse reactions. Patients may not think of these agents as drugs and may fail to mention them when questioned. Patients may not associate an "all-natural" product with potential for harm.

When approaching a patient with a possible drug rash, it is essential to establish a careful medication timeline. Morbilliform drug eruptions typically occur about 7–10 days after initiation of a new medication. Onset of drug hypersensitivity syndrome with eosinophilia and systemic symptoms (DRESS) is usually within the first 6 weeks of therapy. Drug-induced lichenoid eruption, pemphigus, and angiotensin inhibitor-induced angioedema may occur 1 month or longer after beginning the drug.

Certain classes of medication have a higher incidence of drug eruptions (Box 23-1). These include beta-lactam antibiotics in the setting of morbilliform eruptions and drugs such as tetracyclines in the setting of phototoxic reactions (Figure 23-3). Some drugs, such as penicillamine, unmask latent lupus erythematosus in much the same way that corticosteroids unmask latent diabetes. In such cases, the eruption may not resolve when the drug is discontinued.

Because the topic of drug eruptions is quite extensive, this chapter will be presented mainly as charts, tables, and key points bullets. Entities will be presented in alphabetical order to make them easy to locate.

Evaluation of timing of administration

- New exposures require 1–2 weeks to become sensitized for typical morbilliform drug exanthem
- Re-exposures usually reproduce the exanthem within 1–2 days

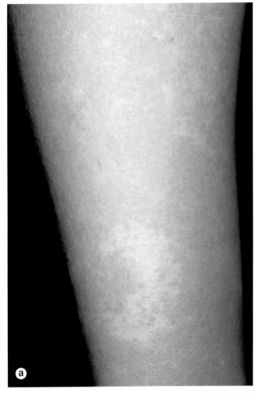

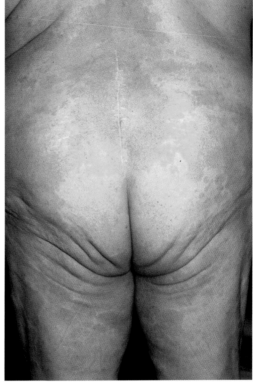

Figure 23-2 Urticarial drug eruption

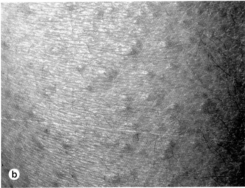

Figure 23-1 a Morbilliform drug eruption. b Phenytoin
hypersensitivity (drug reaction with eosinophilia and
systemic symptoms (DRESS) syndrome) demonstrates
follicular prominence.

- Drug reaction with eosinophilia and systemic
  symptoms (DRESS) syndrome usually occurs
  within the first 6 weeks of therapy

Management of adverse drug reactions

- The offending drug must be discontinued;
  most morbilliform reactions will resolve within
  2 weeks
- Treat symptomatically as needed (topical
  antipruritic agents, sedating antihistamines for
  itching and sleep)

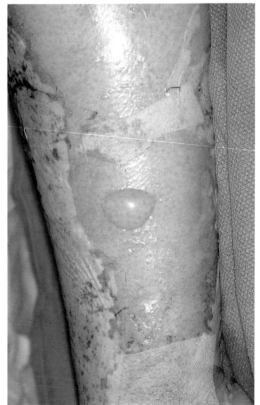

Figure 23-3 Phototoxic reaction

BOX 23-1

List of adverse drug reactions

Acanthosis nigricans (AN)	Linear immunoglobulin A disease
Acne	Livedo reticularis
Acral erythema	Lupus-like reaction
Acute generalized exanthematous pustulosis (AGEP)	Nail pigmentation
Allergic contact dermatitis (ACD)	Nephrogenic systemic fibrosis (NSF)
Alopecia	Neutrophilic eccrine hidradenitis
Anaphylaxis	Patch medication dermatitis
Angioedema	Pellagra
Black hairy tongue	Pemphigus
Black tongue	Photoallergic reaction
Bullous pemphigoid (BP)	Photo-onycholysis
Chemotherapy-associated cutaneous reactions	Phototoxic reaction
Drug exanthem	Pigmentation
Drug reaction with eosinophilia and systemic symptoms (DRESS)	Pityriasis rosea-like reaction
Epidermal growth factor receptor inhibitor (EGFR) folliculitis and paronychia	Pseudoepitheliomatous hyperplasia with pustules (halogenoderma)
	Pseudolymphoma
Erythema annulare centrifugum (EAC)	Pseudoporphyria
Erythema multiforme (EM)	Psoriasiform eruption
Erythema nodosum (EN)	Raynaud's phenomenon
Exfoliative erythroderma	Retinoid dermatitis
Fixed drug eruption (FDE)	Serum sickness-like reaction
Flagellate pigmentation	Subacute cutaneous lupus erythematosus (SCLE)
Fluorouracil dermatitis (5-fluorouracil; 5-FU)	Sweet's-like reaction
Gingival hyperplasia	Toxic epidermal necrolysis (TEN)/Stevens–Johnson syndrome (SJS)
Hair color change	
Heparin necrosis	Trichomegaly (long eyelashes)
Hypersensitivity vasculitis (leukocytoclastic vasculitis; LCV)	Ultraviolet recall
Hypertrichosis	Urticaria
Ichthyosis, acquired	Warfarin necrosis
Leukoderma	Xerotic dermatitis
Lichenoid drug	

- Antihistamines for urticaria, prednisone for severe urticaria
- Prednisone for severe AGEP and DRESS
- Specific treatment for select reactions (example: intravenous immunoglobulin (IVIg) for toxic epidermal necrolysis (TEN))

Acanthosis nigricans (AN)

Key Points

- AN types include hereditary benign, benign, pseudoacanthosis nigricans, malignant and drug-associated

- Drug-associated AN is uncommon (Box 23-2)
- Clinical: velvety, hyperpigmented plaques in flexural areas (neck, axillae, groin); skin tags may overlie these areas
- Histology: mamillated, acanthotic epidermis with basket-weave keratin; hyperpigmentation of basal layer, minimal inflammation

Acne/acneiform eruptions (Box 23-3)

Key Points

- Clinical: rapid onset of monomorphic follicular papules and pustules (comedones are absent in steroid acne) on face and upper torso (Figure 23-4)

Drugs associated with acanthosis nigricans

Nicotinic acid

Glucocorticoids

Insulin

Diethylstilbesterol

Oral contraceptives

Androgens

Growth hormone

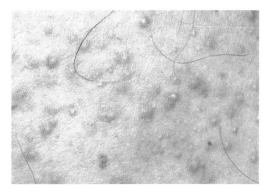

Figure 23-4 Steroid acne

Drugs associated with acne/acneiform eruptions

Corticosteroids

Adrenocorticotropic hormone

Androgens

Progesterone

Iodides

Bromides

Lithium

Cyclosporine

Anticonvulsants

Antituberculosis agents

Vitamins B_2, B_6, and B_{12}

* Standard acne treatments may speed resolution
* Histology: follicular plugging, comedones, perifollicular inflammation

Acral erythema (Acral erythrodysesthesia)

Key Points

* Clinical: erythema, pain and dysesthesia with edema of the hands and, sometimes, feet (Figure 23-5) over several days during course of chemotherapy (Box 23-4)
* Resolves with desquamation approximately 1 week after chemotherapy is discontinued
* Histology: epithelial disorder, vacuolar interface change, necrosis, and inflammation of eccrine glands

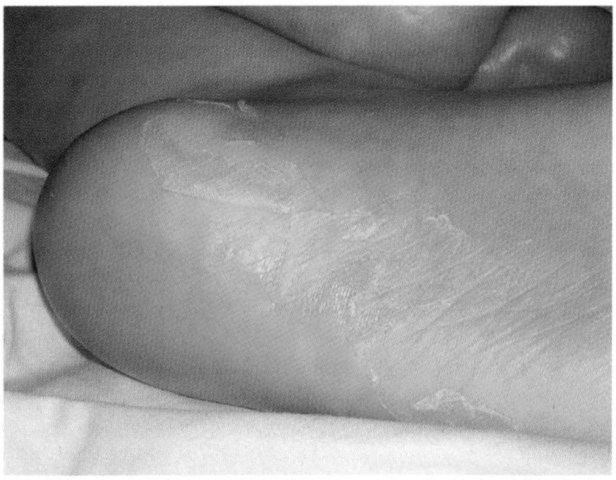

Acute generalized exanthematous pustulosis (AGEP)

Key Points

* Clinical: erythematous plaques studded with pustules, often begins on face or intertriginous areas then generalizing (Figure 23-6)

Figure 23-5 Acral erythema (Acral erythrodysesthesia)

Drugs commonly associated with acral erythema (although others can cause this reaction)

Cytarabine (ARA-C)

Doxorubicin

Fluorouracil (5-fluorouracil)

* May have associated fever and high white blood cell count and may be misdiagnosed as infection
* Occurs early into therapy, usually within 1–2 days (Box 23-5)
* Lasts 1–2 weeks
* If severe, consider use of oral or intravenous corticosteroids
* Histology: subcorneal pustules, epidermal spongiosis, and perivascular mixed inflammation, including neutrophils and eosinophils

Allergic contact dermatitis

Key Points

* Clinical: erythema, vesicles, bullae, sometimes in linear arrays; superficial scaling; pruritus
* May be from topical application of prescription or nonprescription medications (Box 23-6)
* Type IV delayed-type hypersensitivity reaction

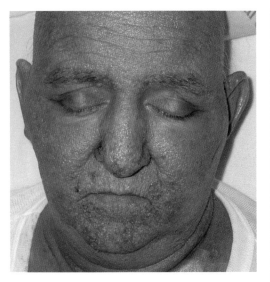

Figure 23-6 Acute generalized exanthematous pustulosis

Drugs associated with acute generalized exanthematous pustulosis

Beta-lactam antibiotics

Macrolide antibiotics

Vancomycin

Drugs (topical) associated with allergic contact dermatitis

Neomycin

Bacitracin

Diphenhydramine

Corticosteroids (either to inert compounding ingredients or to the steroids themselves)

Doxepin

Numerous others

- ACD can be due to medication or vehicle additives (preservatives, fragrances)
- Specific allergen can be confirmed by patch testing
- Histology: parakeratosis and spongiosis (often acute) of the epidermis with a dermal infiltrate that generally includes eosinophils

Alopecia (Box 23-7)

Key Points

- Clinical: usually diffuse hair thinning of scalp (Figure 23-7), rarely other sites involved
- Scalp skin is usually normal
- Females affected more frequently than males

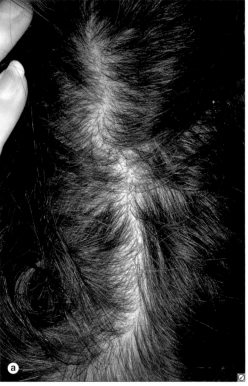

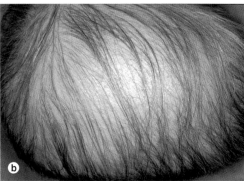

Figure 23-7 a Anagen arrest. b Telogen effluvium. Hair loss secondary to aromatic retinoid

- Anagen arrest from chemotherapy occurs in 2 weeks (Figure 23-7a). Hairs demonstrate tapered fractures
- Telogen effluvium (Figure 23-7b) usually follows the precipitating insult in 3–5 months. Hairs demonstrate nonpigmented club-shaped bulbs
- Hair that regrows can be less pigmented and more curly
- Histology: in telogen effluvium, there is an increased number of telogen hairs, often greater than 20%

Anaphylaxis (Box 23-8)

Key Points

- Clinical: combinations of urticaria, angioedema, bronchospasm, laryngeal or glottic edema, hypotension, and death

BOX 23-7

Drugs associated with alopecia

Chemotherapy (anagen effluvium)

Hormones

Anticoagulants

Anticonvulsants

Amantadine

Amiodarone

Angiotensin-converting enzyme inhibitors

Lipid-lowering agents

Colchicine

Retinoids

Lithium

BOX 23-8

Drugs associated with anaphylaxis

Antibiotics

Angiotensin-converting enzyme inhibitors

Insulin

Blood products

Aspirin

Radiocontrast media

Monoclonal antibodies

BOX 23-9

Drugs associated with angioedema

Antibiotics

Angiotensin-converting enzyme inhibitors (distinct mechanism involving kallikrein–kinin system)

Insulin

Blood products

Aspirin

Radiocontrast media

Opiates (direct histamine release)

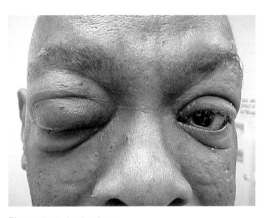

Figure 23-8 Angioedema

- Anaphylaxis is rare, but the most immediate and life-threatening adverse drug reaction
- Immediate recognition and treatment are critical
- Requires sensitization and can occur within minutes of rechallenge
- IgE-mediated immune reaction
- Cascade of enzymatic reactions causing mediator release by mast cells, basophils, and other cells causing dilation and increased permeability of vessels and smooth-muscle contraction
- Histology: sparse to moderate perivascular inflammatory infiltrate of mostly lymphocytes; eosinophils/neutrophils and dermal edema may be present
- Initial treatment is with intramuscular epinephrine, supportive therapy, and transport to an acute care facility

Angioedema (Box 23-9)

Key Points

- Clinical: deep variant of urticaria in which the subcutaneous tissue/mucous membranes are involved (Figure 23-8)

- May be a precursor to anaphylaxis
- Requires sensitization and can occur within minutes of rechallenge
- Most cases are IgE-mediated
- Histology: sparse to moderate perivascular inflammatory infiltrate of mostly lymphocytes; eosinophils/neutrophils and dermal edema may be present

Black tongue (Box 23-10)

Key Points

- Clinical: pigmentation of the lingual papillae (Figure 23-9)
- Direct staining from ingested medications

Black hairy tongue (Box 23-11)

Key Points

- Clinical: black, brown, or yellow pigmentation and hyperplasia of the filiform papillae of the tongue (Figure 23-10)
- Caused by overgrowth of pigment-producing bacteria
- Histology: elongation of filiform papillae with many bacterial colonies between papillae

BOX 23-10

Drugs associated with black tongue

Bismuth

Antibiotics

Monoamine oxidase inhibitors

Tricyclic antidepressants

Griseofulvin

BOX 23-11

Drugs associated with black hairy tongue

Antibiotics

Tobacco

Monoamine oxidase inhibitors

Tricyclic antidepressants

Corticosteroids

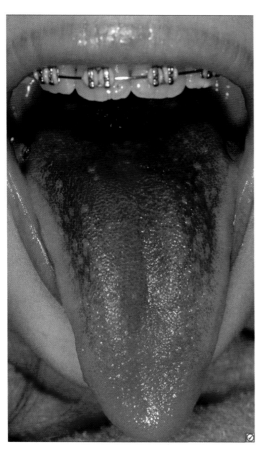

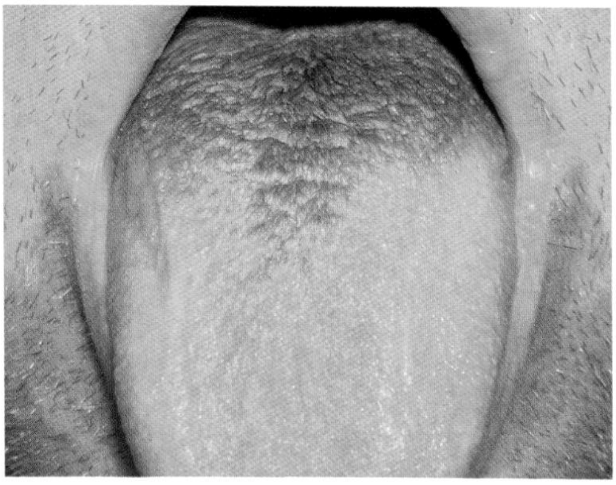

Figure 23-10 Black hairy tongue

BOX 23-12

Drugs associated with bullous pemphigoid

Furosemide

Angiotensin-converting enzyme inhibitors

Sulfasalazine

Penicillin

Penicillamine

Nalidixic acid

Figure 23-9 Black tongue

Bullous pemphigoid (BP)

Key Points

- Clinical: tense blisters on erythematous or normal skin affecting trunk/extremities; urticarial lesions may be present and may precede onset of bullae
- Direct immunofluorescence patterns similar to nondrug-related (idiopathic) BP
- Indirect immunofluorescence may show antibody to 230 kDa BP1 antigen
- Rare drug-associated condition (Box 23-12)
- Histology: subepidermal clefting with eosinophils at base

Chemotherapy-associated cutaneous reactions

Key Points

- Chemotherapy drugs commonly cause skin reactions
- Several unusual or unique reactions are seen only with chemotherapy
- General chemotherapy reactions often involve rapidly growing tissue in a nonspecific manner, affecting skin, mucosa, hair, and nails
- See individual reactions listed, including: acral erythema, neutrophilic eccrine hidradenitis, "flag sign" hair banding, flagellate hyperpigmentation, and epidermal growth factor receptor (EGFR) inhibitor folliculitis and paronychia

Drug exanthem

Key Points

- Clinical: erythematous macules and papules in a confluent measles-like pattern that begins on torso or head and neck and migrates peripherally
- Pruritus, low-grade fever, lymphadenopathy, and eosinophilia may be present
- Resolves without sequelae over 1–2 weeks
- Most common drug reaction involving the skin
- Requires initial exposure for sensitization
- Can occur with first exposure often 8–10 days into treatment
- Exanthem recurs within 24 hours after subsequent exposure
- Often worsens over several days, even if medication has been discontinued
- Treat symptomatically if pruritic
- Antibiotics are by far the drugs most commonly associated with exanthem, especially beta-lactam antibiotics and sulfa drugs (Box 23-13). Beta-lactam reactions are more common. Sulfa reactions tend to be more severe
- Histology: perivascular lymphocytes and variable presence of eosinophils

Drug reaction with eosinophilia and systemic symptoms

Key Points

- Clinical: skin findings often resemble a nonspecific drug exanthem; may progress to generalized erythroderma; follicular prominence and facial edema are common
- Patients may also have fever, adenopathy, leukocytosis, eosinophilia, atypical lymphocytes, and multiorgan involvement, particularly hepatitis and thyroiditis
- Treat with oral or parenteral corticosteroids
- Timing can be days to years after drug administration, but usually occurs in 2–6 weeks
- Increased incidence in African American population
- Often undiagnosed for months because of the unusual timing of rash in relation to drug administration, lack of resolution with discontinuation of suspected drug (Box 23-14), and unsuspected cross-reaction with other medications (with aromatic antiseizure medications phenytoin, barbiturates, and carbamazepine most commonly)
- Should be included in the differential diagnosis of fever with a rash
- Increased mortality if unrecognized
- Treat with corticosteroids, often for months. Symptoms and signs recur if discontinued too early
- For patients in whom the suspected medication is an aromatic anticonvulsant, drugs that may cross-react include carboxamides (carbamazepine and oxcarbazepine), barbiturates (phenobarbital and primidone), phenytoin, lamotrigine, valproate and tricyclics
- Can present with clinical hypothyroidism several months after resolution of symptoms
- Histology: most commonly perivascular lymphocytes and eosinophils (for patients presenting with an exanthem)

BOX 23-13

Drugs associated with exanthem

Beta-lactam antibiotics

Sulfonamides

Erythromycin

Gentamicin

Anticonvulsants

Gold salts

Many others

BOX 23-14

Drugs associated with drug reaction with eosinophilia and systemic symptoms

Anticonvulsants

Allopurinol

Dapsone

Nonsteroidal anti-inflammatory drugs

Sulfonamides

Tricyclics

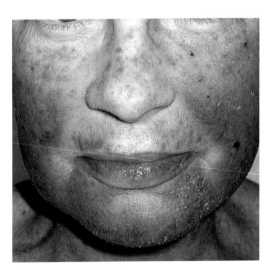

Figure 23-11 Epidermal growth factor receptor folliculitis

Epidermal growth factor receptor inhibitor folliculitis and paronychia

Key Points

- Clinical: acneiform eruption of face (Figure 23-11) and upper torso occurring early into therapy
- Generalized pruritus can occur
- Paronychia involving many nails (Figure 23-12) can occur several months into therapy

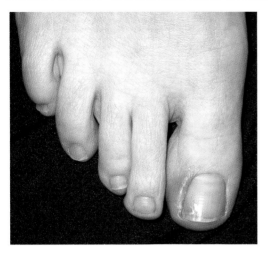

Figure 23-12 Epidermal growth factor receptor paronychia

BOX 23-15

Drugs associated with epidermal growth factor receptor inhibitor folliculitis

Erlotinib

Gefitinib

Cetuximab

Trastuzumab

- Occurs with several injectable or oral agents given chronically for nonsmall cell lung cancer, colorectal cancer, or breast cancer (Box 23-15)
- Eruption predictive of chemoresponsive tumor and is associated with improved outcome
- Treatment similar to acne, but may need to avoid drying agents (retinoids or benzoyl peroxide)
- Histology: folliculitis and perifolliculitis

Erythema annulare centrifugum (EAC)

Key Points

- Clinical: annular erythema with trailing scale
- Rare drug-associated reaction (Box 23-16)
- Histology: tight perivascular cuffing of lymphocytes

Erythema multiforme (EM)

Key Points

- Clinical: variable, with macular, papular, urticarial, targetoid lesions; sometimes vesicles, bullae, or purpura
- Rapidly progresses over 7–10 days, then resolves over 2 weeks
- Rarely a drug-associated finding (up to 10%: Box 23-17); most cases are associated with herpes simplex infection rather than drug

BOX 23-16

Drugs associated with erythema annulare centrifugum

Penicillamine

Penicillin

Cimetidine

Salicylates

Thiazides

Antimalarials

Hormones

BOX 23-17

Drugs associated with erythema multiforme

Allopurinol

Antibiotics

Anticonvulsants

Hormones

Nonsteroidal anti-inflammatory drugs

Penicillamine

- Histology: interface dermatitis with vacuolar change of the dermoepidermal junction, necrotic cells in the epidermis, basket-weave stratum corneum; perivascular to sometimes lichenoid inflammatory infiltrate of lymphocytes
- Drug induced EM presents with atypical targets or features that overlap with TEN

Erythema nodosum (EN: Box 23-18)

Key Points

- Clinical: tender red subcutaneous nodules usually over the anterior lower leg
- More common in young females
- Cannot clinically distinguish from nondrug EN
- Histology: septal panniculitis with fibrosis and variable infiltrate of neutrophils and eosinophils (more often in early lesions) and giant cells (more often in later lesions)

Exfoliative erythroderma (Box 23-19)

Key Points

- Clinical: generalized redness and scaling (Figure 23-14) without involvement of palms and soles
- No bullae like that seen in Stevens–Johnson syndrome (SJS)/TEN (more like erythrodermic psoriasis)
- Patient may be febrile with malaise, chills, and lymphadenopathy

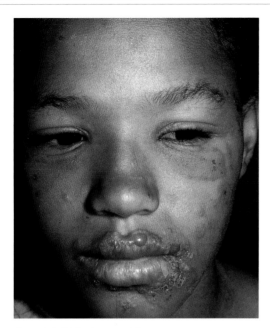

Figure 23-13 Erythema multiforme

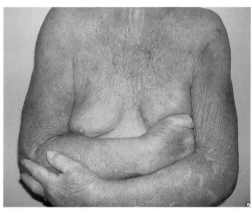

Figure 23-14 Erythroderma

- High-output cardiac failure may occur in compromised patients
- Histology: may be similar to cutaneous T-cell lymphoma

Fixed drug eruption (FDE)

Key Points

- Clinical: one or more tender red plaques that may blister (Figure 23-15) and resolve with postinflammatory hyperpigmentation (Figure 23-16)
- Half occur on genital or oral mucosa
- Onset occurs rapidly within 1–8 hours of drug ingestion
- Recurs in same location with re-exposure
- Less common in United States since phenolphthalein is no longer available as laxative
- Pseudoephedrine can cause a nonpigmenting FDE
- Baboon syndrome is a variant of FDE involving buttocks, groin, and axilla
- If offending agent is not discontinued, the FDE intensifies and may generalize

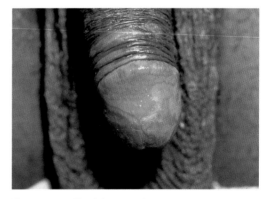

Figure 23-15 Fixed drug eruption

- Some drugs are more likely to affect genitalia (tetracycline, ampicillin) and others face, limbs, or trunk (aspirin: Box 23-20)
- Histology: interface dermatitis with perivascular to lichenoid mixed inflammatory infiltrate that often includes eosinophils and pigment incontinence; sometimes a deeper perivascular infiltrate is present as well. Acute stratum corneum paired with chronic dermal changes

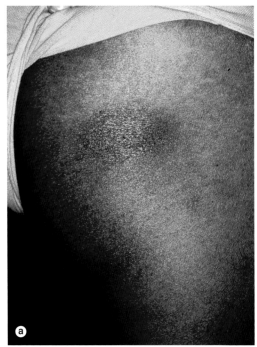

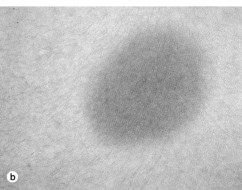

Figure 23-16 a, b Fixed drug eruption

Flagellate pigmentation

* Whipmark-like pigmentation on the trunk (Figure 23-17)
* Associated with bleomycin

Fluorouracil dermatitis (5-fluorouracil (5-FU) Box 23-21)

* Clinical: erythematous, inflamed papules, erosions, rarely ulcerations at sites of actinic keratoses
* Extension of therapeutic effect
* May also cause hyperpigmentation over blood vessels used for infusion

Gingival hyperplasia

* Clinical: starts as diffuse swelling of interdental papillae
* Is dose-dependent and occurs with chronic therapy, but can start as early as 3 months (phenytoin: Box 23-22)
* More common in the young, especially females
* Can occur with painful bleeding of gums
* Secondary bacterial gingivitis can occur

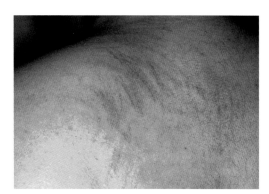

Figure 23-17 Bleomycin pigment

BOX 23-20

Drugs associated with fixed drug eruption

Antibiotics

Nonsteroidal anti-inflammatory drugs

Hormones

Sulfonamides

Trimethoprim

Pseudoephedrine

Drug or food dyes

Acetaminophen

Aspirin

BOX 23-21

Drug associated with fluorouracil dermatitis

5-Fluorouracil (both topical and intravenous)

BOX 23-22

Drugs associated with gingival hyperplasia

Phenytoin

Cyclosporine

Calcium channel blockers

Drugs associated with hair color change

Methotrexate ("flag sign" hair banding)

Tars (darkening)

Anthralin (darkening)

Minoxidil (darkening)

Chloroquine (whitening in red and blond hair)

Imatinib (loss of color/gray)

Interferon (whitening)

Diazoxide (reddish tint)

Hair color change (Box 23-23)

Key Point

* Changes in pigment metabolism or staining

Heparin necrosis

Key Points

* Clinical: local necrosis at subcutaneous injection site, but can occur systemically from intravenous heparin
* Occurs 6–12 days into heparin therapy
* Antibody-induced thrombocytopenia
* Switch anticoagulation to oral warfarin

Hypersensitivity vasculitis (leukocytoclastic vasculitis)

Key Points

* Clinical: macular or palpable purpura (Figure 23-18), often on lower extremities, but may be generalized
* Type III immune complex-mediated reaction
* More common in hospitalized patients
* 10% associated with drugs (Box 23-24)
* Discontinue the implicated drug
* Assess for renal involvement
* Treat with oral corticosteroids if indicated
* Histology: leukocytoclasia around vessels, fibrin thrombi within vessel lumens, inflammatory cells within vessel walls

Hypertrichosis (Figure 23-19; Box 23-25)

Key Point

* Mechanism unknown

Ichthyosis, acquired (Box 23-26)

Key Points

* Clinically similar to ichthyosis vulgaris (Figure 23-20)
* Histology: hyperkeratosis, decreased to normal granular layer

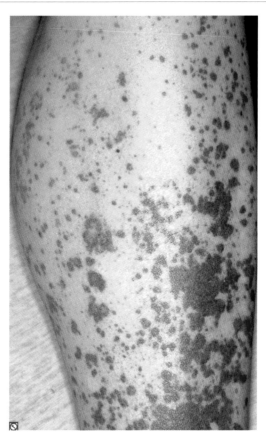

Figure 23-18 Hypersensitivity vasculitis (leukocytoclastic vasculitis)

Drugs associated with leukocytoclastic vasculitis

Antibiotics

Angiotensin-converting enzyme inhibitors

Thiazides

Nonsteroidal anti-inflammatory drugs

Leukotriene receptor antagonists (Churg–Strauss syndrome)

Leukoderma (Box 23-27)

Key Points

* Clinical: hypopigmented or depigmented patches and/or macules
* Most commonly from topical chemical exposure
* Mechanisms include decreased melanin production and melanocyte destruction
* Histology: decreased keratinocyte melanin pigment (compared to unaffected skin); may see pigment incontinence and/or decreased melanocytes

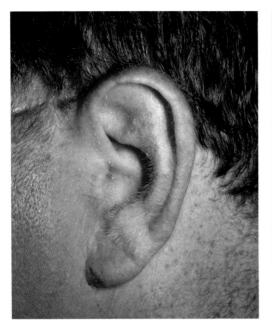

Figure 23-19 Hypertrichosis

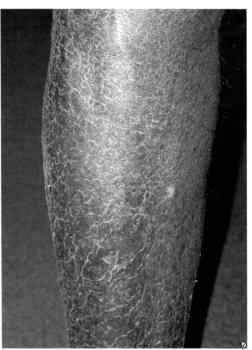

Figure 23-20 Acquired ichthyosis

BOX 23-25

Drugs associated with hypertrichosis

Cyclosporine

Minoxidil

Anabolic steroids

Phenytoin

Penicillamine

Epidermal growth factor receptor inhibitors

BOX 23-26

Drugs associated with acquired ichthyosis

Niacin

Butyrophenones (haloperidol)

Lipid-lowering agents

Retinoids

Lithium

Cimetidine

BOX 23-27

Drugs associated with leukoderma

Carbolic acid

Corticosteroids (intralesional)

Imiquimod

Azelaic acid

Hydroquinone

Monobenzone

Antimalarials

Interferon

Interleukin-2

Retinoids

---

occurs months into therapy and takes months to resolve
• Histology: hyperkeratosis and parakeratosis are common; epidermal acanthosis and hypergranulosis with saw-toothing of the dermoepidermal junction; lichenoid infiltrate that often includes eosinophils

Lichenoid drug eruption (Box 23-28)

Key Points

• Clinical: pruritic lichenoid papules
• Involvement of trunk more common with lichenoid drug reactions than in lichen planus, which more commonly affects extremities; often

Linear IgA disease

Key Points

• Clinical: tense blisters, sometimes in an annular arrangement
• Less (or no) mucosal involvement than linear IgA disease not associated with drugs
• Uncommon drug-associated finding (Box 23-29)

BOX 23-28

Drugs associated with lichenoid drug eruption

Nonsteroidal anti-inflammatory drugs

Antimalarials

Beta-blockers

Angiotensin-converting enzyme inhibitors

Gold

BOX 23-29

Drugs associated with linear immunoglobulin A disease

Vancomycin

Angiotensin-converting enzyme inhibitors

Lithium

Nonsteroidal anti-inflammatory drugs

- Immunofluorescence findings similar to nondrug linear IgA disease
- Indirect immunofluorescence shows low-titer IgA antibody with antibasement membrane zone specificity in a minority of cases
- Can have IgA antibodies to 97-, 180-, and/or 230-kDa antigen
- Histology: subepidermal cleft, often with neutrophils at the base

Livedo reticularis (Box 23-30)

Key Points

- Clinical: mottled or reticular red or bluish discoloration usually affecting the lower extremities

Lupus-like reaction

Key Points

- Clinical: skin findings less common than in lupus erythematosus not associated with drugs
- Occurs primarily in older persons and males > females
- Systemic symptoms similar to lupus erythematosus (polyarthritis, pleuritis, pneumonitis, myalgias, fever)
- Often dose-related (Box 23-31)
- Antinuclear antibody positive and antihistone positive (90%)
- Often begins months or years after medication started
- Clinical signs and symptoms resolve within several days to weeks after discontinuation of medication, although serologies resolve slowly
- Penicillamine can unmask latent lupus erythematosus

BOX 23-30

Drugs associated with livedo reticularis

Amantadine

Quinidine (may have photosensitive component)

Minocycline

BOX 23-31

Drugs associated with lupus-like reaction

Anticonvulsants

Hydralazine

Isoniazid

Lithium

Minocycline

Minoxidil

Hormones

Procainamide

Propylthiouracil

Quinidine

Beta-blockers

BOX 23-32

Drugs associated with nail pigmentation

Chemotherapeutic agents

Antimalarials

Minocycline

Gold

Zidovudine

5-Fluorouracil

Nail pigmentation (Box 23-32)

Key Point

- Various colors (Figure 23-21)

Nephrogenic systemic fibrosis (NSF)

Key Points

- Clinical: thickening/induration of skin, often starting over extremities, leading to joint contractures; skin becomes bound down; yellowish scleral plaques may be seen
- Recent reports implicate gadolinium contrast agents used for magnetic resonance angiography (MRA) in setting of renal impairment (Box 23-33)
- Gadolinium contrast media approved for use in United States in 1993

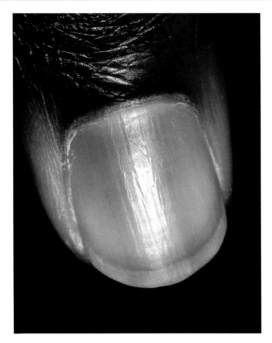

Figure 23-21 Minocycline pigment

BOX 23-34

Drugs associated with neutrophilic eccrine hidradenitis

Bleomycin

Cytarabine

Zidovudine

Acetaminophen

BOX 23-35

Drugs associated with patch medication dermatitis

Clonidine

Estrogens

Testosterone

Scopolamine

Narcotics

BOX 23-33

Drugs associated with nephrogenic systemic fibrosis

Gadolinium-based contrast agents

* NSF first reported shortly after gadolinium available for use (1997)
* No cases of NSF reported before gadolinium use
* Histology: increased fibrocytes and mucin in the reticular dermis and subcutaneous tissue; fibrocytes are procollagen- and CD34-positive

Neutrophilic eccrine hidradenitis

Key Points

* Clinical: tender red papules, nodules, or plaques with or without hyperpigmentation
* Can involve upper trunk, face, extremities, and palms
* Patient can be febrile, thus mimicking infection
* Skin biopsy helpful
* Usually occurs within 3 weeks of starting chemotherapy (Box 23-34)
* Clears 1–4 weeks after discontinuation of offending agent
* Does not always recur with rechallenge (60%)
* Likely a cytotoxic effect on eccrine cells from chemotherapeutic agent in sweat
* Can continue chemotherapy
* Treatments can include corticosteroids, nonsteroidal anti-inflammatory drugs, dapsone
* Histology: perieccrine neutrophils

Patch medication dermatitis

Key Points

* Clinical: erythema and scaling, sometimes with vesiculation/bullae, in an area of an applied patch medication
* Can occur with any medication administered transdermally by patch application (Box 23-35)
* Can be allergic or irritant contact dermatitis
* Allergy can be to the medication or components of the drug delivery system
* Usually oral/systemic form of medication can be administered without complication
* Avoid oral/systemic medication if rash extends beyond applied patch
* Histology: spongiotic dermatitis with eosinophils

Pellagra (Box 23-36)

Key Points

* Clinical: photosensitivity, perineal lesions, thickening, and pigmentation over bony prominences and seborrheic dermatitis-like eruption on face
* Casal's necklace is the photosensitive rash on the upper chest, but same rash can occur on other sun-exposed sites
* Deficiency of niacin (nicotinic acid, vitamin B_3) or precursor amino acid tryptophan
* Pyridoxine (vitamin B_6) deficiency often coexists (needed for conversion of tryptophan to niacin)
* Histology: classic histology shows parakeratosis/necrosis of the upper stratum spinosum

Pemphigus

Key Points

- Clinical: erosions and flaccid bullae, often involving trunk and mucous membranes; may be generalized
- Rare drug-associated finding (Box 23-37)
- Immunofluorescence findings similar to nondrug-associated pemphigus
- Histology: suprabasilar acantholysis, tombstoning of basal layer

Photoallergic reaction

Key Points

- Clinical: erythema and scaling, sometimes with vesicles, in a photo-distributed pattern (Figure 23-22)
- May occur in setting of chronic actinic dermatitis
- Associated with topical more than systemic agents (Box 23-38)
- Topical sunscreens and fragrances are most common causes
- Confirm with photopatch testing
- If due to sunscreen, should use physical blockers (sunscreens containing zinc oxide or titanium dioxide)
- Histology: epidermal spongiosis often with perivascular eosinophils

Photo-onycholysis (Box 23-39)

Key Points

- Clinical: painless separation of nail plate from nail bed
- Variant of a phototoxic reaction

Phototoxic reaction (Box 23-40)

Key Point

- Clinical: erythema and scaling in a photo-distributed pattern that is similar to a sunburn

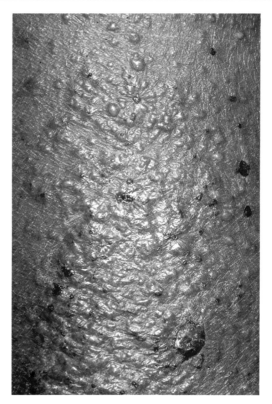

Figure 23-22 Photoallergic reaction to piroxicam

- Associated with systemic more frequently than topical agents
- Ultraviolet (UV) A light in presence of drug creates free radicals causing mitochondrial damage with clinical symptom of burning and, if exposure is long enough, erythema, edema, and bullae
- Reaction is purely dose-related (both drug and UVA light), thus occurs more frequently during days in which ambient UVA radiation is highest (near and around the first day of summer) and when drug is at peak levels in skin
- May avoid by withholding the drug before anticipated greater than normal UV exposure
- Histology: variable epidermal spongiosis; apoptotic cells within the epidermis, perivascular lymphocytes

Pigmentation

Key Points

- Usually related to chronic administration of pigment-associated drug (Box 23-41)
- May or may not be reversible
- Can affect skin, mucous membranes (Figure 23-23), hair, or nails from drug deposition, increased melanin synthesis, increased lipofuscin synthesis, or postinflammatory

Pityriasis rosea (PR)-like reaction (Box 23-42)

Key Points

- Clinical: red-orange thin plaques with fine inner scale, sometimes following lines of cleavage; herald patch characteristic of postviral PR is not usually present (Figure 23-24)
- Does not always follow "Christmas-tree pattern"; may be in atypical distribution (i.e., more on extremities than trunk)
- Histology: mounds of parakeratosis, variable epidermal spongiosis, perivascular lymphocytes, and possibly eosinophils

Pseudoepitheliomatous hyperplasia with pustules (halogenoderma)

Key Points

- Macerated heaped-up plaques and pustules (Figure 23-25)
- Related to ingestion of iodide, bromide, or fluoride compounds
- May occur after iodinated contrast studies in patients with renal failure
- Iododerma favors the face
- Fluoroderma favors the legs

The acute stage of a halogenoderma demonstrates intraepidermal spongiform pustules, follicular pustules, and underlying LCV. Pneumonitis may be present. The lesions respond to systemic

---

BOX 23-41

Drugs associated with pigmentation

Minocycline

Quinacrine

Amiodarone

Clofazimine

Zidovudine

Cytotoxic agents (bleomycin flagellate hyperpigmentation)

Heavy metals (especially gold)

Hormones

Phenothiazines

Hydroxychloroquine

Chloroquine

---

corticosteroids. The later stage demonstrates verrucous lesions studded with pustules. Scarring is common.

Pseudolymphoma (Box 23-43)

Key Points

- Clinical: one or several cutaneous nodules
- Occur alone or in setting of DRESS
- Resolves with discontinuation of offending agent
- Histology: atypical, often dense, inflammatory infiltrate of lymphocytes; keratinocyte necrosis and dermal edema may help suggest a drug-induced etiology

Pseudoporphyria (Box 23-44)

Key Points

- Clinical: tense blisters in photodistributed pattern (especially dorsal hands; Figure 23-26)
- No urine porphyrins or fluorescence like in porphyria cutanea tarda
- A variant of a phototoxic reaction
- Histology: noninflammatory subepidermal cleft with thickening of the basement membrane/vessels

Psoriasiform eruption

Key Points

- Clinical: erythematous plaques with silvery scale (Figure 23-27)
- Uncommon drug-associated finding
- Can occur in patient without history of psoriasis or can represent an exacerbation of existing psoriasis
- Acronym for drugs is "PLAN B" (Box 23-45)
- Histology: confluent parakeratosis with neutrophils in the cornified layer, regular acanthosis, dilated papillary dermal vessels, perivascular lymphocytes and eosinophils

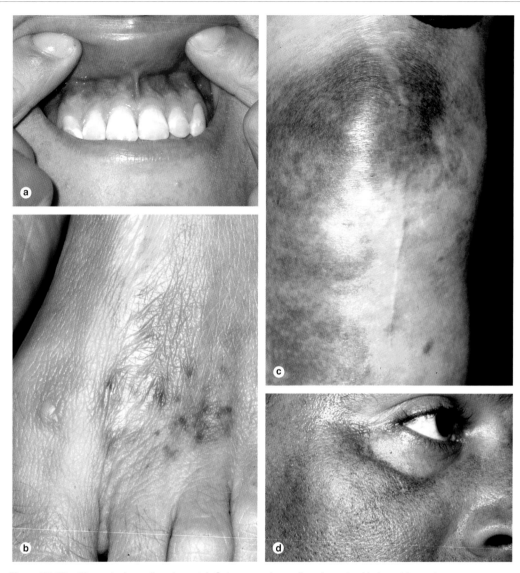

Figure 23-23 a Mucosal minocycline pigment. **b** Cutaneous minocycline pigment. **c** Hydroxychloroquine hyperpigmentation. **d** Ochronotic pigment secondary to hydroquinone

Drugs associated with pityriasis rosea-like reaction

Beta-blockers

Bismuth

Angiotensin-converting enzyme inhibitors

Griseofulvin

Gold

Isotretinoin

Metronidazole

Penicillin

Raynaud's phenomenon

Key Points

- Clinical: change in skin color (from normal to blue/red/white) of digits and/or other acral sites
- Pharmacologic properties influence unstable peripheral vascular system, causing symptomatic vasoconstriction with typical color change in distal digits (Box 23-46)
- Paroxysmal extremity pain associated with cold-associated vasoconstriction
- More common in females
- Digits involved can be white, blue, or red compared to digits with normal circulation

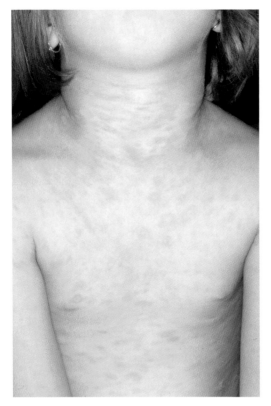

Figure 23-24 Pityriasis rosea-like reaction

* Digital ulcers may occur if vasoconstriction is chronic, prolonged, or following trauma

Retinoid dermatitis

Key Points

* Clinical: coarseness, dry scaling, and minimal erythema of skin
* More common in cold climates with low humidity
* Occurs with both systemic (Box 23-47) and topical agents
* Resolves with discontinuation of treatment or ceramide containing moisturizers

Serum sickness-like reaction
(Box 23-48)

Key Points

* Clinical: skin findings often nonspecific
* Fever, urticaria (Figure 23-28), adenopathy, and polyarthritis
* Neuritis and glomerulonephritis associated with nondrug serum sickness
* Occurs 4–14 days after exposure to a new antigen
* Anaphylaxis reported to be more common following re-exposure to drug within 1 year
* Histology: often nonspecific

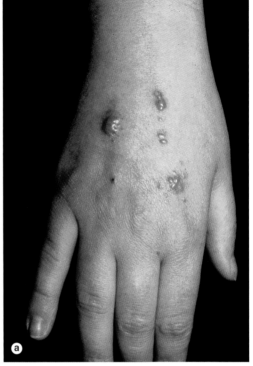

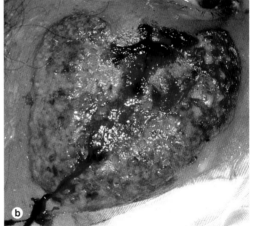

Figure 23-25 a, b Iododerma

Stevens–Johnson syndrome
(see TEN below)

Subacute cutaneous lupus erythematosus (SCLE: Box 23-49)

Key Points

* Clinical: erythematous scaly plaques, often in an annular configuration
* Photosensitive eruption
* May or may not be have autoantibodies against SSA (Ro)

- May represent "unmasking" of pre-existing SCLE or actual induction
- Histology: apoptotic keratinocytes, vacuolar change to lichenoid infiltrate at dermoepidermal junction

---

BOX 23-43

Drugs associated with pseudolymphoma

Anticonvulsants

Sulfonamides

Thiazides

Dapsone

Antidepressants

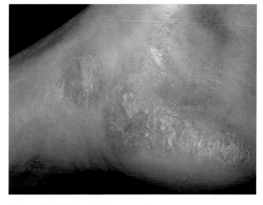

Figure 23-27 Psoriasiform eruption

BOX 23-44

Drugs associated with pseudoporphyria

Furosemide

Nonsteroidal anti-inflammatory drugs

Tetracyclines

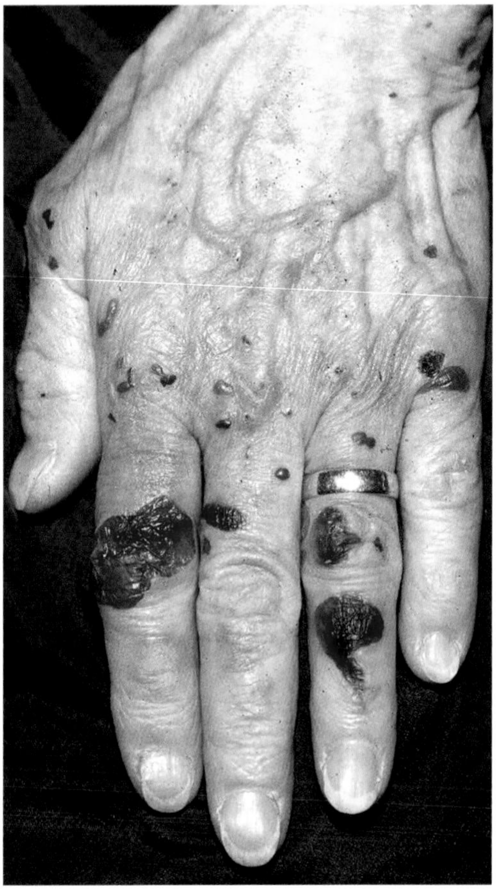

BOX 23-45

Drugs associated with psoriasiform eruption

Prednisone

Lithium

Antimalarials

Nonsteroidal anti-inflammatory drugs

Beta-blockers

BOX 23-46

Drugs associated with Raynaud's phenomenon

Beta-blockers

Ergot alkaloids

Sympathomimetic agents

BOX 23-47

Drugs associated with retinoid dermatitis

Acitretin

Isotretinoin

Tretinoin

BOX 23-48

Drugs associated with serum sickness-like reaction

Antibiotics (especially cefaclor)

Anti-thymocyte globulin

Figure 23-26 Pseudoporphyria

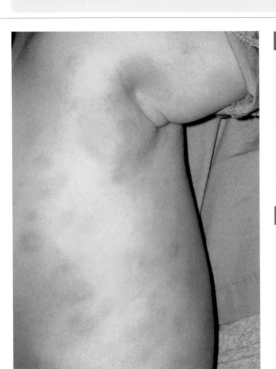

Figure 23-28 Serum sickness-like reaction

BOX 23-50

Drugs associated with Sweet's syndrome

Granulocyte colony stimulating-factor

Tretinoin (*all*-transretinoic acid) oral

Oral contraceptives

Minocycline

Trimethoprim-sulfamethoxazole

BOX 23-51

Drugs associated with toxic epidermal necrolysis

Anticonvulsants

Sulfonamides

Nonsteroidal anti-inflammatory drugs

Allopurinol

Others

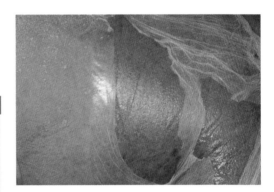

Figure 23-29 Toxic epidermal necrolysis

BOX 23-49

Drugs associated with subacute cutaneous lupus erythematosus

Thiazides

Angiotensin-converting enzyme inhibitors

Calcium channel blocker

Interferons

Statins

Griseofulvin

Terbinafine

Spironolactone

Piroxicam

Antitumor necrosis factor agents

Sweet's-like reaction (Box 23-50)

Key Point

* Clinically and histologically similar to Sweet's syndrome

Toxic epidermal necrolysis (Box 23-51)/ Stevens–Johnson syndrome

Key Points

* Clinical: rare, potentially life-threatening, acute exfoliative bullous eruption of the skin and mucous membranes (Figure 23-29)
* SJS and TEN are thought to be ends of a spectrum of adverse drug reaction, often classified by percentage of skin with epidermal detachment:
  * < 10% body surface area SJS
  * 10–30% body surface area SJS–TEN overlap
  * > 30% TEN
* Rapid onset of symmetrical, painful eruption that progresses quickly, peaking within 3 days
* Skin pain/tenderness is characteristic
* Affected skin exhibits positive Nikolsky sign
* Associated systemic symptoms are common, including fever
* Immune and metabolic pathogenesis

- High risk for sepsis and metabolic problems
- More common in HIV infection
- Mortality of TEN higher than SJS
- Early diagnosis and intervention critical
- TEN is a medical emergency with a high mortality rate
- Patients should be admitted or transferred to burn or critical care unit, where supportive care is essential (fluid resuscitation, nutritional support, pain control, sepsis prevention)
- Avoid adhesives on skin
- Ophthalmology and gynecology consults are important when respective organs are involved
- Survivors are at risk for permanent corneal scarring/vision loss
- Discontinuation of potential offending drug(s) is critical
- IVIg 1 g/kg per day × 2–4 days may be beneficial, although data are mixed; appears to work by blocking Fas-mediated keratinocyte apoptosis
- Thalidomide worsens outcome
- Anecdotal data on a variety of other agents, including biologics and cyclosporine
- Conflicting data regarding corticosteroids (some data suggest use for > 48–72 hours associated with increased risk of septic death)
- Histology: basket-weave stratum corneum overlying confluent epidermal necrosis with detachment of epidermis from the dermis; often minimally inflamed

Trichomegaly (long eyelashes: Box 23-52)

Key Points

- Eyelashes longer and curlier
- Likely associated with immune dysregulation (occurs in HIV infection)

Ultraviolet recall (Box 23-53)

Key Points

- Clinical: drug recalls erythema in "normal" areas exposed to UV light within the previous 5 days
- Reaction subsides with or without discontinuation of treatment

Urticaria

Key Points

- Clinical: urticarial pruritic plaques that arise within 36 hours of offending agent
- A specific urticarial plaque rarely lasts longer than 24 hours

- May occur alone or in combination with angioedema, serum sickness, or anaphylaxis
- Occurs as long as offending agent is given (Box 23-54)
- Treat with antihistamines
- If severe or associated with angioedema or pulmonary symptoms, treat with epinephrine or systemic corticosteroids
- Histology: neutrophils within vessels, perivascular mixed inflammatory infiltrate

Warfarin necrosis

Key Points

- Clinical: areas of cutaneous infarction, often with overlying ulceration, often over fatty areas (e.g., outer thighs, buttocks, Figure 23-30)
- 1:10,000 incidence
- Timing 3–5 days into therapy
- Occurs in patients with protein C deficiency
- When warfarin is started, protein C is lowered (shorter half-life than clotting factors), allowing thrombosis to occur due to an acute state of reduced thrombolysis
- Fully anticoagulate with intravenous heparin, after which warfarin may be safely started
- Histology: necrosis of epidermis and dermis with thrombi within vessels

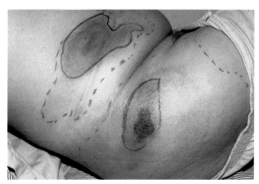

Figure 23-30 Coumadin necrosis

Xerotic dermatitis (Box 23-55)

Key Points

- Clinical: coarse, scaling skin with minimal erythema
- Secondary to topical medications with drying effect
- Oral medications affecting skin lipid barrier/ hydration
- More common in the elderly and in dry/cold climates

BOX 23-55

Drugs associated with xerotic dermatitis

Benzoyl peroxide

Retinoids

Hydroxymethylglutaryl coenzyme A reductase inhibitors

Further reading

Callen JP. Newly recognized cutaneous drug eruptions. Dermatol Clin 2007;25:255–261.

Cham PM, Warshaw EM. Patch testing for evaluating drug reactions due to systemic antibiotics. Dermatitis 2007;18:63–77.

Knowles SR, Shear NH. Recognition and management of severe cutaneous drug reactions. Dermatol Clin 2007;25:245–253.

Mittmann N, Chan BC, Knowles S, et al. IVIG for the treatment of toxic epidermal necrolysis. Skin Ther Lett 2007;12:7–9.

Monti M, Motta S. Clinical management of cutaneous toxicity of anti-EGFR agents. Int J Biol Markers 2007;22(Suppl 4):S53–S61.

Anatomy and basic nail data **24**

David Doyle Jr. and Richard Devillez

Anatomy

Key Points

- Basic anatomy of the nail includes the nail plate, the nail folds, the matrix, the nail bed, and the hyponychium
- The proximal nail fold (PNF) overlies the proximal nail matrix
- Nail bed is beneath the nail plate and functions primarily in adherence of the nail plate to the bed
- The proximal nail matrix forms the dorsal nail plate
- The distal nail matrix (lunula) forms the ventral nail plate

The basic units of anatomy of the nail unit are the nail folds, the matrix, the nail bed, and the hyponychium. These structures each contribute to the formation of the nail plate, which is a hard, convex, translucent structure covering the distal, dorsal surfaces of the fingers and toes.

The PNF is a wedge-shaped fold of skin contiguous with the distal, dorsal digit. The PNF overlies and protects the matrix, which is the structure that generates the nail plate. The distal aspect of the nail matrix is sometimes visible underneath the PNF and is called the lunula. The lateral nail folds are extensions of the PNF which lend support and guidance to the nail plate.

The nail bed underlies the nail plate. The nail bed has a very thin, fragile epithelium arranged in longitudinal, tongue-in-groove fashion. The nail bed attaches to the nail plate by way of these grooves, and therefore one of the nail bed's primary functions is adherence of the nail plate. Although the matrix forms the predominant portion of the nail plate, a small contribution of cells to the ventral surface of the nail plate is made by the nail bed. The direction of nail plate growth is determined by the nail bed.

Where the nail bed ends beneath the nail plate is termed the hyponychium. The hyponychium marks the end of the nail bed and the beginning of the normal volar epidermis. The hyponychium is also the "water-tight" barrier, preventing moisture from entering the nail bed. The nail plate is many times more permeable to water than the normal, intact epidermis.

The proximal aspect of the matrix gives rise to the dorsal aspect of the nail plate, and the distal aspect of the matrix gives rise to the ventral aspect of the nail plate. Defects in the proximal matrix will result in abnormalities of the dorsal nail plate such as pitting and longitudinal ridging/fissuring. Defects in the distal nail matrix will result in abnormalities of the ventral nail plate such as leukonychia (white spots). Defects in the nail bed result in abnormalities such as nail plate separation (onycholysis) and splinter hemorrhages (Table 24-1).

The nail plate is colorless and its apparent color comes from structures beneath the nail plate. The nail plate appears white over the distal nail matrix (seen as the lunula) and pinkish over the nail bed.

The thickness of the nail plate is determined by the length of the nail matrix. In males the nail plate is approximately 0.6 mm thick, and in females the nail plate is approximately 0.5 mm thick.

Table 24-1 Defects of the nail and associated anatomy

Defect in	Clinical manifestation
Proximal matrix	Pitting
	Longitudinal ridging/fissuring
	Beau's lines
Distal matrix	Leukonychia
Nail bed	Onycholysis
	Splinter hemorrhages
	Apparent leukonychia
Nail plate	True leukonychia

Although nail growth rates are influenced by many factors and differ from person to person, as a guideline fingernails grow approximately 2–3 mm per month, and toenails grow approximately 1 mm per month. Some of the factors influencing nail growth are shown in Table 24-2, and a glossary of nail terms is provided in Table 24-3.

Nail Abnormalities

Koilonychia

Key Points

- Defined as spoon-like changes in the nail plate
- May be hereditary
- Acquired causes include hypothyroidism, anemia, trauma, infections, psoriasis, lichen planus

Table 24-2 Factors influencing nail growth

Faster growth	Slower growth
Third digit	First and fifth digit
Male gender	Female gender
Youth	Aging
Pregnancy	Lactation
Increased temperatures (summer)	Decreased temperatures (winter)
Minor trauma (typing, nail biting)	Smoking
Increased blood flow (shunts)	Decreased blood flow (vascular disease)
Dominant hand	Acute infection
Premenses	Chronic disease
Psoriasis	Malnutrition
Hyperthyroidism	Hypothyroidism

Table 24-3 Glossary of nail terms

Term	Meaning
Anonychia	Absence of nail plate
Beau's line	Transverse depression in the nail plate.
Brachyonychia	Short nail plate, most commonly on the thumbs (aka "racquet thumbs")
Chromonychia	Color change of the nail plate (usually translucent)
Elkonyxis	Loss of nail plate in the lunula only (associated with syphilis)
Hyponychium	Epidermis distal to the nail bed
Koilonychia	Spoon-like changes of the nail plate (Figure 24-1)
Leukonychia	White discoloration of the nail plate
Lunula	Half-moon-shaped, distal nail matrix which is often visible
Macronychia	Unusually large nail – most often wider than normal
Median canaliform dystrophy	Median nail plate canal or split, most commonly on thumbs (Figure 24-2)
Melanonychia	Brown dyschromia of the nail (Figure 24-3)
Nail bed	Supporting structure of nail plate, extending from matrix to hyponychium
Nail folds	Two lateral and one proximal – outline, support, and guide growth of the nail
Nail matrix	Structure generating the nail plate – distally seen through the nail plate as the lunula
Onychauxis	Localized nail plate thickening
Onychogryphosis	Ram's horn nail – hypertrophy of nail plate
Onycholysis	Abnormal separation of the nail plate from the nail bed
Onychomadesis	Proximal nail plate shedding
Onychomycosis	Fungal infection of the nail unit
Onychorrhexis	Brittle nails with superficial longitudinal ridges and split distal edges
Onychoschizia	Separation of the nail plate from the nail bed
Pachyonychia	Thickening of the entire nail plate
Paronychia	Inflammation/infection of the nail folds
Pincer nail	Increased curvature of nail compressing nail bed (Figure 24-4)
Pitting	Shallow depressions in the nail plate
Pterygium	Scarring between the nail bed and the proximal nail fold, aka a dorsal pterygium (Figure 24-5)
Pterygium inversus unguium	Ventral pterygium
Trachyonychia	Rough, longitudinally ridged nail plate.

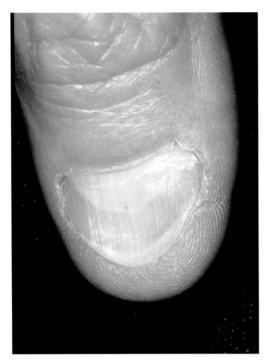

Figure 24-1 Koilonychia

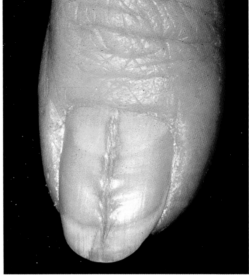

Figure 24-2 Medial canaliform dystrophy

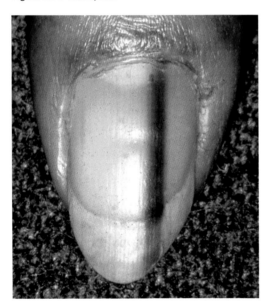

Figure 24-3 Melanonychia striata

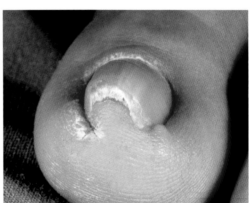

Figure 24-4 Pincer nail

Koilonychia describes spoon-like changes in the nail plate. Koilonychia is present when the lateral edges of the nail plate are elevated above the depressed center of the nail plate. When viewed laterally the nail plate with koilonychia resembles a spoon, hence the common name "spoon nails." Petaloid nail describes flattening of the nail plate, which is an early stage of koilonychia.

The causes of koilonychia can be broadly divided into congenital/hereditary and acquired/traumatic forms. The most common causes of the acquired form of koilonychia are hypothyroidism, anemia, and traumatic/occupational forms. Patients who suffer repeated, occupationally related microtrauma to the nail matrix and/or repeated contact with chemicals/solvents are most likely to develop the traumatic/occupational forms of koilonychia. Koilonychia can also be seen in association with infections (such as syphilis and fungus), psoriasis, and lichen planus. Koilonychia may be physiological in children.

Clubbing

Key Points

- Defined as an increase in Lovibond's angle
- Normal angle is ~160°
- Associated with cardiopulmonary disease, sarcoidosis, cirrhosis, gastrointestinal disease, toxin exposures, trauma

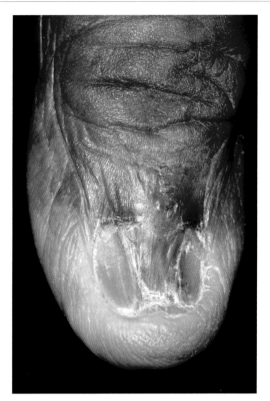

Figure 24-5 Lichen planus, pterygium

Clubbing is defined as an increase in the unguophalangeal angle to 180° or greater. The unguophalangeal angle, also known as Lovibond's angle, is formed by the meeting of the PNF and the nail plate. The normal nail plate proceeds away from the PNF at an angle of approximately 160°.

Clubbing is most commonly noted bilaterally on the thumb and index fingers, and is frequently associated with cardiopulmonary diseases such as lung/mediastinal neoplasms, chronic bronchitis, and congestive heart failure. Other less common causes of bilateral clubbing include sarcoidosis, cirrhosis, gastrointestinal disease, and toxic exposures (arsenic, mercury, and asbestos, for example). Clubbing limited to one hand is most commonly associated with a vascular lesion in the affected area, and clubbing of one finger is usually associated with trauma.

Splinter hemorrhage

Key Points

* Defined as a sliver of extravasated blood visible beneath nail plate
* Associated with trauma
* Systemic associations include endocarditis, diabetes, hypertension, and lupus, as well as many others

Splinter hemorrhages are formed from the extravasation of blood from the nail bed. The longitudinal, tongue-in-groove arrangement of the nail bed is the reason that splinter hemorrhages appear as darkly colored, splinter-like longitudinal lines. Splinter hemorrhages do not blanch with pressure. They usually move distally with the nail plate, when the blood attaches to the ventral surface of the nail plate, although they can attach to the nail bed and appear fixed.

Trauma is the most common cause of splinter hemorrhages, especially when noted in one or two nails with an accompanying history of trauma. When they appear simultaneously in several proximal nails (closer to the lunula), they are likely to be associated with systemic disease. The most common systemic illness associated with splinter hemorrhages is bacterial endocarditis. They have also been noted with diabetes, hypertension, and lupus, to name just a few.

Leukonychia

Key Points

* Defined as a white area of the nail
* True leukonychia does not disappear with pressure
* Apparent leukonychia disappears with pressure
* Mees' lines are a true leukonychia that have been traditionally associated with arsenic toxicity
* Muehrcke's lines are an apparent leukonychia associated with hypoalbuminism
* Lindsay's nails (half-and-half nails) are white proximally and brown-red distally and are associated with renal disease, psoriasis, and chemotherapy
* Terry's nails are white proximally with 1 mm to several millimeters of brown-red distally and are associated with cirrhosis, congestive heart failure, diabetes, and aging

Leukonychia means "white nail," and is the most common nail dyschromia. Leukonychias can be broadly divided into true leukonychias and apparent leukonychias. True leukonychias are caused by white discoloration of the nail plate itself due to dyskeratinization at the matrix, and cannot be hidden by pressing the nail plate down on to the nail bed. Apparent leukonychias are caused by nail bed changes. If one presses the nail plate down on to the nail bed, apparent leukonychias will become hidden. The term "pseudoleukonychia" refers to a defect which is exogenous to the nail unit, such as fungal infection (onychomycosis).

Although most true leukonychias are caused by trauma, true leukonychias appearing as Mees' lines can be an important indicator of systemic disease. There are four characteristics of a true leukonychia that would warrant consideration of systemic disease versus trauma as the cause:

1. Appearance on several nails simultaneously – trauma-induced leukonychias are more often isolated to one or two nails
2. Leukonychia involving the entire width of the nail – trauma-induced leukonychias less commonly span the entire width of the nail
3. Contour similar to that of the lunula – trauma-induced leukonychias tend to be more linear or have a contour similar to the PNF
4. Lack of history of sufficient trauma to cause nail changes – aggressive manicuring is often sufficient trauma to cause a true leukonychia

Mees' lines were originally described as being an indicator of arsenic intoxication; however we now know that many systemic diseases and medications can be the cause of Mees' lines. Patients with true leukonychias that involve the entire width of the nail of several fingers warrant a thorough physical examination, medications review, and query about possible toxic exposures.

Muehrcke's lines are an apparent leukonychia which appears as twin transverse lines across the nail. There is no nail surface irregularity; Muehrcke's lines can be seen, but not felt. Since they represent an apparent leukonychia, they will temporarily disappear when pressure is applied to the nail. Since Muehrcke's nails are an important marker for hypoalbuminism, their presence warrants evaluation for hypoalbuminism. Cancer patients receiving chemotherapy may also have Muehrcke's lines.

Lindsay's nails or half-and-half nails appear as nails that have a normal-colored or whitish proximal portion, and a markedly brownish distal portion. Half-and-half nails are an important marker of chronic renal insufficiency. Their most common mimickers are those seen in patients with psoriasis and patients taking systemic chemotherapy such as 5-fluorouracil.

Terry's nails appear as an apparent leukonychia involving most of the nail, with a thin (0.5–3.0 mm) band of pink or brown distally. They have been associated with cirrhosis, congestive heart failure, diabetes, and age. This finding in a young patient should warrant a work-up for systemic disease.

Beau's lines

* Defined as transverse depressions of the nail plate, secondary to disruption of nail plate formation by the nail matrix
* Usually induced by systemic illness/insult

Beau's lines typically occur as transverse linear depressions or furrows of several nail plates. Severe systemic illnesses/trauma and some chemotherapy agents may cause disruption of nail formation by the matrix, which leads to Beau's lines. They are a common but nonspecific nail finding which hints at a systemic illness/insult, especially when found in several nails the same distance from the PNF. Traumatic changes to one or two nail plates can mimic Beau's lines.

The longitudinal width of Beau's lines is an indication of, and directly proportional to, the duration of the illness which caused the lines. Given that the nail plate grows approximately 0.1–0.15 mm per day, the distance between the PNF and the Beau's line can give an indication of when the insult occurred that caused these lines.

The ultimate expression of Beau's lines is proximal detachment of the nail plate, also known as onychomadesis. Onychomadesis results from prolonged inactivity of the nail matrix due to severe systemic illness/insult, and usually involves most or all the nail plates.

Habit tic deformity

Key Points

* Defined as grooving of the nail plate secondary to chronic manipulation
* Lunula is enlarged

Habit tic deformity results from rubbing and otherwise manipulating the PNF and/or cuticles, and is most often seen on thumb nail plates. These deformities typically involve the entire length of the nail plate and occur in a washboard pattern affecting the middle but sparing the medial and lateral edges of the nail plate. Patients will commonly deny manipulating their nails and indeed many patients may be unconscious of the fact that they are rubbing their nails. Treatment of habit tic deformity may pose a unique challenge and it is often necessary to consult these patients to a qualified psychiatrist for assistance. Habit tic deformities reliably resolve once the causative behavior is corrected.

Median nail dystrophy

Key Point

* Defined as a pattern of grooving in the nail, from the PNF to the distal edge of the nail plate, in a Christmas-tree pattern (Figure 24-2)

Median nail dystrophy is also called "medial canaliform dystrophy" and "dystrophia unguium mediana canaliformis." The findings are nails with a median canal or split in the nail plate and appear as an inverted Christmas-tree pattern. The canal or split extends from the cuticle to the distal edge of the nail plate. Median nail dystrophy is often idiopathic, and is most commonly present on the thumb nails.

Trachyonychia

Key Points

- Defined as nails with a rough, ridged surface
- Associated with alopecia areata, lichen planus, psoriasis, eczema

Trachyonychia is also known as twenty-nail dystrophy, and describes nails with a rough, longitudinally ridged surface. It is most commonly seen in patients with alopecia areata; however it may also occur in patients with lichen planus, psoriasis, and eczema. Trachyonychia is reliably non-scarring and tends to improve spontaneously over time, and therefore treatment is unnecessary.

Onychorrhexis

Key Points

- Defined as splitting of the distal nail plate
- Assocated with lichen planus/trauma

Onychorrhexis describes nails that appear abnormally brittle and have superficial longitudinal ridges and splitting of the distal nail plate. Onychorrhexis is often idiopathic. It is also seen in patients with lichen planus, or may be seen as a result of occupational exposure to gasoline or other industrial solvents.

Onychoschizia

Key Points

- Defined as distal superficial splitting (horizontally) of the nail plate
- Generally secondary to trauma

Onychoschizia describes distal, superficial separation or splitting of the layers of the nail plate. This common condition is usually caused by frequent exposure to detergents, water, and other solvents. Treatment consists of avoidance of frequent handwashing or exposure to other chemicals/solvents, and regular use of a petroleum-based lubricant such as Vaseline jelly.

Pterygium

Key Points

- Defined as a growth of tissue from the PNF to the nail bed
- Associated with trauma and lichen planus and some connective tissue disorders

Focal loss of nail plate growth due to a matrix abnormality can lead to scar formation between the PNF and the nail bed, which is called a dorsal pterygium. Dorsal pterygium (Figure 24-5) is most commonly associated with lichen planus, although it may develop after trauma and in some connective tissue disorders.

Pterygium inversus unguium

Key Points

- Defined as a growth of tissue from the ventral nail plate to the nail bed
- Associated with systemic sclerosis and lupus erythematosus

Pterygium inversus unguium is the term given to abnormal attachment of the ventral surface of the nail plate to the distal nail bed, resulting in abnormal nail bed growth past the normal point of nail plate and nail bed separation (hyponychium). These ventral pterygiums are commonly associated with systemic sclerosis and systemic lupus erythematosus. The first symptom of pterygium inversus unguium is most often pain caused by cutting the nails.

Onycholysis

Key Points

- Defined as detachment of the nail plate from the nail bed
- Secondary to trauma, drug effects, psoriasis, lichen planus

Onycholysis refers to the abnormal distal detachment of the nail plate from the nail bed. It can occur as the result of localized trauma, systemic drugs/disease/infection, or primary skin disorders such as psoriasis and lichen planus. It most commonly occurs as a result of contact irritants and allergens, and usually occurs on fingernails. Treatment consists of strict avoidance of irritants and allergens, avoidance of trauma, and keeping the nails trimmed short.

Paronychia

Key Points

- Defined as inflammation/infection of the nail folds
- Acute paronchyia is usually bacterial in origin
- Chronic paronychia is usually secondary to chronic irritation or *Candida* and treatment with topical steroids is effective

Paronychia is inflammation or infection of the nail folds. For paronychia to occur there must be a breach created in the attachment of the nail fold to the nail plate. Acute paronychia is one of the most common hand infections, and is usually caused by *Staphylococcus*, *Streptococcus*, and *Pseudomonas* species. Treatment of the infection (i.e., draining and other local wound care and antibiotics) should be combined with exploration of the cause(s) of the loss of cuticle attachment which led to the infection. Chronic paronychia is more common than acute paronychia and is commonly associated with repeated trauma, frequent exposure to water, other solvents and detergents, and primary skin disorders such as psoriasis and eczema. The primary organism involved is *Candida albicans*.

Pitting

* Defined as small circular defects in the nail plate
* Associated with alopecia areata ("scotch-plaid" design) and psoriasis and eczema

Nail plate pits result from pathology of the proximal matrix, and occur as shallow depressions in the nail plate surface. It can be subtle on just one nail plate and it can also be widespread and very obvious. Pitting is commonly associated with alopecia areata and psoriasis, as well as eczema. "Scotch-plaid nails" describe nails with geometric pitting patterns, and is most associated with alopecia areata. Nail pits may be the only cutaneous finding in patients with psoriatic arthritis, or they may be associated with distal onycholysis and salmon patches in the nail bed (Figure 24-6).

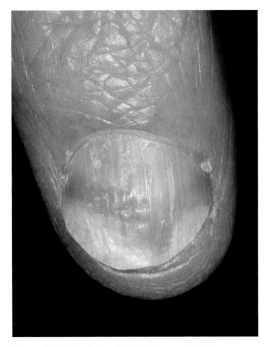

Figure 24-6 Psoriatic nail with pitting and distal onycholysis

Pachyonychia

* Defined as thickening of the entire nail plate
* Seen in pachyonychia congenita, an inherited disease with "door-wedge"-shaped nails

Pachyonychia refers to thickening of the entire nail plate. Onychauxis refers to localized thickening of the nail plate. Both terms refer to increased thickness of the nail plate due to nail bed hyperkeratosis, with loss of translucency of the nail plate. Pachyonychia congenita is a condition in which there is tremendous thickening and upward growth of the nail plates. Onychauxis, especially of the great toe nail, may be a normal variant in elderly patients.

Melanonychia

* Defined as brown dyschromia of the nail plate
* Many causes, although most commonly in patients with pigmented skin, it is a normal variant
* Hutchinson's sign, the extension of pigment on to the nail folds and/or hyponychium, raises the concern for melanoma

Melanonychia refers to longitudinal brown dyschromia of the nail plate. There are many causes of melanonychia, including systemic diseases, topical and systemic medications and, most importantly, melanoma. Evaluation of melanonychia can be a challenge for even very experienced providers. Melanonychia can be a normal variation of nails of African Americans, especially when present on multiple nails. In all races, involvement of a single nail is more suggestive of a neoplastic process than is involvement of several nails. A well-defined, single, thin longitudinal band is more reassuring, whereas multiple, poorly defined, thick longitudinal bands are more concerning for melanoma. Patients with recent change(s) in their longitudinal melanonychia, for instance change in thickness or color, should be evaluated for a neoplastic process. Hutchinson's sign refers to pigmentation of the nail fold (proximal or lateral) and/or the hyponychium. Although a nevus may cause a Hutchinson's sign, the presence of a Hutchinson's sign necessitates a biopsy to rule out melanoma. Microscopic evaluation of a pigmented band can be performed with a hand lens or dermatoscope. Streaks within the band that vary in width are particularly worrisome for melanoma.

Yellow-nail syndrome

* Defined as yellow discoloration of the nails
* Associated with pulmonary disease
* May sometimes be a normal variant

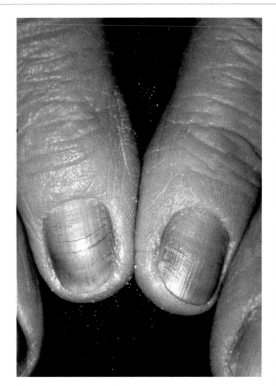

Figure 24-7 Yellow nails

The yellow-nail syndrome (Figure 24-7) is most commonly associated with pulmonary disease, although there are many possible systemic causes, including malignancies. In this syndrome all 20 nail plates appear diffusely yellow and thickened, and the cuticles and the lunula are absent. Patients with yellow-nail syndrome will also describe slow growth of the nail plate. It may be a congenitally acquired condition; however, patients describing nail changes consistent with yellow-nail syndrome warrant evaluation for systemic disease, especially pulmonary disease.

Onychomycosis

Key Points

- Defined as fungal infection of the nail
- Most commonly caused by *Trichophyton rubrum*
- Four basic patterns: (1) distal subungual; (2) white superficial; (3) proximal subungual; and (4) candidal onychomycosis
- Proximal subungual onychomycosis (PSO) is associated with immunosuppression/human immunodeficiency virus (HIV) infection

Fungal infection of the nail unit is known as onychomycosis. Onychomycosis is the most common nail disorder, and represents approximately 50% of all nail disorders. Approximately 90% of all cases of onychomycosis are caused by dermatophyte fungi such as *Trichophyton rubrum* and *T. mentagrophytes*. Yeasts and nondermatophyte molds account for the cause of approximately 10% of cases of onychomycosis. It is much more common on toenails than on fingernails. Fungal infection of the skin of the feet (tinea pedis) commonly leads to onychomycosis; however, onychomycosis does not commonly lead to tinea pedis.

There are four basic patterns of onychomycosis: (1) distal lateral subungual onychomycosis (DLSO); (2) white superficial onychomycosis (WSO); (3) PSO; and (4) *Candida* onychomycosis.

DLSO is the most common pattern of onychomycosis, characterized by distal and/or lateral onycholysis, yellowish-brown discoloration of the nail plate, and hyperkeratosis of the nail bed. DLSO can lead to total dystrophic onychomycosis wherein the whole nail plate and nail bed are involved. *T. rubrum* and *T. mentagrophytes* are the most common causes of DLSO.

WSO (Figure 24-8) is most commonly caused by *T. mentagrophytes*, which has the ability to digest and infect the nail plate directly. WSO appears first as dull white or speckled lesions on the nail plate which often coalesce to involve the entire nail plate. It can be discerned from leukonychia by the crumbled, plaster-like consistency of the nail plate affected by the fungus.

PSO (Figure 24-9) is an uncommon pattern of onychomycosis. It appears clinically as a white discoloration under the proximal nail plate, and the distal nail plate remains unaffected. It is most commonly caused by *T. rubrum* and *T. mentagrophytes*, and may be the first clinical sign of HIV infection or immunosuppression.

Candida species act as opportunistic pathogens to cause onychomycosis. They typically invade nail units previously affected by trauma, dermatophyte infections, or other skin diseases, and cause a yellow, thickened appearance of the nail plate.

Eradication of onychomycosis requires systemic antifungal therapy with azoles (such as fluconazole or itraconazole) or allylamines (such as terbinafine). Before initiating systemic therapy, it is important that laboratory diagnosis of onychomycosis be obtained. If a potassium hydroxide (KOH) preparation is positive, treatment may be initiated; however, a confirmatory fungal culture should be obtained. If a KOH preparation is negative or not available, results of a fungal culture should be obtained before systemic treatment is initiated. If the fungal culture is negative and the diagnosis of onychomycosis is still suspected, nail clippings should be submitted for periodic acid–Schiff staining to confirm the presence of hyphae.

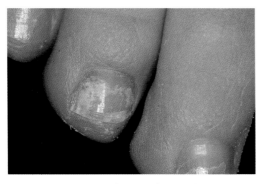

Figure 24-8 White superficial onychomycosis

Nail–patella syndrome

* An autosomal-dominant genetic syndrome with triangular lunulae, absent patellae, and iliac horns
* Associated with renal abnormalities

Nail–patella syndrome is an autosomal-dominant disorder, and is also called "hereditary osteoonychodysplasia" and "Fong's syndrome." It is characterized by dysplasia of the patella and renal abnormalities which may progress to renal failure. The nail findings in the syndrome are hypoplasia or frank aplasia of the nails and triangle-shaped lunulae, most often noted on the thumbs.

Onychocryptosis

* Defined as ingrown nails
* Generally caused by improper nail clipping

Onychocryptosis, known as ingrown nails, typically shows inflammation, is tender to palpation, and is painful upon ambulation. It is caused in most cases by improper nail clipping and/or improperly fitting footwear. It occurs when the lateral nail plate grows into and penetrates the lateral nail fold. The resulting granulation tissue, which commonly appears to sit on top of the nail plate, is sometimes referred to as "proud flesh."

Patients with onychocryptosis should be counseled to cut their nails straight across, which allows the lateral edges of the nail plate to grow out beyond the distal lateral nail fold. Patients with onychocryptosis should also be counseled to avoid improperly fitting footwear, especially footwear that pinches or squeezes the toes together.

Overcurvature of the nail plate can also cause onychocryptosis. Overcurvature of both edges of the nail plate can lead to pincer nails – a painful

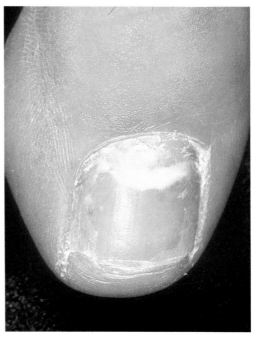

Figure 24-9 White proximal subungual onychomycosis

condition in which the soft tissue beneath the nail plate is "pinched" in between the down-curving nail plate edges.

Treatment for onychocryptosis is partial or full nail plate avulsion, although the condition tends to recur in individuals prone to this condition.

Pincer nail

* Overcurvature of the distal nail plate
* Can be hereditary or acquired

Acrodermatitis continua

* Form of pustular psoriasis
* Nails are shed
* Pustules form in nail bed

Acrodermatitis continua (Figure 24-10) is a form of pustular psoriasis that affects the nail beds and distal digits. It may be associated with generalized flares of pustular psoriasis.

Treatment is difficult, and most patients do not respond to topical therapy. Intralesional injections of triamcinolone can be performed after a digital nerve block. Systemic agents such as acitretin, methotrexate, and newer biologicals are variably effective.

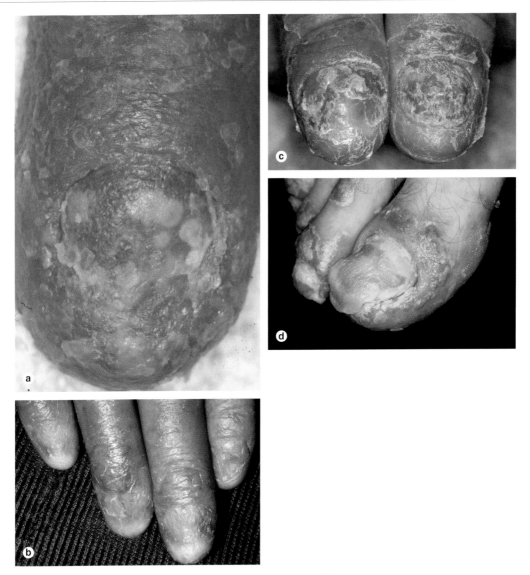

Figure 24-10 a, c, d Acrodermatitis continua. b Acrodermatitis continua with scar

Further reading

Braun RP, Baran R, Le Gal FA, et al. Diagnosis and management of nail pigmentations. J Am Acad Dermatol 2007;56:835–847.

Iorizzo M, Piraccini BM, Tosti A. New fungal nail infections. Curr Opin Infect Dis 2007;20:142–145.

Jellinek NJ. Nail surgery: practical tips and treatment options. Dermatol Ther 2007;20:68–74.

Jiaravuthisan MM, Sasseville D, Vender RB, et al. Psoriasis of the nail: anatomy, pathology, clinical presentation, and a review of the literature on therapy. J Am Acad Dermatol 2007;57:1–27.

Murdan S. 1st meeting on topical drug delivery to the nail. Exp Opin Drug Deliv 2007;4:453–455.

Sehgal VN. Twenty nail dystrophy trachyonychia: an overview. J Dermatol 2007;34:361–366.

Hair disorders

Dirk M. Elston

Clinical presentation

Key Points

- Patients may present because of hair shedding or hair thinning
- A sudden increase in shedding most commonly represents telogen effluvium
- Hair thinning is more likely to represent pattern alopecia
- Scarring alopecia generally requires a biopsy for diagnosis

Diagnosis

Key Points

- Effective treatment depends on accurate classification
- Evaluations should be cost-effective
- Panels of expensive endocrine tests seldom affect management
- Most diagnoses can be made by history and physical examination (Figure 25-1)
- A scalp biopsy is critical to guide therapy in scarring alopecia

Steps in the evaluation of alopecia

1. Determine if a hair shaft abnormality exists

Ask if hairs break. Examine the scalp for patches of short hair. Use a contrasting background to look for evidence of shaft damage. Examine abnormal hair shafts under polarized light or dissecting microscope.

2. Determine if anagen or telogen effluvium exists

Examine hairs obtained via a gentle hair pull, 1-minute combing, or the bag of hair the patient has brought in. The patient *wants* you to look at the bag of hair. He or she will not be satisfied until you do. Tell the patient you are going to examine the hairs microscopically. Leave the room and examine the hairs in the lab. It only takes a minute or two. Pull the hair apart and see if broken fragments fall out. Examine the bulbs to determine if they represent loose-anagen (pigmented bulb with rumpled sock cuticle; Figure 25-2) or telogen (nonpigmented club; Figure 25-3) hairs. Tapered fracture suggests diffuse alopecia areata, chemotherapy, or heavy-metal poisoning.

Telogen effluvium is by far the most common diagnosis in this category. It commonly follows an illness, surgery, delivery, or crash diet by 3–5 months. A full discussion of types of telogen effluvium is presented later in the chapter.

3. Determine if lab tests are necessary

Most patients with hair loss need only limited testing or none at all. Thyroid disorders and iron deficiency are common. Testing for them is relatively inexpensive. A thyroid-stimulating hormone (TSH) test is the preferred screen for thyroid disorders. Microsomal antibody tests seldom affect management. A blood count is a poor screen for iron deficiency. The human body will sacrifice hair long before it stops making blood. Whereas iron supplementation has not been shown to alter the course of idiopathic chronic telogen effluvium, iron deficiency often complicates other causes of hair loss. It is also an indicator of overall nutritional status. A low ferritin proves iron deficiency. Ferritin behaves as an acute-phase reactant, so a normal ferritin does not rule out iron deficiency. Ferritin, serum iron, iron-binding capacity, and saturation should be measured if iron deficiency is suspected.

Patients with *new onset* of virilization need imaging studies and a total testosterone to rule out an ovarian or adrenal tumor. Those with signs of Cushing's disease need a 24-hour urine cortisol. Most

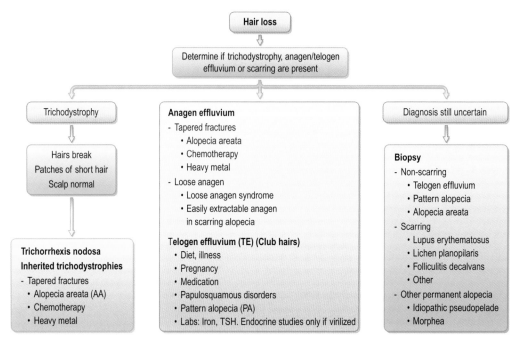

Figure 25-1 Diagnostic algorithm. TSH, thyroid-stimulating hormone

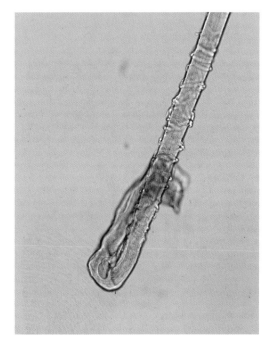

Figure 25-2 Loose-anagen syndrome

patients with *chronic* virilization have polycystic ovarian syndrome (PCOS). The diagnosis is established clinically by the presence of hirsutism, acne, or pattern alopecia together with evidence of anovulation (fewer than 9 periods per year or cycles longer than 40 days). Hormonal testing is relatively insensitive for the diagnosis of PCOS. Imaging for cysts seldom affects management.

Patients with connective tissue disease need an antinuclear antibody (ANA) and urinalysis. Those with signs and symptoms of systemic lupus erythematosus need more extensive laboratory studies to include complement, extractable nuclear antigens, anticardiolipin, and antinative DNA.

Syphilis can mimic alopecia areata clinically and histologically (Figure 25-4). Serologic testing can be helpful in this setting. Beware of prozone reactions, as they may occur in patients with syphilitic alopecia. If the physical examination suggests syphilis and the blood test is negative, serial dilutions of the serum may be required.

4. Determine if a biopsy is necessary

A biopsy is necessary if history and physical examination do not establish a diagnosis and the alopecia is progressive. The combination of vertical and transverse sections increases the diagnostic yield. This requires two biopsies from an involved area. One-half of the vertically bisected specimen can be sent for immunofluorescence. When only a single biopsy specimen is obtained, serial vertical sections are superior for the evaluation of scarring alopecia and may also be preferred for alopecia areata. Transverse sections are superior for pattern alopecia and telogen effluvium.

A scalp biopsy should be performed with a 4-mm punch placed parallel to the direction of hair growth. Gel foam and gentle pressure stop bleeding rapidly, and it is seldom necessary to suture.

The active evolving edge of an alopecic patch typically shows only nonspecific findings. A well-established active area of inflammation is preferred. In the case of lupus, immunofluorescence, basement membrane thickening, follicular plugging, deep infiltrates, and mucin are not reliably present in lesions of less than 3–6 months' duration.

A biopsy of an end-stage scarred area can give information regarding the potential for regrowth. The elastic pattern can also distinguish lupus from lichen planopilaris, pseudopelade and folliculitis decalvans.

5. Determine if a treatable cause of nonscarring alopecia exists

Telogen effluvium commonly resolves spontaneously. In those with pattern alopecia, each episode of telogen effluvium will accelerate the evolution of the pattern alopecia. It is important to control for factors causing the telogen effluvium such as diet and papulosquamous diseases of the scalp. The pattern alopecia itself can be treated with minoxidil and antiandrogens (see below).

6. Determine if a treatable cause of scarring alopecia exists

Unfortunately, many forms of scarring alopecia are difficult to manage and some physicians are hesitant to use potent medications. Complacency can do real harm in this setting. Slowly evolving scarring alopecia marches on. The end-result can be devastating for the patient.

The most important diagnoses to distinguish are lupus erythematosus (Figure 25-5), infection, dissecting cellulitis (Figure 25-6), acne keloidalis (Figure 25-7) and folliculitis decalvans (Figure 25-8), as these are managed differently from other forms of scarring alopecia.

Examinination of the scalp and skin

Important initial steps in the evaluation are to determine if the hair loss is *scarring versus non-scarring* and *patchy versus diffuse*. Nonscarring

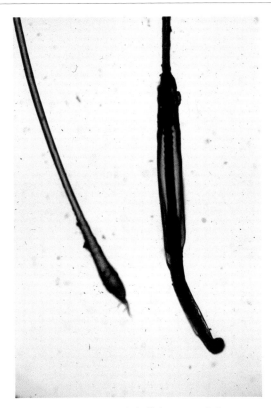

Figure 25-3 Left, telogen hair. Right, anagen hair

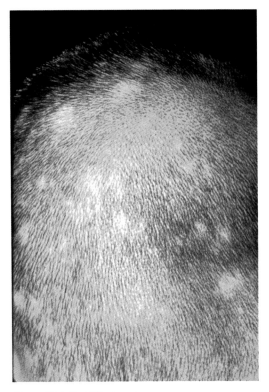

Figure 25-4 Syphilitic alopecia

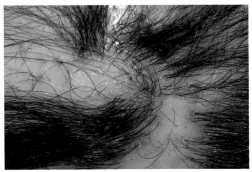

Figure 25-5 Lupus erythematosus

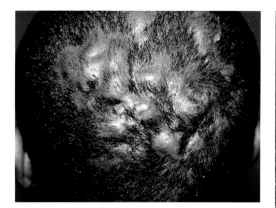

Figure 25-6 Dissecting cellulitis of the scalp

alopecia preserves the follicular openings (ostia). Patchy alopecia may present with circumscribed areas of complete hair loss, or localized areas of hair thinning. Look for erythema, follicular keratin spines, and evidence of papulosquamous disease. Look in the external ears, mouth, and remainder of the skin for evidence of lupus or lichen planopilaris. Ask about oral and genital lesions. Patients may have oral or genital lichen planus, but not mention it because they do not associate the genital lesions with their hair loss. Monilithrix (an inherited trichodystrophy with beaded, easily factured hairs; Figure 25-9) often demonstrates follicular papules on the scalp and eyebrow skin (Figure 25-10).

SPECIFIC FORMS OF ALOPECIA

Shaft fracture/trichorrhexis nodosa

Key Points

* Most common cause of hair loss in African American females
* Related to overprocessing of the hair

The most common form of trichodystrophy is trichorrhexis nodosa. It is most common in African American patients and is a sign of overprocessed hair. Trichorrhexis nodosa is characterized by a frayed node along the hair shaft that resembles two broomsticks pushed together. Patients can be reassured that the hair *follicles* are healthy, although the hair *shafts* are damaged. They should adopt gentle hair care practices to reduce shaft fracture while the healthier hair regrows. A reduced frequency of hair relaxing by an experienced professional is generally acceptable. Most patients will ignore the physician if told to stop relaxing the hair altogether.

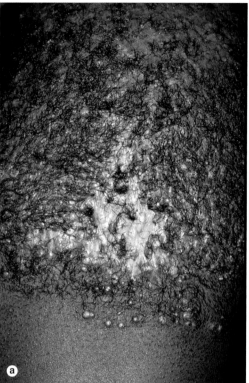

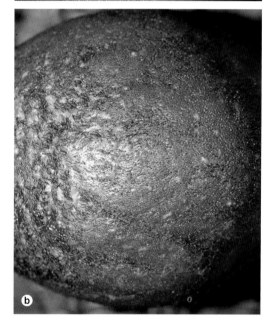

Figure 25-7 a Acne keloidalis. **b** Acne keloidalis with associated folliculitis decalvans

Some inherited trichodystophies are associated with genetic syndromes. An accurate diagnosis is established by microscopic examination of involved hair shafts by an experienced clinician or dermatopathologist using polarized microscopy or a dissecting microscope.

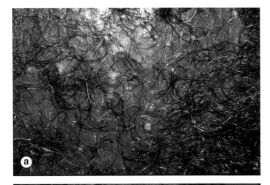

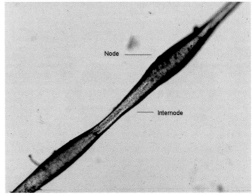

Figure 25-9 Monilithrix

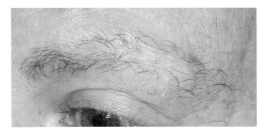

Figure 25-10 Monilithrix

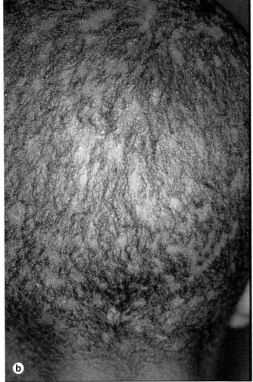

Figure 25-8 a, **b** Folliculitis decalvans

Pattern alopecia

Key Points

- Male pattern shows temporal recession with or without crown thinning
- Female pattern shows diffuse thinning of the crown, worse anteriorly, but with relative sparing of the frontal hair line
- Women with a male pattern should be carefully evaluated for virilization

Pattern alopecia in women presents with central hair thinning. In males; vertex thinning is generally accompanied by recession in temples. Balding in men is mediated by dihydrotestosterone (DHT).

Men with pattern alopecia may be treated with topical 5% minoxidil (Rogaine) or oral finasteride (Propecia) at a dose of 1 mg daily.

In women, the frontal hairline is usually preserved, but the part is distinctly wider anteriorly. The pathogenesis of female-pattern alopecia is complex, and adrenal androgens may play a larger role. Finasteride (Propecia) is of no benefit to the majority of women with pattern alopecia, but minoxidil and spironolactone can be of benefit. Spironolactone (Aldactone) is given at a starting dose of 100 mg twice daily. In women of child-bearing potential, spironolactone should be used in conjunction with an oral contraceptive. Side-effects include urinary frequency, nausea, irregular periods, and the potential for potassium retention. It is contraindicated in those with renal impairment. In patients with normal renal function, the potassium increases slightly, but the increase is rarely of clinical significance.

Patients with pattern alopecia should always be evaluated for causes of telogen effluvium. Telogen effluvium is common and, when present, accelerates the course of pattern alopecia. Common causes include diet and seborrheic dermatitis.

Women with PCOS are at increased risk for heart disease and possibly uterine cancer. Their risk factors should be addressed medically. Serum lipids and a fasting blood sugar should be checked. Hormonal cycling can be useful to prevent endometrial hyperplasia and reduce the risk of cancer. The primary care physician and gynecologist play important roles in the management of these patients.

Patients with PCOS typically have mildly increased testosterone and may have an increased prolactin, but these tests seldom affect management. Only 50% of patients have an elevated luteinizing hormone (LH)/follicle-stimulating hormone (FSH) ratio. *Hormonal studies only rarely affect management, whereas serum lipids commonly affect management.*

Telogen effluvium

Key Points

- Synchronous loss of telogen hairs
- Usually follows surgery, delivery, or a crash diet by 3–5 months
- Self-limited

Telogen effluvium is characterized by active shedding of hairs with a nonpigmented club-like bulb. A gentle pull on a large tuft of hair or combing for 1 minute generally results in the easy extraction of numerous club hairs.

The average adult has approximately 100,000 scalp hairs. At any given time, 90% of these are in the actively growing anagen phase. Approximately 10% are in the resting telogen phase. Telogen hairs rest for 3–5 months, then are shed. During times of stress, the body converts large numbers of hairs to telogen. Three to 5 months later, the patient will notice shedding of large numbers of telogen hairs. Three to 5 years later, the cycle will repeat itself to a lesser degree as the synchronous anagen hairs cycle through telogen and are shed again.

Generalized telogen effluvium commonly occurs 3–5 months after major surgery, pregnancy, or a crash diet. Patchy telogen effluvium is usually related to seborrheic dermatitis or psoriasis. Prolonged generalized telogen effluvium may be related to nutritional deficiency or a thyroid disorder.

Patients should be asked about heavy periods, frequency of periods, and dietary habits, particularly the frequency of meat consumption. Unexplained iron deficiency should prompt the testing of stool for occult blood. An inadequate diet, heavy periods, or other sources of blood loss result in iron deficiency as well as general nutritional deficiency. Iron is a critical nutrient for hair growth, and serves as a good screen for overall nutritional status. Supplementation with iron is important but does not substitute for an adequate diet.

A directed history and physical examination should address signs and symptoms of thyroid disease.

Table 25-1 Treatment of tinea capitis

Antifungal agent	Dose	Usual duration of therapy
Griseofulvin	Usually higher than labeled dosing, 10 mg/kg and up	1 month or more
Fluconazole	5–6 mg/kg per day	1 month or more
Itraconazole	3–5 mg/kg per day	1 week, repeated monthly until cured
Terbinafine	Patient < 20 kg: 62.5 mg/day Patient 20–40 kg: 125 mg/day Patient > 40 kg: 250 mg/day	1 month or more

Tinea

Key Points

- May present as kerion or "seborrheic" scale with hair loss
- Potassium hydroxide exam usually establishes the diagnosis

Tinea capitis is often overlooked in adults. It can complicate discoid lupus, especially if immunosuppressive agents or topical steroids are used. Tinea can present as a boggy kerion, as an alopecic patch with black dots, or as patchy alopecia with minimal gray scale. Black dot and "seborrheic" tinea are best diagnosed by rubbing the scalp with a moist gauze pad (Table 25-1). Short broken hairs will adhere to the gauze and will contain chains of large sphere-like spores.

Alopecia areata

Key Points

- Distinct, smooth patches of hair loss
- Positive pull test with tapered fractures
- Diffuse alopecia areata may mimic pattern alopecia or telogen effluvium
- Treat with intralesional or topical steroids, minoxidil, topical contact sensitizers, psoralen with ultraviolet A, or anthralin

Diagnosis

Alopecia areata (Figure 25-11) is a common form of hair loss, affecting about 0.1% of the population. Patients typically present with the sudden onset of hair loss in an isolated area. Lesions are typically round or oval and completely smooth. A slight pink hue and itching may be present. Exclamation hairs may be noted. In those with salt-and-pepper hair, gray hairs are spared. Close

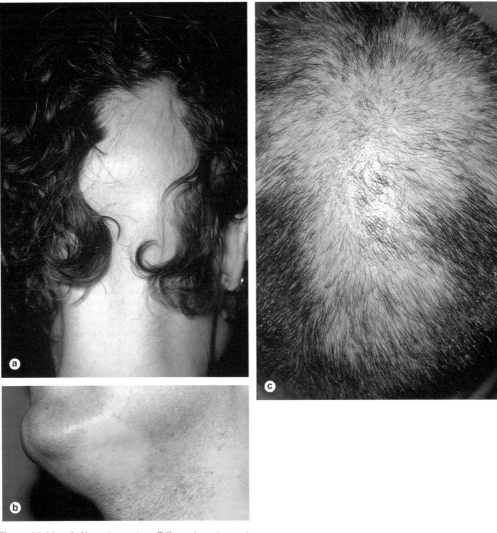

Figure 25-11 a, b Alopecia areata. c Diffuse alopecia areata.

inspection may reveal exclamation-point hairs. The ophiasis pattern consists of a band of hair loss in the occipital and temporal regions.

Alopecia totalis means total scalp alopecia and alopecia universalis means total body hair loss.

Nail changes are present in up to half of patients with alopecia areata. Pits are typically arranged in rows. Rough surfaced nails (trachyonychia), longitudinal splitting of the nail (onychorrhexis), and separation or shedding of the nail (onychomadesis) may be seen. Red spots may be seen in the lunulae.

Differential diagnosis

Trichotillomania (trichotillosis) will show irregular borders, a spared peripheral fringe of hair when the hairline is involved, and regrowth of hairs of different lengths. The pull test will be negative, and there will be absence of nail abnormalities.

Isolated eyebrow and eyelash loss in the absence of scalp hair loss suggests trichotillomania. A punch biopsy can be helpful.

Diffuse alopecia areata may be difficult to distinguish clinically from pattern alopecia or telogen effluvium. Nail findings, the finding of tapered fractures, and sparing of gray hair may help establish the diagnosis. Biopsy may also be helpful.

Pathogenesis

There is strong evidence that alopecia areata is an autoimmune process mediated by Th1 lymphocytes. Patients and family members may have other autoimmune conditions, especially vitiligo, thyroid disease, pernicious anemia, and type 1 diabetes mellitus. Testing is recommended when the review of systems suggests one these entities.

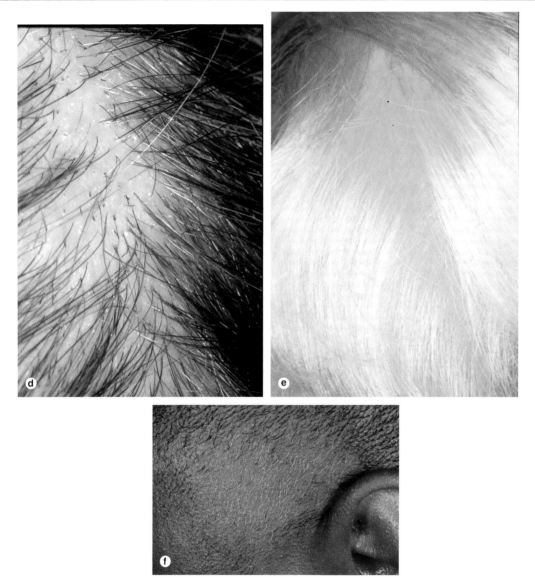

Figure 25-11, cont'd **d** Exclamation-point hairs. **e** Retained white hair in alopecia areata. **f** Migratory poliosis may represent a forme fruste of alopecia areata

Treatment

No treatment is consistently effective in alopecia areata. For localized patches, intralesional injections of triamcinolone (2.5–5 mg/mL) are typically effective. About 0.1 mL/cm^2 is injected into the dermis of active alopecic areas, with a maximum of 3 mL during any one session. The injections are repeated at intervals of 4–6 weeks. Some reversible atrophy may result. Intradermal injections are generally more effective than subcutaneous injections and are associated with a lower risk of atrophy. Superpotent topical steroids may be used for large surface areas or for patients who will not tolerate injections.

Minoxidil solution produces slow regrowth in some patients. Anthralin (Dritho-Scalp 0.5%) has been used to treat alopecia areata with some success. It is applied about 30 minutes prior to showering. Side-effects include staining of skin and clothing, irritation, folliculitis and lymphadenopathy. Topical immunotherapy may be performed with dinitrochlorobenzene (DNCB), squaric acid dibutyl ester (SADBE), or diphenylcyclopropenone (DPCP). DNCB is mutagenic on Ames testing. A 2% solution of the sensitizer in acetone is used to induce sensitization on the forearm. This is repeated at 2-week intervals until a poison ivy-like rash is obtained. A dilute solution, usually about 0.001%, is then applied weekly to the areas of alopecia with a cotton-tipped applicator, to perpetuate a low-grade contact dermatitis. Results are mixed. A total of 20–60% of patients have responded to this regimen in various studies.

Photochemotherapy with psoralen with ultraviolet A and oral cyclosporine have been reportedly effective. Biologic agents have been disappointing.

Information for patients is available from the National Alopecia Areata Foundation (www.naaf.org).

Intentional hair pulling (Trichotillosis, Trichotillomania)

Key Points

- Compulsive pulling of hair and eyelashes
- Young children have a good prognosis
- Adolescent and adults have a poorer prognosis
- Bizarre patterns of hair loss

Infants and preschoolers twist and pull their hair out of habit or for tactile stimulation while they are falling asleep. The prognosis is good for spontaneous resolution. School-age children and adults usually pull in reaction to stress (Figure 25-12). Some respond to simple behavior modification, whereas others require medication as for other compulsive disorders.

Diagnosis

Often, there is denial on the part of the patient and parents. Adults may describe a crescendo of tenderness at the base of the hair that can only be relieved by pulling out the hair. The alopecia is usually subtotal with an irregular outline. The scalp has a rough, stubbly feel, totally unlike the smoothness of alopecia areata. Some patients also exhibit trichophagia with bezoar formation (Figure 25-13).

Differential diagnosis

Alopecia areata presents with smooth, sharply marginated patches of hair loss and tapered fractures, and may have nail changes.

Pathogenesis

In younger children, hair pulling is simply a habit or soothing behavior. In older individuals, it is a compulsive disorder.

Treatment

The diagnosis should be presented in a non-judgmental fashion. Referral to a psychologist or psychiatrist is typically necessary for older patients.

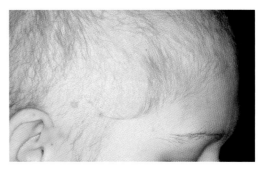

Figure 25-12 Trichotillomania

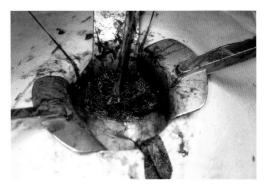

Figure 25-13 Bezoar (courtesy of Wilford Hall Medical Center teaching file)

Triangular alopecia

Triangular alopecia usually involves the temple, but may be seen above the ears. It may be present at birth but parents generally first notice the thinning at about 2–4 years of age. Normal hair density is present, but the majority of hairs are fine, vellus hairs. Treatment is generally not needed, but topical minoxidil may be of some value.

Other localized forms of alopecia

Traction alopecia occurs when the hair is pulled into very tight braids or corn rows. Postoperative pressure alopecia may occur after prolonged immobilization, especially after open-heart surgery. Aplasia cutis congenita is a developmental defect. The smooth atrophic alopecic patch is commonly surrounded by a collar of long dark hair.

Loose-anagen syndrome

Key Points

- Young, blonde girls
- Scalp hair is thin and seldom needs to be cut
- Hair pulls out easily and painlessly
- Rumpled-sock cuticle

Loose-anagen syndrome is characterized by easily extracted hairs and is caused by an abnormally soft cuticle.

Scarring alopecia

Key Points

- Follicular openings lost
- Biopsy necessary to guide treatment
- Systemic therapy often needed

Diagnosis

The skin at the base of hairs at the periphery of the alopecic patch often shows erythema at the base. Hairs may be grouped into tufts, resembling doll's hair. During the active inflammatory phase, intact anagen hairs with a pigmented bulb are often easily extracted from the involved areas. This can be used to monitor response to therapy. Inflamed areas gradually evolve into smooth, hairless patches with no follicular ostia.

Pathogenesis

Key Points

- Inflammatory alopecia may be lymphoid or suppurative
- Lymphoid forms include lupus erythematosus and lichen planopilaris
- Suppurative forms include folliculitis decalvans, infection, and dissecting cellulitis

Follicular stem cells reside in the bulge area, located in the superficial portion of the permanent follicle where the arrector pili muscle attaches to the external root sheath. Destruction of the bulge area results in permanent alopecia. The mesodermal follicular papilla is also necessary for hair regrowth. Sebaceous glands may be required for dissociation of the normal hair shaft and internal root sheath and mice with hypoplastic sebaceous glands develop progressive scarring alopecia.

Chronic cutaneous lupus erythematosus

Key Points

- Biopsy and direct immunofluorescence (DIF) help establish diagnosis
- Use intralesional or systemic steroids acutely, then transition to antimalarials or other steroid sparing therapy

Diagnosis

Clinical features range from typical erythematous, indurated, and hyperkeratotic plaques to patches that appear noninflammatory despite the presence of deep dermal inflammation histologically. Helpful diagnostic features include: follicular plugging, telangiectasia, atrophy, and mottled hyper- and hypopigmentation. Well-developed lesions demonstrate characteristic features on biopsy, but evolving lesions are commonly nonspecific. Diagnostic changes include hyperkeratosis, follicular plugging, basilar vacuolar degeneration, thickening of the basement membrane zone, a patchy perivascular and periadnexal lymphoid infiltrate, and dermal mucin. DIF of established lesions demonstrates a "full house" of all immunoreactants (immunoglobulin (Ig) G, C3, IgM, IgA, C1q) in a continuous granular pattern and shaggy fibrin at the basement membrane of the epidermis and follicle.

Differential diagnosis

A lichenoid tissue reaction may be present in lupus erythematosus, but the remaining features will help distinguish lupus erythematosus from lichen planopilaris.

Treatment

Early aggressive therapy can reduce the incidence of permanent alopecia. Corticosteroids are a mainstay of treatment for active lesions of cutaneous lupus. Topical corticosteroids are occasionally effective. Intralesional corticosteroids are a good choice for localized lesions. Oral corticosteroids are effective, but once initial control has been achieved, it is often best to switch to topical or intralesional steroids or a steroid-sparing agent for maintenance therapy. Osteoporosis, aseptic bone necrosis, cataracts, and glucose intolerance are a few of the many possible complications of systemic steroids. Alternative therapies include antimalarials, retinoids, dapsone, and thalidomide. I generally begin treatment with hydroxychloroquine (400 mg/day in an adult). Patients should be monitored for side-effects, especially ocular toxicity (corneal deposits and retinal damage), although these are very uncommon at usual doses. Other potential side-effects include thrombocytopenia, agranulocytosis, gastrointestinal intolerance, pruritus, lichenoid dermatitis, and toxic psychosis. If a 3-month trial of hydroxychloroquine proves ineffective, chloroquine , quinacrine, or a combination may be used.

Isotretinoin has been effective in some cases of discoid lupus refractory to other treatments. Retinoids are potent teratogens and should be used with due caution.

Dapsone, at a dose of 100 mg/day for an adult, may also be effective. Patients should first be screened for glucose-6-phosphate dehydrogenase deficiency. Potential side-effects include hemolysis, methemoglobinemia, and neuropathy. Thalidomide has been used effectively for the treatment of discoid lesions of lupus erythematosus at doses of 50–100 mg/day (200 mg in refractory cases). Sulfasalazine, mycophenolate mofetil, biologic agents, and methotrexate have also been useful in some patients.

End-stage cicatricial alopecia is best treated by surgical intervention, but the disease can flare in response to surgery. A tapered course of prednisone can prevent the flare.

Lichen planopilaris

> **Key Points**
>
> * May have lichen planus elsewhere
> * Corticosteroids are effective
> * Retinoids are generally the best steroid-sparing agents

Diagnosis

Lichen planopilaris (Figure 25-14) presents with perifollicular erythema with scarring and acuminate keratotic plugs at the margins. Evidence of lichen planus may be present elsewhere. Biopsy may show typical changes of lichen planus (interface dermatitis, sawtooth rete ridges, hypergranulosis, and Civatte bodies) or only perifollicular fibrosis with hyperkeratosis and follicular plugging. Late lesions demonstrate a wedge-like superficial scar.

Differential diagnosis

Deeper follicular involvement, basement membrane zone thickening, lymphoid aggregates in eccrine coils, dermal mucin, and aggregates of lymphoid cells within the subcutis favor a diagnosis of lupus erythematosus. DIF can be helpful, as a continuous granular pattern is typical of lupus, while the DIF in lichen planopilaris demonstrates numerous superficial globular cytoid bodies and shaggy linear deposits of fibrin at the basement membrane zone.

Treatment

Corticosteroids are the mainstay of treatment for lichen planopilaris. There are few controlled trials specific to lichen planopilaris, and retinoids are used largely based on data in other forms of lichen planus and consensus of opinion. Thalidomide and hydroxychloroquine have been reported as effective.

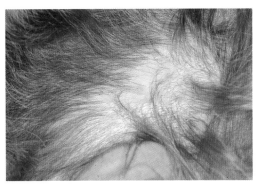

Figure 25-14 Lichen planopilaris

Graham–Little–Piccardi–Lassueur syndrome

> **Key Points**
>
> * Variant of lichen planopilaris
> * Alopecia of the eyebrows, axillary and pubic regions

Frontal fibrosing alopecia

> **Key Points**
>
> * Variant of lichen planopilaris
> * Alopecia of the frontal hair line (Figure 25-15)

Pseudopelade of Brocq

> **Key Points**
>
> * Discrete, smooth, white alopecic patches without follicular hyperkeratosis or perifollicular inflammation (Figure 25-16)
> * Slow progression
> * Most cases represent lichen planopilaris
> * True idiopathic pseudopelade appears to be the same condition as "hot-comb alopecia," central elliptical alopecia, and idiopathic central alopecia in African American women

The idiopathic variant has a diagnostic histology, including a contracted dermis and broad fibrous tract

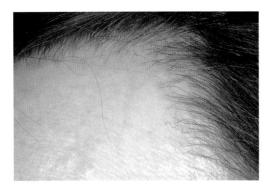

Figure 25-15 Frontal fibrosing alopecia (courtesy of Jeff Miller, MD)

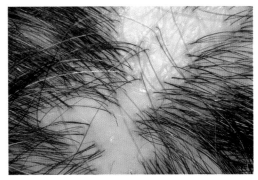

Figure 25-16 Inflammatory pseudopelade

remnants in the absence of dermal scarring. It is slowly progressive and responds poorly to therapy.

Central centrifugal cicatricial alopecia (Figure 25-17)

Key Points

- Term that encompasses a number of conditions, including lichen planopilaris, folliculitis decalvans, and idiopathic pseudopelade
- It is best to make a specific diagnosis when possible, as the treatment varies between some of these conditions

Scarring variants of keratosis pilaris

Key Points

- Keratosis pilaris-like disorders accompanied by a permanent alopecia
- Often involve the cheeks or lateral eyebrows
- Keratosis follicularis spinulosa decalvans is a rare X-linked disorder, with gene localization to Xp21.2-p22.2

Folliculitis decalvans

Key Points

- Recurrent crops of suppurative folliculitis with progressive hair loss
- Staphylococci often present
- Some cases merely represent chronic smoldering infection
- Other cases may represent hypersensitivity to various organisms
- Topical steroids and chronic suppression of staphylococci are often effective

Diagnosis

Folliculitis decalvans, erosive pustular dermatosis of the scalp, and folliculitis necrotica represent a group of scarring disorders that share a suppurative phase.

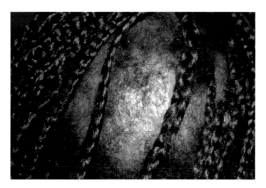

Figure 25-17   Central centrifugal cicatricial alopecia

Each crop of pustules results in progression of hair loss. Infectious agents may be noted with special stains and cultures, most commonly *Staphylococcus aureus*. Some authors have suggested that folliculitis decalvans is merely a chronic staphylococcal infection, but short courses of antibiotic therapy are invariably disappointing. Some evidence suggests that the alopecia involves an altered immunological response to a variety of organisms.

Treatment

Treatment generally requires prolonged use of antistaphylococcal antibiotics such as tetracyclines, cephalosporins, trimethoprim/sulfamethoxazole, clindamycin, or dicloxacillin, with or without rifampin. Topical steroids, selenium sulfide, and zinc pyrithione are used as adjunctive therapy. Tetracyclines may act partly through their antineutrophil effects. Zinc sulfate 400 mg daily for 6 months has been reported as effective. Zinc competes with copper metabolism and chronic therapy can result in a severe refractory anemia.

Dissecting cellulitis (Perifolliculitis capitis abscedens et suffodiens of Hoffman)

Key Points

- Similar to nodulocystic acne
- May occur as part of the follicular occlusion triad

Diagnosis

Dissecting cellulitis is often grouped with acne conglobata and hidradenitis suppurativa, and the term "follicular occlusion triad" has been used for the three conditions. Pilonidal cyst may be added, forming a tetrad. Dissecting cellulitis presents with tender nodules that progress and coalesce into dermal abscesses with draining sinus tracts.

Treatment

Antibiotics and intralesional corticosteroids may be helpful. Isotretinoin and oral zinc can also be effective. Anti-tumor necrosis factor-alpha biological medications appear promising.

Acne keloidalis (Dermatitis papillaris capillitii, keloidal folliculitis)

Key Points

- Ingrown hairs and hypertrophic scars on the nape of the neck

- Some patients develop a progressive alopecia with crops of pustules resembling folliculitis decalvans

Treatment

Mild cases may respond to intralesional and topical corticosteroids. Thick scars with sinus tracts may respond to chloramphenicol 500 mg in 30 g of fluocinonide cream, applied three times daily. Some patients require surgical intervention. Progressive alopecia with pustules is best treated as folliculitis decalvans.

Hirsutism

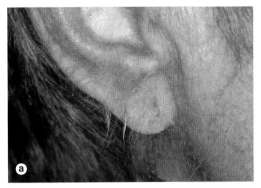

Key Points

- Distinguish hirsutism from hypertrichosis (Figure 25-18)
- Hirsutism occurs only in females and consists of a male pattern of hair growth
- Hirsutism is under hormonal influence
- Hypertrichosis may be familial or may relate to a metabolic disorder, tumor, or syndrome, but is rarely hormonal in origin
- The vast majority of women with medically significant hirsutism have PCOS

Normally, androgens in women are derived almost equally from the adrenal glands and ovaries, by way of theca cells and peripheral conversion. Sex hormone-binding globulin is elevated by estrogen and thyroid hormone, resulting in less free testosterone. It is decreased by androgen excess, obesity, and growth hormone excess. Virilizing tumors are typically suggested by history and physical exam. Patients with *new onset* of virilization need imaging studies and a total testosterone to rule out an ovarian or adrenal tumor. A total testosterone > 200 ng/dL or dehydroepiandrosterone - S > 8000 ng/dL suggests tumor. Imaging studies are needed when a tumor is suspected. Those with signs of Cushing's disease need a 24-hour urine cortisol. The diagnosis of PCOS is established clinically by the presence of hirsutism, acne, or pattern alopecia together with evidence of anovulation (fewer than 9 periods per year or cycles longer than 40 days). Hormonal testing is relatively insensitive for the diagnosis of PCOS and seldom affects management. Serum lipids and other cardiac risk factors should be addressed. PCOS accounts for most patients with severe hirsutism. In PCOS, muscle and adipose are resistant to insulin, but the ovaries are not resistant. Ovarian theca cells produce androgens that, together with a decrease in sex hormone-binding globulin, largely account for the hirsutism. LH/FSH ratio is elevated in only 50% of patients and is an insensitive screen. Hyperprolactinemia may be present in up to 30% of patients. Testosterone is normal to increased.

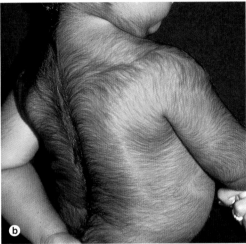

Figure 25-18 a Malignant hypertrichosis. **b** Congenital hypertrichosis

Risks largely relate to hyperlipidemia, obesity, and endometrial cancer. Patients with PCOS should be screened for diabetes and hypertension. A multidisciplinary approach involving the primary care physician, gynecologist, or endocrinologist is generally appropriate. Treatment is generally with epilation, eflornithine, and/or spironolactone, but other options include insulin sensitizers, flutamide, metformin, cyproterone acetate, and luprolide plus estrogen. Better antiandrogens and 5-alpha-reductase inhibitors are on the horizon.

Nonclassic 21-hydroxylase deficiency accounts for up to 10% of our patients with severe hirsutism. Screening with a baseline morning 17-hydroxy (OH)-progesterone leads to many false-positive results. A stimulated 17-OH-progesterone is more specific, but some would argue that testing is of limited clinical benefit, as outcomes with dexamethasone therapy may be no better than empiric treatment with spironolactone. For those with familial, long-standing hirsutism, no laboratory evaluation is needed. Treatment options include laser epilation, waxing, bleaching, shaving, chemical depilatories, spironolactone, and oral contraceptive pills.

Further reading

Elston DM, McCollough ML, Angeloni VL. Vertical and transverse sections of alopecia biopsy specimens: combining the two to maximize diagnostic yield. J Am Acad Dermatol 1995;32:454–457.

Elston DM, McCollough ML, Warschaw KE, et al. Elastic tissue in scars and alopecia. J Cutan Pathol 2000;27:147–152.

Elston DM, Ferringer T, Dalton S, et al. A comparison of vertical versus transverse sections in the evaluation of alopecia biopsy specimens. J Am Acad Dermatol 2005;53:267–272.

Lowenstein EJ. Diagnosis and management of the dermatologic manifestations of the polycystic ovary syndrome. Dermatol Ther 2006;19:210–223.

Olsen EA, Bergfeld WF, Cotsarelis G, et al. Summary of North American Hair Research Society (NAHRS)-sponsored workshop on cicatricial alopecia, Duke University Medical Center, February 10 and 11, 2001. J Am Acad Dermatol 2003;48:103–110.

Olsen E, Stenn K, Bergfeld W, et al. Update on cicatricial alopecia. J Invest Dermatol Symp Proc 2003;8:18–19.

Olsen EA, Hordinsky MK, Price VH, et al. Alopecia areata investigational assessment guidelines – Part II. National Alopecia Areata Foundation. J Am Acad Dermatol 2004;51:440–447.

Sehgal VN, Srivastava G. Trichotillomania trichobezoar: revisited. J Eur Acad Dermatol Venereol 2006;20:911–915.

Sperling LC. Hair and systemic disease. Dermatol Clin 2001;19:711–726.

Sperling LC, Cowper SE. The histopathology of primary cicatricial alopecia. Semin Cutan Med Surg 2006;25:41–50.

Yun SJ, Kim SJ. Hair loss pattern due to chemotherapy-induced anagen effluvium: a cross-sectional observation. Dermatology 2007;215:36–40.